Johan Bellemans

Michael D. Ries

Jan M. K. Victor

Total Knee Arthroplasty

A Guide to Get Better Performance

Johan Bellemans (Editor)

Michael D. Ries (Editor)

Jan M. K. Victor (Editor)

Total Knee Arthroplasty

A Guide to Get Better Performance

With 323 Figures, 137 in Color, and 39 Tables

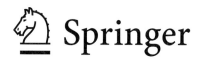 Springer

Johan Bellemans, Professor
Universitair Ziekenhuis
Weligerveld 1
3212 Pellenberg-Leuven
BELGIUM

Michael D. Ries, Professor
Chief of Arthroplasty
Department of Orthopedic Surgery
San Francisco Medical Center
500 Parnassus Ave., MU 320-W
San Francisco, CA 94143
USA

Jan M. K. Victor, M. D.
AZ St-Lucas Hospital
Sint-Lucaslaan 29
8310 Brugge
BELGIUM

ISBN 10 3-540-20242-0 Springer Berlin Heidelberg New York
ISBN 13 978-3-540-20242-4 Springer Berlin Heidelberg New York
Springer Medizin Verlag Heidelberg

Cataloging-in-Publication Data applied for
A catalog record for this book is available from the Library of Congress

Bibliographic information published by Die Deutsche Bibliothek
Die Deutsche Bibliothek lists this publication in the Deutsche Nationalbibliografie;
detailed bibliographic data is available in the internet at <http://dnb.ddb.de>

Springer Medizin Verlag.
A member of Springer Science+Business Media
springer.de

© Springer Medizin Verlag Heidelberg 2005
Printed in Germany

SPIN 10964880
Cover Design: design & production gmbH, Heidelberg, Germany
Typesetting: Goldener Schnitt, Sinzheim, Germany
Printing and Binding: Stürtz, Würzburg, Germany

Printed on acid-free paper 18/5141 – 5 4 3 2 1 0

Preface

Few domains in orthopedics have evolved so dramatically over the past decades as our knowledge and understanding of knee physiology and knee replacement surgery.

Long ago are the days that hinged knees or unconstrained flat on flat components with gamma irradiated in air polyethylene were the standard. Since those days, an unstoppable evolution has taken place towards refinement and better results. Some designs and theories have thereby withstood the test of time better than others, while some debates have been significant. Cemented or uncemented fixation, resurfacing of the patella and mobile or fixed bearings, are some of the issues that are still open today. Despite the fact that some issues have dominated the literature and the public forum during the eighties and nineties, most of us have realised in the meantime that these issues are less fundamental in our quest towards optimal knee joint restoration.

In addition, we have discovered previously neglected or unknown aspects. New terminology and technology has emerged. Paradoxical motion, lateral lift off, asymmetrical roll-back were never heard of during the nineties, and are public domain in today's knee forum. Computer assisted surgery, minimal invasive technology, cross-linked polyethylene and ceramics have entered the world of knee surgeons. All with the same goal in mind; to optimize the performance of the knees we treat.

This book attempts to assemble all these evolutions and new insights into a standard work, in an attempt to provide the reader with a current update on the most modern views on knee arthroplasty.

Experts from all over the world have contributed to achieve this goal. All have published extensively in peer-reviewed journals, and have taken the opportunity to bundle their knowledge in the allocated chapter in this book, thereby providing the reader with a unique work summarising the current scientific knowledge on knee arthroplasty.

The editors are grateful to them for their excellent contributions to this work, and hope with all of those who were involved, that this book may serve as a modern basis for achieving better performance in knee arthroplasty.

Finally, the editors would like to express their special and sincere gratitude to the publishing editor Thomas Guenther from Springer Verlag for his competent and professional support, which allowed us to present this work according to the highest standards available today in medical literature. Thomas Guenther, who always spoke about this work as his baby, suddenly passed away from us during the finalizing weeks of this work.

This book will therefore be the last book that Thomas made. Together with many surgeons who published for Springer-Verlag, Thomas will stay in our minds as a hard and dedicated worker, with a perpetual drive towards perfection. The success of this work is therefore also a last homage to Thomas Guenther.

The Editors

Johan Bellemans   Michael D. Ries   Jan M. K. Victor
May 2005

Short Biography of the Editors

Professor Johan Bellemans
Professor Dr. Johan Bellemans is Professor of Orthopedic Surgery at the Catholic University Leuven, Belgium, and Chief of the Knee and Sports Orthopaedic Department at the Catholic University Hospitals Leuven and Pellenberg, Belgium. His practice is exclusively dedicated to knee and sports related pathology. Professor Bellemans has been involved in the development and design of several innovations in the field of knee arthroplasty, ligament surgery, and arthroscopy. He has published over 60 peer reviewed papers and has lectured over the whole world. Professor Bellemans is founding president of the Belgian Knee Society.

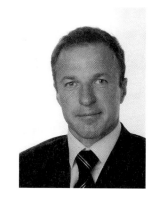

Professor Michael Ries
Dr. Michael Ries is a Professor of Orthopedic Surgery and Chief of Arthroplasty at the University of California, San Francisco, and Professor of Mechanical Engineering at the University of California, Berkeley. His clinical practice is dedicated to Total Joint Arthroplasty and research interests include biomaterials and clinical outcomes related to Total Joint Arthroplasty. Dr. Michael Ries has published over 100 peer reviewed journal articles. He is a member of the American Knee Society.

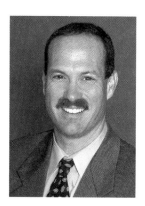

Dr. Jan M. K. Victor
Dr. Jan Victor is Orthopedic Surgeon in the St-Lucas Hospital in Brugge. His clinical practice is focused on knee surgery. He is past-president of the Belgian Orthopedic Association and Coordinator of the Postgraduate Knee Surgery teaching program. He is founding member of the Belgian Knee Society and active member of several European Orthopedic Societies. He has been lecturing and publishing in the field of Total Knee Arthroplasty for more than ten years. He is member of the American Knee Society.

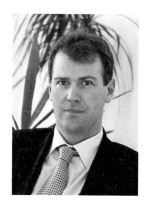

Sections

Table of Contents

IX   Future Perspectives

Editors

Bellemans, Johan,
Professor, M.D., Ph.D.
Universitair Ziekenhuis
Weligerveld 1
3212 Pellenberg-Leuven
BELGIUM

Ries, Michael D.,
Professor, M.D.
Chief of Arthroplasty
Department of Orthopedic Surgery
San Francisco Medical Center
500 Parnassus Ave., MU 320-W
San Francisco, CA 94143
USA

Victor, Jan M.K.,
M.D.
AZ St-Lucas Hospital
Sint-Lucaslaan 29
8310 Brugge
BELGIUM

Authors

Aglietti, P.
Universita' di Firenze
Clinica Ortopedica
Largo Palagi 1
60139 Firenze
ITALY

Akagi, M.
Department of Orthopaedic
Surgery
Kinki University School of
Medicine
377-2 Ohno-Higashi
Osaka-Sayama City
Osaka, 589 - 8511
JAPAN

Anbari, K. K.
Department of Orthopaedic
Surgery
University of Pennsylvania Health
System
3400 Spruce Street, 2 Silverstein
Philadelphia, PA 19104 - 4271
USA

Andriacchi, T. P.
Stanford University
Department of Mechanical
Engineering
Durand Building 225
Stanford, CA 94305 - 4038
USA

Argenson, J. N.
Service de Chirurgie Orthopédique
Hôpital Sainte Marguerite
270, Blvd. de Sainte Marguerite
130009 Marseille
FRANCE

Baldini, A.
Universita' di Firenze
Clinica Ortopedica
Largo Palagi 1
60139 Firenze
ITALY

Banks, S. A.
Assistant Professor
Department of Mechanical &
Aerospace Engineering
University of Florida
318 MAE-A, P.O. Box 116.250
Gainesville, FL 32611 - 6250
USA
and
Technical Director
The Biomotion Foundation
Palm Beach, FL 33480-0248
USA

Baré, J. V.
London Health Science Centre
University Campus
339 Windermere Road
London, Ontario N6A 5A5
CANADA

Beksac, B.
SSK Goztepe Educational Hospital
Department of Orthopaedics and
Traumatology
Istanbul
TURKEY

Bellare, A.
Assistant Professor of Orthopaedic
Surgery (Biomaterials)
Harvard Medical School
Department of Orthopaedic
Surgery
Brigham & Women's Hospital,
MRB 106
75 Francis Street
Boston, MA 02115
USA

Bellemans, J.
Universitair Ziekenhuis
Weligerveld 1
3212 Pellenberg-Leuven
BELGIUM

Booth, R. E. Jr.
Booth Bartolozzi Balderston
Orthopaedics
Pennsylvania Hospital
800 Spruce Street
Philadelphia, PA 19107
USA

Bourne, R. B.
London Health Science Centre
University Campus
339 Windermere Road
London, Ontario N6A 5A5
CANADA

Bozic, K. J.
University of California
Department of Orthopedic Surgery
San Francisco Medical Center
500 Parnassus Ave., MU 320-W
CA 94143, San Francisco
USA

Bozic, V.
University of Southern California
Center for Arthritis and Joint
Implant Surgery
1450 San Pablo Street, 5th Floor,
Suite 5100
Los Angeles, CA 90033
USA

Cameron, H. U.
Orthopaedic & Arthritis Institute
43 Wellesley Street East Suite 318
Toronto, Ontario, M4Y 18H1
CANADA

Cartier, P.
Clinique Hartmann
26 Blvd. Victor Hugo
92200 Neuilly sur Seine
FRANCE

Chaudhari, A. M.
Stanford University
Department of Mechanical
Engineering
Durand Building 201
Stanford, CA 94305 - 4038
USA

Christen, B.
Salem Spital Hirslanden
Abteilung Orthopädie
Schanzlistrasse 39
3013 Bern
SWITZERLAND

Clarke, H.
Insall Scott Kelly
Institute for Orthopaedics and
Sports Medicine
170 East End Ave., 4th Floor
New York, NY 10128 - 7603
USA

Colwell, C. W. Jr.
Orthopaedic Research Laboratories
Scripps Clinic Center
for Orthopaedic
Research and Education
11025 North Torray Pines Road,
Suite 140
La Jolla, CA 92037 - 1027
USA

Connolly, C.
North Sydney Orthopaedic and
Sports Medicine Center
286 Pacific Highway
Crows Nest, Sydney, NSW 2065
AUSTRALIA

Cook, S.
2620 West 111th Terrace
Olathe, KS 66061
USA

Cuomo, P.
Universita' di Firenze
Clinica Ortopedica
Largo Palagi 1
60139 Firenze
ITALY

Deckmyn, T.
AZ Sint-Lucas Hospital
Department of Anaesthesiology
Sint-Lucaslaan 29
8310 Brugge
BELGIUM

Dennis, D. A.
Colorado Joint Replacement
2425 S. Colorado Blvd., Suite 270
Denver, CO 80222
USA

Deshmukh, R. D.
Brigham and Women's Hospital
New England Baptist Hospital
125 Parker Hill Ave.
Boston, MA 02120
USA

D'Lima, D. D.
Orthopaedic Research Laboratories
Scripps Clinic Center
for Orthopaedic
Research and Education
11025 North Torray Pines Road,
Suite 140
La Jolla, CA 92037 - 1027
USA

Dowell, S. T.
Norfolk and Norwich
University Hospital
Colney Lane
77, New Market Road
Norwich, NR4 7UY
U.K.

Dye, S. F.
45 Castro Street, #117
San Fransisco, CA 94114 - 1019
USA

Dyrby, C. O.
Stanford University
Department of Mechanical
Engineering
Durand Building 225
Stanford, CA 94305 - 4038
USA

Eckhoff, D. G.
Department of Orthopaedics
(Adult Reconstruction)
University of Colorado Health
Science Center
Anschutz Outpatient Building,
Room 4111
1635 Ursula Street 4100
Aurora, CO 80010
USA

Galante, J. O.
Ruhs-Presbyterian-St.Luke's
Medical Center
Rush University
1725 W. Harrision - Suite 1055
Chicago, IL 60612 - 3824
USA

Garino, J. P.
Department of Orthopaedic Surgery
University of Pennsylvania Health
System
3400 Spruce Street, 2 Silverstein
Philadelphia, PA 19104 - 4271
USA

Garvin, K. L.
University of Nebraska Medical Center
Department of Othopaedics
600 South 42nd Street
Omaha, NB 68198 - 1080
USA

Glasgow, M. M.
Norfolk & Norwich University
Hospital
Colney Lane
77, New Market Road
Norwich, NR4 7UY
U.K.

Greenwald, A. S.
Orthopedic Research Laboratories
Lutheran Hospital
1730 West 25th Street
Cleveland, OH 44113
USA

Haaker, R. G.
St. Vincenz-Krankenhaus
Danziger Str. 17
33034 Brakel
GERMANY

Haas, S. B.
The Hospital for Special Surgery
535 East 70 Street
New York, NY 10021
USA

Haman, J. D.
Ruhs-Presbyterian-St.Luke's
Medical Center
Rush University
1725 W. Harrision - Suite 1055
Chicago, IL 60612 - 3824
USA

Heim, C. S.
Orthopedic Research Laboratories
Lutheran Hospital
1730 West 25th Street
Cleveland, OH 44113
USA

Hernigou, P.
Centre Hospitalier Henri Mondor
51, Avenue de Lattre de Tassigny
94000 Créteil
FRANCE

Hille, E.
Allgemeinkrankenhaus Eilbek
Abteilung Orthopädie
Friedrichsberger Str. 60
22081 Hamburg
GERMANY

Hungerford, D. S.
Johns Hopkins School of Medicine
Department of Orthopedic Surgery
Good Samaritan Hospital
10715 Pot Spring Rd.
Cockeysville, Baltimore, MD 21030
USA

Hungerford, M. W.
John Hopkins School of Medicine
Department of Orthopedic Surgery
Good Samaritan Hospital
10715 Pot Spring Rd.
Cockeysville, Baltimore, MD 21030
USA

Hunter, G.
8394 Drury Lane
Germantown, TN 38139
USA

Incavo, S.
University of Vermont Medical
School
Department of Orthopaedics
Stafford Hall
95 Carrigan
Burlington, VT 05405
USA

Jacofsky, D.
The CORE Institute
14420 West
Meeker Blvd.
Suite #300
Sun City West, AZ 85375
USA

Jenny, J.-Y.
Chirurgie Orthopédique
et Traumatologique
Centre de Traumatologie
et d'Orthopédie Strasbourg
10, avenue Baumann
67400 Illkirch-Graffenstaden
FRANCE

Jones, W. M.
Emory University
Department of Rehabilitation
Medicine
1441 Clifton Road, Suite 118
Atlanta, GA 30322
USA

Kader, D.
North Sydney Orthopaedic and
Sports Medicine Center
286 Pacific Highway
Crows Nest, Sydney, NSW 2065
AUSTRALIA

Khefacha, A.
Clinique Hartmann
26 Blvd. Victor Hugo
92200 Neuilly sur Seine
FRANCE

Komistek, R. D.
Rocky Mountain Musculoskeletal
Research Laboratory
2425 S Colorado Blvd., Suite 280
Denver, CO 80222
USA

Konermann, W. H.
Orthopädische Klinik
Am Mühlenberg
37235 Hessisch-Lichtenau
GERMANY

Krackow, K. A.
Department of Orthopaedic Surgery
The State University of New York
at Buffalo
Kaleida Health System /
Buffalo General Hospital
100 High Street, Suite B-276
Buffalo, NY 14203 - 1126
USA

Lampe, F.
Allgemeinkrankenhaus Eilbek
Abteilung Orthopädie
Friedrichsberger Str. 60
22081 Hamburg
GERMANY

Laskin, R. S.
Hospital for Special Surgery
Weill Medical College of Cornell
University
535 East 70th Street
New York, NY 10021 - 4892
USA

Lehmann, A. P.
The Hospital for Special Surgery
535 East 70 Street
New York, NY 10021
USA

Lonner, J. H.
Booth Barolozzi Balderstone
Orthopaedics
Pennsylvania Hospital
800 Spruce Street
Philadelphia, PA 19107
USA

Lüdemann, M.
Orthopädische Klinik
Universitätsklinikum Tübingen
Hoppe-Seyler-Str. 3
72076 Tübingen
GERMANY

Luyten, F. P.
Universitair Ziekenhuis
Department of Rheumatology
Weligerveld 1
3212 Pellenberg-Leuven
BELGIUM

Mahoney, C., R.
Iowa Orthopaedic Center
Mercy Center for Joint Replacement
Mercy Hospital
2004 South 40th CT
West Des Moines, IA 50265
USA

McGuan, S.
2730 Camino Capistrano, Suite 7
San Clemente, CA 92672
USA

McKinnon, B. W.
3290 Broadway St.
Bartlett, TN 38133
USA

Mihalko, W.M.
Department of Orthopaedic
Surgery
Orthopaedic Research Lab.
Ferber 162
Buffalo, NY 14214
USA

Munjal, S.
The State University of New York
at Buffalo
Department of Orthopaedic Surgery
Kalcida Health System
Buffalo General Hospital
100 High Street, Suite B276
Buffalo, NY 14203
USA

Murray, D. G.
Nuffield Orthopaedic Centre
Old Road
Headington, Oxford
Oxfordshire, OX3 7LD
U.K.

Myers, P. T.
Brisbane Orthopaedic & Sports
Medicine Center
Level 5, Arnold Janssen Centre
259 Wickham Terrace
Brisbane, QLD 4000
AUSTRALIA

Nasser, S.
Department of Orthopaedic
Surgery
School of Medicine
Department of Biomedical
Engineering
College of Engineering
Wayne State University
Department of Orthopaedic
Surgery
Wayne State University School
of Medicine
Hutzel Warren Medical Center
28800 Ryan Road, Suite 220
Warren, MI 48093
USA

Nogier, A.
Centre Hospitalier Henri Mondor
51, Avenue de Lattre de Tassigny
94000 Créteil
FRANCE

Otto, J. K.
408 S Front St. 305
Memphis, TN 38103
USA

Phillips, C.
Chelsea & Westminster Hospital
369 Fulham Road
London SW10 9NH
U.K.

Pinczewski, L.
North Sydney Orthopaedic and
Sports Medicine Center
286 Pacific Highway
Crows Nest, Sydney, NSW 2065
AUSTRALIA

Poignard, A.
Centre Hospitalier Henri Mondor
51, Avenue de Lattre de Tassigny
94000 Créteil
FRANCE

Pruitt, L. A.
Department of Bioengineering and
Mechanical Engineering
5134 Etcheverry Hall
UC Berkeley
Berkeley, CA 94720
USA

Rand, J. A.
Mayo Clinic
13400 East Shea Blvd.
Scottsdale, AZ 85259 - 5404
USA

Rauh, M. A.
Department of Orthopaedic Surgery
The State University of New York
at Buffalo
Kaleida Health System –
Buffalo General Hospital
100 High Street, Suite B2
Buffalo, NY 14203 - 1126
USA

Rasmussen, G. L.
Orthopaedic Department
5848 South Fashion Blvd.
Salt Lake City, UT 84107
USA

Reichel, H.
Universitätsklinik und Poliklinik
für Orthopädie und Physikalische
Medizin
Universität Ulm
Oberer Eselsberg 45
89081 Ulm
GERMANY

Ries, M. D.
Department of Arthroplasty
Orthopaedic Surgery
San Francisco Medical Center
500 Parnassus Ave., MU 320-W
San Francisco, CA 94143
USA

Scott, R. D.
Brigham and Women's Hospital
New England Baptist Hospital
125 Parker Hill Ave.
Boston, MA 02120
USA

Scuderi, G. R.
Insall Scott Kelly
Institute for Orthopaedics and
Sports Medicine
170 East End Ave., 4th Floor
New York, NY 10128 - 7603
USA

Sikorski, G. M.
Suite 8 Hollywood Specialist Center
95 Monash Avenue
Nedlands, WA 6009
AUSTRALIA

Spector, M.
Department of Orthopaedic Surgery
Havard Medical School
Brigham & Women's Hospital,
MRB 106
Tissue Engineering
VA Boston Healthcare System
75 Francis Street
Boston, MA 02115
USA

Stiehl, J. B.
Orthopaedic Hospital of Wisconsin
575 West Riverwood
Parkway, Suite 204
Milwaukee, WC 53212
USA

Swanson, T. V.
Desert Orthopaedic Center
2800 E. Desert Inn Rd., # 100
Las Vegas, NV 89121
USA

Taelman, V.
Universitair Ziekenhuis
Department of Rheumatology
Weligerveld 1
3212 Pellenberg-Leuven
BELGIUM

Thornhill, T. S.
New England Baptist
Bone & Joint Institute
125, Parker Hill Avenue
Boston, MA 02115
USA

Victor, J. M. K.
AZ St-Lucas Hospital
Sint-Lucaslaan 29
8310 Brugge
BELGIUM

Vince, K.
University of Southern California
Center for Arthritis and Joint
Implant Surgery
1450 San Pablo Street, 5th Floor,
Suite 5100
Los Angeles, CA 90033
USA

Walker, P. S.
Department of Orthopaedic
Surgery
New York University Medical
Center
Veterans Administration Medical
Center
Annex Building 2, Room 206-A
423 East 23rd Street
New York, NY 10010
USA

Wehrli, U.
Kantonspital Bern Ziegler
Abteilung Orthopädie
Morillonstrasse 75
3001 Bern
SWITZERLAND

Westhovens, R.
Universitair Ziekenhuis
Department of Rheumatology
Weligerveld 1
3212 Pellenberg-Leuven
BELGIUM

Whiteside, L. A.
Missouri Bone and Joint Center
Biomechanical Research
Laboratory
14825 Sugarwood Trail
St.-Louis, MO 63014
USA

Williams, A.
Chelsea & Westminster Hospital
369 Fulham Road
London SW10 9NH
U.K.

Williams, T. J.
New England Baptist Bone & Joint
Institute
125, Parker Hill Avenue
Boston, MA 02 115
USA

Wilton, T. J.
Consultant Orthopaedic Surgeon
81 Friar Gate
Derby, DE1 1FL
U.K.

Wimmer, M. A.
Ass. Professor & Director,
Section of Tribology
Department of Orthopaedics
Rush-University Medical Center
1653 W. Congress Parkway,
Suite 1417
Chicago, IL 60612 - 3824
USA

Wülker, N.
Orthopädische Klinik
Universitätsklinikum Tübingen
Hoppe-Seyler-Str. 3
72076 Tübingen
GERMANY

Wymenga, A. B.
Orthopedisch Chirurg
Sint Maartenskliniek
Afdeling Orthopedie
Postbus 9011
6500 GM Nijmegen
THE NETHERLANDS

I   Essentials

1   Arthritis of the Knee: Diagnosis and Management

F. P. Luyten, R. Westhovens, V. Taelman

Summary

In this chapter, an algorithm for the diagnosis of a painful and swollen knee is presented. Arthritis of the knee can be restricted to a monoarticular clinical manifestation, or it may be part of an oligo- or polyarticular disease. A careful anamnesis and clinical examination will allow the clinician to classify the clinical presentation of arthritis of the knee into disease groups such as osteoarthritis, rheumatoid arthritis, spondyloarthropathy, or miscellaneous arthritic diseases. These disease entities are briefly discussed and their therapeutic approaches reviewed. Finally, the case is made for a more routine use of synovial biopsies in daily clinical practice, for diagnosis and to evaluate targeted therapies.

Introduction

Appropriate treatment of arthritis of the knee starts with correct diagnosis of the underlying disease and identification of the causes of the condition. Therefore, in the first part of this chapter we propose a comprehensive and practical algorithm for dealing with "arthritis of the knee", typically with signs and symptoms of pain, swelling, and loss of motion and function, separately or in combination. Subsequently, we discuss clinically important separate disease entities such as osteoarthritis, knee involvement in the major groups of chronic inflammatory arthritis – rheumatoid arthritis and the spondyloarthropathies –, and some miscellaneous forms of arthritis of the knee, perhaps less frequent but certainly clinically relevant, such as crystal-induced arthritis, septic arthritis, and Lyme disease. In these discussions we highlight the predominant clinical features and recent advances in therapeutic options. Special attention is given to the concept of spondyloarthropathies, since this has still apparently not entered the daily practice of many physicians. Finally, we discuss in more detail the synovium of the knee, as this is easily accessible and has received increased attention from rheumatologists. Indeed, through the study of synovial biopsies we have gained increasing insight into the pathophysiology of chronic arthritis.

Major advances in our understanding of the molecular basis of arthritic diseases has led to the development of new targeted therapies with a profound impact on the management of patients with rheumatoid arthritis and the spondyloarthropathies.

Algorithm for Diagnosis of the Arthritic Knee

When one is confronted with a patient who has a painful, swollen knee, a well-structured approach is helpful for forming a working hypothesis and ultimately critical for arriving at the most likely diagnosis.

The most important tool we have in a diagnostic workup is the *clinical history*, which must be as complete as possible. A patient can say what brings him to your office, but in most cases precise and well-directed questions are needed to obtain critical information. Taking a complete history is a demanding task, but a lot of circumstantial evidence can evolve from a full history of the current problem, past medical conditions, and the family history.

The nature of the pain belongs to "the basics", whether it be mechanical, inflammatory, neuropathic, or poorly defined. *Mechanical pain* occurs when the joint is used: walking becomes difficult, and especially climbing stairs causes problems. On resting, there is less pain. Starting pain and stiffness are very characteristic of a more advanced mechanical pain pattern.

Inflammatory pain typically presents at night. More specifically, the second part of the night is troublesome, and patients need to get out of bed and move. They experience morning stiffness for at least 1 h, and this stiffness diminishes progressively as the patient begins to move.

When *pain is neuropathic* in origin, a typical distribution pattern corresponding to the innervation is found.

Psychosomatic pain has no typical presentation or distribution. Complaints are always more impressive than the clinical findings.

Additional questions can help the clinician to identify the problem as *acute/subacute* or a *chronic* arthritis.

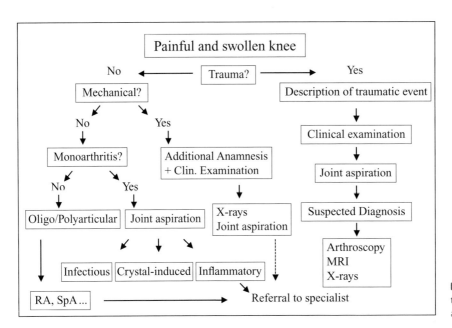

```
                    ┌──────────────────────────────┐
                    │     Painful and swollen knee  │
                    └──────────────────────────────┘
```

Fig. 1-1. Algorithm flow chart for the patient presenting with a painful and swollen knee

How long has the knee problem existed? When pain and swelling have been present for less than 6 weeks, the problem is acute. Beyond 6 weeks' duration, the term chronic is used and implies that spontaneous healing of the arthritis is unlikely. How acutely did the problem occur? Suddenly, as seen in trauma, within hours, which is more likely in septic and crystal-induced arthritis, or over days or weeks, as in rheumatoid arthritis?

Ask the patient whether this is the first time he has experienced arthritis of the knee or if he has had knee or other joint problems in the past. This may provide hints as to whether it is a problem in a single joint or an oligo/polyarticular disease.

It is also important to look for circumstantial evidence. Did trauma occur just before the knee swelling began? Did the patient have an episode of fever? Did the patient experience an infection such as angina, gastroenteritis, or urethritis? Does the patient have other clinical conditions that could be linked to the knee arthritis, such as skin problems (psoriasis, erythema nodosum), chronic diarrhoa as seen in inflammatory bowel disease, eye problems such as uveitis or scleritis? In this setting a complete familial history can also add useful information.

Thereafter, a clinical workup including a complete joint assessment and a *full clinical examination*, evaluating all the peripheral joints and the axial skeleton, can provide further clues to the diagnosis and help to localize the problem to the joint, periarticular structures, or muscle. *It is not always trivial to distinguish a synovitis from joint pain by intra-articular swelling, the distinction being crucial for the diagnosis.* For instance, a diagnosis of rheumatoid arthritis requires a (poly)synovitis; inflammatory polyarthralgia is not sufficient.

When the knee is swollen and the presence of intra-articular joint fluid is suspected, *arthrocentesis* should be performed. The results of the white blood cell count and cell differentiation, Gram staining, bacterial culture, and detection of crystals of urate or pyrophosphate are diagnostic in case of infectious arthritis, gout, or pseudo-gout. The white blood cell count in the synovial fluid differentiates between a non-inflammatory problem (<2000 WBC/mm³), an inflammatory picture (2000–20 000 WBC/mm³), a strongly inflammatory picture such as in crystal arthritis (20 000–50 000), and a most probable septic arthritis (WBC >50 000 with >75% PMN).

Finally, it is important to establish whether the knee problem is a genuine *monoarthritis* or rather one where multiple joints are involved. The latter is classified as *oligoarthritis* when fewer than five joints are involved, or as *polyarthritis* when five or more joints are inflamed. In addition, assessments of *symmetrical* or *asymmetrical* joint involvement are performed.

A few typical clinical entities, most frequent in daily clinical practice, are briefly presented.

Monoarthritis, Mechanical in Origin

Once the knee pain is recognized as mechanical, the most likely diagnosis in the older patient is osteoarthritis with or without a meniscal or ligamentous pathology. Further investigations can be limited to standard weight-bearing X-rays.

In younger people, mechanical pain will more likely be associated with a meniscal or chondral/osteochondral problem or defect. Further investigations include MRI, CT-arthrography, and arthroscopy.

Chapter 1 · Arthritis of the Knee: Diagnosis and Management – F.P. Luyten et al.

5   1

Acute Inflammatory Monoarthritis of the Knee

With inflammatory knee pain and swelling the differential diagnosis is far more complex. Acute monoarthritis of the knee is infectious until proven otherwise. Previous arthrocentesis, skin wounds, typically on lower leg regions or the feet, should be asked about and looked for. Fever is not always present, certainly not in the immunocompromised patient. Arthrocentesis is mandatory for bacterial examination and culture. Gram staining and the white blood cell count can be quickly obtained and are mostly sufficient to begin antibiotic treatment. Arthroscopic lavage and intravenous antibiotic treatment must be started as soon as possible.

In older patients, a crystal-induced arthritis such as gout or pseudogout is the most likely explanation for acute monoarthritis of the knee. Again, arthrocentesis is the key to the correct diagnosis, demonstrating the presence of urate or pyrophosphate crystals.

Chronic Monoarthritis of the Knee

Monoarthritis of the knee is often a presenting feature of spondyloarthropathy. This group of diseases is marked by inflammatory back pain, asymmetrical synovitis of peripheral joints, and enthesopathy (see "Spondyloarthropathies", below). Again, the importance of a complete history for detecting related conditions of the skin, eyes, or bowels should be stressed.

Less frequently, chronic monoarthritis of the knee is the result of a low-grade infection (*Mycobacteria*), sarcoidosis, Lyme disease, villonodular synovitis, or algodystrophy.

Chronic Polyarthritis, with Knee Arthritis as First Symptom

On clinical examination, so-called monoarthritis often turns out to be polyarthritis. This can be the onset of spondyloarthropathy. Monoarthritis of the knee as the presenting manifestation of rheumatoid arthritis is less common; more typically, rheumatoid arthritis shows a picture of symmetrical polyarthritis, including smaller joints of the hands and feet. In this setting, a blood examination with biochemical testing for inflammatory parameters and rheumatoid factor is helpful.

Osteoarthritis of the Knee

The clinical history and examination typically reveal a chronic noninflammatory, mono- or oligoarticular presentation (both knees, hands) in middle-aged and older individuals. The signs and symptoms are usually local and restricted to one or both knees, sometimes associated with hand OA or more generalized OA. Pain is by far the predominant symptom, relieved by rest and without night pain or morning stiffness, but, especially in more advanced disease, there is pronounced pain at the beginning of movement. It is still unclear what causes the pain in OA. Most probably it is caused not by the cartilage, as this tissue has no nerve supply, but rather by the subchondral bone and other intra- and periarticular structures such as synovium, menisci, and ligaments. Acute flares with an inflammatory component and swelling of the joint may occur, frequently caused by crystals, which may indicate the possible association with calcium pyrophosphate crystal arthritis (CPPD).

The *clinical examination* reveals pain on passive and active motion, together with local tenderness, and crepitus in the more advanced stages. Joint swelling can be seen and may be the result of hydrops, synovitis, and osteophytosis or bone remodeling. Muscle atrophy, typically of the quadriceps, is secondary to disuse in the more advanced cases or in patients with more chronic synovitis, and is an additional reason to look for crystal-induced arthritis. Advanced loss of articular cartilage in one compartment, predominantly the medial one, will be associated with secondary axis deviations such as genu vara or valga. Retropatellar OA can be presented as a single compartmental involvement, particularly in younger patients, evolving in some cases from the so-called chondromalacia patellae. In these cases, the pain is localized around the patella and is typically aggravated by climbing stairs.

The *diagnosis of OA* is confirmed by *radiographic imaging*. For diagnostic purposes, since OA involves three compartments, anteroposterior, mediolateral, and skyline views are recommended. X-ray findings typically show joint space narrowing (JSN), subchondral bone sclerosis, and osteophytosis. The subchondral bone reaction, and especially osteophytosis, appears most often earlier than JSN. However, JSN is more significant and sensitive to change. In some cases of knee OA, JSN is more striking and can be present without any osteophytosis. Most importantly, there is a poor correlation between clinical symptoms, clinical outcome, and X-ray changes. It is impossible to predict the outcome of knee OA in individual patients based on radiographic appearance alone.

Laboratory findings are usually normal, although sometimes a slight elevation of C-reactive protein and some elevation of the erythrocyte sedimentation rate can be seen, especially in patients with more generalized OA, with combined erosive osteoarthritis of the hands or in patients with associated crystal arthropathy. Synovial fluid reveals minimal abnormalities, with a cell count usually below 2000 cells/mm³. Calcium pyrophosphate or apatite crystals are seen quite frequently. Scintigraphy is of little or no use in the diagnosis. Despite the advances that have been made in the development of sensitive assays, serological markers for diagnostic or prognostic purposes remain investigational.

Newer imaging modalities such as computed tomography (CT) and magnetic resonance imaging (MRI) provide additional insight into the degree or nature of damage to the cartilage, subchondral bone, and soft tissues. MRI shows great promise for detecting early changes in OA, especially with regard to the articular cartilage soft-tissue involvement and bone narrow abnormalities.

Treatment modalities have recently been presented and discussed, and this has resulted in recommendations and guidelines proposed by both the American College for Rheumatology [1] and the European League Against Rheumatism [2]. The treatment algorithm includes *nonmedical* approaches, with education, weight loss, and restoring muscle strength as the most critical parameters. The *medical* approach focuses mainly on treating pain, the major symptom of OA, and on pain-relieving drugs. Paracetamol preparations in doses of up to 4 × 1 g/day remain the first-line treatment for mild and moderate gonarthritis. The addition of non-steroidal anti-inflammatory drugs (NSAIDs) is recommended when insufficient pain relief is achieved with proper doses of analgesics alone. Topical anti-inflammatory treatments appear reasonably efficacious and should be tried. The place in the treatment algorithm of nutritional supplements such as glucosamine and chondroitin sulfate is still not clear. The position of intra-articular treatments with corticosteroids and hyaluronic acid remains controversial, and it is clear that we lack convincing predictors of response to identify those patients likely to benefit from these treatments.

Surgical treatments include tissue-repair approaches, arthroscopic lavage and débridement, osteotomy, and unicompartmental and total knee replacement. There is little or no evidence that surgical reconstruction of torn cruciate ligaments or the meniscus prevents the development of knee OA. It remains to be seen whether cartilage repair procedures prevent or slow down knee OA. The combination of tissue repair, such as the repair of cartilage defects, with an osteotomy, performed on the right patient and by a trained surgeon, may delay the need for knee replacement and will most likely benefit the younger patient population (below 50 years). Indeed, OA in the young and active population remains a largely unsolved problem. Developments of new structure-modifying drugs together with tissue-engineering approaches are the hope for the near future.

Knee Involvement in Rheumatoid Arthritis

In rheumatoid arthritis (RA), knee arthritis is frequently just one component of symmetrical polyarthritis. Especially when the symmetrical polyarthritis of small joints of the hands and feet is mild and/or overlooked in the clinical examination, a late diagnosis can lead to considerable damage from this disease.

Signs and Symptoms

The classical presentation of RA is that of a gradually developing symmetrical polyarthritis of the hands and feet, with a peak incidence in women in their fourth and fifth decades of life. Although we know a good deal about the epidemiology and immunologic and genetic aspects of RA, it is still unclear what initiates and perpetuates the process. At present, RA is still best described and depicted by the 1987 revised classification criteria of the American Rheumatism Association [3] (◙ Table 1-1).

It must be remembered that RA not only involves joints and tendon sheets, but is also a systemic disease affecting the body as a whole (fatigue, extra-articular features such as nodules, serositis, vasculitis, anemia, interstitial lung disease). It has a major impact on every patient's physical and psychosocial life.

Involvement of the knee in RA is common and usually obvious. Minor inflammation in the knees should not be overlooked. Examination of the "bulge" sign and loss of the "cool patella" sign can contribute to an adequate diagnosis. When the knee synovitis is important, a Baker's cyst is a frequent finding. Ruptures of Baker's cysts can mimic acute thrombophlebitis.

Joint Damage and Destruction

Early disease is not synonymous with mild disease. Although it is still unpredictable whether patients with early disease will eventually develop a malignant rheumatoid course, a number of prognostic factors should be looked for:
- High persisting disease activity and early joint damage
  - Persistently elevated levels of CRP and ESR
  - Uncontrolled persisting polyarthritis
  - Early X-ray damage (joint erosion and JSN) and joint deformity
  - Functional disability (as measured by the HAQ – health assessment questionnaire)
- Extra-articular features as RA nodules, vasculitis
- Rheumatoid factor positivity, especially at high levels, CCP positivity (antibodies to cyclic citrullinated peptides)
- Psychosocial problems, low level of education

Chapter 1 · Arthritis of the Knee: Diagnosis and Management – F.P. Luyten et al.

7

1

◻ Table 1-1. American Rheumatism Association revised criteria for the classification of rheumatoid arthritis

Criteria	Definition
1. Morning stiffness	Morning stiffness in and around the joints, lasting at least 1 h before maximal improvement
2. Arthritis of three or more joint areas	At least three joint areas (out of 14 possible areas; right or left PIP, MCP, wrist, elbow, knee, ankle, MTP joints) simultaneously have had soft-tissue swelling or fluid (not bony overgrowth alone) as observed by a physician
3. Arthritis of hand joints	At least one area swollen (as defined above) in a wrist, MCP or PIP joint
4. Symmetrical arthritis	Simultaneous involvement of the same joint areas (as defined in 2) on both sides of the body (bilateral involvement of PIPs, MCPs, or MTPs without absolute symmetry is acceptable)
5. Rheumatoid nodules	Subcutaneous nodules over bony prominences or extensor surfaces, or in juxta-articular regions as observed by a physician
6. Serum rheumatoid factor	Demonstration of abnormal amounts of serum rheumatoid factor by any method for which the result has been positive in less than 5% of normal control subjects
7. Radiographic changes	Radiographic changes typical of rheumatoid arthritis on posteroanterior hand and wrist radiographs, which must include erosions or unequivocal bony decalcification localized in, or most marked adjacent to, the involved joints (osteoarthritis changes alone do not qualify)

[a] For classification purposes, a patient has RA if at least four of these criteria are satisfied (criteria 1–4 must have been present for at least 6 weeks)

Persisting disease activity is associated with increased mortality.

Joint damage occurring within the first year of disease activity is assessed by standard X-rays. X-rays of the hands and feet show early periarticular osteoporosis; at the later stage joint erosions and JSN can be seen, followed by the presence of joint subluxation or even dislocation. Joint damage in the hands, and even earlier damage detectable in the feet, is correlated with involvement of other joints and with general disease severity and shows continuous progression without appropriate treatment. Standard X-rays of the knee do not contribute to the early diagnosis of RA. Ultrasound techniques can reveal joint effusion, synovial hypertrophy, and vascularity. MRI techniques additionally reveal aspecific bony edema in early disease. These examinations contribute little, however, when an adequate clinical examination is performed.

Eventually, destruction of the knee by RA will lead to functional disability. The loss of cartilage and the presence of ligament laxity at the level of the collateral and cruciate ligaments further contribute to difficulties in walking and climbing stairs.

A classical valgus deformity is the late outcome of RA knee arthritis, marked by posterior subluxation of the tibia, resulting in a fixed flexion contracture of the knee.

Treatment

Comprehensive management of RA involves pharmacological but also a variety of nonpharmacological interventions to improve and maintain function, such as patient education, physical therapy, surgery, and occupational therapy. *Early disease control is mandatory*, as

there seems to be a window of opportunity to prevent joint damage. Therefore, the classical therapeutic pyramid is reversed with early use of so-called disease-modifying antirheumatic drugs (DMARDs) such as methotrexate and sulfasalazine. A fast control of inflammation, even using temporary oral steroids, is of benefit.

The study of the etiopathogenesis of the disease has provided insights into the immunological reactions between the antigen-presenting cells and the T and B lymphocytes, as well as into the cytokine imbalance resulting from this disease process. This has led to the development of new targeted treatments such as blocking antibodies or soluble receptors of TNFα. These novel treatments appear to exert a more profound disease control in patients refractory to standard DMARDs, and the data even suggest an arrest in joint tissue damage. The use of these powerful but expensive treatment options in early disease should be carefully weighed, also in view of the still unknown possible long-term side effects.

Involvement of the Knee in Spondyloarthropathy

In spondyloarthropathy, knee arthritis can present as acute inflammatory monoarthritis, as chronic inflammatory monoarthritis, or as a first sign of chronic inflammatory oligo- or polyarthritis. The spondyloarthropathies [4,5] comprise a number of related diseases with common clinical, radiological, biological, genetic, and therapeutic features and include the following entities:
1. Ankylosing spondylitis (AS)
2. Reactive arthritis

Table 1-2. Characteristics of spondyloarthropathies

1. Absence of rheumatoid factor and rheumatoid nodules
2. Inflammatory peripheral arthritis
3. Spinal inflammation: inflammatory back pain, sacroiliitis with or without spondylitis
4. Inflammatory enthesopathy
5. Clinical overlap between the different clinical entities of the group
6. Familial aggregation
7. Association with HLA B27

3. Psoriatic arthritis
4. Idiopathic acute anterior uveitis
5. Inflammatory bowel disease-related arthritis
6. Undifferentiated spondyloarthropathy
7. Late-onset pauciarticular juvenile chronic arthritis

The characteristics of spondyloarthropathies (SpA) are listed in ■ Table 1-2.

Characteristics of Spondyloarthropathies

According to the respective clinical diagnosis (see above), inflammatory knee involvement in SpA can present in different ways, usually as part of oligoarthritis, less frequently as monoarthritis or as part of an asymmetrical polyarthritis.

Oligoarthritis is seen in undifferentiated spondyloarthropathy, psoriatic arthritis, inflammatory bowel disease (IBD)-associated arthritis, late-onset pauciarticular juvenile arthritis, and, to a lesser extent, in AS and reactive arthritis. Peripheral arthritis is a key feature in these SpA and is generally asymmetrical, nonerosive,

and self-resolving. It involves the large weight-bearing joints of the lower limbs, most frequently the knees and ankles. Knee monoarthritis may be the presenting feature. Some patients develop a chronic erosive mono- or oligoarthritis. In psoriatic arthritis, the asymmetrical oligoarthritis subtype is the most prevalent and affects predominantly the joints of the lower limbs. This implies that the knee is often affected. In 2%–20% of patients with IBD, peripheral joint involvement is present and can fluctuate with the activity of the bowel inflammation. A *monoarticular* presentation is found in reactive arthritis and AS. AS has predominantly axial involvement, but 25% of patients with AS also develop peripheral arthritis. The hip and shoulder are frequently involved, and, to a lesser extent, knee involvement is seen in these patients. Knee arthritis as a first symptom of *polyarthritis* is seen in psoriatic arthritis and in IBD-related SpA.

Knee pain in patients with SpA must be differentiated from knee arthritis with or without synovitis and enthesitis at the insertions of the patellar ligament on the patellar apex and the tubercle of the tibia. In patients with late-onset pauciarticular juvenile chronic arthritis, enthesitis of the tuberositas tibiae is seen as the presenting sign in about 10% of patients. Although in SpA calcaneal enthesitis is the most frequent enthesopathy, enthesitis of the patellar ligament and the quadriceps insertion can be present as well.

The *enthesitis* frequently causes pain but can be asymptomatic as well. Soft-tissue swelling is sometimes present and can be shown by ultrasound (US), conventional radiography, and MRI. Enthesitis of the patellar ligament is often mistaken for osteonecrosis or traction apophysitis (Osgood-Schlatter and Sinding-Larsen disease). Enthesitis can be differentiated by ultrasound from bursitis, which is omnipresent in the vicinity of enthesis as well.

Table 1-3. Differences in characteristics of peripheral arthritis in SpA and in RA

Characteristics	Peripheral arthritis in SpA	Rheumatoid arthritis
Age	Younger (av 30 years)	Older (av 50 years)
Sex predominance	No	Female
Onset	Abrupt	Gradual
Behavior	Migratory	Nonmigratory
Affected joints	Mono- to pauciarticular	Polyarticular
	Asymmetrical	Symmetrical
	Lower limbs	Hands and feet >hip and knees
Course	Non deforming	Deforming
Enthesitis	Often	No
Rheumatoid factor	Absent	Present
Radiology	No erosions	Erosive
Prior symptoms	Urogenital or enterogenic infection	None
Extra-articular manifestations	Psoriasis	Rheumatoid nodules
	Bowel inflammation	Vasculitis
	Urethritis	
	Uveitis	

Chapter 1 · Arthritis of the Knee: Diagnosis and Management – F.P. Luyten et al.

9   1

Imaging. MRI and US can be of value in diagnosing SpA, especially in cases where peripheral arthritis is the only clinical manifestation. Knee synovitis in SpA differs from that in RA due to the involvement of adjacent enthesopathy [6]. MRI detects both perienthesial fluid or edema and bone marrow edema at the enthesial insertions in the knees of spondyloarthropathy patients, while the latter is absent in the knees of RA patients. US demonstrates the relationship between enthesial abnormalities and bone edema at the cortex–enthesis interface. A recent study suggests that enthesitis of the adjacent entheses is always present in peripheral synovitis of spondyloarthropathy in contrast to its absence in RA, an observation which has important implications for diagnosis.

Differential Diagnosis. Other arthritides such as RA need to be excluded. The main differences between peripheral arthritis in SpA and RA are listed in ◻ Table 1-3.

Differences in Characteristics Between Peripheral Arthritis in SpA and RA

Young patients with a swollen knee in the absence of trauma must be suspected of having a spondyloarthropathy. The possibility of spondyloarthropathy must be considered if, in addition to the knee arthritis, certain particular symptoms are present. The clinical characteristics of these associated symptoms must be evaluated, e.g., synovitis of other joints, dactylitis (sausage toe or finger), inflammatory axial disease, and extra-articular manifestations such as uveitis or conjunctivitis, urethritis or cervicitis, bowel inflammation, skin lesions such as psoriasis, and endocarditis. The patient must be repeatedly interviewed for family history of SpA and episodes of urogenital and enterogenic infection prior to the arthritis.

Detailed characteristics of the symptoms reported by the patients are in most cases sufficient to strongly suggest the diagnosis. If not, two additional investigations can be helpful: testing for HLA-B27 and pelvic radiographs.

The final diagnosis is made on the basis of concordance of the clinical manifestations and the physician's personal experience in the field. There are no diagnostic criteria available, but the available classification criteria can be used to examine the specific manifestations. If these criteria are fulfilled the diagnosis can be made, but even if a patient does not fulfill the classification criteria, he can still suffer from an incomplete or unusual form of spondyloarthropathy.

Treatment of Knee Arthritis in SpA

Suitable rest is advisable for patients with arthritis of the weight-bearing joints. The further therapeutic approach is decided depending on the clinical presentation such as an nonarthritis, or of the knee arthritis is part of an oligo- or polyarticular disease.

Acute monoarthritis is treated with NSAIDs for 6 weeks. If the first-line treatment fails, other therapeutic options are introduced. The indications for NSAID use are pain and morning stiffness. No controlled data are available regarding the efficacy of NSAID treatment in peripheral arthritis in SpA, but in clinical practice it appears that NSAIDs can be efficacious, especially in reactive arthritis. Patients should be treated for 6 weeks at the optimal dose. The use of NSAIDs is less desirable, and in some cases contraindicated, if concomitant IBD is present.

A single intra-articular injection of corticosteroids in spondyloarthropathy patients with monoarthritis may have a beneficial effect and last for some time. Such an injection can be repeated at a maximum frequency of 3–4 injections in the same joint during a 1-year period.

Physiotherapy is helpful in maintaining the function of the affected joint. Mobilization exercises and strengthening of the quadriceps without weight-bearing are useful. However, physiotherapy appears to have no effect on the inflammatory process.

If monoarthritis persists, or knee involvement is part of chronic oligo- or polyarticular disease, disease-modifying antirheumatic drug (DMARD) therapy is started. Sulfasalazine and methotrexate are frequently used as DMARDs in SpA.

Sulfasalazine is the only "second-line" drug with proven efficacy in prospective controlled trials for the treatment of peripheral arthritis in SpA. It is considered a safe and well-tolerated treatment for persistent, chronic peripheral synovitis in SpA. The effect is greater when it is started at an early stage of the disease than in patients with already existing joint deformities. Incremental dosages starting at 0.5 g twice daily and increasing to 1.5 g twice daily are used. The clinical effect must be evaluated at 3 months. Although sulfasalazine has a good safety profile, biochemical evaluation of liver enzymes and white cell blood counts must be performed on a regular basis. Sperm count can be reduced in men but is particularly a problem in men with pre-existing fertility problems. However, sulfasalazine is a safe drug for women contemplating pregnancy.

In daily practice, methotrexate is used on a regular basis in SpA, in analogy to its use in RA. Methotrexate is started at a weekly dose of 10–15 mg on a fixed day in combination with folic acid 1 mg OD. No placebo-controlled data are available, however, addressing the efficacy of methotrexate in peripheral spondyloarthropathy.

Pamidronate and thalidomide have shown some efficacy in open studies for AS patients with refractory disease. Although designed for refractory spinal disease, patients with concomitant peripheral arthritis also experience a beneficial effect in the peripheral joints.

Recent advances in biological therapies with cytokine-blocking strategies are promising. TNFα blockade is efficacious in the treatment of axial disease in AS and peripheral synovitis, and in patients with psoriatic arthritis. In open studies TNFα blockade also showed a beneficial effect on the peripheral manifestations of SpA and on the articular manifestations of Crohn's disease.

Finally, arthroscopic lavage can be of use in chronic monoarthritis for individual patients, but it's effect is usually only temporary.

Crystal-induced Arthritis

The clinical presentation of crystal-induced arthritis is predominantly acute inflammatory monoarthritis, or recurrent episodes of inflammatory mono- or oligoarthritis. Crystal arthritis comprises a group of acute and chronic arthritides caused by the deposition of different types of crystals in the joint tissues. Monosodium urate crystals in gout and calcium pyrophosphate dihydrate (CPPD) crystals in pseudogout are the clinically most frequent crystal deposition diseases. Correct diagnosis is made by the identification of crystals in the synovial fluid. Pain relief during the acute event and prevention of recurrent attacks is the goal of the treatment.

Gout occurs as a result of hyperuricemia, although asymptomatic hyperuricemia is common. In early stages of gout, the clinical manifestation is an acute attack of inflammatory monoarthritis in the MTP joint, but the knee is also frequently involved. Subsequent attacks can occur more frequently, and may become oligo- to polyarticular and persist longer. *Radiographic* features are soft-tissue swelling, the presence of tophi (soft-tissue densities which occasionally are calcified) and bony erosions (punched-out lesions) with sclerotic margins and overhanging edges. In contrast to other inflammatory arthritides, the joint space is preserved. NSAIDs and colchicine are effective in the treatment of gout. Drugs that alter serum acid levels (allopurinol, probenecid) should be started after more than two or three attacks have occurred, not at the time of the acute attack, but once started they should never be stopped.

Pseudogout is an acute inflammatory crystal mono- or oligoarthritis, and frequently seen with chondrocalcinosis, a radiographic diagnosis associated with deposition of CPPD in cartilage. The release of CPPD crystals in the joint space causes the inflammation, and diagnosis is made by polarized light microscopy of the joint fluid, identifying weakly positively birefringent blunt or square crystals. NSAIDs are preferentially used as treatment. In some cases, differentiating CPPD disease and other forms of polyarthritis, such as RA, can be difficult. Some patients display a pseudo-rheumatoid pattern, with involvement of multiple joints, particularly the knees, wrists, and elbows. Lack of erosions, low RF titers, and the presence of synovial fluid crystals help to establish the correct diagnosis.

Crystals are also commonly found in osteoarthritis of the knee. Distinguishing osteoarthritis from CPPD arthritis is therefore not always easy, but this is usually of little consequence, as there are no "dramatic" therapeutic implications. In primary OA, the medial compartment is more involved, while the pseudo-osteoarthritis caused by CPPD deposition is more in the lateral compartment. Radiographs typically show chondrocalcinosis in the latter case.

Miscellaneous Forms of Arthritis of the Knee

Infectious Arthritis

Infectious arthritis presents typically as an (sub)acute inflammatory monoarthritic disease. Up to 90% of infectious arthritis cases present as monoarthritis. The only exception is gonococcal arthritis, which presents more commonly as a migratory polyarthritis. If the condition is unrecognized, joint destruction will occur rapidly.

In any acute joint disease, infection must be suspected. However, infectious arthritis is an uncommon condition; the incidence in the developed world is estimated to be about six cases per 100 000 per year [7]. The knee is indeed the most commonly involved joint. The pathogenic process starts when the synovium or the synovial fluid becomes a culture medium for bacteria. Usually, the microorganisms reach the joint via bacteremia, although spreading from adjacent tissues or direct inoculation through the skin also occurs. Whether a clinically relevant infection develops depends on the virulence of the infecting organism, the size of the bacterial inoculum, and the resistance of the host. The most likely causative organism is *Staphylococcus aureus*, but many other organisms have been isolated from septic joints, including streptococci and Enterobacteriaceae. Age-specific organisms are *Haemophilus influenzae* type b in children and *Neisseria gonorrhoeae* in adults. Rare pathogens such as fungi are more often found in case of immunodeficiency, the presence of penetrating wounds, or intravenous substance abuse. Most patients suffer from an underlying medical condition such as diabetes mellitus, or an underlying joint condition such as RA.

Fever is common but can be absent. The only definitive *diagnostic test* is the demonstration of bacteria in the

Chapter 1 · Arthritis of the Knee: Diagnosis and Management – F.P. Luyten et al.

11   **1**

synovial fluid or in the synovium, or recovery of bacteria from a synovial fluid/synovium biopsy culture. When a joint is suspected of being infected, arthrocentesis should be performed prior to the initiation of any antimicrobial therapy. This procedure is not yet sufficiently practiced. The fluid should be subjected to a cell count, Gram staining, and culture, preferably in blood culture medium. A count of more than 50 000 cells/mm^3, of which more than 90% are polymorphonuclear leukocytes, makes infection highly likely.

Treatment requires both adequate drainage of purulent joint fluid and appropriate antimicrobial therapy. Following aspiration of the joint, and after blood, oral, and genital swabs have been obtained for culture, antibiotics should be administered on an "educated/best-guess" basis, considering the patient's age and history and the results of the Gram stain. The choice and the appropriate dosage should be adjusted when an etiological agent is identified and its antibiotic sensitivity is determined. There is no need to inject antimicrobials into the joint. Irrigation of the joint is recommended to evacuate bacterial products and debris associated with infection. The optimal duration of treatment is controversial, as is the route of administration of the antibiotic drug. An empirical period of 4–6 weeks of intravenous antibiotic treatment is commonly suggested. In case of gonococcal arthritis, treatment for 7 days is believed to be sufficient.

Lyme Arthritis

Arthritis in Lyme disease can present as chronic inflammatory monoarthritis or as migratory polyarthritis. Lyme arthritis is one of many possible features of Lyme disease (LD), a complex multisystem and infectious disease, resulting from infection with species of the spirochete *Borrelia burgdorferi* sensu latu, which is spread in Europe by the bite of infected *Ixodes ricinus* ticks [8] (in North America by Ixodes scapularis). LD occurs in endemic pockets with an incidence of 50–300 cases per 100 000 per year. Lyme manifestations can be grouped in three stages: an early localized stage in which a pathognomonic skin feature, erythema migrans, usually occurs; an early disseminated stage in which spirochetemia causes seeding of many organs, which leads to a wide spectrum of clinical manifestations; and the late disseminated stage when mainly neurological and musculoskeletal symptoms are reported. Clinical presentation of LD in the later stages is not uncommon. Of the untreated patients, 50% develop migratory polyarthritis, while 10% develop chronic, intermittent monoarthritis, usually of the knee, characterized by large inflammatory articular effusions. The *diagnosis* is based on the characteristic clinical findings and a history of exposure in an area where LD is endemic, and it can be confirmed by serological testing (ELISA). A positive result of the ELISA test should be confirmed by Western blot. *Borrelia burgdorferi* can be detected in joint fluid or synovial tissue by polymerase chain reaction. LD is usually cured by antibiotic treatment at any stage of the disease. *Treatment* is easier and more successful the earlier it is given. In the case of Lyme arthritis, either oral or intravenous regimens are usually effective. If accompanying neuroborreliosis is suspected, intravenous regimens are indicated.

Pigmented Villonodular Synovitis/Synovial Chondromatosis

Pigmented villonodular synovitis (PVNS) and synovial chondromatosis are two types of proliferative disorders affecting the synovial lining of joints. The clinical presentation is typically chronic inflammatory monoarthritis. In PVNS, histology is characterized by hypercellular synovial connective tissue containing hemosiderin-laden macrophages. In synovial chondromatosis the synovial mesenchymal cells mature into chondroblasts that form nodules of cartilage. Both conditions are uncommon. The incidence of PVNS is estimated to be approximately 1.8/1 million. The presentation is usually monoarticular, affecting mainly the knee. All age groups can be affected, although PVNS occurs more frequently in young adults, whereas the average age of synovial chondromatosis is in the fifth decade of life. In both conditions patients present with slowly progressive joint pain and swelling. Plain radiographic investigation often shows only increased soft-tissue density. MRI usually demonstrates key diagnostic features. The diagnosis is confirmed by biopsy, and the *treatment* of choice is synovectomy [9].

The Knee and the Study of the Synovium: From Research to Clinical Practice

The knee synovium is easily accessible and has provided an excellent tool for diagnosis, but most importantly for studying the pathogenesis of the disease processes. It is anticipated that synovial biopsies will also be routinely used in evaluating treatment response.

The classical clinical indication for taking a synovial biopsy is chronic (>6 weeks) nontraumatic inflammatory (synovial fluid WBC count >2000 cells/mm^3) arthritis limited to one or two joints in which the diagnosis remains unclear after an appropriate noninvasive diagnostic workup, including synovial fluid analysis with culture for fungi and mycobacteria. There has never been much discussion about the usefulness of synovial biopsies for the diagnosis of atypical chronic infections (e.g., fungi, mycobacteria), plant-thorn and other foreign-body synovitis, all kinds of synovial tumors, chronic sarcoidosis, and some infiltrative and deposition diseases (e.g., amyloidosis, hemochromatosis).

Although the synovium is also an important target tissue of RA and the SpA, the examination of synovial biopsies for clinical reasons has never been popular in these prototypical chronic arthritides, probably because their diagnosis does not depend so much on histology.

Given the fact that it is impossible to obtain access to the target tissue without an invasive procedure, most of our knowledge of synovial histology in chronic arthritis has come from postmortem studies or from studies of synovial biopsies taken during curative orthopedic procedures in end-stage disease. The popularity of synovial biopsies for differential diagnosis in chronic arthritis has suffered greatly from the lack of disease-specific light-microscopic characteristics at this late stage of the disease, and this for a very long time [10].

The introduction of arthroscopy, and particularly of the minimally invasive needle arthroscopy technique under local anesthesia, has made it possible to take synovial biopsy samples at every stage of the disease, and even repetitively, in an office-based setting. This evolution has led to a renewed interest in the synovium. Since the beginning of the 1990s, numerous studies based on the analysis of synovial biopsies obtained by needle arthroscopy have provided better insight into the pathophysiology of the chronic arthritides. Thanks to the use of immunohistological techniques and molecular biology, the analysis of synovial biopsy material has been carried beyond the structural level. A closer identification of the cells infiltrating the synovium by their cell surface molecules and receptors, together with an analysis of their protein products, has given us a better understanding of the driving forces and the dynamics of synovial inflammation. We now know that what we call early arthritis from a clinical point of view reflects an already chronic disease stage at the histological level, and that an asymptomatic phase precedes the onset of clinical signs and symptoms of arthritis [11]. The signs and symptoms of arthritis have been correlated with the production of specific key cytokines such as TNFα and IL1-β in the synovium by macrophages [12]. In chronic arthritis, synovial macrophages are part of a well-organized cellular network together with lymphocytes and synovial fibroblasts. Communication between these cells takes place via direct cell–cell contact but also via the production of growth factors, cytokines, and chemokines. Thanks to both in vivo and in vitro research based on synovial biopsy material, we are beginning to understand this complex network [13]. The process of bone destruction in RA has been much elucidated, and destructive factors such as RANK Ligand, TNF-α, and IL1-β have been found in the synovium, as well as protective factors such as osteoprotegerin

(OPG) [14]. Matrix metalloproteinases, enzymes produced at the cartilage–pannus interface, have been shown to be responsible for cartilage degradation and are counterbalanced by inhibitory proteins [15]. It appears that the synovial tissue itself sometimes has, especially at later disease stages, an invasive, tumor-like nature [16].

Much effort has been made to differentiate the chronic arthritides from one another at the synovial level. Quantitative differences have been found in the different inflammatory cell types infiltrating the synovium and in the balances of several cytokines and growth factors [17]. Moreover, at both the macroscopic and the microscopic level, the synovial vascularity has been postulated to be specifically increased in SpA in comparison to RA [18]. Looking for the origin of the perinuclear factor, an old but very specific blood test for RA, researchers have identified specific serum antibodies against certain citrullinated proteins, which in turn have been traced back to the synovium and are very specific for RA [19]. The more new specific markers are found, the more we can expect synovial biopsies to become an attractive differential diagnostic tool in daily practice.

During the past decade, the benefit of an earlier and more aggressive treatment of chronic arthritis has become clear. Better knowledge of the pathophysiology of chronic arthritis has led to the development of new, more targeted treatment strategies such as blocking of TNFα and IL1-β. Sequential synovial biopsies are increasingly being used for disease monitoring and for the rapid evaluation of new treatment modalities, which are themselves often based on the identification of new candidate targets in the synovium [20]. The high cost and the considerable risk of severe side effects of these new therapies will make it necessary to look for predictive drug-response markers, and most probably these will be found in the synovium too. We are only beginning to realize how informative the study of the synovium will become.

Acknowledgements. We thank our colleagues for their generous assistance in preparing this chapter, especially to K. de Vlam, F. Lensen, P. Verschueren.

References

1. American College of Rheumatology Subcommittee on Osteoarthritis Guidelines (2000) Recommendations for the medical management of osteoarthritis of the hip and knee: 2000 update. Arthritis Rheum 43:1905–1915
2. Pendleton A et al (2000) EULAR recommendations for the management of knee osteoarthritis: report of a task force of the Standing Committee for International Clinical Studies Including Therapeutic Trials (ESCISIT). Ann Rheum Dis 59:936–944
3. Arnett FC et al (1988) The American Rheumatism Association 1987 revised criteria for the classification of rheumatoid arthritis. Arthritis Rheum 31:315–324
4. Wright V (1978) Seronegative polyarthritis. A unified concept. Arthritis Rheum 21:619–633

Chapter 1 · Arthritis of the Knee: Diagnosis and Management – F.P. Luyten et al.

13

1

5. Miceli-Richard C et al (2003) Spondyloarthropathy for practicing rheumatologist: diagnosis, indication for disease-controlling antirheumatic therapy, and evaluation of response. Rheum Dis Clin N Am 29:449–462

6. Mc Gonagle D et al (1998) Characteristic magnetic resonance imaging entheseal changes of knee synovitis in spondylarthropathy. Arthritis Rheum 41:694–700

7. Nade S (2003) Septic arthritis. Best Practice Res Clin Rheumatol 17:183–200

8. Franz J, Krause A (2003) Lyme disease (Lyme borreliosis). Best Practice Res Clin Rheumatol 17:241–264

9. Ruddy S, et al (2001) Kelley's textbook of rheumatology. W.B. Saunders, Philadelphia

10. Schulte E et al (1994) Differential diagnosis of synovitis. Correlation of arthroscopic biopsy to clinical findings (in German). Pathologe 15:22–27

11. Kraan MC et al (1998) Asymptomatic synovitis precedes clinically manifest arthritis. Arthritis Rheum 41:1481–1488

12. Tak PP et al (1997) Analysis of the synovial cell infiltrate in early rheumatoid synovial tissue in relation to local disease activity. Arthritis Rheum 40:217–225

13. Firestein GS (2003) Evolving concepts of rheumatoid arthritis. Nature 423:356–361

14. Haynes DR et al (2003) Osteoprotegerin expression in synovial tissue from patients with rheumatoid arthritis, spondyloarthropathies and osteoarthritis and normal controls. Rheumatology 42:123–134

15. Seemayer CA et al (2003) Cartilage destruction mediated by synovial fibroblasts does not depend on proliferation in rheumatoid arthritis. Am J Pathol 162:1549–1557

16. Zvaifler NJ, Firestein GS (1994) Pannus and pannocytes. Alternative models of joint destruction in rheumatoid arthritis. Arthritis Rheum 37:783–789

17. Baeten D et al (2000) Comparative study of the synovial histology in rheumatoid arthritis, spondyloarthropathy, and osteoarthritis: influence of disease duration and activity. Ann Rheum Dis 59:945–953

18. Fearon U et al (2003) Angiopoietins, growth factors, and vascular morphology in early arthritis. J Rheumatol 30:260–268

19. Baeten D et al (2001) Specific presence of intracellular citrullinated proteins in rheumatoid arthritis synovium: relevance to antifilaggrin autoantibodies. Arthritis Rheum 44:2255–2262

20. Smeets TJ et al (1999) Analysis of serial synovial biopsies in patients with rheumatoid arthritis: description of a control group without clinical improvement after treatment with interleukin 10 or placebo. J Rheumatol 26:2089–2093

2   Knee Arthroplasty to Maximize the Envelope of Function

S. F. Dye

Summary

The knee functions as a type of biological transmission whose purpose is to accept and transfer a range of loads between and among the femur, patella, tibia, and fibula without causing structural or metabolic damage. Arthritic knees are like living transmissions with worn bearings that have limited capacity to safely accept and transmit forces. A new method of representing the functional capacity of the knee and other joints is the "envelope of function", a load and frequency distribution that delineates the range of loads a given joint can sustain while still maintaining homeostasis of all tissues. The purpose of joint replacement surgery, therefore, is to maximize the envelope of function for a given joint as safely and predictably as possible.

A fundamental principle of all orthopedic treatment is to restore, as much as possible, normal musculoskeletal function. Following minor trauma to a previously normal joint such as the knee (e.g., contusion, mild medial collateral ligament sprain), the process of healing – the result of over 400 million years of vertebrate evolutionarily designed molecular and cellular mechanisms [1] – is most often accomplished without the necessity of any therapeutic intervention. True restoration to the full pre-injury functional status is expected and most often occurs. With more substantial trauma to the knee, such as occurs with a complete rupture of the anterior cruciate ligament treated with a reconstruction, restoration to the full pre-injury physiological functional status is more problematic and often does not occur despite modern surgical techniques [2–4]. Even well-reconstructed knees have unfortunately demonstrated the development of early arthrosis if the joint is exposed to sufficiently high levels of loading, such as occurs with soccer and other similar pivoting sports. One can say that the pre-injury functional capacity of such an anterior cruciate ligament reconstructed knee has not been fully restored.

In the case of knees with advanced degenerative arthrosis which undergo joint replacement surgery, the principle of functional restoration may be more properly stated as maximization of the functional capacity of the knee. As effective as current joint replacement techniques
are at achieving pain relief and often associated increases in muscle strength and control, knees that have had joint replacement surgery do not replicate the functional status of a healthy, uninjured, adult joint. No one with a total knee replacement, for example, should run marathons or play tackle football. Since the goal of total knee replacement surgery is to maximize joint function, what, then, is the function of the knee?

The Knee as Biological Transmission

Over the past decade or so, a new concept of joint function has been developed that appears to provide a better theoretical description and therefore understanding of the function of the knee, and, by extension, of all diarthroidal joints. In a leap of insight, Menschik of Vienna communicated to me (A. Menschik (1988), personal communication) that the knee could be best conceptualized as a type of "step-less transmission", the purpose of which is to accept and redirect repeated biomechanical loads between the femur, patella, tibia, and fibula, and eventually through the ankle and foot, into the ground. Following much consideration and discussion with other individuals within the international knee community, it became clear that this view of the function of the knee as a kind of biological transmission was not only accurate, but represented a substantial advance in conceptual thinking with potential implications for the entire field of orthopedic surgery [5]. In this analogy of the knee as biological transmission, the ligaments can be visualized as sensate, nonrigid, adaptive linkages, articular cartilage as bearings, and the menisci as mobile, sensate bearings [6]. The patellofemoral joint can be seen as a large slide bearing within the biological transmission that is exposed to the greatest forces, both in compression and in tension, of any component of human joints. The muscles in this analogy can be conceptualized as cellular engines that, in concentric contraction, provide motive forces across the knee and, in eccentric contraction, act as brakes and dampening systems, absorbing shock loads. The importance of eccentric contraction to knee function has been demonstrated by Winter [7], who has shown that the muscles about the knee actually absorb more than three times the energy that is generated in motive forces. The various components of a living joint are constantly metabolically active, with the presence of complex molecular and cellular mechanisms that are designed to maintain and restore tissue homeostasis under normal and injurious biomechanical conditions [8]. The concept of musculoskeletal function should therefore include the capacity not only to generate, transmit, absorb, and dissipate loads, but also to maintain *tissue homeostasis* while doing so.

The Envelope of Function

Mechanical transmissions are complex systems designed to differentially accept and redirect loads/torque between components. The functional capacity of a mechanical transmission can be represented by the range of torque that can be safely managed without structural failure or over-heating of the components. This range of loading can be represented by a torque envelope. Similarly, the functional capacity of the knee can be represented by a load and frequency distribution that I have termed the "envelope of function". The envelope of function was developed as a simple method to incorporate and connect the concepts of load transference and tissue homeostasis in order to visually represent the functional capacity of the knee. It defines a range of loading that is compatible with and inductive of the overall tissue homeostasis of a given joint or musculoskeletal system. The envelope of function, in its simplest form, is a load and frequency distribution that defines a safe range of loading for a joint (◘ Fig. 2-1).

The upper limit of the envelope represents a threshold between loads that are inductive of tissue homeostasis and loads that initiate the complex biological cascade of trauma-induced inflammation and repair (◘ Fig. 2-2). The area within the envelope can be termed the *zone of homeostasis*, or the *zone of homeostatic loading*. Loads that are beyond the threshold of the envelope but are lower than those that induce macrostructural failure of a joint component are in the area that can be termed the *zone of supraphysiological overload*. Loading in this region can induce the painful osseous remodeling associated with the initial stages of a stress fracture, which is manifested as increased activity on technetium bone scans before any structural changes are noted on radiographs. These sites of increased osseous metabolic activity may return to documented homeostasis as shown by normal bone scans following nonoperative treatment, primarily involving a reduction of loading. If more energy is placed across a joint, a second threshold is reached – the lower limit of the *zone of structural failure*. Such high loads result in overt structural failure of at least one

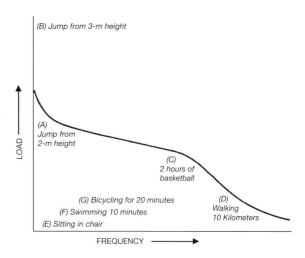

◘ Fig. 2-1. The envelope of function for an athletically active young adult. The letters represent the loads associated with different activities. All of the loading examples, except B, are within the envelope for this particular knee. The shape of the envelope of function represented here is an idealized theoretical model. The actual loads transmitted across an individual knee under these different conditions are variable and due to multiple complex factors, including the dynamic center of gravity, the rate of load application, and the angles of flexion and rotation. The limits of the envelope of function for the joint of an actual patient are probably more complex. (Reprinted with permission from [5])

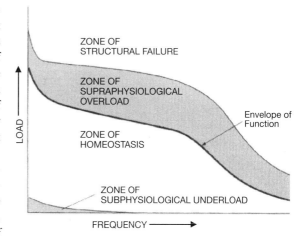

◘ Fig. 2-2. The four different zones of loading across a joint. The area within the envelope of function is the zone of homeostasis. The region of loading greater than that within the envelope of function but insufficient to cause macrostructural damage is the zone of supraphysiological overload. The region of loading great enough to cause macrostructural damage is the zone of structural failure. The region of decreased loading over time resulting in loss of tissue homeostasis is the zone of subphysiological underload. (Adapted from [3], reprinted with permission)

component of a joint or musculoskeletal system, such as a rupture of the anterior cruciate ligament or a fracture of the tibial plateau. An extended period of decreased loading, such as may occur with prolonged bed rest, can result in loss of tissue homeostasis, as evidenced by osteopenia and muscle atrophy associated with disuse. This lower threshold demarcates the *zone of subphysiological underload.* It appears that most, if not all, musculoskeletal systems respond to differential loading as depicted in these four regions.

Frost's extensive work regarding homeostatic properties and principles of tissues, particularly bone, independently corroborates and complements the concept of the envelope of function [9, 10]. Frost's view of excessive microdamage corresponds to the loading of tissues within the zone of supraphysiological overload [11]. Too little loading over time, resulting in disuse osteopenia, is reflected in his concept of minimum effective strain or minimum effective signal as a lower threshold limit [12]. Virtually all symptomatic knees with radiographically identifiable arthrosis sufficient to be considered for joint replacement surgery will also manifest loss of osseous homeostasis with technetium scintigraphy [13] (◘Fig. 2-3a,b – left knee). Following well-performed total knee replacement surgery, the inflamed subchondral osseous tissue that is the source of abnormal scintigraphic activity (and, one also presumes, much of the nociceptive output from the arthritic knee) has been operatively removed. The components of a total knee are thus placed against (without cement) or near (with cement) living bone that was in most cases formerly homeostatic. A new level of meta-bolic activity of the living bone under the components needs to be achieved following total knee replacement surgery [14]. Postoperative technetium scintigraphy is an excellent method of objectively tracking this process. The desired outcome is for the scintigraphic activity under the components to eventually become minimal and indefinitely remain so (◘ Fig. 2-3a,b – right knee). Findings of increased uptake in one or more geographical regions indicates loss of osseous homeostasis and can be an indicator of current or eventual overt radiographically identifiable loosening [15, 16] (◘ Fig. 2-4a,b – left knee).

Knees that have undergone joint replacement surgery do not necessarily have all of the possible nociceptive sources of pain removed or addressed at the time of surgery. Tissues such as inflamed synovium often remain following total knee replacement surgery, and can thus be a possible source of persistent pain, effusion, and dysfunction, despite well-placed components. The goal of treatment is to maximize the load transference capacity of a knee that has had joint replacement surgery, in other words, to maximize the postoperative envelope of function for that joint. The indicators that a joint is being loaded within its postoperative envelope of function are the absence of pain, swelling, and warmth, an excellent

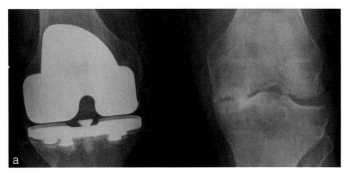 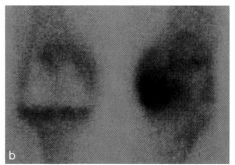

◘**Fig. 2-3a, b.** *a* A technetium 99m methylene diphosphonate 3-h delayed bone scan of a 78-year-old man, 6 years following total joint replacement of the right knee and advanced degenerative arthrosis on the left knee, manifesting minimal subcomponent activity indicative of relative homeostasis of the right knee. The marked increased activity noted in the left knee corresponds to the pathophysiological metabolic activity associated with the advanced degenerative arthrosis. *b* Radiographs of the same patient showing a total knee replacement on the right and advanced degenerative arthrosis on the left knee

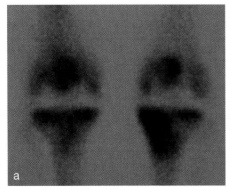 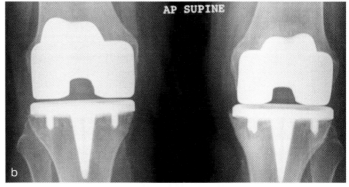

◘ **Fig. 2-4a, b.** *a* A technetium bone scan of a 68-year-old woman, 9 months following joint replacement surgery on the right knee and 3 years following joint replacement surgery on the left knee, manifesting expected low-level metabolic activity associated with the right knee components and increased metabolic activity under the medial aspect of the tibial component of the left knee, consistent with possible loosening. *b* Radiograph of the same patient, manifesting acceptable total knee replacement on the right and evidence of possible loosening under the medial aspect of the tibial component on the left knee

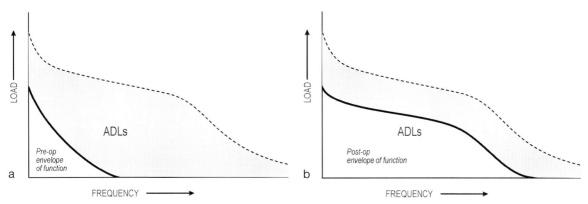

Fig. 2-5a,b. *a* Example of a preoperative envelope of function of a patient with symptomatic knee arthrosis, showing severe restrictions of functional capacity. ADLs, Activities of daily living. *b* Example of a postoperative envelope of function, showing substantial increases in the functional capacity following successful total knee replacement, but not restoration to full physiological function of an asymptomatic normal knee

range of motion and muscle control, and a minimal level of subcomponent scintigraphic activity.

I have often found it valuable to draw out both the preoperative and expected postoperative envelopes of function for patients prior to surgery (■ Fig. 2-5a,b). Most patients can readily grasp the concept of the envelope, and therefore can have a better understanding of what function is to be expected postoperatively. By this method, they can more readily understand that joint replacement surgery is not designed to restore a knee to full, normal physiological function. Patients have a responsibility, as well, to do all that they can (by participating in pre- and postoperative physical therapy, for example) to maximize their envelope and, once this is achieved, to not exceed the functional capacity of the joint following surgery by avoiding activities associated with supraphysiological loading. For most total knee patients, this information is much appreciated and is well within their expectations.

Conclusion

Joint replacement surgery is designed to expand the envelope of function of symptomatic arthritic knees as safely and predictably as possible. Properly utilized, total knee replacement surgery is capable of substantial increases in the functional capacity of a given arthritic joint, but it is not designed to restore the full physiological function of a normal, uninjured adult knee. Future developments in the therapeutic management of arthritic knees may eventually involve biological approaches that could result in further improvements in maximizing the post-treatment envelope of function over what can be achieved with the current technique of using artificial components. By tracking the loss of osseous homeostasis in knees starting at a time prior to the development of overt radiographically identifiable degenerative changes, an improved understanding of the natural history of arthrosis

could be achieved. Such an improved understanding of the natural history of knee arthrosis could have broad implications for the early detection, control, and ultimately prevention of arthrosis in all joints.

References

1. Dye SF (1987) An evolutionary perspective of the knee. J Bone Joint Surg 7:976–983
2. Daniel DM, Stone ML, Dobson BE, Fithian DC, Rossman DJ, Kaufman KR (1994) Fate of the ACL-injured patient. A prospective outcome study. Am J Sports Med 22:632–644
3. Dye SF, Wojtys EM, Fu FH, Fithian DC, Gillquist J (1998) Factors contributing to function of the knee joint after injury or reconstruction of the anterior cruciate ligament. J Bone Joint Surg 80A:1380–1393
4. Garrick JG, Requa RK (2003) Sports fitness activities: the negative consequences. J Am Acad Orthop Surg 11:439–443
5. Dye SF (1996) The knee as a biologic transmission with an envelope of function. Clin Orthop Rel Res 325:10–18
6. Dye SF, Vaupel GL, Dye CC (1998) Conscious neurosensory mapping of the internal structures of the human knee without intra-articular anesthesia. Am J Sports Med 26:773–777
7. Winter DA (1983) Energy generation and absorption at the ankle and knee during fast, natural, and slow cadences. Clin Orthop 175:147–154
8. Guyton AC, Hall JE (1996): Textbook of medical physiology. W.B. Saunders, Philadelphia
9. Frost HM (1989) Some ABCs of skeletal pathophysiology. I: Introduction to the series [editorial]. Calcif Tissue Int 45:1–3
10. Frost HM (1989) Some ABCs of skeletal pathophysiology. II: General mediator mechanism properties [editorial]. Calcif Tissue Int 45:68–70
11. Frost HM (1989) Some ABCs of skeletal pathophysiology. IV: The transient/steady state distinction [editorial]. Calcif Tissue Int 45:134–136
12. Frost HM (1983: A determinant of bone architecture. The minimum effective strain. Clin Orthop 175:286–292
13. Dye SF (1994) Comparison of magnetic resonance imaging and technetium scintigraphy in the detection of increased osseous metabolic activity about the knee of symptomatic adults. Orthop Trans 17:1060–1061
14. Brand RA, Stanford CM, Swan CC (2003) How do tissues respond and adapt to stresses around a prosthesis? A primer on finite element stress analysis for orthopedic surgeons. Iowa Orthop J 23:13–22
15. Henderson JJ, Bamford DJ, Noble J, Brown JD (1996) The value of skeletal scintigraphy in predicting the need for revision surgery in total knee replacement. Orthopedics 19:295–299
16. Smith SL, Wastie ML, Forster I (2001) Radionuclide bone scintigraphy in the detection of significant complications after total knee joint replacement. Clin Radiol 56:221–224

D. G. Eckhoff

Summary

The purpose of this chapter is to identify the functional anatomy that impacts the reconstruction of the arthritic knee with a prosthetic implant. This work does not attempt to review all the detailed soft-tissue anatomy of the knee that is covered more expansively both in description and illustration in other resources. It focuses instead on bone morphology of the knee. The conclusion is that morphological features of the knee are largely asymmetrical, and these features are related in both linear and angular relationships to one another in a way that will impact the function of the prosthetic replacement.

Introduction

The knee is defined in this chapter as composed of two parts, the soft-tissue sleeve and the underlying bony architecture. The soft-tissue sleeve extends from hip to ankle and invests the bony architecture. The bony architecture, both normal and pathological, is the focus of this anatomical review of the knee.

Soft-tissue Sleeve

Protection and nutritional support of the knee are provided by skin, fat, capsule, and synovium. Located in these soft tissues is a network of vessels (arteries, veins, lymphatics) and nerves. In general terms, the vessels and nerves pass from the hip to the ankle along the posterior aspect of the limb and send branches both medial and lateral around the knee to meet near the anterior midline. This anatomical feature allows surgical exposure of the knee from the anterior aspect with minimal risk to neurovascular structures. A full appreciation of the three-dimensional location and relationship of the nerves and vessels to each other as well as to other soft tissues of the knee is beyond the scope of this dissertation, and is best obtained by inspection of the Visible Human (http://www.visiblehuman.org).

Muscle-tendon units lie in the soft-tissue sleeve and are a significant component of the functional anatomy of the knee. The quadriceps (rectus femoris, vastus lateralis, vastus intermedius, vastus medialis) and articularis genu lie anterior to the femur. They arise from the pelvis (rectus femoris), the proximal femur (vastus lateralis, vastus intermedius, vastus medialis), and distal femur (articularis genu), and attach by way of a conjoined tendon to the tibia to form the extensor mechanism of the knee. Invested in the conjoined tendon is the body's largest sesamoid bone, the patella. Retinaculum and synovium attaching to the patella and its tendon pass around the medial and lateral aspects of the knee to the distal femur and proximal tibia. Surgical approaches to the knee discussed in later chapters all violate the retinacular and synovial investments of the extensor mechanism, and to a lesser extent the muscles and tendons just described.

The muscle-tendon units lying posterior to the femur are referred to collectively as the hamstrings. The lateral hamstring (biceps femoris) and the medial hamstrings (sartorius, gracilis, semitendinosis, semimembrinosis) arise from the pelvis and attach to the fibular head and medial aspect of the tibia, respectively. These muscles function collectively in knee flexion. They also function in rotating the knee, with the lateral hamstrings rotating the tibia external relative to the femur and the medial hamstrings rotating the tibia internal relative to the femur. In the arthritic knee, discussed below and elsewhere in this text, these muscle-tendon units become unbalanced in their effect on the knee, producing angular and rotational contractures.

Also implicated in knee contractures are the gastrocnemius muscles, the popliteal muscle, and the iliotibial band. The gastrocs originate just proximal and posterior to the femoral condyles and insert through the Achilles tendon on the calcaneus. The popliteal muscle arises from the posterior lateral femur and attaches to the posterior lateral tibia. The iliotibial (IT) band arises from the lateral pelvis and attaches to the anterolateral tibia at Gerde's tubercle. The latter structure, the IT band, is implicated in an external rotation of the tibia and secondary lateral tracking of the patella in the pathological knee. Planned sequential release and balancing of these soft tissues, discussed in later chapters, are integral steps in the performance of total knee arthroplasty.

Ligaments joining the femur and tibia are four in number, two cruciates and two collaterals. The medial collateral ligament (MCL) can be separated into two components, superficial and deep. The deep MCL originates from the area of the medial femoral epicondyle and inserts on the mid body of the medial meniscus and the proximal medial tibial plateau, forming a confluence with the coronary ligament attaching the meniscus to the tibia. The superficial MCL has an origin similar to that of the deep MCL but lacks any attachment to the meniscus and inserts more distally along the medial tibia. The MCL slopes from posterior proximally to anterior distally. The lateral collateral ligament originates from the area of the lateral epicondyle and inserts on the fibular head. It slopes opposite the MCL, passing from anterior proximally to posterior distally. The origins of the collaterals (MCL and LCL) lie on a line joining the femoral epicondyles, also known as the epicondylar line.

There are two cruciate ligaments. The anterior cruciate ligament (ACL) originates from the lateral wall of the femoral intercondylar notch and inserts on the mid tibia between the articular surfaces, passing from posterior proximally to anterior distally. Passing in the opposite direction, from anterior proximally to posterior distally, is the posterior cruciate ligament (PCL), which arises from the medial wall of femoral intercondylar notch and inserts over an area approximately 2 cm in vertical length on the posterior aspect of the tibia. The origin of the cruciates (ACL and PCL) is not on the same line as the origins of the collaterals, i.e., the epicondylar line. The cruciate origins lie on a line passing through the center of the condyles, a line equidistant from points on the posterior articular surface of the condyles. The location and clinical significance of this line will be discussed in more detail in relation to femoral condylar geometry below, but it is important to recognize for the purpose of balancing the soft tissues and restoring the kinematics of a knee that the origins of the cruciates and collaterals are not on the same line.

Another anatomical feature of these knee ligaments worth noting is the opposite slope of the cruciates (ACL and PCL) and collaterals (MCL and LCL) described above. The clinical significance of this observation is that in the absence of the ACL, the collaterals will uncross or unwind to become more closely parallel. This occurs because the tibia rotates internally relative to the femur in the absence of restraint from the ACL and/or the PCL [1]. In the course of knee replacement, one or both cruciates are removed, permitting this relative rotation of the tibia to the femur to occur, i.e., the collaterals unwind, potentially altering the contact pattern of the femoral and tibial components in the prosthetic knee. This issue of contact pattern and the associated issue of wear in a pros-

thetic knee are dependent on bone morphology or bony architecture of the knee, which will now be addressed.

Bony Architecture (Bone Morphology)

The distal femur has a unique three-dimensional shape marked by asymmetry. The two rounded asymmetrical prominences that articulate with the tibia, referred to as condyles, are separated by a space referred to as the intercondylar notch. The condyles are joined proximally by the femoral trochlear groove, the site of articulation between the patella and the femur. The trochlear groove is characterized as a trough with its lowest point, called the sulcus, set between medial and lateral anterior projections. These anterior projections, or ridges, are confluent with the condyles distally while the sulcus of the trochlear groove ends in the intercondylar notch. These morphological features of the distal femur are covered anterior, posterior, and distal by articular cartilage.

These morphological characteristics of the distal femur have been a source of both historical and contemporary interest [2–8]. More than a dozen linear dimensions and half a dozen angular dimensions of the distal femur have been repeatedly measured [4,5]. These measurements will not be recounted here in detail, but several documented relationships of functional anatomy will be highlighted. Specifical-

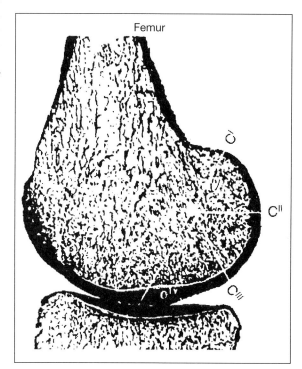

❑ **Fig. 3-1.** The Weber brothers created cross-sectional images of the femoral condyles by cutting cadaveric specimens, coating them with ink, and pressing them to paper. They found radii C1, C11, and C111 to be equal. This technique was the first to illustrate the circular profile of the condyles

ly, the shape of the posterior femoral condyles, the location and orientation of the trochlear groove, and the spatial relationship of the tibia to the femur need to be reviewed, since these are issues of functional anatomy that are integral to the practice of contemporary total knee arthroplasty.

The circular contour of the posterior condyles was first documented by the Weber brothers [2] (◘ Fig. 3-1). This perception of circular geometry of the posterior condyles was challenged by Fick [3], who proposed that the condyles were more helical in shape; i.e., he argued for a changing radius of curvature producing an instant center of flexion and extension. Fick's interpretation still commands a large following of engineers who find it difficult to reconcile the biomechanical data regarding knee motion with circular condyles. Nevertheless, abundant data now support the earlier Weber work [6]. A recent study suggests this controversy arises because authors of biomechanical studies beginning with Fick have repeatedly selected a flexion axis perpendicular to the sagittal plane of the knee [7]. While it is perhaps intuitive that the limb stays in the sagittal plane through a range of flexion and extension, there are no anatomical or kinematic data to support this idea, or the corollary that the axis of flexion and extension is perpendicular to the sagittal plane. The controversy can be resolved by allowing the knee to flex about an axis not perpendicular to the sagittal plane [7]. This axis not perpendicular to the sagittal plane permits motion to occur about a single axis centered in the condyles and supports the concept of circular condyles. Based on these observations, morphological studies have been conducted using modern computer techniques that confirm the circular profile of the posterior condyles, establishing a single axis for flexion and extension of the knee through an arc of 10°–120° [8, 9]. This work demonstrates with careful sizing and positioning of cylinders within the condyles that the two condyles are circular in shape. It also demonstrates that the condyles share a single axis of rotation but display differing radii of curvature, with medial greater than lateral (◘ Fig. 3-2).

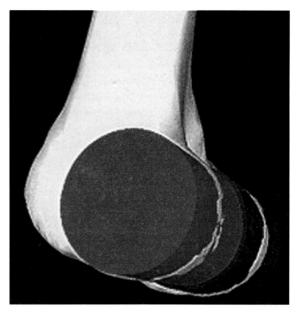

◘ **Fig. 3-2.** The cylindrical profile of the condyles can be demonstrated using computer techniques to create three-dimensional reconstructions of the distal femur from CT images with cylinders fit into the condyles. The medial cylinder (blue) is slightly larger than the lateral cylinder (red) but they share the same cylindrical axis

This work documents that the center of the cylinder is different from the line joining the epicondyles (◘ Fig. 3-3a, b). Further, the data presented in this work demonstrate that the cylindrical axis, corresponding to the center of each condyle, passes through the origins of the cruciate ligaments. As noted above, the epicondylar line incorporates the origins of the collateral ligaments, but not the origins of the cruciate ligaments. The work cited here documents that the epicondylar line and the line joining the center of the condyles are not the same. These observations of the relative relationship between the epicondylar line and the cylindrical axis based on the circular profile of the posterior condyles represent an important functional anatomical feature of the distal femur.

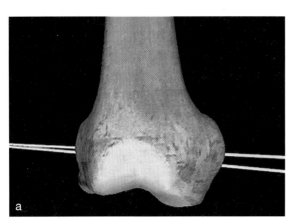

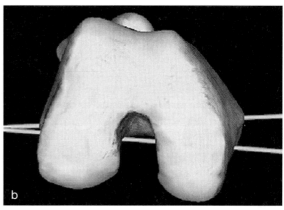

◘ **Fig. 3a, b.** The epicondylar (upper) and cylindrical (lower) axes do not lie in a single plane and are not parallel or collinear in the coronal plane (*a*) or the transverse plane (*b*)

It should be noted again that the foregoing discussion of circular condyles applies to the posterior femoral condyles, i.e., that portion of the distal femur articulating with the tibia from 10° to 120° of knee flexion. The condyles articulating with the tibia in the last 10° of extension have a curvature different from that of the posterior condyles [4,6]. Further, the anterior or trochlear portion of the distal femur demonstrates yet another curvature different from the condyles. It is not the curvature of the trochlea, however, but the location and orientation of its sulcus that plays a role in functional anatomy and merits further attention.

The location and orientation of the sulcus have been carefully documented both in cadavers [10] and on radiographs [11]. The sulcus of the trochlear groove lies lateral to the midplane of the distal femur and is oriented between the anatomical and mechanical lines of the femur in the coronal plane (◘ Fig. 3-4).

The anatomical line of the femur passes up the femoral shaft from the center of the distal femur to the greater trochanter (Fig. 4a). The mechanical line passes from the center of the distal femur to the center of the femoral head (Fig. 4b). Relative to these femoral references there is 2° deviation of the sulcus to the anatomical line and 4° deviation of the sulcus to the mechanical line

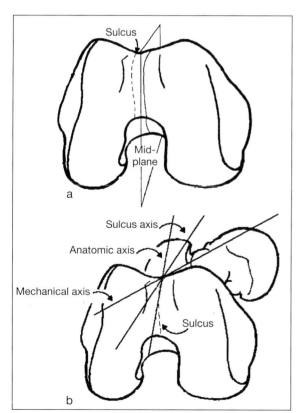

◘ **Fig. 3-4a, b.** *a* The trochlea is offset to the lateral side of the distal femur and its lowest point, the sulcus, is lateral to the midplane. *b* The orientation of the sulcus (sulcus axis) lies between the mechanical and anatomical axes of the femur

[10]. In both normal and arthritic Caucasian knees measured radiographically, the sulcus lies 5±1 mm lateral to the midline of the knee [11]. In a cadaveric collection from Africa the sulcus was measured by micrometer as 2.4±2.1 mm lateral to the midline [10]. The discrepancy in degree but not direction of displacement between studies is attributed to racial variation, an opinion supported by earlier work documenting that black femora are longer and narrower than Caucasian femora [10]. This issue of population differences in functional anatomy of the knee will be revisited below.

Like the distal femur, the proximal tibia can be characterized as an asymmetrical three-dimensional structure. Its medial surface is concave with its periphery, covered by the medial meniscus. The lateral surface is convex with its periphery, covered by the lateral meniscus. The menisci function in conjunction with the ligaments in the kinematics of the normal knee by guiding the femoral condyles over the surface of the tibia in flexion and extension. They are routinely excised along with the ACL in the process of placing a prosthetic knee, however, playing no role in the functional anatomy of the knee from the perspective of total knee arthroplasty. For this reason, the functional significance of the proximal tibia anatomy lies less in its topological features and soft-tissue attachments, and more in its spatial position relative to the femur.

The intuitive notion that the tibia centers below the femur is depicted repeatedly in anatomical illustrations and surgical manuals. This important feature of functional tibia anatomy is misrepresented in these illustrations, however. The center of the tibia – defined as the point equidistant from the front to back and side to side – is not centered below the center of the femur. Studies of both normal and arthritic knees performed with three-dimensional computed tomography demonstrate that the center of the tibia is offset posterior (4±6 mm) and lateral (5±4 mm) to the femur center (◘ Fig. 3-5c) [12]. The clinical significance of this relationship is that surgeons seeking to align implants congruently are often misled into centering the tibia component on the tibia and centering the femoral component on the femur with the expectation that the two components will then align or center with each other. However, the anatomical offset of the femur and tibia centers leads to translation between the two prosthetic components. This problem is compounded by the fact that engineers are designing implants with increasing conformity to limit wear without the recognition that most implants are translated in application. The combination of conformity and anatomical translation likely leads to increased, not decreased wear, a topic revisited below.

Most anatomical representations and surgical manuals also depict the tibia and femur as rotationally aligned. This depiction of the functional anatomy appears consistent with studies of the normal knee but inconsistent with

3

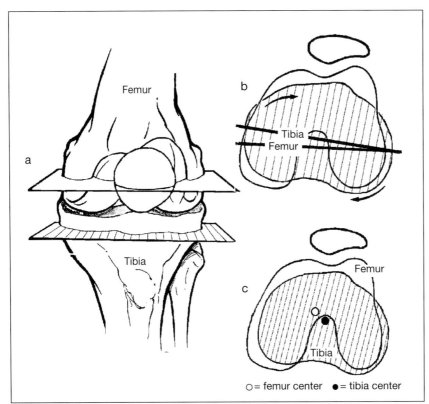

○ = femur center   ● = tibia center

◘ Fig. 3-5a–c. Femoral-tibial rotation (*b*) and offset (*c*) are illustrated on cross-sections of the femur (*a*, solid plane) and tibia (*a*, hatched plane) superimposed on each other. The tibia is externally rotated to the femur in pathological knees (*b*), and the center of the tibia is posterior and lateral to the center of the femur in both normal and pathological knees (*c*)

studies of the pathological or arthritic knee (◘ Fig. 3-5b). Knees demonstrating a history of anterior knee pain and early patella-femoral arthritis were found to have an external malrotation of the tibia to the femur (7±1°) [13]. Knees undergoing total knee arthroplasty for medial compartment osteoarthritis were also found to have an external malrotaton of the tibia to the femur (5±1°) [14]. Unlike the translation discussed above, which reflects the normal morphology of the knee, this malrotation is not present in the normal knee [13, 14] but reflects a rotational contracture of soft tissues (hamstrings, IT band, etc.) associated with the pathological conditions of anterior knee pain and osteoarthritis.

The anatomical significance of this observation from a functional perspective is again related to the placement of components in the process of total knee arthroplasty. A study of the rotational alignment of components in total knee arthroplasty found that the tibial component was externally malrotated 5° relative to the femoral component when the component was referenced to the transtibial axis, and not to the femoral component [15]. Retrieval studies of failed total knee implants document a consistent pattern of external malrotation and translation in the wear of the tibial polyethylene [16, 17]. These studies documenting component malposition and patterns of abnormal wear reflect differences in kinematics between the normal and the replaced knee using conventional surgical techniques and currently available implants.

Another significant difference between the position of a total knee tibial component and functional anatomy occurs as a result of intentionally or unintentionally altering the slope of the joint line. When referenced to the mechanical line of the tibia, the articular surface slopes approximately 3° down from lateral to medial and 5° down from front to back. Historically, methods of total knee arthroplasty recreated this functional anatomy by making an anatomical cut of the proximal tibia to position the tibial component parallel to the joint line. However, contemporary techniques of total knee arthroplasty often replace this sloped surface with an implant placed perpendicular to the mechanical line, the so-called classical cut of the tibia. This alteration in functional morphology necessitates additional compensatory cuts that remove relatively more lateral than medial femur, both distal and posterior, to create rectangular spaces for the implant and to balance the soft tissues. The rationale and methods of these cuts are discussed in later chapters and they are raised here only to illustrate the normal morphology and the potential to alter it, intentionally or unintentionally, in the process of performing a total knee arthroplasty.

The last morphological feature of the knee to address in this review is the patella. As previously stated, it is the largest sesamoid bone in the body, measuring 2.0–2.5 cm ventral to dorsal. When viewed from the ventral surface it is a convex oval bone. Viewed from the dorsal or artic-

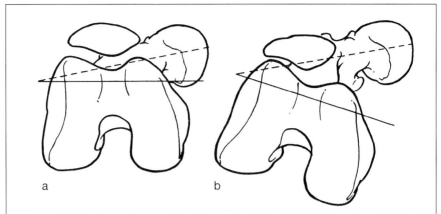

⬛ Fig. 3-6a, b. The patella sits lateral on the distal femur, consistent with the location of the sulcus of the trochlea (*a*). The patella tilts relative to the femur in the face of altered femoral anteversion (*b*) but maintains a constant relationship to the proximal femur and the coronal plane of the body when the foot is in the sagittal plane

ular side, there is a cartilage cap covering the surface with a ridge separating a large lateral facet from a smaller medial facet. A small cartilage reflection lies along the far medial side and is referred to as the odd facet.

When viewed in relationship to the femur, the patella appears to sit lateral to the midplane (⬛ Fig. 3-6a). This observation is consistent with the documented shape of the trochlea and the location of the sulcus of the femur [10] (see Fig. 4a). This relationship of the patella to the femur is present in both normal and osteoarthritic knees [11] and should be taken into account when positioning these components in total knee arthroplasty.

The patella may tilt relative to the femur, reflecting underlying femoral pathology. In the context of the normal knee, i.e., in the absence of pathology, the patella lies parallel to the coronal plane of the femur (Fig. 6a). In the pathological knee, e.g., the osteoarthritic knee and the knee with anterior pain, the patella tilts relative to the femur. Traditional illustration of the tilted patella places the coronal plane of the femur parallel to the horizon and the plane of the patella inclined relative to the femur. An alternative representation is that the patella is tethered by the extensor mechanism in the coronal plane of the body and it is the distal femur that assumes a tilted orientation relative to the patella and the body (⬛ Fig. 3-6b). This representation reflects an appreciation of the normal hip morphology and the variable degrees of distal femoral anteversion that are associated with the pathological knee [13, 18]. This appreciation of abnormal anteversion leads to the intuitive notion that surgical correction of patellar tilt in total knee arthroplasty is achieved in part by addressing the rotation of the femoral component in total knee arthroplasty. Failure to appreciate the presence of abnormal femoral anteversion leads to malrotation of the femoral component with an adverse effect on patella tracking, an outcome well documented in the arthroplasty literature [19]. These issues of surgical correction of femoral rotation and patella tilt will be addressed elsewhere in this book, but it is important here to appreciate that the functional anatomy of the knee varies with

pathology, shaping the perception of the problem and dictating the surgical approach to correction.

All architectural components of the knee, i.e., femur, tibia, and patella, have now been addressed along with the investing soft-tissue sleeve. However, several caveats are in order before concluding. This review addresses normal functional anatomy, but it does not address in any detail the wide range of normal, both in size and in shape, occurring in the human population [20]. There is also significant morphological variation in the knees of subpopulations, reflecting racial differences [20]. Morphological variation also occurs in the context of disease, e.g., the osteoarthritic knee is different from the normal knee [18]. Recognition of this anatomical variation is necessary to appreciate the art of total knee arthroplasty and to understand the surgical techniques described in subsequent chapters of this text.

References

1. Kapandji I (1987) The physiology of the joints. Churchill-Livingston, New York
2. Weber W, Weber F (1992) Mechanics of the human walking apparatus. Sect 4: The knee. Springer-Verlag, Berlin Heidelberg New York
3. Fick R (1911) Mechanik des Kniegelenkes. In: von Bardeleben K (ed) Handbuch der Anatomie des Menschen, Band 2, 1, vol 3. Gustav Fischer, Jena
4. Mensch J et al (1975) Knee morphology as a guide to knee replacement. Clin Orthop Rel Res 112:231–241
5. Yoshioka Y et al (1987) The anatomy and functional axes of the femur. J Bone Joint Surg 69-A:873–880
6. Pinskerova V et al (2001) Tibial femora movement. 1: The shapes and relative movements of the femur and tibia in the unloaded cadaver knee. J Bone Joint Surg 82-B:1189–1203
7. Hollister A et al (1993) The axes of rotation of the knee. Clin Orthop Rel Res 290:259–268
8. Eckhoff D et al (2001) Three-dimensional morphology and kinematics of the distal part of the femur viewed in virtual reality, part I. J Bone Joint Surg 83-A [Suppl 2]:43–50
9. Eckhoff D et al (2003) Three-dimensional morphology and kinematics of the distal part of the femur viewed in virtual reality, part II. J Bone Joint Surg 85-A [Suppl 4]:97–104
10. Eckhoff D et al (1996) Sulcus morphology of the distal femur. Clin Orthop Rel Res 331:23–28
11. Eckhoff D et al (1996) Location of the femoral sulcus in the osteoarthritic knee. J Arthroplasty 11:163–165

12. Eckhoff D et al (1999) Femorotibial offset. A morphologic feature of the natural and arthritic knee. Clin Orthop Rel Res 368:162–165
13. Eckhoff D et al (1997) Knee version associated with anterior knee pain. Clin Orthop Rel Res 339:152–155
14. Eckhoff D et al (1994) Version of the osteoarthritic knee. J Arthroplasty 9:73–79
15. Eckhoff D et al (1995) Malrotation associated with implant alignment technique in total knee arthroplasty. Clin Orthop Rel Res 321:28–31
16. Lewis P et al (1994) Posteromedial tibial polyethylene failure in total knee replacements. Clin Orthop Rel Res 299:11–17
17. Wasielewski R et al (1994) Wear patterns on retrieved polyethylene tibial inserts and their relationship to technical considerations during total knee arthroplasty. Clin Orthop Rel Res 299:31–43
18. Eckhoff D et al (1994) Femoral anteversion and arthritis of the knee. J Pediatr Orthop 14:608–610
19. Figgie H et al (1989) The effect of alignment of the implant on fractures of the patella after condylar total knee arthroplasty. J Bone Joint Surg 71-A:1031–1039
20. Eckhoff D et al (1994) Variation in femoral anteversion. Clin Anat 7:72–79

3

4 Alignment of the Normal Knee; Relationship to Total Knee Replacement

D. S. Hungerford, M. W. Hungerford

Summary

There is an interplay between the anatomy of the articular surfaces, their relationship to the axes of rotation of the normal knee, and the four principle ligaments that stabilize the knee that gives the knee its complex and spectacularly successful kinematics. These kinematics are complex, but now are well understood owing to clinical and biomechanical research. With resurfacing total knee replacement comes the possibility of altering this complex interplay to the detriment of both function and survival of the prosthetic reconstruction. It is imperative that the surgeon understand this interplay and seek to reproduce it through the replacement surgery. Moreover, it is also important to understand the specific consequences of the common malalignments so they can be detected and corrected prior to finishing the arthroplasty.

Introduction

The alignment parameters of the normal knee have been understood for a long time and are not really a source of controversy [5, 9]. Moreover, their relationship to the kinematic function of the normal knee has also been well documented. Although the kinematic function of the knee is quite complex, the relationship of ligament structure to the normal anatomy of the knee has been understood since the early studies of Brantigan and Voshell [1]. Within the parameters of the normal knee, it is the ligament function which has received the greatest attention in terms of the overall knee function. The reason for this is that the ligaments are much more vulnerable to injury than are the normal aspects of alignment. However, in the case of total knee replacement (TKR) with resection of the articular portions of the joint and their replacement by artificial parts, the reconstitution of normal alignment is not guaranteed. The authors believe that the relationship between the alignment of the component parts and subsequent function has been oversimplified. It is the purpose of this chapter first to define the normal alignment of the knee, second to define the relationship between alignment and ligament balance in TKR, and

finally to outline the consequences of malalignment in relationship to failure of TKR.

The ultimate goal of all TKRs is to produce a well-aligned prosthesis with good ligament balance. One without the other is unacceptable. Although it is possible to achieve excellent overall alignment and still fail to achieve ligament balance, if the ligament imbalance has been created by malalignment, balance can seldom be achieved by the common techniques of ligament loosening or tightening. In addition, the arthritic process, and its attendant deformity can result in significant loosening or stretching of ligaments. It is also unacceptable for the surgeon to balance that instability by producing malalignment. By understanding the normal alignment of the human knee, its relationship to normal ligament function and kinematics, and the consequences of malalignment, the surgeon will be well positioned to achieve a high degree of accuracy in both alignment and balance.

Normal Alignment

Although the relationship of the joint line to the common reference axes varies slightly with the length of the femur and the breadth of the pelvis, for most individuals the joint line is horizontal when the leg is positioned for single-leg stance (○ Fig. 4-1). In single-leg stance the ankle must be brought directly under the center of gravity. This means that the lower leg and the mechanical axis are inclined toward the midline by 3°. This can vary by as much as ±1.5° depending on the breadth of the pelvis and the length of the femur. The relationship of the distal femoral joint line to the femoral shaft averages 9° and varies from 7° to 11°. In our experience of measuring this relationship in thousands of patients we have seen only one patient in whom the joint line was actually perpendicular to the mechanical axis. The tibial shaft is normally parallel to the mechanical axis and is therefore 87° to the joint line and *not* perpendicular to the joint line. This relationship of the joint line to the mechanical and anatomical axes leads to several difficulties in describing deviations from the normal. For example, it is common to describe the 87° angle between the joint line and the tibial shaft as being in 3° of varus, indicating that the 87° is on the medial side and 3° from perpendicular. If that relationship were 85°, then it would be logical to describe this as 5° of varus but it would be only 2° of varus *deformity*. This becomes even more confusing because the vast majority of TKRs today are implanted with a tibial cut that is perpendicular to the mechanical axis and therefore is actually implanted with 3° of valgus malalignment. We will come back to this point in discussing alignment in regards to TKR.

Much of the focus in the literature concerning alignment in both the normal and the replaced knee is placed only on alignment in the coronal plane. However, in both instances, alignment in all three planes needs to be addressed (◘ Fig. 4-2).

Femoral Rotational Alignment

The distal femur has a characteristic relationship to the coronal plane (◘ Fig. 4-3). With the posterior aspect of the medial and lateral femoral condyles defining the coronal plane, the femoral shaft is in neutral rotation vis-à-vis the hip and the knee. In this position, the lateral epicondyles can be seen to be more posterior than the medial epicondyle. The angle between a line connecting the epicondyles and a line defining the posterior plane of the condyles is about 3°. Some authors have used the epicondylar axis as the rotational reference of choice for determining femoral rotation in TKR. The rotational reference that is used is less important at this point in the discussion than the relationship between the position of the posterior condyles in space to that rotational reference.

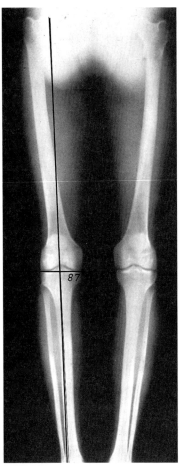

◘ **Fig. 4-1.** Long standing X-ray with normal alignment. With the ankles together, single-leg stance is simulated. The mechanical axis is 87° to the joint line, which is horizontal in the stance position

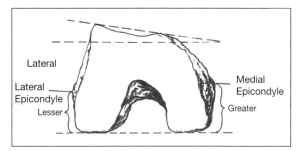

◘ **Fig. 4-3.** The distal femur and the three anatomical references for femoral rotation. Posterior femoral condyles define the coronal plane; transepicondylar axis – often used as a surrogate reference for the coronal plane; trochlear anatomy bears a characteristic relationship to the coronal plane. This will be distorted with severe patellofemoral disease

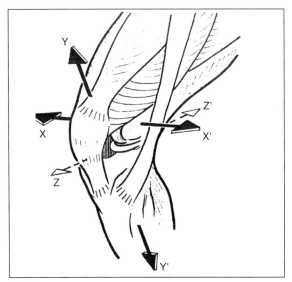

◘ **Fig. 4-2.** All three axes of rotation for the knee (redrawn from Kapandji)

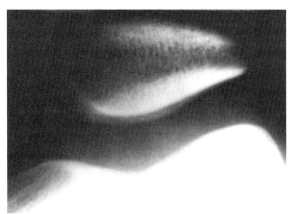

◘ **Fig. 4-4.** Skyline view of the typical PF joint, showing the relationship of the trochlea to the coronal plane

There is no question that the posterior lateral condyle is closer to the epicondylar axis than the posterior medial condyle (see Fig. 3). Another feature of the anatomy of the distal femur is the relationship of the trochlea to the rotational axis of the femur. The lateral facet of the trochlea is projected more anterior than the medial facet. This relationship is seen on the typical patellar skyline view, and its relationship is also a good secondary check for rotational alignment of the femoral component in TKR (◘ Fig. 4-4).

Tibial Rotational Alignment

The rotational alignment of the tibia is best seen when the entire tibial plateau is exposed (◘ Fig. 4-5). When the entire tibial plateau can be seen, the transverse axis passes between the midpoint of the medial and lateral plateaus. The neutral rotation of the tibial plateau places the tibial tubercle just lateral to the midline of the tibia. The axis between the medial and lateral maleoli is not reliable. The tibial tubercle alone is also not a reliable rotational reference because it is a single point and it takes two points to define a plane. Finally, the posterior margins of the tibial plateau are not reliable references either, because the medial tibial plateau characteristically projects more posteriorly than the lateral tibial plateau.

Sagittal Plane Alignment

Femur

The distal portions of the femoral condyles are somewhat flattened, particularly on the lateral side (they have a much larger radius of curvature distally than posteriorly). That portion of the femoral condyles that makes contact with the tibial plateaus with the knee in full extension

is the distal reference plane and is perpendicular to the coronal plane of the thigh. Although this is roughly the same plane as the femoral shaft, it is not exactly the same plane, because of the anterior bow of the femur. A more technically accurate reference plane would be the plane that connects the middle of the greater trochanter and the lateral epicondyle. In using an extramedullary alignment system, these are the references. Most TKR instrumentation systems in use today provide for an intramedullary rod placed in the femoral canal. Although this risks placing the femoral component in a few degrees of flexion, it is a generally reliable reference. Evolving computer navigation will likely resolve the inaccuracies of both the extra- and intramedullary reference methods for the distal femoral cut.

Tibia

The tibial plateaus are sloped posteriorly 7°–10°, referable to the coronal plane of the lower leg (◘ Fig. 4-6). It should be noted that the lower leg is conical from proximal to distal and the coronal plane does *not* parallel the anterior tibial shaft. The fibula is a more reliable coronal plane reference. TKR instrumentation systems frequently offer both intra- and extramedullary alignment references. Both can be effective for flexion/extension alignment of the tibial component.

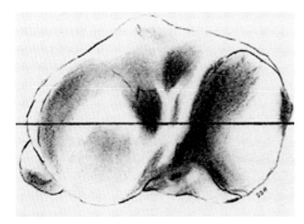

◘ **Fig. 4-5.** Fully exposed tibial plateaus, showing the transverse axis (coronal plane) and the relationship of the tibial tubercle and the posterior margins of the medial and lateral plateaus

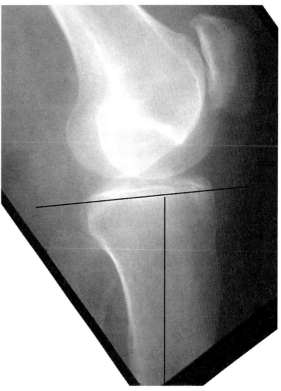

◘ **Fig. 4-6.** Lateral X-ray of the tibia clearly shows the posterior slope of the plateaus

Relationship of Alignment to Kinematic Function of the Knee

Kinematic function of both the normal and the replaced knee is the subject of other chapters, but the relationship of ligament function and component placement to alignment parameters must be understood in both the normal and the replacement scenarios. Kapandji has best illustrated these concepts [5]. The collateral and cruciate ligaments of the knee function normally *only* when they bear a normal relationship to the anatomy of the normal knee. The axes around which flexion/extension occurs encompass the epicondyles, which are located within the concavity of a line connecting the instant centers of rotation of the knee (◘ Fig. 4-7). Because of this location, the collaterals are taut in extension and become relaxed as flexion proceeds. This relaxation is a function of both the position of attachment and the posterior slope of the tibial plateaus. Imagine that the attachment point of the MCL were picked up and physically moved anterior to its anatomical attachment (◘ Fig. 4-8). It can now be seen that the ligament would be tightened in flexion, a condition that would actually block flexion. In the natural knee the articular surfaces cannot practically be repositioned, but in total knee replacement it is very easy to do so. In other words, it should be possible to perfectly align the components with the alignment references that have been outlined above and thereby maintain the relationship of the ligaments to the articulating surfaces of the new construct. Alignment references for the normal knee consist of rotational alignment *around* the x-, y-, and z-axes. However, in TKR, alignment also includes position *along* the alignment axes. ◘ Table 4-1 outlines *all* of the alignment parameters that are important to TKR. It is only when all of these parameters are addressed and successfully fulfilled that a total knee replacement can function in a kinematically normal way. If the surgeon is willing to use a totally constrained prosthesis, most of the alignment parameters can be ignored. Varus/valgus alignment has an obvious cosmetic component and would not be ignored, nor would flexion/extension alignment. The less constrained the prosthesis, the more important the align-

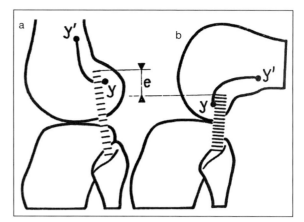

◘ **Fig. 4-7a, b.** (*a*) Medial view, (*b*) lateral view. The attachments of the collateral ligaments to the epicondyles lie within the line connecting the instant centers of rotation. Because of this anatomical location, and because of the decreasing radii of curvature of the condyles and the posterior slope of the plateaus, the ligaments are under less tension in flexion than in extension. (After Kapandji)

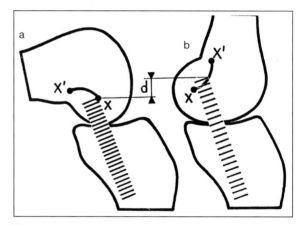

◘ **Fig. 4-8a, b.** The attachment of the medial collateral ligament has been physically moved anterior to the line connecting the instant centers. In flexion, the attachment points are becoming further apart. With continuing flexion, such a phenomenon would either block flexion or stretch out the ligament, which would produce instability

ment. Whenever prosthetic constraint is substituted for alignment and ligament balance, stress is transferred to the interfaces and to the prosthetic components. Posterior cruciate substituting prostheses will be less sensitive to flexion instability caused by malalignment, but ignoring flexion stability will produce post wear, and even post fractures have been reported [7].

Alignment Issues in TKR

From the beginning of the history of TKR, alignment has been oversimplified. Interest has focused mainly on varus/valgus alignment, which is mostly what the patient sees. However, the femur can be perfectly aligned with the tibia, and the components can be even severely

◘ **Table 4-1.** All of the alignment parameters that are important to total knee replacement

	X-axis	Y-axis	Z-axis
Malalignment *around* axis	Flexion/ extension	Internal/ external rotation	Varus/ valgus
Malalignment *along* axis	Medial/ lateral translation	Proximal/ distal dis- placement	Anterior/ posterior displacement

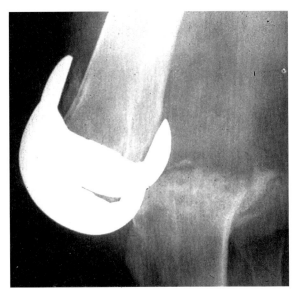

Fig. 4-9. Although this patient's leg is neutrally aligned and the mechanical axis passes through the center of the prosthesis, the femoral component is displaced anteriorly, producing instability in flexion and leading to the dislocation seen here

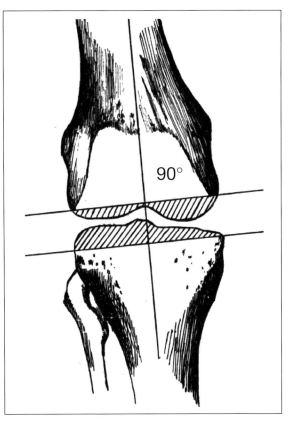

Fig. 4-10. The tibial resection line is perpendicular to the mechanical axis in the 'classic' alignment method of Insall and Freeman, producing over-resection of the lateral plateau. To avoid lateral instability in flexion, the femur must be externally rotated, producing a compensatory sunder-resection of the lateral posterior femoral condyle

malaligned (Fig. 4-9). In fact, the most common form of TKR alignment, introduced by Freeman [2] and Insall [4] in the late 1960s and early 1970s, produces minor offsetting malalignments of the femoral and tibial components.

This has been referred to as the 'classic' alignment method as opposed to the 'anatomical' alignment method introduced by Hungerford, Kenna, and Krackow [3]. The 'classic' method makes tibial and femoral cuts to place the joint line perpendicular to the mechanical axis. However, from Fig. 1 it can be seen that the normal joint line is *not* perpendicular to the mechanical axis. The classic alignment therefore produces a 3° varus malalignment of the femoral component that is offset by a 3° valgus malalignment of the tibial component. These produce a balanced knee in full extension. However the valgus cut on the tibia over-resects the lateral tibial plateau, and this produces lateral instability in flexion (Fig. 4-10). Most systems using the classic alignment system recommend externally rotating the femoral component to compensate for this lateral instability in flexion [11]. Romero et al. compared the consequences of the two alignment systems in normal cadaver knees and found that both systems produce indistinguishable ligament balance throughout the whole range of flexion [10]. There is one particular advantage of the classic system. The tibial cut is perpendicular to the mechanical axis, and therefore a stem attached at 90° to the tibial base plate is lined up with the medullary canal. A long stem attached to a base plate used for an anatomical cut would have to be at 87° to the base plate, and this would necessitate separate components for right and left knees. This is not an issue for most primary knees, since a 90° standard-length stem is easily accommodated within the metaphysis (Fig. 4-11).

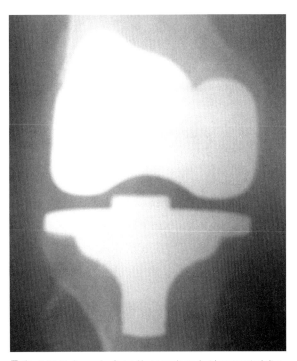

Fig. 4-11. Radiograph of a total knee implanted with anatomical alignment references. The short stem points toward the lateral cortex but is easily accommodated within the tibial metaphysis

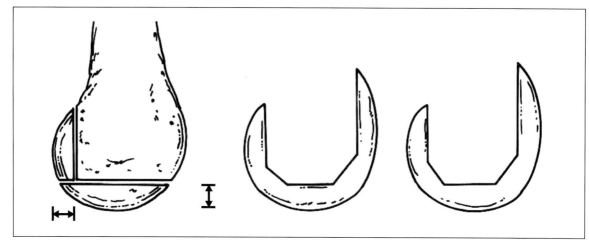

◨ **Fig. 4-12.** Measured resection resects that amount of bone that will reestablish the level of the articular surfaces at their original pre-disease level. One intact surface is necessary as a reference for the resection level

Measured Resection

The concept of measured resection was introduced by Hungerford, Kenna, and Krackow in 1978 [3] and is currently incorporated to some degree in most instrument systems. The concept involves resecting that amount of the distal and posterior femur that will be replaced by the prosthetic components (◨ Fig. 4-12). Following this concept will place the articular surfaces of the replaced knee at the same level as they were in the natural knee. This is usually possible for a primary total knee replacement, because there is generally at least one intact reference point for both the distal and posterior joint lines. If a normal knee is replaced in this way, the replaced knee functions kinematically identical to the normal knee.

Of course, one argument could be that the knee that is a candidate for replacement is not a 'normal' knee. However, most of the kinematic abnormalities that afflict the arthritic knee are due to lost cartilage and bone that takes place during the arthritic process. This loss will be replaced through the proper implantation of the prosthetic components and kinematic balance will be restored. The ultimate goal of TKR must include both normal alignment and ligament balance. One without the other is unacceptable. Martin and Whiteside have shown that it is possible to achieve ligament stability in both full extension and 90° of flexion in spite of malpositioning the femoral component proximally and an equal amount anteriorly (theoretically offsetting malalignments) and using a correspondingly thicker tibial spacer [6]. However, doing so produces mid-flexion instability.

Consequences of Malalignment

Malalignment has four basic consequences, three due to the overload conditions that are imposed. Interface over-

load produces aseptic loosening. Plastic overload accelerates wear. Ligament overload produces pain and/or limits motion. Malalignment may also produce instability. Of the 275 revision total knee replacements performed at the Good Samaritan Hospital in Baltimore between 1983 and 1993, one or more malalignments contributing to failure were identified [8].

A comprehensive review of the subject of malalignment is beyond the scope of this chapter. However, the importance of the subject to the success of TKR can be illustrated by dissecting the cause of an undesirable finding at the time of trial reduction: lateral patellar subluxation. The 'knee-jerk' response to such a finding is to perform a lateral retinacular release and move on. However, unless the patella was subluxing prior to the arthroplasty, something was done during the arthroplasty that has produced this condition, and that 'something' should be discovered and corrected.

Reasons for Patellar Subluxation

There are nine malalignments that produce patellar subluxation:

- Femoral component malalignment. This comprises internal rotation, medial displacement, and valgus malalignment. These three reorient, or displace the trochlear grove to increase the 'Q' angle, increasing the tendency toward lateral patellar subluxation.
- Anterior displacement/femoral component oversizing: These both displace the trochlea, and hence the patella, anteriorly, tightening the lateral retinaculum and increasing the tendency toward lateral subluxation.
- Tibial component malalignment. This comprises internal rotation, medial displacement, and valgus malalignment. These three displace the tibial tubercle

laterally, increasing the 'Q' angle, and increasing the tendency toward lateral patellar subluxation.
- Patellar component malalignment:
    a) Under-resection of the patella displaces the ligament attachment to the patella more anteriorly, tightening the lateral retinaculum and increasing the tendency to lateral subluxation.
    b) Lateral displacement of the patellar component laterally displaces the center of the patellar articulating surface, requiring medial translation to interface with the trochlea. This increases the 'Q' angle and increases the tendency to subluxation.

There is no patellar subluxation in the majority of the knees presenting for replacement. Therefore, if there is patellar subluxation at the end of the procedure, it is more logical to look for a cause rather than simply jump to a lateral retinacular release.

Similar circumstances apply to fixed flexion contracture, medial-lateral instability or imbalance, instability in flexion, instability in extension, global instability, and limited flexion. All of the above can be associated with the presurgical pathology, or all of them can be produced by component malalignment. It is the surgeon's responsibility to eliminate these adverse conditions prior to closing the knee, and in order to do so he/she must understand the origins of the problems, including the possible role of malalignment. Significant malalignment is usually revealed during the trial reduction by imposing the abnormal kinematics that are characteristic of it.

References

1. Brantigan OC, Voshell AF (1941) The mechanics of the ligaments and menisci of the knee joint. J Bone Joint Surg 23:44–66
2. Freeman MA, Swanson SA, Todd RC (1973) Total replacement of the knee using the Freeman-Swanson knee prosthesis. Clin Orthop 94:153–170
3. Hungerford DS, Kenna RV, Krackow KA (1982) The porous-coated anatomic total knee. Orthop Clin North Am 13:103 0150122
4. Insall J, Ranawat CS, Scott WN, Walker P.Insall J, Ranawat CS, Scott WN, Walker P (1976) Total condylar knee replacment: preliminary report. Clin Orthop120:149–154
5. Kapandji IA (1990) The physiology of the joints, vol II. Churchill Livingstone, New York
6. Martin JW, Whiteside LA (1990) The influence of joint line position on knee stability after condylar knee arthroplasty. Clin Orthop 259:146–156
7. Mauerhan DR J (2003) Arthroplasty. Fracture of the polyethylene tibial post in a posterior cruciate-substituting total knee arthroplasty mimicking patellar clunk syndrome: a report of 5 cases. J Arthroplasty 18:942–945
8. Mont MA, Fairbank AC, Yammamoto V, Krackow KA, Hungerford DS (1995) Radiographic characterization of aseptically loosened cementless total knee replacement. Clin Orthop 321:73–78
9. Moreland JR, Bassett LW, Hanker GJ (1987) Radiographic analysis of the axial alignment of the lower extremity. J Bone Joint Surg [Am] 69:745–749
10. Romero J, Duronio JF, Sohrabi A, Alexander N, MacWilliams BA, Jones LC, Hungerford DS (2002) Varus and valgus flexion laxity of total knee alignment methods in loaded cadaveric knees. Clin Orthop 394:243–253
11. Worland RL, Jessup DE, Vazquez-Vela Johnson G, Alemparte JA, Tanaka S, Rex FS, Keenan J (2002) The effect of femoral component rotation and asymmetry in total knee replacements. Orthopedics 25:1045–1048

5 Functional In Vivo Kinematic Analysis of the Normal Knee

A. Williams, C. Phillips

Summary

The concept of tibiofemoral "roll-back" driven by tension in the cruciate ligaments (the "four-bar linkage" theory) as a model of tibiofemoral motion during knee flexion has dominated thinking for the past 30 years. Some obvious flaws have been overlooked, however. An interventional MRI scanner has been used to allow study, for the first time, of the weight-bearing living knee during a squat, in three dimensions. Results show that during knee flexion the lateral femoral condyle does move posteriorly, whereas in the active range of flexion the medial femoral condyle does not move significantly. This differential motion equates to femoral external rotation (or tibial internal rotation). It is proposed that this axial rotation is driven by the shapes of the articular surfaces, and not the ligaments. The findings have far-reaching implications for arthroplasty and the understanding of ligament function.

Introduction

The biomechanics of the normal knee has been a subject of on-going speculation since 1836. Different theories as to how the tibia, femur, and patella articulate have developed as a result of research involving cadaveric and living subjects. One of the biggest challenges still encountered is how to study *functional* kinematics of the knee, taking into consideration how muscle contraction, movement, and loading affect joint position.

Methods of Investigating Knee Motion

The majority of methods incorporate either invasive or irradiating techniques or sometimes both, therefore reducing acceptability to the volunteers being studied. In addition there can be problems in analysis such as the phenomenon of "cross-talk" in Röntgen Stereophotogrammetric Analysis (RSA) [1]. Magnetic Resonance Imaging (MRI) is an attractive tool, being a noninvasive technique that does not involve ionizing radiation and

which produces high-resolution images in any plane, thereby allowing accurate three-dimensional analysis of the knee joint. However, due to the space constraint in conventional MRI scanners, studies have been non-weight bearing and involve a small range of knee motion.

"Interventional" Magnetic Resonance Imaging

Although many different types of "open" scanner are regularly used in the clinical setting, few vertical-access "interventional" scanners exist worldwide. One is based at St. Mary"s Hospital, London, UK. This model design incorporates a 0.5-T magnet housed in two vertical coils spaced 56 cm apart (◘ Fig. 5-1).

Despite the magnet"s field strength being a third of that encountered in conventional scanners, the images produced are of satisfactory resolution, enabling dynamic analysis of bony and soft-tissue structures within the knee. As a result of the space, subjects can be scanned during active movement from full extension through to full flexion in both non-weight-bearing (seated) and physiological weight-bearing positions.

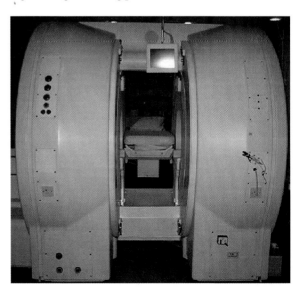

◘ **Fig. 5-1.** 0.5 Tesla interventional MR scanner

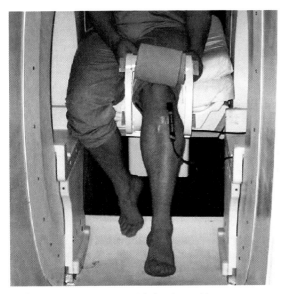

Fig. 5-2. Scanning in non-weight-bearing position

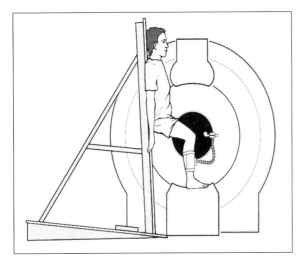

Fig. 5-3. Diagram of scanning in full weight-bearing position

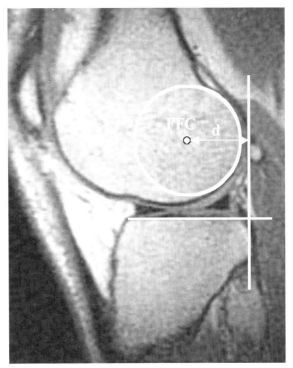

Fig. 5-4. Measurement of the position of the posterior femoral condyles relative to the tibia *FFC*, Flexion Facet Center; *d*, distance measured to ipsilateral posterior tibial cortex. (after [2])

This scanner design incorporates two methods of image registration, known as "Flashpoint Tracking" and "MR Tracking", which allow images to be continually obtained from one chosen plane in the knee joint, irrespective of significant movement between consecutive scans. Either of these "tracking" devices and a receiver coil are attached to the subject"s knee (■ Figs. 5-2 and 5-3).

This facility makes it easy to accurately assess relative movement of femur on tibia, during a full range of motion, while analyzing medial and lateral compartments simultaneously but individually. To achieve this, the position of the posterior femoral condyles relative to the tibia are measured in the sagittal plane at mid-medial and mid-lateral positions of the knee, according to the method of Iwaki et al. [2]. On individual scan images of the medial and lateral compartments in increasing increments of flexion, the centres of the posterior circular surfaces of the femoral condyles were identified and used as fixed femoral reference points [2,3]. The distance between these and a vertical line drawn from the ipsilateral posterior tibial cortex was measured for each position with a Vernier caliper and corrected for magnification (■ Fig. 5-4). Changes in this distance, with progressive increments of knee motion, thus represent relative motion of the femur on the tibia occurring with knee flexion.

Recent cadaveric studies have established the sagittal contours of the medial and lateral joint surfaces [1]. Through several dynamic MR studies, the consequence of this articular geometry on knee kinematics has become apparent [3–5].

Weight-bearing Tibiofemoral Motion Using Open-access MRI

The use of this technique has produced some dramatic findings. Through collaborative work, our findings have been compatible with results of other studies employing conventional MRI of cadaveric specimens [2, 6], horizontal access open MRI of the non-weight-bearing living knee [3, 7], and RSA [8]. Primary results from the St. Mary"s Interventional MRI Unit, analyzing weight-bearing knees in living subjects, have now been reproduced in a number of studies [3–5,9]. Knees have been scanned at 10° increments from hyperextension to 140°. The results of the most detailed study of normal tibiofemoral motion are

5

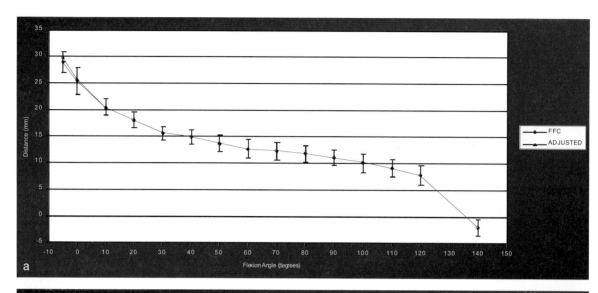

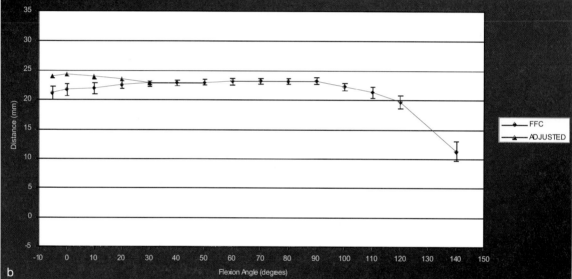

☐ **Fig. 5-5a, b.** Mean AP translation of lateral (*a*) and medial (*b*) femoral condyles from extension to deep flexion

summarized in the graphs of mid-medial and mid-lateral compartments [4] (☐ Fig. 5-5a, b).

In the lateral compartment the femur moves posteriorly – fairly rapidly at first, then steadily until 120° (producing about 20 mm of displacement), and thereafter rather abruptly (a further 10 mm) into a deep squat. Medially the situation is very different. In the range of flexion to 120° there is little anteroposterior movement of the femur on the tibia, but from this point to full flexion there is a modest sharp posterior displacement akin to the lateral side (9 mm). The limit of active knee flexion is 120°, and the kinematics from here to a deep squat are a passive phenomenon and distinct from that occurring in earlier flexion.

The differential medial and lateral motion equates to longitudinal axial rotation with knee flexion; internal tibial rotation/external femoral rotation occurs around a medial axis. For an average-sized male knee this produces 20° of rotation.

Recent fluoroscopic studies have also confirmed this finding of longitudinal rotation with flexion [10]. It is this axial rotation which, when viewed as a lateral projection of the knee fluoroscopically, gives the "illusion" of femoral "roll-back", since the lateral femoral excursion, but not the medial, is appreciated at first glance.

Knee flexion can be divided into three arcs: the screw-home arc, the functional active arc, and the passive deep-flexion arc.

Screw-Home Arc

The screw-home arc is the movement of the knee between approximately 20° of flexion to terminal extension. Little is known about this arc and its functional significance. In contrast to the functional active arc there is profound asymmetry between the shapes of the medial and femoral condyles articulating with the tibia [1] (see below). The medial femoral condyle articulates with the upward sloping anterior tibial surface. This contributes to the posterior part of the medial femoral condyle rising 1–2 mm with progressive terminal extension. As the lateral femoral condyle rotates internally when it moves forward in extension, it rolls down over the anterior edge of the lateral tibial plateau to compress the anterior horn of the lateral meniscus; hence, presumably, the presence of a recess in the lateral tibial plateau and the sulcus terminalis of the lateral femoral condyle. It is not yet known if the terminal rotation observed with screw-home is obligatory and it is the subject of on-going study.

Functional Active Arc

The functional action arc from approximately 20° to 120° of flexion is influenced by neuromuscular control. During this phase longitudinal rotation with flexion is not obligatory and can, to a large extent, be reversed by voluntarily externally rotating the tibia during flexion, allowing the knee to function almost as a uniaxial hinge [3]. Knee motion can vary within an "envelope" of kinematic boundaries [11]. The mechanisms responsible for axial rotation with flexion are not defined and do not appear to be simply under the control of the cruciate ligaments as was previously thought. As well as voluntary control, the different shapes of the articulations are very important in this regard (see below).

Passive Deep-Flexion Arc

In the arc of 120°–140° of deep flexion, tibiofemoral motion is passive, as a result of external force (usually body weight) allowing extra flexion. Medially the femoral condyle rises about 2 mm as it moves posteriorly, riding up on the posterior horn of the medial meniscus. This may explain why degenerate posterior horn tears of the medial meniscus often occur in deep flexion. On the lateral side of the knee there is extreme movement of the lateral femoral condyle, which drops approximately 2 mm as it nearly subluxes off the tibia. Therefore, in a deep squat both medial and lateral condyles now move backwards close to subluxation, largely balanced, presumably, by extensor mechanism tension and posterior anatomical impingement.

Articular Contact Points

It is natural to assume at first that relative motions of the medial and lateral tibiofemoral articular surface contact points will "mirror" the motion of the bones in terms of direction and in magnitude [12]. If the sagittal profiles of the femoral condyles were single radius curves (i.e., a circle) or "J"-shaped (closing helix) curves and the tibial surfaces flat, this would have to be true. The situation for a circle would be analogous to the wheel of a car moving on the road: Whether sliding or rolling, the contact point would lie on a line perpendicular to the road passing through the center of the wheel. Hence, as the wheel moved, so, correspondingly, would the contact point. In the knee, however, the situation is different and the actual anatomy present "disassociates" the movements of the articular contact points and of the bones. Through detailed study of cadaveric specimens the sagittal shapes of the medial and lateral joint surfaces have been established [1]. The medial tibia is flat for its posterior half, leading anteriorly to an "up-slope". With the well-fixed and therefore relatively immobile posterior horn of the medial meniscus [13], the distal articular surface is significantly concave, thereby stabilizing the femur. Laterally the tibia presents a broadly convex surface to the femur. In this much less stable arrangement the lateral meniscus is highly mobile [13] to provide important load sharing with the articular surfaces. The medial femoral condyle surface describes arcs of two circles. The more anterior is shorter and has a larger radius than the posterior. Laterally the anterior arc is very small or even absent, so that the articular surface is effectively described by the arc of a single circle (□ Fig. 5-6a, b).

In the lateral joint compartment, the femoral surface moves posteriorly by a combination of rolling and sliding and, akin to a wheel, takes the articular contact point back with it. Medially the joint surface motion is almost exclusively by sliding (i.e., "spinning on the spot"), initially in the early part of flexion, about the center of the more anterior "extension facet center" and then from about 30°–40° about the center of the more posterior arc (the "flexion facet center"). The shift in position of the "active" center of rotation is quite abrupt. This shift is accompanied by a corresponding posterior change in position of joint surface contact (similar to the change in position of the lateral joint surface contact point), but not a posterior bodily transition of the femur [14]. This phenomenon is possible only due to the shapes of the articulating surfaces.

Implications and Future Developments

While caution is necessary in extrapolating these results of knee motion, observed in a controlled squat, to normal daily activities such as walking and running, the authors

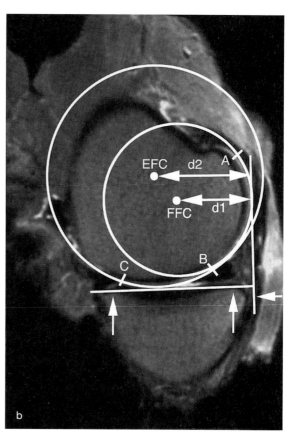

Fig. 5-6a, b. Sagittal MRI images of the lateral (*a*) and medial (*b*) tibiofemoral joints showing the posterior (*FFC*, Flexion Facet Center) and anterior (*EFC*, Extension Facet Center) circular arcs of the femoral condyles

believe the findings of differential compartment motion in the knee to be very important. Primarily, the results challenge the popular concept of femoral "roll-back". It is reasonable to argue that "roll-back" exists laterally. Due to lack of anteroposterior translation medially, in the active range of flexion (up to 120°) this term is not appropriate for the bone itself. However, what of the contact area? First, "rolling" cannot be sensibly applied to change in position of an area. Second, there is no steady transfer of contact through knee flexion provided by "rolling"; rather, as the knee flexes, the medial femur spins only abruptly changing the center about which it rotates and so allowing a change in articular contact position. This is certainly not the description of "roll-back" that has hitherto been popularized.

Furthermore, the kinematics presented here produce the perceived benefits of the "roll-back" model. The posterior shift of joint contact and femoral external rotation with knee flexion increase the extensor mechanism lever arm. Femoral external rotation allows avoidance of posterior bone impingement, thereby maximizing flexion and providing the further benefit of reducing the "Q angle", so aiding patellar kinematics.

Dynamic MRI allows analysis of not only bony structures, but also of the ligaments. Previous mathematical models suggested that, when taut, the cruciate ligaments act as a rigid four-bar link, guiding TF motion. Imaging of knees with both intact and deficient anterior and posterior cruciate ligaments during the full range of flexion, in loaded and unloaded positions [9,15], makes it evident that the ligaments do not tend to play a great role in guiding motion in normal physiological movement of the knee when taut, but rather during excessive application of force, such as that encountered during sporting activity. The ACL assists in controlling the static weight-bearing tibiofemoral position in the lateral compartment and the PCL acts similarly in the medial compartment. Nevertheless, neither ligament influences the *extent* of active motion during weight-bearing flexion of the knee [4]. It would seem likely that the articular surface geometry is a more potent factor driving knee kinematics. The dramatic differences in sagittal shapes of the medial and lateral compartments account for the similarly clear differences in medial and lateral kinematics.

Much of the interest in knee kinematics has been directed towards optimizing prosthetic design. The history of knee replacement shows that improvements in implant performance were associated with the designs becoming closer in shape to the natural knee. Current designs have produced very successful functional outcomes in the 0°–90° range of flexion. Most are designed to produce femoral "roll-back" either by preserving the PCL (PCR) or substituting it for the cam-post mechanisms common to the posterior stabilized (PS) designs. Both types perform well, despite the argument that is raging for and against the two groups. Only the PS designs produce femoral roll-back; in reality, the PCR designs have rather erratic motion, including paradoxical anterior sliding of the femur during flexion [16]. Since no prosthesis, total or unicompartmental, reproduces normal joint geometry, none can rightly claim to restore normal joint kinematics. This is not to say that they do not perform well; many do, but not by restoration of normal kinematics. Rather, their functional success lies in the fact that the changes they impose are well tolerated.

Application of our observed tibiofemoral kinematics might be useful, particularly in restoring physiological knee function, including flexion. However, one must proceed with caution. A simplistic view would be that a prosthesis allowing external femoral rotation about a medial axis during knee flexion, so as to provide more normal kinematics, might produce better results. However, although we do not believe in the four-bar linkage model, there will be some price for sacrificing the cruciate ligaments, and at best the prosthetic articular surfaces in current designs remain far from normal. This means that these designs probably will not confer any advantage over current standard total condylar designs.

Perhaps the next generation of total knee replacements will require articular surfaces shaped in the anatomical manner, to guide more physiological knee motion and achievement of higher levels of function.

Acknowledgements. We thank the English Football Association/Professional Footballers Association for generously funding Miss Carol Phillips" post, and Professor W. Gedroyc, MRCP, FRCR, Director of The Interventional MRI Unit and Consultant Radiologist, St. Mary"s Hospital, London.

References

1. Martelli S, Pinskerova V (2002) The shapes of the tibial and femoral articular surfaces in relation to tibiofemoral motion. J Bone Joint Surg (Br) 84:607–613
2. Iwaki H, Pinskerova V, Freeman M (2000) Tibiofemoral movement. 1: The shapes and relative movements of the femur and tibia in the unloaded cadaver knee. J Bone Joint Surg (Br) 82:1189–1195
3. Hill PF, Vedi V, Williams A, et al (2000) Tibiofemoral movement. 2: The loaded and unloaded living knee studied by MRI. J Bone Joint Surg (Br) 82:1196–1198
4. Johal P et al (2004) Tibio-femoral movement in the living knee: an in-vivo study of weight-bearing and non-weight-bearing knee kinematics, using "interventional" MRI. J Biomechanics (paper accepted; in preparation)
5. Todo S, Kadoya Y, Miolanen T, et al (1999) Anteroposterior and rotational movement of femur during knee flexion. Clin Orthop Rel Res 362: 162–170
6. Pinskerova V et al (2001) The shapes and relative motions of the femur in the unloaded cadever knee. In: Insall JN, Scott WN (eds) Surgery of the knee, chap. 10, 3rd edn. Saunders, Philadelphia, pp 255–283
7. Nakagawa S, Kadoya Y, Todo S, et al (2000) Tibiofemoral movement. 3: Full flexion in the living knee studied by MRI. J Bone Joint Surg (Br) 82:1199–1200
8. Karrholm J, Brandsson S, Freeman M (2000) Tibiofemoral movement. 4: Changes of axial tibial rotation caused by forced rotation at the weight-bearing knee studied by RSA. J Bone Joint Surg (Br) 82:46–48
9. Logan M, Williams A, Lavelle J, et al (2004) What really happens during the Lachmann test? A dynamic MRI analysis of tibiofemoral motion. Am J Sports Med 32:369–375
10. Komistek R, Dennis D, Mahfouz M, et al (2003) In vivo fluoroscopic analysis of the normal knee. Clin Orthop Rel Res 410:69–81
11. Blankevoort L, Huiskes R, De Lange A (1988) The envelope of passive knee joint motion. J Biomech 21:705–720
12. Wretenberg P, Ramsey D, Nemeth G (2002) Tibiofemoral contact points relative to flexion angle measured with MRI. Clin Biomech 17:477–485
13. Vedi V, Williams A, Tennant S, et al (1999): Meniscal movement: an in vivo study using dynamic MRI. J Bone Joint Surg (Br) 181:37–41
14. Pinskerova V et al (2004) Does the femur roll back with flexion? J Bone Joint Surg [Br] 86:925–931
15. Logan M, Dunstan E, Robinson J, et al (2004) Tibiofemoral kinematics of the ACL deficient knee employing vertical access open interventional MRI. Am J Sports Med 32:720–726
16. Komistek R, Scott R, Dennis D, et al (2002) In vivo comparison of femorotibial contact positions for press-fit PS and PCL retaining TKA. J Arthroplasty 17:209–216

6 Gait Analysis and Total Knee Replacement

T.P. Andriacchi, C.O. Dyrby

Summary

The relationship between ambulatory function and the biomechanics of the knee was examined during activities of daily living including walking, stair climbing, and squatting into deep flexion. Each activity was characterized by a unique relationship between the primary motion (flexion) and secondary movements (including internal-external rotation, anterior-posterior displacement) that occur during the weight-bearing and non-weight-bearing phases of each activity. The results demonstrate that the secondary motion of the knee have an important influence on wear, stair climbing function, and the ability to achieve flexion during deep flexion. The short- and long-term outcomes of total knee arthroplasty require a better understanding of the relationship between the primary and secondary motion of the knee during the most common activities of daily living.

Introduction

The primary goals of total knee replacement include restoring function and maintaining the long-term mechanical integrity of the device. An understanding of knee kinematics during ambulatory activities is fundamental to meeting both of these goals. In particular, short-term outcome will be dependent on restoring ambulatory function during activities of daily living. Long-term failure modes such as wear, fatigue failure, and loosening will be influenced by the kinematics of the joint, since the cyclic mechanical demands on the joint are dependent on ambulatory function. This chapter examines the relationship between knee kinematics, patient function, and the mechanical factors that influence long-term failure modes of primary total knee replacement.

Defining Knee Motion (Kinematics)

As total knee arthroplasty (TKA) designs evolve there is a need to precisely define a method for describing knee motion. The motion of the knee is complex and involves rotations and translations with six degree of freedom during most ambulatory activities. The material presented in this chapter is defined by the relative six degree of freedom motions between the femur and tibia. A joint coordinate system was defined on the basis of a coordinate system embedded in the femur and tibia [6]. The origin of the femoral coordinate system is located at the midpoint of the transepicondylar line (◘ Fig. 6-1a). The origin of the tibial coordinate system is located at the midpoint of a line connecting the medial and lateral tibial plateaus.

Projection angles [1] were used to define relative rotations of the femur with respect to the tibia (◘ Fig. 6-1b). Angles were determined by projecting an axis from the femoral coordinate system onto a plane created by two axes in the tibial coordinate system. For example, projecting the anterior-posterior (AP) axis of the femur onto a plane created by the AP and superior-inferior axis of the tibia was done to calculate the flexion-extension of the knee, femur relative to the tibia. This system allows for a consistent way to determine relative rotations at all flexion angles. Translation of the femur was determined by projecting the femoral origin onto one of the tibial axes and determining the distance between that and the tibial origin (◘ Fig. 6-1a). For example, projecting the femoral origin on the AP axis of the tibia allows calculation of AP translations, projection onto the tibial medial-lateral axis to determined medial-lateral translations, and the inferior-superior axis determined inferior-superior translations.

Primary and Secondary Motions of the Knee (Passive vs Active Function)

While the primary motion of the knee is flexion, the secondary motions, including AP translation, internal-external (IE) rotation, and abduction-adduction (AA), play an important role in the overall function of the knee joint [8]. During passive motion of the knee, the secondary motions are coupled to knee flexion [16]. Certain passive motions of the knee (screw-home; external tibial rotation with extension [9] and femoral roll-back [3] (◘ Fig. 6-2); posterior movement of the femur with flexion) have been characterized and regarded as fundamental to

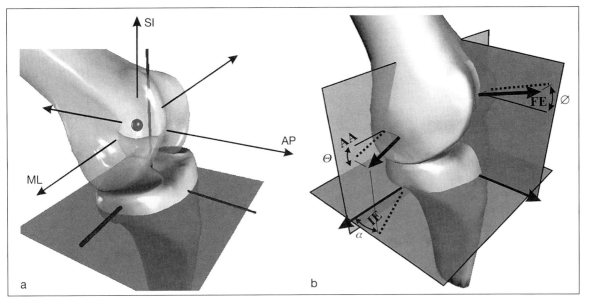

■ **Fig. 6-1.** The anatomical coordinate systems used to describe the motion of the femur with respect to the tibia. Flexion-extension (*FE*), abduction-abduction (*AA*), and internal-external rotation (*IE*) were defined by the projection of the anatomical femoral or the axes onto planes fixed in the tibial coordinate system. The anterior-posterior (*AP*) displacement of the tibia was determined by the projection of the origin of the tibial coordinate system on the AP axis of the femur

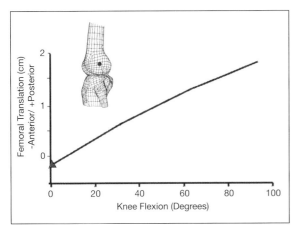

■ **Fig. 6-2.** Femoral roll-back during flexion to 90∞. The femur starts in the anterior position at full extension then moves posteriorly as the knee flexes

weight-bearing motion of the knee described as roll-back (Fig. 6-3). During walking the position of the femur at heel strike (HS) is posterior. This is consistent with the extensor mechanisms pulling the tibia forward during the final portion of swing phase. After HS, the femur translates in an anterior direction through midstance to terminal extension. Similarly, the femur externally rotates while extending from HS to terminal extension (the reverse of the passive screw-home movement). Again, this external rotation is caused by forces generated by muscle contraction and the inertia of the upper body rotating the femur while the foot is planted on the ground. Interest-

normal knee function. The passive characteristics of the secondary motions of the knee have been related to the shape of the articular surfaces and ligament function [16]. The secondary motions are contained within an envelope of passive limits of the joint [4]. However, when extrinsic forces, such as muscle forces, are present the secondary motions are driven by the magnitude and direction of these forces, since secondary motions such as AP translation or IE tibial rotation require relatively low forces to displace the joint from a neutral position [14, 15]. Thus, during weight-bearing activities the secondary motions of the knee are dependent on extrinsic forces acting during a particular activity [1].

The AP motion of the knee during walking (■ Fig. 6-3) provides an interesting contrast to the passive non-

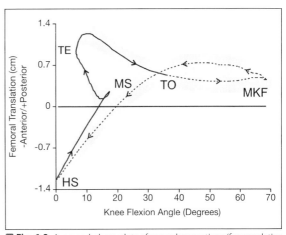

■ **Fig. 6-3.** Averaged phase plots of secondary motions (femur relative to the tibia) versus knee flexion angle during walking for anterior-posterior translation. *Arrows* indicate direction of motion. *Solid curve* indicates stance phase while *broken curve* indicates swing phase. *Shaded areas* indicate the confidence interval. *HS* heel strike, *MS* midstance, *TE* terminal extension, *TO* toe off, *MKF* maximum knee flexion [6]

ingly, no significant offset in AP translation or IE rotation was found during the active leg extension. The AP motion of the knee demonstrated that the femur and tibia are not guided solely by the bony and ligamentous structures during ambulation. The secondary motions during weight bearing cannot necessarily be predicted from passive characteristics such as screw-home movement or femoral roll-back. The secondary motions occur within a range that depends on the angle of knee flexion, the activity performed, and muscle activation. Therefore, under weight-bearing conditions, secondary knee motions are dependent on the type of activity.

The secondary motions of the knee during activities of daily living are extremely important in restoring normal function following TKA. The following provides specific examples of the influence of knee kinematics during stair climbing, squatting, and walking on the outcome of TKA.

Activities of Daily Living and TKA Outcome

Stair Climbing

The ability to step up or down is required for restoring normal function following total knee replacement. The AP translation (secondary to flexion) of the knee has been shown to influence the ability of patients to ascend stairs in a normal manner [2]. Abnormal roll-back was one explanation given for the reduced quadriceps moment associated with cruciate sacrificing, because reduced roll-back would shorten the lever arm of the quadriceps muscle [2]. However, a recent study [1] demonstrated that the femur does not simply roll back with flexion during stair climbing. AP translation of the femur was dependent on the phase of the stair-climbing cycle. During the early swing phase, the femur moves forward with flexion as a result of the hamstring muscle producing knee flexion (◨ Fig. 6-4). The femur begins moving posteriorly at approximately 45° of flexion, probably as tension in the posterior cruciate ligament (PCL) increases.

The importance of understanding the unique characteristics of AP translation during stair climbing was illustrated in a study of patients with posterior stabilized (PS) TKA, cruciate retaining (CR) TKA, and aged-matched controls during stair climbing (◨ Fig. 6-5). General patterns of AP translation for all three groups were similar but large differences were seen in the position of the femur at foot strike on the step. The PS design was more anterior relative to the CR design or to the control subjects. The PS design group reaches a maximum anterior position at approximately 70°, compared with 40° in the control group and 55° in the CR group. The cam-post mechanism for this particular PS design engaged at

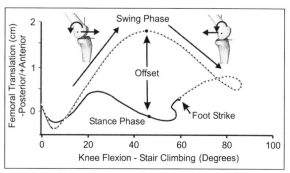

◨ Fig. 6-4. Averaged normal phase plot of femoral translation versus knee flexion during stair climbing. During early swing phase the femoral reference point (midpoint of transepicondylar axis) translates anterior with flexion. During late swing phase, the femoral reference point translates posterior with flexion. During support phase, there is minimal translation of the femoral reference point [1]

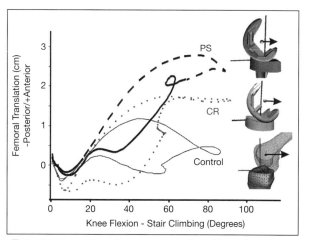

◨ Fig. 6-5. Comparison of averaged phase plots of femoral translation versus knee flexion during stair climbing for normal subjects, patients with a cruciate retaining design (CR) and patients with a cruciate sacrificing, i.e., posterior stabilizing (PS) design. The PS group maintained an anterior location of contact until approximately 70° of flexion where normally the cam engages. The CR group was also more anterior than the normal group. The swing phase anterior-posterior motion prior to stair climbing appears to be dependent on the function of the PCL [1]

approximately 70°. The results of this study suggest that restoring or replacing PCL function near 45° of flexion is an important consideration in total knee replacement, since PCL tension at 45° of flexion is needed to maintain the normal lever arm of the quadriceps during stair climbing.

A recent study [7] of 21 bilateral TKR with CR designs in one knee and PS designs in the contralateral knee supported the conclusion regarding the function of the PCL during stair climbing. With the PS design, the maximum external knee flexion moment (sustained by net quadriceps contraction) was significantly reduced compared with the CR side and matched controls. There was a significant increase in hip flexion, with the PS design, which could be associated with a forward lean. Forward lean would allow the individual to move his or her center of mass in front of the knee, suggesting a compensation for reduced quadriceps efficiency (reduced lever arm). With the CR design, there could possibly be more normal femoral roll-back that would increase the lever arm, and therefore the mechanical advantage of the quadriceps. This would allow a greater moment to be produced for the same amount of quadriceps activation.

Squatting into Deep Flexion

The capacity for deep flexion is essential for activities of daily living, especially for Indian, Middle Eastern, and Japanese cultures. However, even in Western cultures there are a wide range of activities (recreational and occupational) that require deep flexion. For example, recent studies [1, 5, 11] of deep flexion indicate the importance of IE rotation during squatting into deep flexion. Squatting from a standing position requires approximately 150° of flexion to a resting squat. Flexion between 0° and 120° is accompanied by approximately 10° of external rotation of the femur. However, between 120° and 150° flexion, the femur externally rotates an additional 20°. Therefore, beyond 120° flexion, the knee requires substantial external rotation to achieve deep flexion [5]. Currently, most designs of total knee arthroplasty can achieve only 120° flexion. However, patients requiring deeper flexion will need the capacity for substantial tibial rotation beyond 120° flexion.

Walking Kinematics and Wear

Implant wear is the primary mechanical factor limiting the long-term outcome of total knee replacement. The kinematics of the knee are a critical factor influencing wear at the joint [17,18]. Again, the secondary motions are an important consideration in the outcome of total knee replacement since these motions will have a substantial influence on wear. For example, subtle variations in rolling, tractive rolling, and sliding motion and the direction of the pathway of motion can have substantial effects on the production of wear debris or cyclic fatigue of the ultra-high-molecular-weight polyethylene [18]. The degree of rolling and sliding can be quantified by the slip velocity. The magnitude of the interfacial slip velocity provides quantification of the rolling versus sliding behavior of the tibiofemoral joint when relative motion occurs. For pure rolling, the interfacial slip velocity will approach zero [12, 13]. The absolute maximum slip velocities occur during swing phase just before heel strike. A previous knee simulator study [12] showed that the maximum wear rate was significantly greater when these slip velocities were incorporated as input to the simulator relative to studies where the slip velocities were not applied. Therefore, the high slip velocities during heel strike and during

swing phase indicate the potential for sliding motion that can produce a greater volume of abrasive wear debris.

The considerable differences in the wear scar formation between retrieved and simulator tested implants [10] can be explained by differences between in vivo kinematics and the type of kinematics used in wear simulators. In addition, the variability of in vivo wear scar formation has been related to the variability of human gait following TKR [19]. Most of the variability in worn contact area may be explained by gait abnormalities of TKR patients. These abnormalities cause larger wear areas contributing to possibly higher wear rates. Since most TKR patients walk with an abnormal gait pattern, knee simulator input parameters should be reconsidered.

Conclusion

Motion of the knee is very complex and cannot be described by a single motion path. Typical activities of daily living: walking, stair climbing, and increasingly deep knee flexion, show that knee motion is activity dependent. There is also evidence of different motion patterns in a single activity due to muscle activity or knee replacement designs. In order for advancements to be made in the design of total knee replacement, one must understand not only the forces and moments, but also the six degree of freedom of motion of the knee. Internal-external rotations and anterior-posterior translations play an important role in determining the longevity of knee replacements. The successful outcome of TKA is dependent on the kinematics of the knee during activities of daily living.

References

1. Andriacchi TP, Dyrby CO, Johnson TS (2003) The use of functional analysis in evaluating knee kinematics. Clin Orthop 410:44–53
2. Andriacchi TP, Galante JO, Fermier RW (1982) The influence of total knee replacement design on walking and stair climbing. J Bone Joint Surg 64-A:1328–1335
3. Andriacchi TP, Stanwyck TS, Galante JO (1986) Knee biomechanics and total knee replacement. J Arthroplasty 1:211–219
4. Blankevoort L, Huiskes R, Delange A (1988) The envelope of passive knee-joint motion. J Biomech 21:705–720
5. Dyrby CO, Andriacchi TP (1998) Deep knee flexion and tibio-femoral rotation during activities of daily living. In: Trans Orthop Res Soc, New Orleans
6. Dyrby CO, Andriacchi TP (2004) Secondary motions of the knee during weight-bearing and non-weight-bearing activities. J Orthop Res 22:794–800
7. Dyrby CO, Tria F, Johnson R, et al (2004) Bilateral posterior stabilized and cruciate retaining total knee replacements compared during stair-climbing. In: Trans Orthop Res Soc, San Francisco
8. Fukubayashi T, Torzilli PA, Sherman MF, Warren RF (1982) An in vitro biomechanical evaluation of anterior-posterior motion of the knee. Tibial displacement, rotation, and torque. J Bone Joint Surg 64-A:258–264
9. Hallén LG, Lindahl O (1966) The "screw-home" movement in the knee-joint. Acta Orthop Scand 37:97–106

10. Harman MK, DesJardins JD, Banks SA, et al (2001) Damage patterns on polyethylene inserts after retrieval and after wear simulation. In: Trans Orthop Res Soc, San Francisco

11. Hefzy MS, Kelly BP, Cooke TD (1998) Kinematics of the knee joint in deep flexion: a radiographic assessment. Med Eng Phys 20:302–307

12. Johnson T, Andriacchi T, Laurent M (2000) Development of a knee wear test method based on prosthetic in vivo slip velocity profiles. In: Tran Orthop Res Soc, Orlando

13. Johnson T, Andriacchi T, Laurent M, et al (2001) An in vivo based knee wear test protocol incorporating a heel strike slip velocity transient. In: Trans Orthop Res Soc, San Francisco

14. Markolf KL, Bargar WL, Shoemaker SC, Amstutz HC (1981) The role of joint load in knee stability. J Bone Joint Surg 63-A: 570–585

15. Markolf KL, Graff-Radford A, Amstutz HC (1978) In vivo knee stability. A quantitative assessment using an instrumented clinical testing apparatus. J Bone Joint Surg 60-A:664–674

16. Wilson DR, Feikes JD, Zavatsky AB, O'Connor JJ (2000) The components of passive knee movement are coupled to flexion angle. J Biomech 33:465–473

17. Wimmer MA, Andriacchi TP (1997) Tractive forces during rolling motion of the knee: implications for wear in total knee replacement. J Biomech 30:131–137

18. Wimmer MA, Andriacchi TP, Natarajan RN, et al (1998) A striated pattern of wear in ultra high-molecular-weight polyethylene components of Miller-Galante total knee arthroplasty. J Arthroplasty 13:8–16

19. Wimmer MA, Nechtow WH, Kleingries M, et al (2003) TKR wear scar formation is influenced by the host's gait pattern. Trans Orthop Res Soc, New Orleans

6

7 The Polyethylene History

A. Bellare, M. Spector

Summary

Our understanding of the wear behavior of polyethylene (PE) components has deepened over the past few years as the adverse effects of gamma irradiation (in air) sterilization have become understood. This understanding has led to methods to improve the wear performance of the polymer using cross-linking. However, it will still be several years before the clinical benefits of new methods of processing PE are clear and the benefit-risk ratio is established.

Introduction

Ultra-high-molecular-weight polyethylene (UHMWPE) is one of the principal materials employed in total knee arthroplasty. While the lubrication and friction of the metal-on-PE articulation provides the low-friction arthroplasty that Sir John Charnley sought, the wear of PE yields particulate debris that potentiates an osteolytic response, which remains a significant problem. The often rapid and extensive destruction of bone attributable to PE wear particles is so dramatic, and so challenges revision arthroplasty, that it has commanded the most attention in recent years. However, the actual incidence of this problem remains somewhat in question. This point notwithstanding, the prevalence of PE wear particle-induced osteolysis is great enough to warrant changes in how the material is processed so as to improve its resistance to wear. Extrinsic factors that contribute to the wear of polyethylene are also being addressed: prosthetic designs that reduce stresses in the polymer; prosthetic designs and manufacturing processes that reduce the number of particles released from modular junctions, which can participate in three-body wear of polyethylene; and materials that may allow the production of more scratch-resistant metallic counterfaces.

It is well known that PE components of total joint replacement prostheses undergo processes that produce PE wear debris due to the articulation of the harder metallic component, usually a cobalt-chromium alloy, against the softer PE component. The generation of wear debris not only damages the surface of the PE component but is also known to elicit a biological response that often results in bone resorption. This bone loss (referred to as osteolysis) can eventually lead to loosening of the prosthetic device. The location and size of PE particle-induced osteolytic lesions often greatly complicate revision surgery. Work in recent years has focused on processing parameters that serve as the determinants of the resistance of PE to wear. The reduction of the amount of wear debris from, and surface damage to, PE would prolong the lifetime of such prostheses.

The objective of this chapter is to review the history of the use of polyethylene in total joint arthroplasty, as a basis for understanding the methods being employed to improve its performance. There are several prior reviews [26, 27] of this subject that can be accessed for useful reference.

Polyethylene Molecular Structure

UHMWPE has a very low frictional coefficient against metal and ceramics and is therefore used as a bearing surface for joint replacement prostheses. Moreover, the wear resistance of UHMWPE is greater than that of other polymers investigated for this application. Low strength and creep, however, present potential problems.

The term polyethylene refers to plastics formed from the polymerization of ethylene gas. The possibilities for structural variation of molecules formed by this simple repeating unit for different molecular weight (e.g., crystallinity, branching, and cross-linking) are so numerous and dramatic, with such a wide range of attainable properties, that the term polyethylene refers to a wide array of materials. The earliest type of polyethylene was made by reacting ethylene at high (20 000–30 000 pounds per square inch) pressure and temperatures of 200°–400°C with oxygen as catalyst. Such material is referred to as low-density polyethylene. A great amount of polyethylene is produced now by newer, low-pressure techniques using aluminum-titanium (Ziegler) catalysts. This is called linear polyethylene due to the linearity of its molecules, in contrast to the branched molecules produced by high-pressure processes. The linear polymers can be used to make high-density polyethylene by means of the higher degree of crystallinity attained with the regularly shaped molecules. Typically, there is no great difference in molecular weight between the low- and high-density varieties, e.g., 100 000–500 000. However, if the low-pressure process is used to make extremely long molecules, i.e., UHMWPE, the result is remarkably different. This material, with a molecular weight between 1 and 10 million, is less crystalline and less dense than high-density polyethylene and has exceptional mechanical properties. It is extremely tough and remarkably wear resistant; a 0.357 magnum bullet fired from 25 feet bounces back from a l-inch thick slab of UHMWPE. The material is used in very demanding applications (e.g., ore chutes in mining equipment) and is by far the most successful polymer used in total joint replacements. It far outperforms the various acrylics, fluorocarbons, polyacetals, polyamides, and polyesters which were tried for such purposes.

Processing of Polyethylene

Implants of polyethylene are usually manufactured by the machining of components from bulk stock fabricated from as-synthesized polyethylene powder using mainly ram extrusion or compression molding. These processes involve application of heat and pressure to consolidate the powder into bulk components, followed by machining of the implant components, packaging, and sterilization.

Various grades of UHMWPE resins have been available for orthopedic implant application, primarily from Ruhrchemie AG, which later changed its name to Hoechst, and is currently called Ticona. The early UHMWPE resin used by John Charnley was called RCH-1000 for (R)uhr (CH)emie. This resin is similar to the current GUR 1020 UHMWPE resin. RCH-1000 was classified as a form of HDPE (high-density polyethylene), which is why earlier papers refer to UHMWPE as HDPE [26]. Later, the orthopedic grade of polyethylene was called CHIRULEN. Since the 1990s, the UHMWPE resin used in implants has been called GUR or (G)ranular (U)HMWPE (R)uhrchemie. Common examples of polyethylene resins used today are GUR 1050 and GUR 1020. The numbers following GUR refer to the following: the first digit refers to approximate or loose density (1); the second digit refers to presence (1) or absence (0) of calcium stearate, which has been used as a lubricant to assist processing; the third digit refers to molecular weight (2=2 million g/mole and 5=5 million g/mole), and the fourth digit (0) refers to the resin grade. Calcium stearate is no longer added to orthopedic-grade polyethylene, since reports showed increased levels of oxidation and fusion defects associated with calcium stearate [24, 40, 43, 46]. Another source of UHMWPE

was Montell (Formerly Himont), which produced the Hi-Fax 1900H, a resin that has different structure and properties compared to the Hoechst resins [45]. However, Hi-Fax is no longer available, and GUR 1050 and GUR 1020 remain the only grades of polyethylene used in orthopedic implants.

The as-synthesized polyethylene resin particles are approximately 100 μm, but can be submicrometer in size as well. The broad size distribution of GUR 4150 (the digit "4" refers to the country code, USA, which was the nomenclature used for GUR resins.) powder particles have been measured by Pienkowski et al. [35, 36]. Each powder particle contains 10- 30-μm diameter aggregates comprising approximately 1-μm diameter nodules connected to each other by fibrils. Olley et al. [34] have shown that voids or defects remain along the resin boundaries even after the powder is "fully" consolidated into bulk components. The likely reason for the presence of defects is the high viscosity associated with the ultra-high molecular weight of the polyethylene that is required for high wear resistance. The incomplete consolidation of high-molecular-weight polyethylene resin compared with low-molecular-weight polyethylenes, however, is not a major concern. Gul et al. showed that there was no correlation between the degree of consolidation of UHMWPE powder particles and the rate of generation of particulate wear debris under the processing conditions that they used [23].

The nascent UHMWPE powder contains extended-chain crystals (thick lamellae) as well as thin lamellae [16]. The high melting temperature of 141°C observed using a differential scanning calorimeter suggests that the powder contains mostly extended-chain crystals, as present in high-pressure crystallized UHMWPE. However, a study utilizing morphological, chemical, and molecular techniques indicated that a dual lamellar structure existed. It is postulated that the fibrils of the polyethylene resin powder contain thick, extended-chain crystalline lamellae, while 20-nm thick lamellae (such as those present in bulk components manufactured using molding or ram extrusion) exist in the spherical domains [16]. It is unclear why the powder morphology contains fibrils connecting spherical domains (sometimes referred to as the "cauliflower" morphology). The presence of fibrils in the powder suggests that the as-synthesized powder has UHMWPE macromolecules trapped in a low-entanglement, aligned state compared with melt-crystallized UHMWPE. This low entanglement would assist in consolidation of powder during molding or ram extrusion processes. A highly entangled state would make it harder to consolidate the powder, since it would require the chains from powder particles to disentangle and then re-entangle with the chains of the adjacent powder particles.

The most common processes used to consolidate polyethylene powder particles into bulk stock are compression molding into thick sheets and ram extrusion into rods. The final implant is usually machined from the bulk stock. These processes involve compaction of UHMWPE nascent powder at elevated temperatures, above melting temperature. They also utilize pressure to assist in consolidation. The final stage of processing involves annealing at elevated temperatures to remove residual stresses associated with processing and to increase the crystallinity of the components. Compression molded sheets of GUR 1020 and GUR 1050 UHMWPE resins 2.5–7.5 cm thick are commercially produced.

Ram extrusion is another common process employed to sinter nascent UHMWPE powder into 2.5- to 30-cm diameter rods that are several meters in length. Like compression molding, the extrusion processes are also followed by annealing at elevated temperatures. The bulk UHMWPE rods and sheets are generally uniform except for small spatial variations in anisotropy due to spatially non-uniform crystallization occurring due to the low thermal conductivity of polyethylene [2].

Direct compression molding of tibial and acetabular components has also been performed in some cases. The primary advantage of direct compression molding of implants is that the articular surfaces of the joint components are smooth, lacking machine marks or grooves. However, by far the common choice for implant manufacture is machining of compression molded sheets and ram extruded, rod stock of UHMWPE.

The Sterilization Issue

During the 1990s, sterilization of polyethylene components received much attention as studies began to show that sterilization can degrade the mechanical and wear properties of UHMWPE [4–11, 13, 18–20, 26, 33, 37–39, 41, 42]. Until the mid 1990s, the common practice was to package UHMWPE components of total joint replacements in air and thereafter sterilize the package using 25–37 kGy of gamma radiation. It is well known that radiation induces cross-linking, chain scission, and long-term oxidative degradation of polyethylene. In the polymer science field, the effects of ionizing radiation on post-irradiation aging of several types of polyethylene, including pressure-crystallized UHMWPE [6], have been studied in great detail, especially by Bhateja et al. [4–9]. Costa and co-workers demonstrated the detailed mechanism of oxidation and have shown that oxidation can also occur in ethylene oxide-sterilized UHMWPE, albeit to a much smaller extent than in gamma radiation-sterilized UHMWPE [14, 17–20]. It is now well established that long-term post-irradiation aging can have detrimental effects on both the morphology and the mechanical properties of UHMWPE [10, 11, 38, 39]. The effects of post-irradiation aging on TKRs have been well documented [42] in analyses of TKR

retrievals. The vast number of studies on gamma sterilization-induced oxidation of UHMWPE have resulted in several reviews that summarize various issues related to sterilization, its chemistry, and its effects on polyethyelene used in joint replacement prostheses [17, 26, 37].

It was originally believed that oxidation was associated primarily with fatigue damage mechanisms such as delamination wear, which occurs in TKRs. However, it is now well established that the rate of particulate wear debris generation can also increase due to the molecular weight reduction and embrittlement in both tibial components and acetabular cups [3, 29]. Initially, gamma radiation increases resistance to wear debris generation due to the low level of cross-linking that accompanies gamma radiation. However, with aging, oxidative effects begin to dominate and negate any initial benefits of gamma radiation, leading to higher wear rates than unirradiated UHMWPE. Orthopedic implant manufacturers have recognized the effect of oxidation on degradation of polyethyelene. Currently, some implant manufacturers sterilize UHMWPE using non-radiation methods, such as ethylene oxide or gas plasma sterilization. Other orthopedic manufacturers have resorted to packaging of components in low oxygen environments, such as vacuum-foil packaging, or packaging in nitrogen or argon gas. These methods should decrease the rate of oxidation during storage. However, it is not yet known whether in vivo oxidation rates would eventually affect the clinical performance of conventional UHMWPE, packaged in low oxygen environments and then sterilized using gamma radiation.

Modified Forms of Polyethylene

The problems associated with wear of PE components in joint replacement prostheses has prompted work directed toward the development of new forms of PE to improve wear resistance.

One approach used to reduce surface damage and sub-surface crack growth in knee components is through development of new prosthetic designs that increase the contact area between components, thereby reducing stress in PE. Such methods, based on measurements and calculations of contact stress on components, have led to the development of thicker and more conformal PE components that are expected to reduce catastrophic failure and delamination wear.

Other approaches to reduce wear rates in PE aim at altering the form of polyethylene through alteration of the number or size of the crystallites or the molecular bonding of the molecular chains in the noncrystalline domains of the polymer. More recent methods that have been used to realize these goals include: (1) processing techniques apply high pressures to the polymer, and (2) the use of cross-linking chemistry.

Carbon-Fiber Reinforced and Heat-Pressed Polyethylene

In the 1980s and early 1990s attempts to improve the performance of polyethylene turned to carbon fiber reinforcement and to heat-pressing. In an effort to reduce creep a fiber reinforced polymer composite was produced by blending carbon fibers with UHMWPE (Poly Two, Zimmer, Warsaw, IN). The composite was directly molded into tibial inserts and patellar components [15]. The material was also used for the fabrication of acetabular cups in total hip replacements [15]. As reported in a review of UHMWPE [27], although the Poly Two devices had a significantly higher creep resistance (p<0.03), "they required extraordinary quality-control measures, had lower fatigue resistance compared with ultra-high molecular weight polyethylene, and demonstrated no clinical improvement in the rate of wear". The use of Poly Two was discontinued approximately 7 years after its introduction into the marketplace.

Heat pressing was another method employed in an attempt to improve the tribology of polyethylene. However, several investigations of retrieved heat-pressed tibial inserts [12, 21, 30] demonstrated delamination. In one study [12], 52% of 33 retrieved components showed severe delamination within 4 years of implantation. Light microscopy revealed a surface layer separated from the insert with a clear line of demarcation 250–580 µm below the articulating surface.

High-Pressure Forms of Polyethylene

In the early 1990s, high-pressure crystallization was employed to produce PE components (Hylamer, DuPont, Wilmington, DE) with an increase in mechanical properties such as yield stress and modulus of elasticity [27]. Two forms of high-pressure PE, which vary in certain mechanical properties (viz., modulus of elasticity), have been introduced into the clinic for total hip and knee arthroplasty. The primary difference in the bulk structure of conventional and high-pressure forms of PE is that in conventional PE the degree of crystallinity is 50%–55% while it is 68%–75% in the high-pressure form. The high-pressure process facilitates thickening of crystallites in PE from 0.025 µm in conventional processes to approximately 0.2 µm in the high-pressure form. While the high-pressure PE is more resistant to deformation by creep and fatigue crack growth, it has never been shown to have a substantially higher wear resistance in laboratory wear tests.

Recent clinical results indicate that the linear wear rate and consequential incidence of osteolysis and revision rate for the high-pressure form of PE are greater than for conventional PE. Why the clinical wear rate for this modification of PE might be greater than for conventional PE, despite the improvement in certain mechanical properties, is not entirely clear. It may be that the high-pressure form is less resistant to oxidation than was previously appreciated. If so, implementation of sterilization methods that do not favor oxidation may result in improved performance of this form of PE. However, the fact that wear of PE devices is as multifactorial as it is indicates that additional laboratory investigations of high-pressure forms of PE will be required before their wear performance can be more fully explained.

Cross-Linked Polyethylene

Cross-linking is currently being used in an attempt to improve the wear performance of PE [26, 28, 31, 32, 44]. Cross-linking of PE converts the otherwise linear, high-molecular-weight PE macromolecule into an interpenetrating network structure of polymer chains. This type of molecular structure is often quantitatively characterized by the molecular weight between cross-links (usually referred to as M_c), i.e., the higher the M_c, the lower the density or degree of cross-linking junctions. Cross-linking of PE can be performed using cross-linking agents such as peroxides and silanes, and by the use of gamma or electron beam radiation. Laboratory hip simulator wear tests have shown that there is a decrease in wear rate with an increase in degree of cross-linking of PE. These studies, and the clinical results of a few trials that employed cross-linked PE acetabular cups several years ago, provide compelling evidence that cross-linking can reduce wear rates in acetabular components.

While cross-linking has been found to improve the performance of PE components in total hip arthroplasty, the trade-off in other mechanical properties has raised questions about the potential problems with such an approach and focused attention on the indications that might best benefit from its use [1, 25]. With an increase in cross-linking density comes an undesirable change in mechanical properties such as reduced elongation-to-failure, which occurs largely in the case of radiation cross-linking but to a lesser extent in the case of peroxide cross-linking. Associated with this reduction in the elongation-to-break is a reduction in the energy required to propagate a crack and the resistance of cross-linked parts to cyclic loading. It is possible that while cross-linking may improve wear resistance it may place components at greater risk of fracture.

There may be a reduction in the degree of crystallinity with increasing cross-link density, which may affect properties such as modulus of elasticity and creep. The modulus can be expected to decrease with decreasing crystallinity, but the effects on creep are less certain. In polymers with little or no crystallinity (namely rubbers), increasing cross-link density decreases creep. The effects of cross-linking on the creep of semi-crystalline polymers such as UHMWPE is less clear; this can be an important issue because the early radiographic studies of highly cross-linked polyethylene in hip prostheses may principally be measuring creep. Cross-linking a crystalline polymer may introduce defects and constraints that can decrease the overall crystallinity since the crystals have to grow around the defects. It has been shown (for example, comparing Hylamer to conventional UHMWPE) that lower crystallinity results in lower resistance to creep deformation. Processing of UHMWPE after cross-linking can be altered to restore the crystallinity (e.g., by annealing after the melting). Alternatively, the melt can be pressurized so that crystallization occurs under pressure, and increases crystallinity compared with melting without any applied pressure. In that case, crystallinity is not lost, and the cross-linking may additionally assist in resisting creep deformation.

Also of interest is the observation using laboratory uniaxial, reciprocating wear tests that cross-linked PE had a larger increase in wear rates compared with non-cross-linked PE when a rougher counterface was used. It is not yet known whether this increased susceptibility to a rough counterface is due to a reduced degree of crystallinity in cross-linked PE or to a reduced elongation-to-failure.

Because of the questions related to the change in certain properties with cross-linking, only an intermediate degree of cross-linking (an equivalent radiation dose of 50–100 kGy rather than 200 kGy) is being employed by many, so that there is a balance between increase in wear resistance and reduction in mechanical properties. Some have shown that, although there is a strong dependence of radiation dose (or cross-link density) on wear resistance in hip simulator tests, similar doses led to less improvements in wear rates using a knee simulator. One reason for lower sensitivity of cross-linking to wear in the knee simulator is that linear wear tracking does not lead to high volumetric wear rates even for conventional PE, and it is difficult to conclude whether cross-linking is appropriate for knee components using smooth counterface, linear tracking; some believe that a low level of cross-linking may be beneficial for the knee prosthesis.

Acknowledgements. M. Spector, Director, Tissue Engineering, VA Boston Healthcare System, was supported by the Department of Veterans Affairs, Veterans Health Administration, Rehabilitation Research and Development Service; M. Spector is a Research Career Scientist.

References

1. Baker DA, Bellare A, Pruitt L (2003) The effects of degree of cross-linking on the fatigue crack initiation and propagation resistance of orthopedic-grade polyethylene. J Biomed Mater Res 66A:146–154

2. Bellare A, Cohen RE (1996) Morphology of rod stock and compression-moulded sheets of ultra-high-molecular-weight polyethylene used in orthopaedic implants. Biomaterials 17:2325–2333

3. Besong AA, Tipper JL, Ingham E, Stone MH, Wroblewski BM, Fisher J (1998) Quantitative comparison of wear debris from UHMWPE that has and has not been sterilised by gamma irradiation. J Bone Joint Surg (Br) 80:340–344

4. Bhateja SK (1982) Changes in the crystalline content of irradiated linear polyethylenes upon ageing. Polymer 23:654–655

5. Bhateja SK (1983) Radiation-induced crystallinity changes in linear polyethylene: influence of aging. J Appl Polymer Sci 28:861–872

6. Bhateja SK (1983) Radiation-induced crystallinity changes in pressure-crystallized ultrahigh molecular weight polyethylene. J Macromolecular Sci - Physics B22:159–168

7. Bhateja SK, Andrews EH (1985) Radiation-induced crystallinity changes in polyethylene blends. J Mater Sci 20:2839–2845

8. Bhateja SK, Andrews EH, Yarbrough SM (1989) Radiation-induced crystallinity changes in linear polyethylenes: long-term aging effects. Polymer J 21:739–750

9. Bhateja SK, Andrews EH, Young RJ (1983) Radiation-induced crystallinity changes in linear polyethylene. J Polymer Sci: Polymer Physics Edition 21:523–536

10. Birkinshaw C, Buggy M, Daly S, O'Neill M (1989) The effect of gamma radiation on the physical structure and mechanical properties of ultrahigh molecular weight polyethylene. J Appl Polymer Sci 38:1967–1973

11. Birkinshaw C, Buggy M, Daly S, O'Neill M (1988) Mechanism of ageing in irradiated polymers. Polymer Degradation Stability 22:285–294

12. Bloebaum RD, Nelson K, Dorr LD, Hofmann AA, Lyman DJ (1991) Investigation of early surface delamination observed in retrieved heat-pressed tibial inserts. Clin Orthop 269:120–127

13. Bostrom MP, Bennett AP, Rimnac CM, Wright TM (1994) The natural history of ultra high molecular weight polyethylene. Clin Orthop 309:20–28

14. Brach del Prever E, Crova M, Costa L, Dallera A, Camino G, Gallinaro P (1996) Unacceptable biodegradation of polyethylene in vivo. Biomaterials 17:873–878

15. Burstein AH (1981) Structural mechanical properties of polyethylene acetabular cups. In: The Hip. Proceedings of the Ninth Open Scientific Meeting of The Hip Society. Mosby, St. Louis, pp 293–297

16. Cook JTE, Klein PG, Ward IM, Brain AA, Farrar DF, Rose J (2000) The morphology of nascent and moulded ultra-high molecular weight polyethylene. Insights from solid-state NMR, nitric acid etching, GPC and DSC. Polymer 41:8615–8623

17. Costa L, Brach del Prever E (eds) (2000) UHMWPE for Arthroplasty: characterisation, sterilisation and degradation. Edizioni Minerva Medica, Turin

18. Costa L, Jacobson K, Bracco P, Brach del Prever EM (2002) Oxidation of orthopaedic UHMWPE. Biomaterials 23:1613–1624

19. Costa L, Luda MP, Trossarelli L, Brach del Prever EM, Crova M, Gallinaro P (1998) In vivo UHMWPE biodegradation of retrieved prosthesis. Biomaterials 19:1371–1385

20. Costa L, Luda MP, Trossarelli L, Brach del Prever EM, Crova M, Gallinaro P (1998) Oxidation in orthopaedic UHMWPE sterilized by gamma-radiation and ethylene oxide. Biomaterials 19:659–668

21. Engh GA, Dwyer KA, Hanes CK (1992) Polyethylene wear of metal-backed tibial components in total and unicompartmental knee prostheses. J Bone Joint Surg (Br) 74:9–17

22. Gomoll A, Wanich T, Bellare A (2002) J-integral fracture toughness and tearing modulus measurement of radiation cross-linked UHMWPE. J Orthop Res 20:1152–1156

23. Gul RM, McGarry FJ, Bragdon CR, Muratoglu OK, Harris WH (2003) Effect of consolidation on adhesive and abrasive wear of ultra high molecular weight polyethylene. Biomaterials 24:3193–3199

24. Hamilton JV, Wang HC, Sung C (1996) The effect of fusion defects on the mechanical properties of UHMWPE. In: Transactions of the 5th World Biomaterials Congress, Toronto, p 511

25. Krzypow D, Bensusan J, Sevo K, Haggard W, Parr J, Goldberg V, Rimnac C (2000) The fatigue crack propagation resistance of gamma radiation or peroxide cross-linked UHMW polyethylene. In: Transactions of the 6th World Biomaterials Congress, Kamuela, Hawaii, p 382
26. Kurtz SM, Muratoglu OK, Evans M, Edidin AA (1999) Advances in the processing, sterilization, and cross-linking of ultra-high molecular weight polyethylene for total joint arthroplasty. Biomaterials 20:1659–1688
27. Li S, Burstein AH (1994) Ultra-high molecular weight polyethylene. J Bone Joint Surg 76-A:1080–1090
28. McKellop H, Shen FW, Lu B, Campbell P, Salovey R (1999) Development of an extremely wear-resistant ultra high molecular weight polyethylene for total hip replacements. J Orthop Res 17:157–167
29. McKellop H, Shen FW, Lu B, Campbell P, Salovey R (2000) Effect of sterilization method and other modifications on the wear resistance of acetabular cups made of ultra-high molecular weight polyethylene. A hip-simulator study. J Bone Joint Surg 82-A:1708–1725
30. Mintz L, Tsao AK, McCrae CR, Stulberg SD, Wright T (1991) The arthroscopic evaluation and characteristics of severe polyethylene wear in total knee arthroplasty. Clin Orthop 273:215–222
31. Muratoglu OK, Bragdon CR, O'Connor DO, Jasty M, Harris WH (2001) A novel method of cross-linking ultra-high-molecular-weight polyethylene to improve wear, reduce oxidation, and retain mechanical properties. Recipient of the 1999 HAP Paul Award. J Arthroplasty 16:149–160
32. Muratoglu OK, Bragdon CR, O'Connor DO, Jasty M, Harris WH, Gul R, McGarry F (1999) Unified wear model for highly cross-linked ultra-high molecular weight polyethylenes (UHMWPE). Biomaterials 20:1463–1470
33. Nusbaum HJ, Rose RM (1979) The effects of radiation sterilization on the properties of ultrahigh molecular weight polyethylene. J Biomed Mater Res 13:557–576
34. Olley RH, Hosier IL, Bassett DC, Smith NG (1999) On morphology of consolidated UHMWPE resin in hip cups. Biomaterials 20:2037–2046
35. Pienkowski D, Hoglin DP, Jacob RJ, Saum KA, Nicholls PJ, Kaufer H (1996) Shape and size of virgin ultrahigh molecular weight GUR 4150 HP polyethylene powder. J Biomed Mater Res 33:65–71
36. Pienkowski D, Jacob R, Hoglin D, Saum K, Kaufer H, Nicholls PJ (1995) Low-voltage scanning electron microscopic imaging of ultrahigh-molecular-weight polyethylene. J Biomed Mater Res 29:1167–1174
37. Premnath V, Harris WH, Jasty M, Merrill EW (1996) Gamma sterilization of UHMWPE articular implants: an analysis of the oxidation problem. Ultra high molecular weight polyethylene. Biomaterials 17:1741–1753
38. Pruitt L, Ranganathan R (1995) Effect of sterilization on the structure and fatigue resistance of medical grade UHMWPE. Mater Sci Eng c3:91–93
39. Roe R-J, Grood ES, Shastri R, Gosselin CA, Noyes FR (1981) Effect of radiation sterilization and aging on ultrahigh molecular weight polyethylene. J Biomed Mater Res 15:209–230
40. Schmidt MB, Hamilton JV (1996) The effects of calcium stearate on the properties of UHMWPE. In: Transactions of the 42nd Annual Meeting of the Orthopaedic Research Society, Atlanta, p 22
41. Shinde A, Salovey R (1985) Irradiation of ultrahigh-molecular-weight polyethylene. J Polymer Sci: Polymer Physics Edition 23:1681–1689
42. Sutula LC, Collier JP, Saum KA, Currier BH, Currier JH, Sanford WM, Mayor MB, Wooding RE, Sperling DK, Williams IR, et al (1995) The Otto Aufranc Award. Impact of gamma sterilization on clinical performance of polyethylene in the hip. Clin Orthop 319:28–40
43. Swarts D, Gsell R, King R, Devanathan D, Wallace S, Lin S (1996) Aging of calcium stearate-free polyethylene. In: Transactions of the 5th World Biomaterials Congress, Toronto, p 196
44. Wang A, Essner A, Polineni VK, Stark C, Dumbleton JH (1998) Lubrication and wear of ultra-high molecular weight polyethylene in total joint replacements. Tribology Int 31:17–33
45. Weightman B, Light D (1985) A comparison of RCH 1000 and Hi-Fax 1900 ultra-high molecular weight polyethylenes. Biomaterials 6:177–183
46. Wrona M, Mayor MB, Collier JP, Jensen RE (1994) The correlation between fusion defects and damage in tibial polyethylene bearings. Clin Orthop 299:92–103

8 Failures with Bearings

K. J. Bozic

Summary

Despite the long-term clinical and radiographic success that has been reported with total knee arthroplasty (TKA), failures related to the articular bearing surface continue to be one of the most significant factors that limit survivorship of TKA implants. Many variables influence wear and bearing surface failure, including factors related to the patient, the surgeon, and the implant. Future efforts should be directed at changes in the materials, implant design, sterilization methods, and surgical technique that could potentially lead to improvements in wear properties and an overall reduction in the incidence of bearing surface failures in TKA.

Introduction

Total knee arthroplasty (TKA) has emerged as one of the most successful and cost-effective interventions in orthopedic surgery. Clinical and radiographic success rates of greater than 90% at 10- to 15-year follow-up have been reported [7, 11]. Despite the high rates of success, however, problems related to the articular bearing surface have been one of the most common causes of failure. Fatigue and delamination are the most frequently reported mechanisms of bearing surface damage in TKA [19, 26]. Factors that influence wear rates and bearing surface damage include factors under the control of the surgeon, including

patient selection, implant selection, and surgical technique, and factors under the control of the manufacturer, including material composition, manufacturing technique, sterilization technique, shelf life, thickness, conformity, and issues related to modularity. The purpose of this chapter is to review the literature regarding the most common causes of bearing surface failure associated with TKA.

Mechanisms of Bearing Surface Failure

Bearing surface failures have been associated with articular wear, osteolysis, and problems related to modularity, including locking mechanism failure and backside wear.

Mechanisms of Wear Debris Generation

McKellop and colleagues have defined four modes of wear debris generation [18] (◘ Table 8-1). *Mode 1* describes wear that occurs between the two primary bearing surfaces, as intended by the designers of the implant. This type of wear occurs when the femoral implant articulates with the polyethylene articular insert. *Mode 2* refers to the condition of a primary bearing surface rubbing against a secondary surface in a manner not intended by the designer, such as when the femoral component wears through the articular insert and wears against the tibial

◘ **Table 8-1.** Modes of wear in prosthetic joints (from [18])

Wear mode	Description	Example
1	Wear that occurs between the two primary bearing surfaces, as intended by the designers of the implant	Femoral component articulating with the tibial insert
2	Primary bearing surface rubbing against a secondary surface in a manner not intended by the designer	Femoral component wears through articular insert and articulates against the metal base plate
3	Third body wear that occurs between the primary bearing surfaces due to particulate debris	PMMA, metallic debris, or bone chips in joint space between femoral component and tibial insert
4	Wear that occurs between two secondary (nonbearing) surfaces	Backsided wear that occurs between the UHMWPE articular insert and the tibial base plate

base plate. *Mode 3* refers to third-body wear that occurs between the primary bearing surfaces due to particulate debris such as polymethylmethacrylate (PMMA) fragments, bone chips, or metallic debris from porous coatings. *Mode 4* refers to wear that occurs between two secondary (nonbearing) surfaces. This would include 'backsided' wear that occurs between the UHMWPE articular insert and the tibial base plate [17, 20, 32].

Wear mechanisms associated with polyethylene articular inserts have been studied extensively in hip and knee replacement [1, 2, 4, 26, 31]. Wear mechanisms that have been associated with hip and knee arthroplasty include *abrasive wear, adhesive wear, third-body wear, delamination, and fatigue. Abrasive wear* results if particles are generated when imperfections in a harder surface (e.g., metal femoral component) plow grooves into a softer material (e.g., UHMWPE articular insert) [15]. This can occur either at the primary articulation or at other secondary surfaces. *Adhesive wear* occurs when small submicron particles adhere to the metallic counterface and are pulled off by the passing of the adjacent articulation surface [15]. *Third-body wear* occurs when third-body particles, such as cement, hydroxyapetite (HA), metal, and/or polyethylene, become embedded in the articulating bearing [26]. Adhesive and abrasive wear are most commonly associated with total hip arthroplasty, leading to biologically active sub-micron particulate wear debris that can result in osteolysis and peri-prosthetic bone loss [18, 28].

The most common mechanisms of wear and polyethylene damage in total knee arthroplasty are *delamination* and *fatigue*, whereby the formation of subsurface cracks leads to the generation of particles that are shed from the bearing surface [15]. Delamination can result in the loss of conformity of the articular bearing, leading to an altered pattern of load distribution and ultimately to failure of the articular bearing surface [19] (◘ Fig. 8-1).

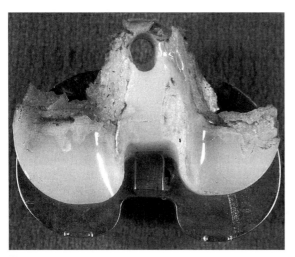

◘**Fig. 8-1.** Explanted tibial insert demonstrating extensive delamination of the articular surface

Factors that Affect Polyethylene Wear in Total Knee Arthroplasty

Ultra-high molecular weight polyethylene (UHMWPE) has been the articular bearing surface of choice for total knee replacement for the past 30 years [5]. Polyethylene wear can occur at both the articular surface and the undersurface of the articular insert at the interface of the tibial base plate (so-called backside wear). Many factors affect bearing surface wear, including factors associated with manufacturing, sterilization and shelf life of the implant, implant design factors, patient factors, surgical technique, and duration of time in vivo.

Manufacturing Technique

Several investigators have examined the effect of specific resins on wear rates associated with articular bearing surfaces in TKA. In a retrieval study, Won et al. examined the effect of resin type and manufacturing method on wear rates of Miller-Galante (M-G) I and II tibial inserts that were gamma irradiated in air [36]. Their analysis revealed that M-G I retrieved inserts, which were made by direct compression molding of Hi-fax 1900 resin, had significantly more wear damage in the form of scratching and embedded metallic debris, whereas M-G II retrievals, which were manufactured by machining from a ram-extruded rod of GUR 415 resin, had significantly more wear damage in the form of delamination. Light-microscopic examination of thin sections of the retrieved implants revealed that delamination of M-G II components occurred through a subsurface region of severely oxidatively degraded UHMWPE, while no such subsurface-degraded region was observed in M-G I retrievals. Based on their findings, the authors concluded that wear of UHMWPE tibial inserts is influenced by both resin type and manufacturing technique.

Sterilization Technique

Numerous in vitro and in vivo studies have been performed to evaluate the impact of sterilization techniques, such as gamma irradiation in air and ethylene oxide (EtO) gas, on wear rates in total knee arthroplasty [5, 8, 16, 22, 33, 35]. White et al. used qualitative and quantitative techniques to evaluate the effects of sterilization methods on the wear and physical and mechanical properties of 29 retrieved UHMWPE tibial inserts [33]. They reported higher rates of delamination, lower toughness, and lower percent elongation in inserts that were sterilized with gamma radiation in air compared with tibial inserts that were sterilized with ethylene oxide. Based on these findings, the authors concluded that EtO sterilization caused less microstructural damage to polyethylene and resulted in significantly less wear than sterilization with gamma radiation in air. Reeves and colleagues used Fourier transform infrared analysis and finite element modeling to compare wear rates between gamma-irradiated in air and gas-plasma sterilized UHMWPE tibial inserts [22]. They found that under high cyclic stresses, delamination occurred in the majority of the inserts gamma-irradiated in air but in none of the gas-plasma-sterilized inserts.

In a retrieval study of 1635 UHMWPE tibial inserts, Williams et al. found that those gamma irradiated in air had a high incidence of delamination and cracking, leading at times to complete wear through of the bearing, while inserts that were sterilized with EtO showed no evidence of fatigue damage, even after in vivo clinical use longer than 15 years [35]. Collier and colleagues used mechanical testing and Fourier transform infrared spectroscopy to study how gamma sterilization leads to degradation of the physical and mechanical properties of UHMWPE tibial inserts [8]. Their results indicated that gamma sterilization in air resulted in elevated oxidation of polyethylene, which reduced static strength and elongation properties and significantly decreased fatigue resistance of polyethylene bearings.

The overwhelming conclusion from most of the in vitro and in vivo studies regarding sterilization technique in total knee arthroplasty has been that gamma irradiation in air has an adverse effect on the physical and mechanical properties, thus leading to higher wear rates of UHMWPE articular bearing surfaces. In fact, in a review article on the subject that was published in 2002, Blunn and colleagues indicated that "delamination of loaded UHMWPE…will not occur in normal use over ten years if the UHMWPE has been well compacted and has not been sterilized by gamma irradiation in air" [5].

Shelf Life

Shelf life is defined as the period of time between when the implant is sterilized and packaged and when it is inserted into the patient [6]. Kurtz et al. examined the effects of shelf aging following gamma irradiation in air on the mechanical properties of UHMWPE tibial and acetabular inserts [16]. Using finite element modeling techniques, they reported that post-irradiation aging during shelf storage of UHMWPE inserts is likely to worsen long-term wear. Similarly, Bohl et al. investigated the effects of shelf aging on the in vivo performance of 188 gamma-sterilized UHMWPE Synatomic tibial inserts [6]. They found clinical failure (defined as component retrieval because of polyethylene degradation) rates ranging from 20.8% for prostheses that had shelf lives before implantation of 8–11 years to 0% for prostheses that had shelf lives of less than 4 years. The authors concluded that longer

shelf life had an adverse effect on the mechanical properties of UHMWPE tibial inserts. Based on these findings, they recommended component expiration dates should be placed on implant packages and that implants that are shelf aged beyond this date should be discarded.

Other Design Factors (Implant Thickness, Conformity, and Type of Polyethylene)

Bartel et al. investigated the effect of conformity and plastic thickness on contact stresses in metal-backed hip and knee implants [4]. Using both analytical and finite element methods, the investigators found that for metal-backed components, minimum thickness of less than 6 mm for non-conforming surfaces and less than 4 mm for nearly conforming surfaces may result in excessively large contact stresses. Furthermore, their results demonstrated that bonding of the plastic to the metal backing decreased the tensile stresses at the edge of the contact zone and the maximum shear stress immediately under the load, suggesting a potential benefit of non-modular metal-backed tibial components.

In a follow-up study from the same research lab, published in 1986, Bartel and colleagues used elasticity and finite element solutions to estimate the effect of conformity, thickness, and material on contact stresses and surface damage in UHMWPE hip and knee implants [3]. They found that stresses associated with surface damage in the tibial component of the total knee replacement were much greater than those in the acetabular component of the total hip replacement. Also, their analysis of contact stresses of the polyethylene insert for tibial components suggested that a thickness of more than 8–10 mm should be maintained whenever possible. Other interesting findings were that contact stresses in the tibial component were reduced most when the articular surfaces conformed in the medial-lateral direction, and were much less sensitive to changes in geometry in the anterior-posterior direction. Finally, they found that the use of carbon-fiber reinforced PE resulted in stresses that were greater by as much as 40%.

In a separate study, Wright and Bartel analyzed surface damage in retrieved TKA tibial inserts and compared these findings with analytical studies to assess the influence of thickness, articular conformity, and type of polyethylene on wear patterns [38]. With respect to these design parameters, they found greater surface damage in thin components (less than 4–6 mm), components with relatively flat tibial articulating surfaces, and carbon-reinforced polyethylene components.

Sathasivam and Walker used computer modeling techniques to simulate static and dynamic loading of tibial inserts in total knee arthroplasty [25]. Their results indicated that much lower contact stresses, and therefore less surface damage, are seen in designs that allow for conformity in the frontal (e.g., medial-lateral) plane.

Patient Factors, Length of Time In Vivo

Several authors have suggested that wear of tibial articular inserts is affected by patient factors, including weight and duration of time in vivo [37, 38]. In 1986, Wright and Bartel observed patterns of surface damage from retrieved total knee polyethylene components and compared their findings with analytical studies of contact stresses in articular inserts [38]. They reported that the amount and severity of surface damage to the tibial insert increased with patient weight and with length of time in vivo.

In a separate study, Wright and colleagues used light microscopy to evaluate surface damage to carbon fiber-reinforced and non-reinforced UHMWPE tibial inserts that had been retrieved from failed posterior stabilized total knee prostheses [37]. They reported that the amount of surface damage was directly proportional to the duration of time in vivo for both types of implants.

Surgical Technique

Wasielewski et al. examined 55 unconstrained polyethylene tibial inserts that were retrieved at revision TKA for evidence of wear [31]. They found the most severe wear patterns in inserts with third-body wear from metal-backed patellar failures and cement debris. Furthermore,

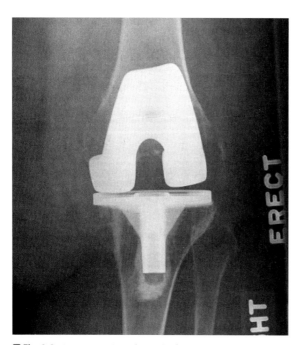

◘ Fig. 8-2. Anteroposterior radiograph of a TKA demonstrating medial compartment wear secondary to incomplete ligament balancing of a varus knee. Note the extensive osteolysis in the proximal tibia

they reported that articular wear and cold flow were greatest in the tightest pre-TKA compartment (e.g., medial in the varus knee and lateral in the valgus knee). The authors concluded that wear associated with unconstrained TKA is affected by clinical and mechanical factors under the surgeon's control, including component size and position, knee alignment, and ligament balance (◘ Fig. 8-2).

D'Lima and colleagues used finite element modeling techniques to assess the effect of malalignment on polyethylene contact stresses in total knee arthroplasty [10]. They found that increased conformity significantly reduced contact stresses in neutral alignment, liftoff significantly increased contact stresses under both low- and high-conformity conditions, and malalignment in rotation was especially detrimental with the high-conformity insert design. Based on these findings, the authors concluded that both implant design and surgical technique can play a critical role in wear rates in TKA, and that mobile bearing designs could result in lower contact stresses by minimizing the effect of rotational malalignment.

Problems Related to Modularity

Another issue that has been debated in the literature is the benefits and drawbacks associated with modular tibial implants [24, 27, 29]. Proponents of modularity cite the ability to alter soft-tissue balancing intra-operatively and the potential for less traumatic revision surgery as benefits of modularity [27, 29]. Opponents of modularity point to potential problems associated with backside wear and incompetent locking mechanism designs as arguments against the use of modular tibial inserts [21, 24].

Backside Wear

Many investigators have demonstrated that in addition to articular surface damage and wear, backside wear between the articular insert and the metal tibial base plate is a major contributor to wear debris in TKA [17, 20, 24, 30] (◘ Fig. 8-3). Li et al. performed an in vitro analysis of 55 retrieved tibial inserts from four different TKA designs [17]. Their results suggested that backside wear of tibial inserts can be a significant contributor to polyethylene wear in TKA, and as a result, surgeons and manufacturers should pay close attention to the fixation of tibial inserts to metal trays.

In a review article on the subject published in 2002, Wasielewski reported that the forces at the undersurface articulation created during physiological loading are influenced by insert type, articular design, and surgical technique [30]. He noted that increasing articular insert constraint, while reducing contact stresses at the point of contact on the articular surface, can actually increase

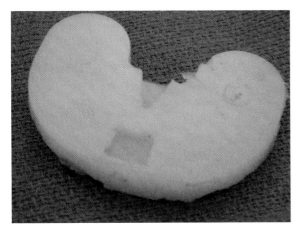

Fig. 8-3. Explanted tibial insert demonstrating backside wear secondary to motion between the tibial insert and the metal base plate

backside wear, due to transfer of forces to the interface between the articular insert and the tibial base plate. Also, designs with a cam-post mechanism, such as posterior cruciate substituting designs, create a significant shear force at this interface (**Fig. 8-4**). Furthermore, he reported that factors under the control of the surgeon, including component alignment and position and ligament balance, may also influence backside wear.

Rao et al. analyzed 29 retrieved modular tibial components from 12 fixed bearing designs with regard to backside wear and relative motion between the polyethylene insert and the metal base plate [20]. Their results suggested that backside wear was correlated with the relative motion between the polyethylene insert and the metal base plate. Based on their findings, the authors concluded that new locking mechanism designs directed toward better securing of the polyethylene insert to the tibial tray are needed to minimize the generation of particular wear debris at the modular interface.

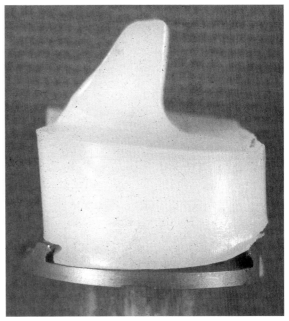

Fig. 8-5. Explanted tibial insert and base plate demonstrating dissociation and displacement of the tibial insert secondary to failure of the base-plate locking mechanism. (Courtesy of Michael Ries)

Dissociation of Tibial Insert

Although rare, several case reports have been published regarding patients who suffered dissociation of the modular tibial insert from the metal base plate in fixed bearing knees [9, 23]. In a report of two cases of dissociation of a modular PCA insert, Davis et al. postulated that anterior liftoff of the insert during knee flexion was the cause of the dissociation [9]. Ries recently reported a case of a constrained condylar insert-base plate dissociation that occurred as a result of anterior cam-post impingement, leading to failure of the posterior locking mechanism and posterior liftoff [23] (**Fig. 8-5**). These authors suggested that use of a modular constrained condylar knee may not be appropriate for patients with a deficient extensor mechanism.

Osteolysis

Osteolysis, although less common in TKA than in total hip arthroplasty (THA), is a major cause of TKA failure leading to the need for revision surgery. The mechanism of periprosthetic bone loss associated with particulate debris has been critically evaluated in both in vitro and in vivo studies [12–14]. Willert and Semlitsch first proposed that wear-particle generation and migration into the joint cavity and periprosthetic space may stimulate macrophage recruitment and phagocytosis [34]. Since that time, further research has revealed that sub-micron wear particles are phagocytosed by macrophages, resulting in the release of various pro-inflammatory factors and

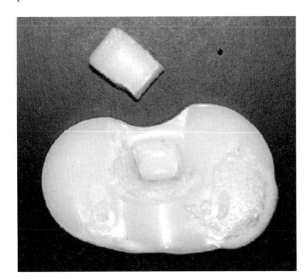

Fig. 8-4. Explanted tibial insert from a posterior stabilized TKA demonstrating fracture of the tibial post. (Courtesy of Steve Haas)

chemical mediators from these activated cells [12]. Cellular mediators that have been studied and are thought to play a significant role in osteolysis are interleukin-1 (IL-1), interleukin-6 (IL-6), tumor necrosis factor-α (TNF-α) and prostaglandin E_2 (PGE_2) [13]. Proliferation of these cellular mediators then leads to stimulation and differentiation of osteoclasts and inhibition of osteoblasts. These factors work synergistically, ultimately leading to the dissolution of bone at the prosthetic interface, allowing for prosthetic micro motion that leads to further generation of wear debris [14].

In vitro studies have demonstrated that many factors influence the biological response to wear debris, including the size, volume, surface chemistry, and material composition of the particles [2]. Many investigators have noted that osteolysis is less common in TKA than in THA [12, 15, 26]. In THA, adhesive and abrasive wear mechanisms dominate, resulting in the formation of high volumes of sub-micron particulate debris. Conversely, in TKA, fatigue and delamination are the most common mechanisms of bearing surface damage. These modes of failure produce wear debris particles that are larger than the wear particles observed around total hip replacements. It has been hypothesized by Ayers and others that the more aggressive biological response seen with THA could be explained by the fact that sub-micron particles provide a greater stimulus to the macrophage to produce inflammatory mediators that result in osteolysis [2].

References

1. Ayers DC (2001) Maximizing ultra high molecular weight polyethylene performance in total knee replacement. Instr Course Lect 50:421–429
2. Ayers DC (1997) Polyethylene wear and osteolysis following total knee replacement. Instr Course Lect 46:205–213
3. Bartel DL, Bicknell VL, Wright TM (1986) The effect of conformity, thickness, and material on stresses in ultra-high molecular weight components for total joint replacement. J Bone Joint Surg [Am] 68:1041–1051
4. Bartel DL, Burstein AH, Toda MD, Edwards DL (1985) The effect of conformity and plastic thickness on contact stresses in metal-backed plastic implants. J Biomech Eng 107:193–199
5. Blunn G, Brach del Preva EM, Costa L, Fisher J, Freeman MA (2002) Ultra high molecular-weight polyethylene (UHMWPE) in total knee replacement: fabrication, sterilisation and wear. J Bone Joint Surg [Br] 84:946–949
6. Bohl JR, Bohl WR, Postak PD, Greenwald AS (1999) The Coventry Award. The effects of shelf life on clinical outcome for gamma sterilized polyethylene tibial components. Clin Orthop 376:28–38
7. Colizza WA, Insall JN, Scuderi GR (1995) The posterior stabilized total knee prosthesis. Assessment of polyethylene damage and osteolysis after a ten-year-minimum follow-up. J Bone Joint Surg [Am] 77:1713–1720
8. Collier JP, Sperling DK, Currier JH, et al (1996) Impact of gamma sterilization on clinical performance of polyethylene in the knee. J Arthroplasty 11:377–389
9. Davis P, Bocell J, Tullos H (1999) Dissociation of the tibial component in total knee replacements. Clin Orthop 272:199–204
10. D'Lima DD, Chen PC, Colwell CW Jr (2001) Polyethylene contact stresses, articular congruity, and knee alignment. Clin Orthop 392:232–238
11. Faris PM, Ritter MA, Keating EM, Meding JB, Harty LD (2003) The AGC all-polyethylene tibial component: a ten-year clinical evaluation. J Bone Joint Surg [Am] 85:489–493

12. Goodman S, Lind M, Song Y, Smith R (1998) In vitro, in vivo and tissue retrieval studies on particulate debris. Clin Orthop 352:25–34
13. Howell G, Bourne R (2000) Osteolysis: etiology, prosthetic factors, and pathogenesis. Instr Course Lect 49:71–82
14. Jacobs J, Rosebuck K, Archibeck M, Hallab M, Glant T (2001) Osteolysis: basic science. Clin Orthop 393:71–77
15. Jacobs J, Shanbag A, Glant T, Black J, Galante J (1994) Wear debris in total joint replacements. J Am Acad Orthop Surgeons 2: 212–220
16. Kurtz SM, Bartel DL, Rimnac CM (1998) Postirradiation aging affects stress and strain in polyethylene components. Clin Orthop 350:209–220
17. Li S, Scuderi G, Furman BD, et al (2002) Assessment of backside wear from the analysis of 55 retrieved tibial inserts. Clin Orthop 404:75–82
18. McKellop H, Campbell P, Park S-H, et al (1995) The origin of submicron polyethylene wear debris in total hip arthroplasty. Clin Orthop 311:3 20
19. Muratoglu OK, Mark A, Vittetoe DA, Harris WH, Rubash HE (2003) Polyethylene damage in total knees and use of highly cross-linked polyethylene. J Bone Joint Surg [Am] 85 [Suppl 1]:S7–S13
20. Rao A, Engh G, Collier M, Lounici S (2002) Tibial interface wear in retrieved total knee components and correlations with modular insert motion. J Bone Joint Surg [Am] 84:1849–1855
21. Rao KS, Siddalinga Swamy MK (1989) Sensory recovery in the plantar aspect of the foot after surgical decompression of posterior tibial nerve. Possible role of steroids along with decompression. Lepr Rev 60: 283–287
22. Reeves EA, Barton DC, FitzPatrick DP, Fisher J (2000) Comparison of gas plasma and gamma irradiation in air sterilization on the delamination wear of the ultra-high molecular weight polyethylene used in knee replacements. Proc Inst Mech Eng [H] 214:249–255
23. Ries MD (2004) Dissociation of the UHMWPE Insert from tibial baseplate in total knee arthroplasty. A case report. J Bone Joint Surg [Am] 86:1522–1524
24. Rodriguez J, Baez N, Rasquinha V, Ranawat C (2001) Metal-backed and all-polyethylene tibial components in total knee replacement. Clin Orthop 392:174–183
25. Sathasivam S, Walker PS (1998) Computer model to predict subsurface damage in tibial inserts of total knees. J Orthop Res 16: 564–571
26. Schmalzried T, Callaghan J (1999) Wear in total hip and knee replacements. J Bone Joint Surg [Am] 81:115–136
27. Shaw J (1992) Angled bearing inserts in total knee arthroplasty. A brief technical note. J Arthroplasty 7:211–216
28. Sinha R, Shanbag A, Maloney W, Hasselman C, Rubash H (1998) Osteoylsis: cause and effect. Instr Course Lect 47:307–320
29. Surace M, Berzins A, Urban R, et al (2002) Backsurface wear and deformation in polyethylene tibial inserts retrieved postmortem. Clin Orthop 40:14–23
30. Wasielewski RC (2002) The causes of insert backside wear in total knee arthroplasty. Clin Orthop 404:232–246
31. Wasielewski RC, Galante JO, Leighty RM, Natarajan RN, Rosenberg AG (1994) Wear patterns on retrieved polyethylene tibial inserts and their relationship to technical considerations during total knee arthroplasty. Clin Orthop 299:31–43
32. Wasielewski RC, Parks N, Williams I, et al (1997) Tibial insert undersurface as a contributing source of polyethylene wear debris. Clin Orthop 345:53–59
33. White SE, Paxson RD, Tanner MG, Whiteside LA (1996) Effects of sterilization on wear in total knee arthroplasty. Clin Orthop 331:164–171
34. Willert H, Semlitsch M (1977) Reactions of the articular capsule to wear products of artificial joint prostheses. J Biomed Mater Res 11:157–164
35. Williams IR, Mayor MB, Collier JP (1998) The impact of sterilization method on wear in knee arthroplasty. Clin Orthop 356:170–180
36. Won CH, Rohatgi S, Kraay MJ, Goldberg VM, Rimnac CM (2000) Effect of resin type and manufacturing method on wear of polyethylene tibial components. Clin Orthop 376:161–171
37. Wright T, Rimnac C, Faris P, Bansal M (1988) Analysis of surface damage in retrieved carbon fiber-reinforced and plain polyethylene tibial components from posterior stabilized total knee replacements. J Bone Joint Surg [Am] 70:1312–1319
38. Wright TM, Bartel DL (1986) The problem of surface damage in polyethylene total knee components. Clin Orthop 205:67–74

9 Failures in Patellar Replacement in Total Knee Arthroplasty

J. A. Rand

Summary

Patellar failure after TKA is often multifactorial. A careful assessment of patient factors, implant design and surgical technique must be performed. If there are major problems with implant design or component positioning, revision of the entire arthroplasty may be necessary to correct the patellar failure and ensure a durable result. Isolated revision of the patellofemoral joint for any reason must be approached cautiously, as a high failure rate is often encountered.

Introduction

In a recent series of revision total knee arthroplasties (TKA), extensor mechanism problems comprised almost 12% of the reasons for reoperation [1]. Reasons for failure in the patellofemoral joint are multifactorial and may be related to patient selection, implant design, surgical technique, or combinations of these factors. Therefore, any discussion of patellar component failures must consider multiple potential reasons for failure. Unfortunately, most studies of patellofemoral complications have not considered the importance of the tibiofemoral joint for the complication. Anterior knee pain, patellar instability, fracture, loosening, wear, extensor mechanism rupture, and a variety of miscellaneous problems affecting the patella can adversely affect the results of a TKA.

The anatomy and kinematics of the patellofemoral joint are complex. There is variability in the orientation of the patellar groove in both the coronal and transverse planes. The patellar groove is oriented approximately perpendicular to the epicondylar axis. Since there are substantial individual variations in alignment and patellar tracking, the design of the femoral component needs to accommodate these variations. The patella undergoes a medial shift in early flexion followed by a lateral shift in deep knee flexion beyond 90°. In deep flexion, the contact area on the patella moves distally on the lateral facet of the patella, resulting in a decrease in contact area. The contact areas and kinematics of the patella are altered in TKA and are affected by implant orientation and design of the femoral and patellar components.

Etiology

Patient selection is an important variable influencing extensor mechanism complications. Patellar complications are increased in patients with a diagnosis of patellofemoral arthritis, obesity, osteoporosis, valgus deformity, post-traumatic arthritis, and prior proximal tibial osteotomy (◘ Fig. 9-1).

A diagnosis of osteoarthritis and obesity has been associated with an increased risk of patellar complications [2]. In the presence of valgus deformity, varying degrees of lateral femoral condyle hypoplasia make rotational positioning of the femoral implant difficult. In knees with

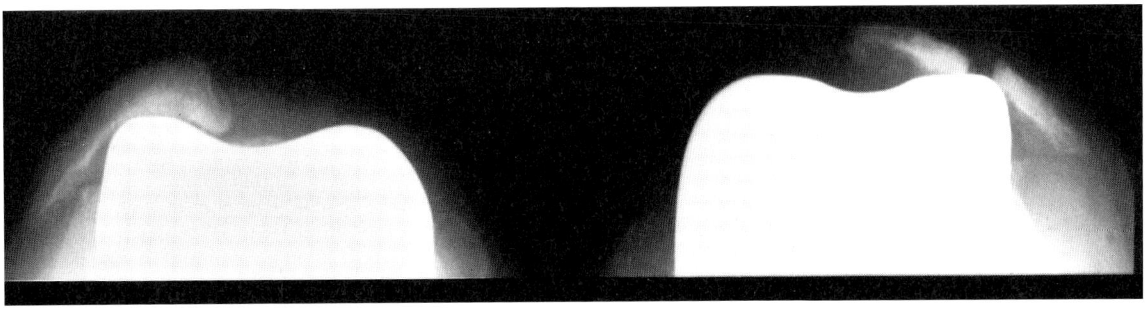

◘ **Fig. 9-1.** Merchant X-ray demonstrating patellar subluxation bilaterally with fracture on the left knee in a patient with preoperative patellofemoral arthritis

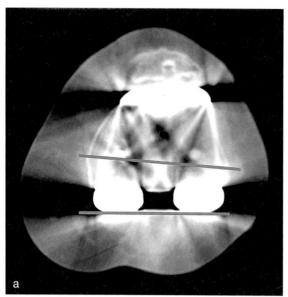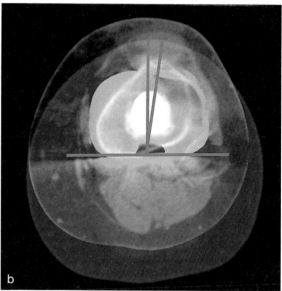

Fig. 9-2a, b. CAT scans of (*a*) femoral and (*b*) tibial component with internal malrotation

preoperative valgus, a lateral retinacular release was necessary in 102 of 134 knees to treat intraoperative patellar subluxation [3]. The presence of patella infera following proximal tibial osteotomy or post-traumatic arthritis can result in impingement between the patella and the tibial component, resulting in pain or patellar instability. The patient with severe osteoporosis is at risk of patellar fracture following patellar resurfacing.

Surgical technique is an important variable influencing patellar complications. A midvastus or subvastus surgical approach results in improved patellar tracking and less frequent need for a lateral retinacular release than does an anteromedial arthrotomy. Using meta analysis, a lateral retinacular release was required in ten of 164 (6%) subvastus approaches compared with 31 of 172 (18%) medial parapatellar approaches [4–6]. Femoral and tibial component position affect patellar alignment and complications. Patellar complications are diminished by maintenance of the joint line and patellar height, lateral placement of the femoral component on the femur, medial placement of the patellar component on the patella, and posterior placement of the tibial component on the tibia. The femoral component should not be flexed on the femur, and the trochlear flange should be aligned with the anterior femoral cortex. If the trochlear portion of the femoral component is prominent, the extensor mechanism will be displaced in an anterior direction, resulting in increased lateral retinacular tension. The result is a potential decrease in knee motion and possible patellar maltracking. In severe cases, the patella may mechanically catch on the trochlear flange of the femoral component. Any deviation of the femoral, tibial, or patellar components from these ideal locations can adversely affect patellar alignment, leading to patellar failure. Internal malrotation of either the tibial or the

femoral component will adversely affect patellar tracking (**□** Fig. 9-2).

Alignment of the femoral component with the epicondylar axis or the AP axis appears to be best. Femoral component rotation parallel to the epicondylar axis resulted in the most normal patellar tracking and decreased shear forces early in flexion [7]. Rotating the femoral component either internal or external to the epicondylar axis adversely affected patellar tracking. There is a close relationship between the femoral epicondylar axis and the patellar axis. Placing the tibial component perpendicular to the epicondylar axis resulted in correct rotation in 73% of cases [8]. In a study of 102 TKAs, there was a mean of 6.2° of internal rotation in the knees with anterior knee pain compared with 0.4° of external rotation in the control knees [9]. In a comparison of 30 TKAs with patellar complications and 20 controls without, combined internal rotation of 1°–4° resulted in lateral patellar tracking and tilt, 3°–8° patellar subluxation, and 7°–17° patellar dislocation or patellar failure [10].

Reproduction of patellar thickness, correct size and position of the patellar component, and balance of the extensor mechanism are necessary for a satisfactory result. A lateral retinacular release was required for 17% with medial compared with 46% with a central placement of the patellar implant [11]. The amount of bone resected from the patella will affect patellar tracking and patellar strain. Resection of excessive patellar bone can result in weakening of the patella, leading to fracture or implant fixation in poor-quality bone predisposing to loosening. Thickening the patella at the time of resurfacing will tighten the lateral retinaculum, resulting in patellar tilt or subluxation. If the patella is resurfaced, the original patellar thickness should be reproduced. Asymmetric resurfacing of the patella should be avoided. In a series of

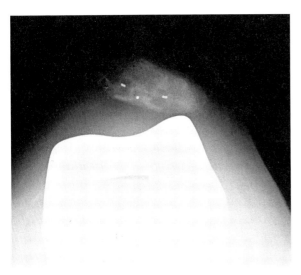

◘ **Fig. 9-3.** Merchant X-ray demonstrating lateral patellar tilt and sub-luxation in a TKA design with a shallow trochlear groove. There is also some internal rotation of the femoral component

knee flexion angles greater than 60° exceeded the yield point of the polyethylene for all designs [17]. Anatomically shaped patellar implants provide increased contact area over dome-shaped implants when aligned correctly but will have a decreased contact area with slight tilt or malrotation. Eighteen of 75 anatomically shaped patellar implants had a complication [18]. For this reason, a dome-shaped patella is preferred to the anatomical shape, as it is more forgiving of minor malalignment. A study of a two-peg anatomical, three-peg dome, and three-peg anatomical patellar component design found improved results with the three-peg designs [19].

Either an inset or onlay patellar design may be used. In an in vitro comparison of an inset to an onlay design, patellar strain was increased by 28% for the inset and 22% for the onlay design over the unresurfaced value [20]. In a retrospective comparison of 135 resurfacing patellae with 116 inset patellae, patellar tilt, subluxation, and lateral retinacular release were less frequent with the inset than with the resurfacing design [21].

Are extensor mechanism complications different in resurfaced and unresurfaced patellae of TKA? Controversy has surrounded the need for patellar resurfacing at the time of TKA. This controversy arises from differing results which are clearly influenced by studies using TKA designs that do not allow congruent tracking of the native patella and surgical techniques that led to patellar malalignment. These results are further complicated by differing rates for reoperation that are influenced by the ease of resurfacing of the painful unresurfaced patella but not treatment of anterior knee pain in the resurfaced patella. Selective resurfacing attempts to identify those individuals who will have an improved clinical result by resurfacing while avoiding the complications of unnecessary resurfacing. The best data regarding the results of patellar resurfacing derive from randomized, prospective studies of patellar resurfacing. Using meta analysis of nine randomized, prospective series, there were 518 resurfaced and 542 unresurfaced patellae followed for 2–10 years [22–30]. Anterior knee pain was present in 38 (7.3%) of the resurfaced and 118 (21.8%) of the unresurfaced patellae. Knee scores were similar in both groups. Patellar complications occurred in 14 (2.7%), leading to reoperation in ten (1.9%) of the resurfaced patellae. This is in contrast to patellar complications in 37 (6.8%) of unresurfaced patellae, leading to reoperation in 36 (6.6%) [22–30]. If anterior knee pain persists in the unresurfaced patella, will pain be relieved by resurfacing? Using meta analysis of 60 knees with secondary patellar resurfacing, 36 (60%) were improved, 12 (20%) unchanged, and 12 (20%) worse after resurfacing [25–29, 31, 32]. Therefore, selective patellar resurfacing may be the best approach considering patient demands, implant design, patellar articular cartilage, and intraoperative patellar alignment.

21 TKAs with asymmetric resurfacing of the patella, 11 knees were revised, recommended for revision, or had anterior knee pain [12]. A lateral retinacular release for patellar maltracking is not innocuous. Patellar complications occurred in 14% of 540 knees with in comparison to 7% of 510 knees without a lateral retinacular release [13]. Complications in the lateral release group consisted of patellar radiolucency in 11, patellar fracture in nine, hematoma in seven, extensor lag in seven, patellar instability in five, and patellar implant loosening in three [13].

Implant design affects patellar alignment and patellar tracking. A trochlear groove that is asymmetric or deep produces a decrease in shear and compressive force on the patella compared with a symmetric or shallow trochlear groove design [14]. Patellar complications occurred in 15 of 148 TKAs with a shallow trochlear groove compared with one of 153 TKAs with a deep trochlear groove [15] (◘ Fig. 9-3).

In a comparison of 150 TKAs performed with a standard design with 150 TKAs with a 3° external rotation built into the femoral component (resulting in a lateralized trochlear groove), the prevalence of lateral retinacular release was decreased from 14% to 5% and patellar maltracking from 12% to 5% [16]. Therefore, selection of a femur with a deep, offset trochlear design is preferable to minimize patellar complications. The patellar implant may be a central dome, offset dome, or anatomical in shape. Failure of the patella due to wear and deformation of patellar components are observed with all polyethylene and metal-backed patellar component designs. All polyethylene dome designs are susceptible to deformation, while metal-backed designs are susceptible to deformation of the polyethylene over the metal or to dissociation of the metal backing. In a study of six different TKA designs, contact pressures in the patellofemoral joint at

Specific Complications and Failure Mechanisms

Patellar instability may manifest as pain and weakness, intermittent giving way, or episodes of patellar dislocation. Patellar tilt and subluxation are frequently encountered on routine radiographs of asymptomatic patients. Why some patients with patellar malalignment are asymptomatic while others are symptomatic remains an enigma. The etiology of patellar instability can be traced to patient selection, implant design, surgical technique, or trauma [33]. Preoperative patellar subluxation, preoperative valgus, or patellofemoral arthritis have been correlated with an increased prevalence of lateral retinacular release and increased postoperative patellar malalignment [3]. Implant designs that have a shallow trochlear groove, fixed axis of rotation, or unrestricted rotation have had a high prevalence of patellar subluxation and dislocation. In a study of 289 TKAs using a design with a shallow trochlear groove and followed up, 14 knees required revision for patellar maltracking [32]. Problems with surgical technique are a frequent reason for patellar instability. Internal malrotation of the femoral or tibial component, excessive valgus knee alignment, lateral placement of a patellar component on the patella, medial translation of the femoral component on the femur, thickening the patella with resurfacing, or oversizing the femoral component onto the anterior surface of the femur may contribute to patellar instability.

Treatment of patellar instability must be directed at the etiology. Implant malposition is best treated by component revision. Soft-tissue imbalance should be treated by a proximal realignment consisting of a lateral retinacular release and vastus medialis advancement. Although distal realignment of the tibial tuberosity can correct patellar instability, it creates a compensatory deformity, alters patellar kinematics, and may predispose to patellar tendon rupture. Most published studies of treatment of patellar instability did not assess implant rotation, making interpretation of the results difficult. In our own series, the etiology of patellar instability was failure to balance the extensor mechanism in nine knees, tibial component malrotation in four, atraumatic medial retinacular tears in four, quadriceps weakness in four, activity-related tears of the medial retinaculum in two, and a traumatic tear of the medial retinaculum in one knee [34]. Recurrent subluxation occurred in four of 14 knees following proximal realignment, while two of nine knees sustained a rupture of the patellar tendon following combined proximal and distal realignment. One of two knees treated by revision had a recurrent patellar subluxation. Two knees developed deep infections. Distal extensor mechanism realignment has been recommended using a tibial tubercle transfer as treatment for patellar instability. However, as distal extensor mechanism realign-

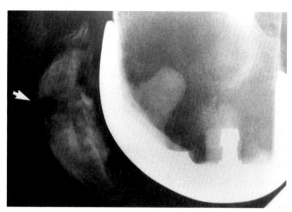

Fig. 9-4. Lateral X-ray demonstrating an asymptomatic patellar fracture with non-union

ment alters knee kinematics and is associated with rupture of the patellar tendon in some patients, proximal realignment is the preferred technique in the absence of implant malposition. Revision of the femoral and tibial components should be considered for those knees with component malposition.

Patellar fractures may present as anything from asymptomatic findings on routine radiographs to acute episodes with disruption of the extensor mechanism (Fig. 9-4).

In a series of 12 464 TKA from the Mayo Clinic there were 85 patellar fractures, for a prevalence of (0.68%) [35]. The prevalence of fracture is greater in men than in women, in resurfaced than in unresurfaced patellae, and in revision than in primary TKA. The etiology of patellar fracture includes trauma, avascularity, implant malalignment, obesity, excessive patellar bone resection, high activity level, large range of motion, inset patellar design, large central fixation lug, revision TKA, and osteoporosis. The position of the tibial and femoral components affects the severity and results of patellar fractures. In a series of 36 patellar fractures, a good or excellent result was achieved in 15 of 16 with minor malalignment as compared with three of 20 with major malalignment [36]. Avascularity of the patella following a medial arthrotomy combined with a lateral retinacular release has been suggested as an etiology of fracture. Another explanation for the association of patellar fracture with lateral retinacular release is abnormal forces on a maltracking patella that necessitated the lateral release. In a series of 1146 TKAs, a patellar fracture occurred in 22 of 406 (5.4%) knees with as compared with 18 of 740 (2.4%) without a lateral retinacular release [37]. There was no significant difference in the prevalence of patellar fracture following lateral retinacular release in which the superior lateral genicular artery was spared or sacrificed [38].

A variety of classification systems have been used for patellar fractures after TKA. Differences in classification make comparison of results from various series difficult.

The easiest classification system is the one from the Mayo Clinic [35]. Fractures are divided into three types based on the stability of the patellar prosthesis and on whether or not the extensor mechanism is intact. A type-I fracture has a stable implant and an intact extensor mechanism. A type-II fracture has a disruption of the extensor mechanism. A type-III fracture has a loose patellar implant and an intact extensor mechanism. The type-III fractures are divided into subtypes A and B, based on the quality of remaining bone stock (A = good and B = poor with <10 mm or marked comminution). For the 38 type-I fractures, non-operative treatment consisted of observation in 27, immobilization in ten, and operative treatment including patellar component removal and patelloplasty in one knee. A fibrous union occurred in 16, non-union in 15, and union in six fractures. Of the 12 type-II fractures, only one was treated without an operation (resulting in a satisfactory outcome). Operative management with open reduction and internal fixation resulted in union of one of six fractures. Partial patellectomy and tendon repair in five knees resulted in complications in three. Of the 12 type-II fractures, six had complications, five a reoperation, and seven either pain or weakness. A type-III fracture occurred in 38 knees. Of the 12 type-IIIA fractures, eight were treated with and four without an operation. Only two of the 12 fractures united. Two of four knees treated without an operation had pain. Complications occurred in five of five fractures treated by resection of the patellar components and internal fixation. Of the 12 type-IIIA fractures, seven knees had complications, three a reoperation, and seven pain or weakness. Of the 16 type-IIIB fractures, a satisfactory result occurred in three of four knees following non-operative treatment. Pain or weakness occurred in seven of 12 knees following operative management. Of the 28 type-III fractures, eight had a complication, three underwent reoperation, and 15 remained symptomatic. Considering the entire group of fractures, there were improved results and fewer complications following non-operative than following operative management. Non-operative treatment of 46 fractures resulted in complications in four knees and in reoperation of one knee. Operative treatment of 32 fractures resulted in complications in 18 and reoperation of 16 knees. The authors concluded that non-operative treatment should be selected for type-I and some type-III fractures. Operative treatment should be used for type-II fractures.

In summary, treatment of patellar fractures must consider the etiology and carefully evaluate the position of the femoral and tibial components. Treatment of most patellar fractures should be non-operative, with an initial period of immobilization. Operative treatment should be reserved for those fractures with an extensor mechanism rupture. Revision of the femoral or tibial components may be required to address implant malrotation or malposition.

Ruptures are the most difficult extensor mechanism problems to manage, with the highest frequency of failure and complications. The location of rupture may be in the patellar tendon, in the quadriceps tendon, or in association with a patellar fracture. At the Mayo Clinic, the prevalence of quadriceps tendon rupture was 24 of 23 800 (0.1%) and patellar tendon rupture was 18 of 8288 (0.17%) TKA [38, 39]. Quadriceps tendon tears are often associated with systemic diseases such as diabetes mellitus or use of systemic corticosteroids [38]. Lateral retinacular release, prior operation, and extensile surgical exposures may result in quadriceps rupture [38]. Finally, trauma from a fall or vigorous activity may rupture the tendon damaged by systemic disease or surgery [38]. The results of treatment of quadriceps ruptures after TKA have been variable. Excision of devitalized tissue and direct suture to the freshened patellar bone bed is recommended [38]. Reinforcement of the repair site with an autograft, allograft, or synthetic material may help to protect the repair. Healing takes precedence over motion. Prolonged immobilization in extension followed by gradual range of motion in a brace is the preferred postoperative management. Partial ruptures of the quadriceps tendon have a better prognosis than complete ruptures. They present with quadriceps weakness but still have active extension. Treatment consists of operative repair and protected rehabilitation.

Patellar tendon rupture is a more difficult problem than a quadriceps rupture as the patellar tendon is poorly vascularized. In a series of 18 patellar tendon ruptures, the etiology was difficult exposure in the stiff knee, extensive release of the patellar tendon at the time of surgical exposure, manipulation for limited motion, revision TKA, and distal extensor mechanism realignment for treatment of patellar maltracking [39]. Direct suture repair alone was unsuccessful in all nine attempts, and staple repair was successful in two of four attempts [40]. For acute ruptures direct repair must be augmented with an autogenous or allogeneic tendon graft or a synthetic ligament. Late reconstruction of a chronic rupture requires an Achilles tendon or whole extensor mechanism allograft. In the presence of a soft-tissue defect over the anterior aspect of the knee, an autogenous gastrocnemius flap may be used. In a series of seven repairs using semitendinosis augmentation, only one knee had a residual extensor lag of 10° [40]. Of nine knees treated with the Achilles allograft, three had a residual extensor lag [41]. Two grafts failed, requiring repeat repair, and there was one infection. The use of a whole extensor mechanism allograft requires careful patient selection, meticulous surgical technique, and carefully supervised rehabilitation. There must be adequate soft-tissue coverage, good motion, a well-aligned or revisable TKA, and adequate tibial bone at the level of the tibial tuberosity. The low-demand patient who is able and willing to cooperate in

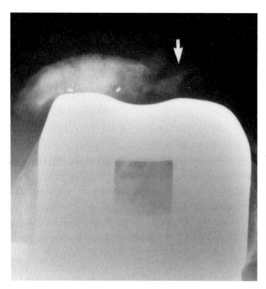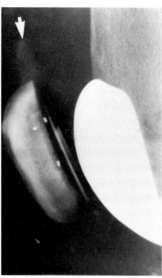

Fig. 9-5. Merchant (left) and lateral (right) radiograph of loose patellar implant. There is lateral subluxation of the patella and a femoral implant design with a shallow trochlear groove

a prolonged rehabilitation program is the best candidate. The results of allograft extensor mechanism reconstruction have been variable. In one report, six revisions were performed in 18 of 27 allografts that were followed [42]. In a report of 40 allograft extensor mechanism reconstructions, 15 had a residual extensor lag and there were eight graft failures [43]. In summary, suture repair with augmentation should be used for acute ruptures while allograft reconstruction is reserved for chronic ruptures. A high prevalence of residual extensor lag and a high complication rate should be anticipated.

Patellar implant loosening and wear are less frequent with modern than with older implant designs. Modern surgical technique with alignment of the implants on the epicondylar axis of the femur has improved patellar alignment and decreased the prevalence of these problems. However, the problem of wear of patellar implants has not been resolved, as the contact stresses in most TKA designs exceed the yield point of the polyethylene of the patellar implant. Patellar failure may present as an incidental finding on radiographs or as symptomatic anterior knee pain and crepitation. The etiology of patellar implant loosening includes fixation in deficient bone, component malposition, patellar maltracking, patellar osteonecrosis, asymmetric bone resection, altered joint line, osteolysis, failure of bone ingrowth in cementless designs, and obesity [44].

Patellar implant loosening was a problem with early implant designs which had a small central fixation keel that was prone to breakage. Loosening occurred in 180 of 4583 (4.2%) TKAs [45]. Loosening was associated with five radiographic findings: bone-cement radiolucency, increased bone density, trabecular bone collapse, fragmentation and fracture of the patella, and lateral subluxation of the patella [45]. Lateral retinacular release was performed in 132 of 180 (73%) TKAs with patellar loosen-

ing as compared with 2320 of 4104 (59%) without. Patellar maltracking with avascular necrosis from the lateral retinacular release were felt to be the reasons for patellar loosening [45]. Patellar implant design was changed to three pegs to improve fixation. A change from a single central fixation peg to three peripheral pegs was adopted by many manufacturers in the late 1980s. The three-peg designs have continued to have problems with loosening, but at a lower rate than some of the single- or two-peg designs. Therefore, implant design and surgical technique can contribute to implant loosening (**❑** Fig. 9-5).

Deformation and wear of patellar components due to high loads in the patellofemoral joint, combined with lack of congruity between the dome-shaped patella and the femoral component design, are commonly seen at the time of revision TKA. In a retrieval study, wear was identified in 65% of metal-backed designs and in 78% of all polyethylene designs [46]. Wear of metal-backed patellar components remains a problem. Revision of the entire arthroplasty may be required. Once the metal backing is exposed, damage to the femoral component occurs with the generation of metal debris. The prevalence of failure of metal-backed patellar components is dependent upon the design, implant alignment, and duration of use. Survivorship of a metal-backed patella at 9 years was 73% for TKAs with a shallow trochlear groove compared with 93% for TKAs with a deep trochlear groove [47]. Inset patellae with metal backing have a low failure rate. In a series of 331 mobile bearing patellae followed up for a mean of 73 months, there were three patellar fractures and one dislocation but no failures from wear [48]. Revision of metal-backed patellar components is recommended in the presence of patellar malalignment, symptomatic crepitation, or significant wear or deformation observed at the time of reoperation for any reason. If there is correct patellar tracking, dome-shaped polyethylene patellar implants may be retained in the presence of mild deformation or wear at the time of revision of a femoral implant. Implant design and surgical technique must be carefully evaluated in the knee with failure of a patellar component.

A variety of miscellaneous soft-tissue complications may affect the patellofemoral joint. A fibrous nodule may develop at the junction of the proximal pole of the patella and the quadriceps tendon. The nodule becomes entrapped in the intercondylar notch of a posterior stabilized design during flexion, resulting in a painful clunk on knee extension [49]. The prevalence of the patellar clunk syndrome was 32 of 900 (3.5%) TKAs [50]. Arthroscopic or open resection of the fibrous nodule is usually successful. Peripatellar fibrosis is a universal finding at the time of revision of a TKA, yet crepitation in the patellofemoral joint of a TKA may or may not be painful. The prevalence of this complication is related to femoral component design being more frequent in those designs with a shallow trochlear groove. Three types of peripatellar fibrosis have been described: circumferential, fibrotic bands, and nodular [51]. Arthroscopic débridement of peripatellar fibrosis resulted in 59% fair or poor results, with five knees having a recurrence of symptoms [51]. Patella infera after TKA can be a source of pain. A change in joint line of less than 8 mm has been found to be one of the variables associated with good results with a posterior stabilized TKA [36]. Both joint line elevation and shortening of the patellar tendon can occur, resulting in patellar impingement against the polyethylene of the tibial component. Since patellar tracking is improved with medial placement of a dome-shaped patellar implant on the patella, a portion of the lateral facet is often left unresurfaced. In the presence of patellar tilt or subluxation, impingement of the unresurfaced lateral facet of the patella against the trochlea of the femur may occur. Resection of the unresurfaced bone is usually curative.

References

1. Sharkey PF, Hozack WJ, Rothman RH, Shastri S, Jacoby SM (2002) Why are total knee arthroplasties failing today? Clin Orthop 303:7–13
2. Healy WL, Wasilewski SA, Takei R, Oberlander M (1995) Patellofemoral complications following total knee arthroplasty. J Arthroplasty 10:197–201
3. Stern SH, Moeckel BH, Insall JN (1991) Total knee arthroplasty in valgus knees. Clin Orthop 273:5–8
4. Dalury DF, Jiranek WA (1999) A Comparison of the midvastus and paramedian approaches for total knee arthroplasty. J Arthroplasty 14:33–37
5. Parentis MA, Rumi MN, Deol GS, Kothari, M, Parrish WM, Pellegrini VD (1999) A comparison of the vastus splitting and median parapatellar approaches in total knee arthroplasty. Clin Orthop 367:107–116
6. White RE, Allman JK, Trauger JA, Dales BH (1999) Clinical comparison of the midvastus and medial parapatellar surgical approaches. Clin Orthop 367:117–122
7. Miller MC, Berger RA, Petrella AJ, Karmas A, Rubash HE (2001) Optimizing femoral component rotation in total knee arthroplasty. Clin Orthop 382:38–45
8. Incavo SJ, Coughlin KM, Pappas C, Beynnon BD (2003) Anatomic rotational relationships of the proximal tibia, distal femur, and patella. J Arthroplasty 18:643–648
9. Barrack RL, Schrader T, Bertot AJ, Wolfe MW, Myers L (2001) Component rotation and anterior knee pain after total knee arthroplasty. Clin Orthop 392:46–55
10. Berger RA, Crossett LS, Jacobs JJ, Rubash HE (1998) Malrotation causing patellofemoral complications after total knee arthroplasty. Clin Orthop 356:144–153
11. Hofmann AA, Tkach TK, Evanich CJ, Camargo MP, Zhang Y (1997) Patellar component medialization in total knee arthroplasty. J Arthroplasty 12:155–160
12. Pagnano M, Trousdale RT (2000) Asymmetric patella resurfacing in total knee arthroplasty. Am J Knee Surg 13:228–233
13. Weber AB, Worland RL, Jessup DE, Van Bowen J, Keenan J (2003) The consequences of lateral release in total knee replacement: a review of over 1000 knees with follow-up between 5 and 11 years. Knee 10:187–191
14. Petersilge WJ, Oishi CS, Kaufman KR, Irby SE, Colwell CW Jr (1994) The effect of trochlear design on patellofemoral shear and compressive forces in total knee arthroplasty. Clin Orthop 309:124–130
15. Theiss SM, Kitziger KJ, Lotke PS, Lotke PA C(1996) omponent design affecting patellofemoral complications after total knee arthroplasty. Clin Orthop 326:183–187
16. Kaper BP, Woolfrey M, Bourne RB (2000) The effect of built-in external femoral rotation on patellofemoral tracking in the Genesis II total knee arthroplasty. J Arthroplasty 15:964–969
17. Takeuchi T, Lathi VK, Khan AM, Hayes WC (1995) Patellofemoral contact pressures exceed the compressive yield strength of UHMWPE in total knee arthroplasties. J Arthroplasty 10:363–368
18. MacCollum MX, Karpman RR (1989) Complications of the PCA anatomic patella. Orthopedics 12:1423–1428
19. Firestone TP, Teeny SM, Krackow KA, Hungerford DS (1991) The clinical and roentgenographic results of cementless porous-coated patellar fixation. Clin Orthop 273:184–189
20. Wulff W, Incavo SJ The effect of patella preparation for total knee arthroplasty on patellar strain. J Arthroplasty (2000) 15:778–782
21. Rand JA, Gustilo RB (1996) Comparison of inset and resurfacing patellar prostheses in total knee arthroplasty. Acta Orthop Belg 62 [Suppl 19:154–163
22. Partio E, Wirta J (1995) Comparison of patellar resurfacing and nonresurfacing in total knee arthroplasty: a prospective, randomized study. J Orthop Rheum 8:69–74
23. Burnett S, Bourne RB (2003) Indications for patellar resurfacing in total knee arthroplasty. J Bone Joint Surg [Am] 85:728–745
24. Feller JA, Bartlett RJ, Lang DM (1996) Patellar resurfacing versus retention in total knee arthroplasty. J Bone Joint Surg [Br] 78:226–228
25. Wood DJ, Smith AJ, Collopy D, White B, Brankov B, Bulsara MK (2002) Patellar resurfacing in total knee arthroplasty. J Bone Joint Surg [Am] 84:187–193
26. Bourne RB, Rorabeck CH Vaz M, Kramer J, Hardie R, Robertson D (1995) Resurfacing versus not resurfacing the patella during total knee replacement. Clin Orthop 321:156–161
27. Waters TS, Bentley G (2003) Patellar resurfacing in total knee arthroplasty. J Bone Joint Surg [Am] 85:212–217
28. Barrack RB, Bertot AJ, Wolfe MW, Waldman DA, Milicic M, Myers L (2001) Patellar resurfacing in total knee arthroplasty. J Bone Joint Surg [Am] 83:1376–1381
29. Barrack RB, Wolfe MW, Waldman DA, Milicic M, Bertot AJ, Myers L (1997) Resurfacing of the patella in total knee arthroplasty. J Bone Joint Surg [Am] 79:1121–1131
30. Schroeder-Boersch H, Scheller G, Fischer J (1998) Advantages of patellar resurfacing in total knee arthroplasty. Arch Orthop Trauma Surg 117: 73–78
31. Muoneke HE, Khan AM, Giannikas KA, Hagglund E, Dunningham TH (2003) Secondary resurfacing of the patella for persistent anterior knee pain after primary knee arthroplasty. J Bone Joint Surg [Br] 85:675–678
32. Campbell DG, Mintz AD, Stevenson TM (1995) Early patellofemoral revision following total knee arthroplasty. J Arthroplasty 10:287–291
33. Rand JA (1994) The patellofemoral joint in total knee arthroplasty. J Bone Joint Surg [Am] 76:612–620

34. Grace JN, Rand JA (1988) Patellar instability after total knee arthroplasty. Clin Orthop 237:184–189

35. Ortiguera CJ, Berry DJ (2002) Patellar fracture after total knee arthroplasty. J Bone Joint Surg [Am] 84:532–540

36. Figgie HE, Goldberg VM, Heiple KG, Moller HS, Gordon NH (1986) The influence of tibial-patellofemoral location on function of the knee in patients with the posterior stabilized condylar knee prosthesis. J Bone Joint Surg [Am] 68:1035–1040

37. Ritter MA, Pierce MJ, Zhou H, Meding JB, Faris PM, Keating EM (1999) Patellar complications (total knee arthroplasty). Clin Orthop 367:149–157

38. Pagnano MW (2003) Patellar tendon and quadriceps tendon tears after total knee arthroplasty. J Knee Surg 16:242–247

39. Rand JA, Morrey BF, Bryan RS (1989) Patellar tendon rupture after total knee arthroplasty. Clin Orthop 244:233–238

40. Cadambi A, Engh GA (1992) Use of a semitendinosis tendon autogenous graft for rupture of the patellar ligament after total knee arthroplasty. J Bone Joint Surg [Am] 74:974–979

41. Crossett LS, Sinha RK, Sechriest VF, Rubash HE (2002) Reconstruction of a ruptured patellar tendon with Achilles tendon allograft following total knee arthroplasty. J Bone Joint Surg [Am] 84:1354–1361

42. Emerson RH (2003) Extensor mechanism allografting in revision total knee replacement. Tech Knee Surg 2:91–98

43. Nazarian DG, Booth RE (1999) Extensor mechanism allografts in total knee arthroplasty. Clin Orthop 367:123–129

44. Lonner JH, Lotke PA (1999) Aseptic complications after total knee arthroplasty. J Am Acad Orthop Surg 7:311–324

45. Berend ME, Ritter MA, Keating EM, Faris PM, Crites BM (2001) The Failure of all-polyethylene patellar components in total knee arthroplasty. Clin Orthop 388:105–111

46. Collier JP, McNamara JL, Surprenant VA, Jensen RE, Suprenant HP (1991) All-polyethylene patellar components are not the answer. Clin Orthop 273:198–203

47. Kraay MJ, Darr O, Salata MJ, Goldberg VM (2001) Outcome of metal-backed cementless patellar components. Clin Orthop 392:239–244

48. Buechel FF, Rosa RA, Pappas MJ (1989) A metal-backed, rotating-bearing patellar prosthesis to lower contact stress. Clin Orthop 248:34–49

49. Hozack WJ, Rothman RH, Booth RE, Balderson RA (1989) The patellar clunk syndrome. Clin Orthop 241:203–208

50. Lucas TS, DeLuca MD, Nazarian DG, et al (1999) Arthroscopic treatment of patellar clunk. Clin Orthop 367:226–229

51. Markel DC, Luessenhop CP, Windsor RE Sculco TA. Arthroscopic (1996) A treatment of peripatellar fibrosis after total knee arthroplasty. J Arthroplasty 11:293–291

10 Experience with Patellar Resurfacing and Non-Resurfacing

H. U. Cameron

Summary

The role of patellar replacement in total knee arthroplasty is controversial. With a modern patella-friendly femoral component design, patellar resurfacing is frequently not necessary. In the revision situation, the most difficult and unresolved question is what to do with an eroded avascular patella following patellar component loosening. This is never an issue if the patella was not resurfaced at the index operation.

The Role of the Trochlear Groove

Femoral component designs in total knee arthroplasty have evolved significantly in the past 10 years. Prior to that, most femoral component trochlear grooves were relatively shallow and patella-unfriendly. Results of knee replacements introduced more than 10 years ago may not be comparable to outcomes with currently available implant designs. Virtually all total knee arthroplasties used with greater than 10-year follow-up required patellar replacement to reduce anterior knee pain and to help stair-climbing ability. What is remarkable, given these patella-unfriendly designs, is that when bilateral cases have been studied, i.e., a replacement in one side versus none in the other, several studies, however flawed, reported no difference in outcome [1]. To some extent this may reflect only the sensitivity of the instrument used, i.e., the Hospital for Special Surgery (HSS) score, and indicates a need to focus more on the outcome measures specific to the patellofemoral joint.

Twelve years ago, in a cohort study, I evaluated the effect of patellar resurfacing and non-resurfacing [2]. The knee system studied was the Tricon (Smith and Nephew, Memphis, Tenn.), which did not have a particularly patella-friendly trochlea. All patellar studies were carried out at 3 years following the index operation, when the knee had reached a steady state and before wear became an issue. There were 68 resurfaced and 43 unresurfaced patellas. The questions asked of these patients were: Was there any anterior knee pain, and was stair-climbing ability adequate? The incidence of anterior knee pain in the replaced knees was 7.6% and in the unreplaced knees 17.6%; 61% of the patients with the replaced patella were able to use the operated limb as the lead leg on stairs without the use of a rail, as opposed to 37% of the unreplaced. The HSS scores, however, were identical.

Given the relatively high incidence of anterior knee pain even in the patients with resurfaced patellas, I questioned the etiology of their symptoms. Anterior knee pain does not necessarily correlate with patellar pathology. Mild anterior knee pain is common in arthritic patients, but severe isolated anterior knee pain associated with patellofemoral arthrosis is surprisingly rare. In 25 years I have performed isolated patellofemoral replacement in less than 50 cases.

Patellar Pain – Postreplacement

If part of the unresurfaced patella makes contact with the metal of the femoral component, this is potentially a source of pain. I evaluated the effect of peripheral patellar bone contact with the femoral component by having a "wing" patella made [3]. The polyethylene wings completely covered the patellar surface and any excess polyethylene was removed during surgery. At 3-year follow-up there were 290 inlay Tricon M patellar components and 171 wing components. The incidence of anterior knee pain was 7% for the inlay and 7.1% for the wings, indicating that contact per se between the femoral component and the unresurfaced area of the patella was not the problem. The question of patellar tilt was also examined. There was tilt of less than 20° in 25% of the inset patella and 10% of the winged patella. Therefore, patellar tilt did not appear to correlate with pain.

My impression has been that maltracking is frequently a source of anterior knee pain following revision total knee arthroplasty, but it is difficult to substantiate this clinical impression.

At 10 years after total knee arthroplasty with a metal-backed patella, wear was present in 75% of cases and was the most common cause of knee revision [4].

Current Experience

In the past, most surgeons felt that patellar replacement was an advantage; what of the present? The Profix knee (Smith and Nephew, Memphis, Tenn.) has a patella-friendly groove. When this became available I cautiously stopped resurfacing the patella. Initially, I replaced the patella in patients who complained preoperatively of anterior knee pain, which is surprisingly uncommon even when bone is exposed and significantly eroded.

A recent review of the records of more than 700 cases showed an incidence of anterior pain of only 3%, a vast reduction from the previous generation of knee-replacement designs. Only three patients felt that their anterior knee symptoms were of sufficient magnitude to justify patellar resurfacing. Of these, two experienced no immediate improvement after patellar resurfacing but 3 years later have no pain. One did experience immediate pain relief, but 4 years later the pain has recurred. These results have encouraged me to completely abandon patellar resurfacing.

I had felt that extending the trochlear groove would support the patella, giving full metal contact through 105° of knee flexion, and would reduce patellar pain. A cruciate-substituting knee requires a box and therefore a relatively short trochlea. After reviewing the results of the Profix cruciate-retaining versus cruciate-substituting knees, however, I found no difference in anterior knee pain. The reason that I chose not to resurface any of the posterior cruciate-substituting knees was my concern that the patellar implant would catch in the box or that the patellar surgery would encourage overgrowth of surrounding tissues to produce the patellar clunk phenomenon. Findings from one knee design, however, cannot be reliably extrapolated to a different knee system. Popovic and Lemair [5] found a 50% incidence of anterior knee pain when the posterior-substituting rotoglide knee was used as opposed to a much lower incidence with the cruciate-retaining version. They hypothesised that the sharp edge of the box was the source of the problem, so it would seem that box geometry can contribute to patellar pain.

Revision Total Knee Arthroplasty

Patellar maltracking is a common problem in revision total knee arthroplasty, particularly since earlier instrumentation seldom allowed control of external rotation of the femoral component. Until recently, the advantage of 3° of external rotation of the femoral component, which leads to lateralization of the trochlear groove and much improved patellar tracking, was not recognized. Even today, posterior referencing instruments oriented along the posterior condylar line will routinely internally rotate the femoral component in the valgus knee, which commonly has lateral femoral condylar dysplasia.

The diagnosis of an internally rotated femoral component can be made by carefully controlled skyline radiographs. If the X-ray is taken with the knee in too much flexion, it may be unhelpful, and some authors have advocated CT scanning [6]. Intra-operative derotation of the femoral component cannot be accomplished by simply trying to manually externally rotate the femoral component, since it will usually return to its original position. Resecting the anterolateral femoral condyle and augmenting the posterior lateral femoral condyle also allows only limited correction, because notching of the femur will occur. My preferred technique is to resect some of the posterior medial femoral condyle and insert a screw into the anterior medial femoral condyle, leaving the head protruding. The screw can be turned in and out, forcing the femoral component into external rotation and thus providing the degree of correction necessary to ensure good patellar tracking. The screw is simply buried in cement during the cementation process.

The Unreplaced Patella

If the patella has been tracking correctly prior to revision surgery, no further treatment is necessary. If it has been maltracking or is laterally subluxed, the articular surface may be grooved. If the groove is small it can be ignored. However, if the groove is deep, further surgery is necessary. If the groove is far lateral, the lateral edge of the patella may be smoothed to produce a convex surface. If it is far medial, as it can be in extreme cases, shaving alone may produce a convex surface. If convexity of the patellar component cannot be restored, either a medial edged resection or a patellar replacement with a large implant may be required.

Replaced Patella – not Loose

Treatment of the patellar replacement during revision total knee arthroplasty is dependent upon the degree of polyethylene wear. If the wear is not gross and the patella component is not metal-backed, it can be retained. The geometry may not completely match the trochlear geometry of the revision femoral component; however, the typical presence of a patellar meniscus around the periphery of the replaced patellar component tends in general to compensate for these discrepancies. The patellar meniscus is aneural and should not be excised if the original patellar component is to be retained.

If there is severe polyethylene wear, particularly if the patellar component is metal-backed, revision should be performed. If the patient is extremely elderly, patellar revision for wear may not be necessary. However, even elderly patients can have a long life expectancy. The patient's age and activity should be considered, as well as the amount of patellar component wear, when the decision is made to retain or revise the component.

In removing a well-fixed patellar component, use of too much force must be avoided since the patella can be fractured or the patellar tendon avulsed. The patella must be stabilized with sharp towel clips proximally and distally to prevent excessive traction on the patellar tendon. If necessary, the implant-cement or implant-bone interface can be loosened with a very small high-speed burr. The membrane is then removed. Unless very little of the patella was resected at the original operation, no further reaming should be done. The implant bed is simply roughened up with a high-speed burr and small holes are drilled transversely or obliquely rather than anteroposteriorly; anteroposterior drilling tends to inadvertently penetrate the anterior surface of the patella, thereby significantly weakening it. A new patellar component, generally biconvex is then cemented in place. In cementing a revision patellar component it is generally better to apply pressure to the implant with one's thumb during the cement-curing process, because if the bone bed is asymmetric, clamps may tend to tilt the patellar component against the remaining bone.

If patellar fracture occurs, internal fixation is necessary, provided bone stock is adequate. Due to the reduced area of bone contact, it is unlikely that simple cerclage wiring will produce adequate stability to ensure union. Additional compression screws should be considered. If a new patellar component is cemented in place, ingress of some of the cement into the fracture gap is almost inevitable, with the increased likelihood of a non-union. It would seem preferable, therefore, not to insert a new patellar component, recognizing that patellar pain is likely at least for the first year. Should the pain persist after sound union, delayed patellar resurfacing can be performed.

Loose Patellar Component

If the patellar component is loose it should be removed. If adequate bone stock remains, a new patellar component can be cemented in place after thorough débridement and removal of all osteolytic cysts and membrane. Frequently, however, the remaining bone is not adequate to support a new prosthesis. The eroded, hollowed-out, thin avascular patella can be very difficult to treat [7]. If a new patellar component is cemented in place under such circumstances, early loosening, at least radiologically, is likely to occur (◘ Fig. 10-1).

In an effort to improve cement fixation, I have used multiple screws inserted transversely across the patella, like rebars. Whether or not this will add to the longevity is not clear. Alternatively, cementless revision with porous

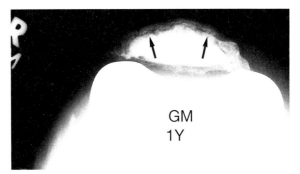

◘ **Fig. 10-1.** During revision total knee arthroplasty, a new patellar component was cemented in place. The radiolucent line between the cement and bone has been present since revision. While this patient's patellar component has not required additional surgery, it is at least radiologically loose

tantalum can be useful. However, cementless tantalum patellar revision has been reported to be associated with a 40% incidence of anterior knee pain. Cementless tantalum patellar revision may be appropriate for cases in which reaming is not possible because of poor patellar bone stock.

Hanssen [8] reported on bone-grafting the defect with morselized allograft and covering it with a membrane to promote bone regeneration. However, bone grafting may not be successful if the bone bed is avascular. If the patella cannot be revised, anterior knee pain should be anticipated at least for 1 or 2 years. The hollowed-out patella often does not fit in the trochlear groove, and patellar instability may result. If so, then the lateral one third of the patella should be removed to produce a reasonable fit in the trochlear groove. However, this procedure may also cause patellar avascular necrosis, due to disruption of the intraosseous blood supply.

Immediate patellectomy is not usually a viable option because immobilization in extension, which would be required for several weeks, would likely result in reduction of range of motion. It may be preferable, therefore, to simply resect the lateral one third of the patella. If avascular necrosis does not occur, the initial severe patellofemoral pain may decrease after 2–3 years. If avascular necrosis occurs, it is occasionally completely asymptomatic. More typically, however, the patella slowly fragments. Since the process is slow, disruption of the extensor mechanism with a quadriceps lag usually does not occur.

Revision Results

For the purpose of this book chapter, I have reviewed my results of revision total knee arthroplasty, concentrating on the patella. The knee designs evaluated included the Tricon II, TCIII, a cruciate-retaining Profix, and a cruciate-substituting Profix. Follow-up of these cases is between 2 and 15 years.

There were 127 Tricon II knees, 12 Profix CR, 38 Profix CS, and 64 TC III-type knees. Of the Tricon II knees, 6.3% have required revision and of the TC IIIs, 3%. The fact that the Tricon has the longest follow-up may have influenced this. Patellofemoral pain (any anterior knee pain at all) was present in 25.6% of Tricon II, 0% of Profix CR, 10.5% of Profix CS, and 20.3% of the TC III knees (◘ Tables 10-1–3).

◘ **Table 10-1.** Overall patellofemoral results of various knee replacement designs

Implant design	Tricon (in %)	Profix (CR, in %)	Profix (CS, in %)	TC III (%)
Re-revised	6.3	0	0	3.0
Fair and poor	20.5	33.3	26.3	60.8
Lateral release	9.5	0	13.6	20.1
Derotated	0	16.7	15.6	5.8
Patellofemoral ache	25.6	0	10.5	20.3
Patellar AVN	14.6	0	5.3	4.5

◘ **Table 10-2.** Patellofemoral pain

Implant design	Tricon (in %)	Profix (CR, in %)	Profix (CS, in %)	TC III (%)
No replacement	11.0	0	9.1	15.8
Original patella	31.1	0	0	9.1
New cemented	16.9	0	0	7.1
New press fit	36.7	Not performed	Not performed	Not performed
Patelloplasty	57.4	0	40.0	100
Patelloplasty and lateral edge resection	81.6	0	0	20

◘ **Table 10-3.** Fair and poor results

Implant design	Tricon (in %)	Profix (CR, in %)	Profix (CS, in %)	TC III (%)
No replacement	22.2	2.5	45.5	42.1
Original patella	12.5	0	0	54.5
New cemented	25.5	25.0	16.6	78.6
New press fit	0	Not performed	Not performed	Not performed
Patelloplasty	57.0 } }68	}25	}37.5	}26.7
Patelloplasty and lateral edge resect	72.7			

It is apparent from these results that there has been a significant reduction in patellofemoral pain following revision surgery using a patella-friendly trochlea and external rotation of the femoral component. The incidence of avascular necrosis has also been reduced significantly.

While the incidence of patellofemoral pain has also been reduced significantly, the cases in which a patelloplasty of the patella with or without a lateral edge resection is required remain a very significant problem, for which there is no satisfactory solution. This problem does not arise if the patella was not replaced at the time of the primary procedure. Surgeons carrying out knee replacement, therefore, should understand the femoral component trochlear geometry of the implant that they are using, and should consider not resurfacing the patella if the femoral component is patella-friendly.

References

1. Barrack RL (2003) All patella should be resurfaced during primary total knee arthroplasty – in opposition. J Arthroplasty 18 [Suppl 1]:35–38
2. Cameron HU: 1991: Comparison between patella resurfacing with an inset plastic button in patellaplasty. Can J Surg 34:49–53
3. Cameron HU (1992) Patella resurfacing in total knee replacement. J Western Pacific Orthop Assoc 29:57–61
4. Cameron HU (1994) Tibial component wear in total knee replacement. Clin Orthop 309:29-32
5. Popovic N, Lemair E (2003) Anterior knee pain with a posterior stabilized mobile bearing knee prosthesis; the effect of femoral component design. J Arthroplasty 18:396–401
6. Berger RA, Crossetts LS, Jacobs JJ, et al (1998) Malrotation causing patello-femoral complications after total knee arthroplasty. Clin Orthop 356:144
7. Neilson CL, Lonne JH, Lakji A, et al (2003) Use of trabecular metal patella for marked patellar bone loss during revision total knee arthroplasty. J Arthroplasty 18:37–41
8. Hanssen AD (2001) Bone grafting for severe patellar bone loss during revision total knee arthroplasty. J Bone Joint Surg [Am] 83:171–176

10

11 Failure in Constraint: "Too Much"

N. Wülker, M. Lüdemann

Summary

Constraint is limitation of motion in a joint, e.g., due to an axis mechanism or to conformity between two articular surfaces. In addition to flexion and extension, the normal knee has some anterior-posterior translation and rotates around a vertical axis. If these motions are impeded by excessive constraint in a prosthetic design, no physiological motion will be possible. Unfavorable long-term results and complications have been reported in this setting. Possible sequels of excessive constraint are fatigue of the bone-prosthesis interface, limitation of motion, patellar displacement, or periprosthetic fracture.

Constraint

Constraint is limitation of motion between two bodies linked by a joint. In human joints, constraint may be normal, i.e., by ligaments, capsules, or articular surface geometry; it may be pathological, i.e., by contractures or arthrosis; and it may be artificial, i.e., by implants.

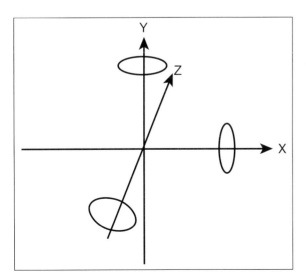

◻ Fig. 11-1. Unconstrained motion has six degrees of freedom: rotations around the x-, y-, z-axes and translations along the x-, y-, z-axes. In a constrained joint, one or more degrees of freedom are diminished or abolished

Unlimited motion has 6° of freedom: three rotations and three translations (◻ Fig. 11-1). In constrained motion, one or more degrees of freedom are diminished or abolished. The ultimately constrained joint is a hinge joint, which has only one rotation and no translation.

In a normal knee joint, rotation around a horizontal axis, i.e., flexion and extension, is by far the most important motion. The usual flexion-to-extension range is approximately 150°-0°. In addition, external tibial rotation during extension, i.e., rotation around a vertical, also occurs and amounts to approximately 15° through the full flexion-to-extension range. This has been referred to as the screw-home mechanism. Translation is mostly along an anterior to posterior axis and may amount to 10-15 mm through the full flexion-to-extension range [15,18]. This is commonly referred to as the roll-back mechanism. It shifts the tibia away from the femoral condyles in maximum flexion, providing additional flexion range. Thus, physiological knee motion has more than one degree of freedom range. Motions in addition to flexion and extension have to be taken into account in knee joint replacement.

Constrained Knee Designs

In knee joint replacements, motion may be constrained with one or more axes built into the implant. Hinged motion around a horizontal axis, i.e., with one degree of motion freedom, was implemented in the first knee replacement designs. They are referred to as first-generation hinge implants.

The Walldius hinge prosthesis was introduced in the 1950s [25] and was originally made of acrylate; this was later changed to cobalt-chromium. Shiers published a preliminary report of his metal hinge prosthesis for use with bone cement in 1954 [21]. In the 1970s, a hinged design with a patellar flange was described by the French Guépar group (Groupe pour l'utilisation et l'étude des prothèses articulaire).

Hinged implants were relatively easy to use because all the ligaments could be resected at the time of the arthroplasty and alignment was determined by the stems. However, some authors reported unfavorable long-term results with these prostheses: e.g., a complication rate of 23% for hinged implants [10], 29% poor results [12], and a 70% complication rate [9] for the Guépar prosthesis, and unfavorable results for the Walldius implant [11]. The probability of the prosthesis remaining in situ after 6 years in osteoarthritis was calculated as 65% for hinged prostheses, compared with 90° for medial unicompartmental prostheses. Also, severe bone loss made salvage by arthrodesis difficult [14]. Better results were reported for Implants that combined hinged motion with a metal-to-polyethylene articulation (slide and hinge principle), such as the St. Georg hinge [7] and the Blauth prosthesis [2], introduced in the 1970s.

In subsequent prostheses, such as the St. Georg rotation knee, introduced in 1979, rotation around a vertical axis was added, giving the joint two degrees of freedom. These joints are generally referred to as second-generation rotating hinge joints and are in common use today.

Other models added some anterior-posterior translation as a second degree of freedom by linking the femoral and the tibial component with a tibial metal post running in a femoral cam, such as the GSB implant [6]. However, this prosthesis yielded unfavorable results after 7.8 years [22].

Another way to constrain knee motion is to vary the contact design between the femoral component and the upper surface of the polyethylene insert. These prostheses are generally referred to as semi-constrained implants. Generally, constraint is proportional to the conformity between the two surfaces: If both surfaces are in total contact, i.e., if the radii of curvature are equal, motion will be pure rotation and no translation will be possible. This is implemented in so-called constrained condylar, total condylar, or deep-dished designs. If the insert is flat, i.e., if the radius of curvature is greater than in the femoral component, some translation will be possible in addition to rotation. Also, polyethylene posts or spines at the upper surface of the insert that engage into a femoral box or cam can prevent certain motions. The cam-spine mechanism is most commonly used to prevent posterior translation of the tibial component in posterior-stabilized total knee designs. Some knees also use the cam-spine mechanism to prevent rotation around a sagittal axis, i.e., medial and lateral instability.

The classic semi-constrained knee is the total condylar constrained knee prosthesis (TCP III), which was introduced in 1977 to provide greater stability and constraint with a non-linked implant. In 1988, the TCP III eventually became the Insall-Burstein II constrained condylar knee prosthesis (CCK), which was modular.

Indications for Constrained Designs

A knee with functional ligaments and with limited axial deviation is now generally considered an indication for an unconstrained condylar prosthesis. The use of constrained designs in this setting has generally been abandoned.

Unstable knees usually necessitate some degree of constraint. The notable exception is the anterior cruciate ligament; it is resected in most bicondylar knee replacements. Therefore, almost all prostheses have sufficient articular surface congruity to compensate for lost anterior ligamentous stability. The posterior cruciate ligament, which may be primarily insufficient or lost due to resection of its tibial insertion, has to be replaced with a posterior constraint, which is usually provided by a polyethylene spine of the insert reaching into a femoral component cam. Medial or lateral collateral ligament insufficiency, if significant, requires a design which eliminates rotation around a sagittal axis. This will most commonly be a rotation hinged knee, which rotates only around a vertical and frontal axis.

Another indication for a constrained knee is significant axis deviation. The maximum accepted deformation for a surface replacement prosthesis is somewhat variable. However, varus or valgus angulation beyond 20° as a rule requires a medial or lateral release and increased height of the polyethylene insert. In axis deviation of more than 20°, this height may exceed 20 mm, which makes it prone to raising the joint line and technical failure. Therefore, a constrained rotation knee design is preferable in this situation. This setting is quite common in patients with rheumatoid arthritis. Bone defects in tumor reconstructions may also require a hinged implant [16].

Constraint Sequels

The ligaments and capsule of a normal knee and of a knee following surface replacement are able to absorb a substantial amount of energy. During normal gait, this energy peaks during push-off at late stance phase and during touchdown of the foot at the beginning of stance. However, forces at the knee joint are created by body weight, by muscle power, and by acceleration and deceleration. Therefore, significant forces occur throughout the entire gait cycle and not just during the stance phase. The soft tissues of the knee joint, in particular the cruciate ligaments, the collateral ligaments, and the joint capsule, serve as shock absorbers, i.e., they absorb energy. If a knee is deprived of this mechanism, stress is transmitted directly from the prosthesis onto the implant-fixation boundary, which may result in fatigue at the prosthesis-bone interface in uncemented implants and at the cement-bone interface or at the cement-prosthesis interface in cemented implants. In addition, significant forces will be present at the hinge or other constraint mechanism of the knee, e.g., a tibial insert polyethylene spine, which may be damaged or may fail [17].

Limitation of motion may be another consequence of excessive constraint. For physiological motion in a normal knee, the roll-back mechanism is necessary. This mechanism moves the tibia anteriorly in maximum flexion, displacing the tibia away from the femoral condyles and thereby preventing impingement between the two posteriorly. If roll-back is prevented by constraint, this may limit motion.

Patellar tracking on the femoral shield depends on physiological motion. Femoral roll-back reduces patellofemoral forces by improving the efficiency of the extensor mechanism. Lack of femoral roll-back may increase pressures at the patellofemoral joint during flexion, with or without surface replacement of the patella. Lack of rotation around a vertical axis may result in patellar displacement, which occurs particularly in a lateral direction.

Knee function during gait significantly differs between hinged prostheses and a standard surface replacement. These differences were clearly demonstrated during gait and stair climbing [4].

Finally, constrained knee designs generally require more bone resection than surface replacements. In hinged or rotation designs, resection must be sufficient to accommodate the hinges or rotation pegs of the implant. With spines at the tibial insert, room for a cam must be created by femoral bone resection. Also, because these implants are generally larger, they may be more prone to infection.

Too Much Constraint

In a knee prosthesis with excessive constraint, forces at the implant and at the interface between implant and bone will be greater than necessary. Without the energy absorption described above, excessive forces may accelerate wear and loosening of the prosthesis.

These considerations have led to a general agreement to implement as little constraint as necessary in knee joint replacements. However, in spite of the logic behind this approach, the available data are still somewhat controversial. Some papers report a significant failure rate with hinged implants [10]. Other authors have repeatedly had good success with hinge and rotation knee replacements, when used in patients with primary arthrosis without deformity [7, 20] and when used in instability, deformity, etc. [5, 13, 19, 24]. Our own clinical data include examples of complications in constrained implants which might have been avoided if a less-constrained implant had been used:

Implant Loosening (■ Fig. 11-2). Loosening with progressive reduction in quality of the arthroplasty was observed in 27% of Guepar prostheses after 1-3 years [12]. In mod-

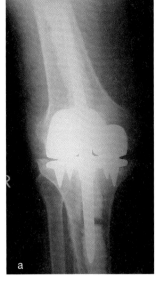
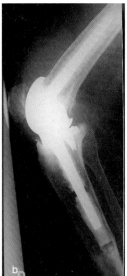
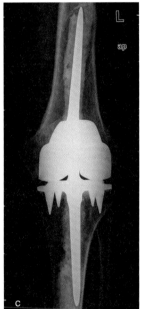
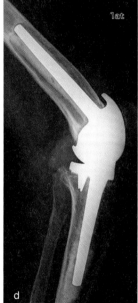

■ **Fig. 11-2a-d.** Implant loosening. *a, b* Radiographs of a 64-year-old male patient with aseptic loosening of the tibial component, 3 years after implantation of a hinged total knee replacement (Blauth prosthesis) because of gonarthrosis of the right knee. The prosthesis had to be removed, a cemented revision-Blauth hinged total knee replacement was implanted. *a* Anteroposterior view, *b* lateral view. *c, d* Radiographs of a 68-year-old male patient with aseptic loosening and migration of the femoral component, 5 years after implantation of a hinged total knee replacement (Blauth prosthesis) because of gonarthrosis of the left knee. The femoral component and the inlay had to be changed. *c* Anteroposterior view, *d* lateral view

ern constrained implants this is much lower. Radiolucent lines may be a precursor of loosening, even though development to true loosening is often not demonstrated, and the occurrence of radiolucent lines is not correlated with the clinical outcome [3].

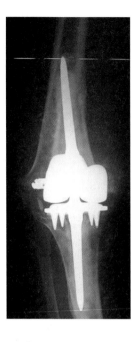

⬛ Fig. 11-3. Implant breakage: Radiograph of an 88-year-old male patient with breakage and dislocation of the axis 11 years after implantation of a Blauth prosthesis in the right knee because of severe gonarthrosis

Implant Breakage (⬛ Fig. 11-3). Prosthetic component breakage occurred in 10% of hinged implants used for complex primary and salvage revision total knee arthroplasty [23]. Breakage may occur as early as 5 months after the initial surgery [26]. The incidence of damage or breakage of modern constrained prostheses is not precisely known, but cases have been reported [17].

Periprosthetic Fracture (⬛ Fig. 11-4). Periprosthetic fractures of the femur or, less commonly, of the tibia, associated with total knee arthroplasty may occur intra- or postoperatively as a constraint-complication. Periprosthetic fracture has been observed in about 0,4 % to 1,25 % of all total knee arthroplasties and may be caused by the limited motion of constrained knee designs. The clinical data from the authors' institution showed 10 periprosthetic fractures (6 of the femoral condyle and 4 of the femoral shaft) in 330 patients (2,4%) using a hinged Blauth prosthesis.

Patellar Maltracking. Patellar complications were reported in 13% of hinged implants after 6 years [23]. Extensor mechanism problems occurred in 16% after 2-13 years. Patellar symptoms were present in 28% of Guépar prostheses [12]. Patellar subluxation and dislocation occurred in 49% of the knees.

Deep Infection. The incidence of deep infection – a serious complication – is generally higher in hinged knee implants than in surface replacements and was between 11% and 14.5% in various studies [1,12,23]. This may be related to the size of the implant and to the amount of bone resection, but it is most likely also due to the fact that these implants were used in complex primary and salvage revision cases.

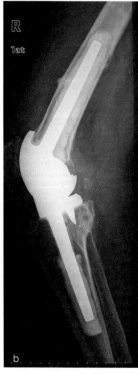

⬛ Fig. 11-4a, b. Periprosthetic fracture. Radiograph of a 78-year-old male patient with a periprosthetic fracture of the femur, 4 months after implantation of a hinged total knee replacement (Blauth prosthesis) because of gonarthrosis with varus angulation. This fracture healed with non-weight-bearing. *a* Anteroposterior view, *b* lateral view

References

1. Benevenia J, Lee FY, Buechel F, Parsons JR (1998) Pathologic supracondylar fracture due to osteolytic pseudotumor of knee following cementless total knee replacement. J Biomed Mater Res 43:473-477
2. Blauth W, Hassenpflug J (1990) Are unconstrained components essential in total knee arthroplasty? Long-term results of the Blauth knee prosthesis. Clin Orthop 258:86-94
3. Cameron HU, Hu C, Vyamont D (1997) Hinge total knee replacement revisited. Can J Surg 40:278-283
4. Draganich LF, Whitehurst JB, Chou LS, Piotrowski GA, Pottenger LA, Finn HA (1999) The effects of the rotating-hinge total knee replacement on gait and stair stepping. J Arthroplasty 14:743-755
5. Easley ME, Insall JN, Scuderi GR, Bullek DD (2000) Primary constrained condylar knee arthroplasty for the arthritic valgus knee. Clin Orthop 380:58-64
6. Gschwend N, Siegrist H (1991) The GSB knee joint: reoperation and infections. Orthopade 20:197-205
7. Heinert K, Engelbrecht E (1988) Long-term comparison of the "St. Georg" knee endoprosthesis system. 10-year survival rates of 2,236 gliding and hinge endoprostheses. Chirurg 59:755-762
8. Hendel D, Garti A, Weisbort M (2003) Fracture of the central polyethylene tibial spine in posterior stabilized total knee arthroplasty. J Arthroplasty 18:672-674
9. Hoikka V, Vankka E, Eskola A, Lindholm TS (1989) Results and complications after arthroplasty with a totally constrained total knee prosthesis (GUEPAR). Ann Chir Gynaecol 78:94-96
10. Hui FC, Fitzgerald RH Jr (1980) Hinged total knee arthroplasty. J Bone Joint Surg [Am] 62:513-519

11. Jones GB (1968) Arthroplasty of the knee by the Walldius prosthesis. J Bone Joint Surg [Br] 50:505-510

12. Jones EC, Insall JN, Inglis AE, Ranawat CS (1979) GUEPAR knee arthroplasty results and late complications. Clin Orthop 140:145-152

13. Jones RE, Skedros JG, Chan AJ, Beauchamp DH, Harkins PC (2001) Total knee arthroplasty using the S-ROM mobile-bearing hinge prosthesis. J Arthroplasty 16:279-287

14. Knutson K, Lindstrand A, Lidgren L (1986) Survival of knee arthroplasties. A nation-wide multicentre investigation of 8000 cases. J Bone Joint Surg [Br] 68:795-803

15. Lee TQ, Yang BY, Sandusky MD, McMahon PJ. The effects of tibial rotation on the patellofemoral joint: assessment of the changes in in situ strain in the peripatellar retinaculum and the patellofemoral contact pressures and areas. J Rehabil Res Dev 2001 38:463-469

16. Mascard E, Anract P, Touchene A, Pouillart P, Tomeno B (1998) Complications from the hinged GUEPAR prosthesis after resection of knee tumor. 102 cases. Rev Chir Orthop Reparatrice Appar Mot 84:628-637

17. Mikulak SA, Mahoney OM, dela Rosa MA, Schmalzried TP (2001) Loosening and osteolysis with the press-fit condylar posterior-cruciate-substituting total knee replacement. J Bone Joint Surg [Am] 83:398-403

18. Most E, Zayontz S, Li G, Otterberg E, Sabbag K, Rubash HE (2003) Femoral rollback after cruciate-retaining and stabilizing total knee arthroplasty. Clin Orthop 410:101-113

19. Rinta-Kiikka I, Alberty A, Savilahti S, Pajamaki J, Tallroth K, Lindholm TS (1997) The clinical and radiological outcome of the rotating hinged knee prostheses in the long-term. Ann Chir Gynaecol 86:349-356

20. Rottger J, Heinert K (1984) St. Georg knee endoprosthesis system (slide and hinge principle). Observations and results following 10 years' experience with over 3,700 operations. Z Orthop Ihre Grenzgeb 122:818-826

21. Shiers LG (1954) Arthroplasty of the knee; preliminary report of new method. J Bone Joint Surg [Br] 36:553-560

22. Sprenger TR, Doerzbacher JF (2002) Long-term follow-up of the GSB II total knee used in primary total knee arthroplasty. J Arthroplasty 17:176-183

23. Springer BD, Hanssen AD, Sim FH, Lewallen DG (2001) The kinematic rotating hinge prosthesis for complex knee arthroplasty. Clin Orthop 392:283-291

24. Walker PS, Manktelow AR (2001) Comparison between a constrained condylar and a rotating hinge in revision knee surgery. Knee 8:269-279

25. Walldius B (1957) Arthroplasty of the knee using an endoprosthesis. Acta Orthop Scand [Suppl 24]:1-112

26. Wang CJ, Wang HE. Early catastrophic failure of rotating hinge total knee prosthesis. J Arthroplasty 2000 15:387-91

12 Failure in Constraint: "Too Little"

F. Lampe, E. Hille

Summary

Implant constraint failures are the consequence of in-adequate balance between the given, intrinsic stability of the implant replacing a joint and the extrinsic stabilization provided by the soft tissues enveloping the joint. Achieving this balance is one of the central challenges in total knee arthroplasty (TKA). The success crucially depends on preoperative assessment of the deformity and the soft-tissue situation (extrinsic stability), the correct choice of implant (intrinsic stability), which also depends on the former, and the adequate intraoperative treatment of the soft-tissue stabilizers. Therefore, this chapter will focus on the aspects of intrinsic implant stability against the background of the functional interaction with the (often pathologically deformed) soft-tissue apparatus of the knee. Our guiding principle will be: "As little implant constraint as possible with the achievable soft-tissue stability." For this reason we start from a systematic classification of knee joint deformities, from which one can derive an algorithm that will facilitate the decision for a certain implant constraint combined with suitable soft-tissue treatment.

Introduction

Knee implants differ by, among other things, the degree of mobility in three-dimensional kinematic modes of movement - varus-valgus angulation (frontal plane), anteroposterior translation (sagittal plane), mediolateral translation (frontal plane), rotation (transverse plane), and roll-and-glide (sagittal plane) – and by the extent to which the intrinsic stability of the implant can substitute or support the extrinsic soft-tissue stabilizers for these modes of movement (□ Table 12-1).

These properties are determined by the extent of implant constraint, in which the so-called kinematic conflict presents a fundamental problem. On the one hand, the implant should enable good mobility and kinematics as physiological as possible, with the soft-tissue envelope preserved. This requires an implant design with relatively little intrinsic constraint. In consequence, internal con-straint forces transmitted to the implant-bone interface and thus the risk of implant-bone fixation failure are reduced to a minimum in such a design. On the other hand, maximum congruency of the femoral and tibial joint surfaces should be realized in order to increase the contact surfaces and thereby minimize the contact stresses, and thus wear, at the bearing surfaces. However, the increased congruency of the bearings restricts their relative mobility and thus causes unfavorably high constraint forces, which might compromise the implant-bone fixation in designs with higher intrinsic constraint. Thus, every implant design aims to resolve this conflict by offering some suitable compromise.

□ **Table 12-1.** Different implant designs with increasing constraint and corresponding level of intrinsic mobility

Implant constraint	A/P trans-lation	M/L trans-lation	Varus/valgus angulation	Rotation
Non-hinged				
Mobile bearings				
Floating platform	+/+	+/+	+/+	+
Rotating platform	+/+	+/+	+/+	+
Fixed bearings				
PCL retaining (PR)	+/+	+/+	+/+	+
PCL substituting (PS)	+/-	-/-	+/+	(+)
Intercondylar stabilization (ICS)	+/-	-/-	(-/-)	(-)
Hinged				
Rotating hinge	-/-	-/-	-/-	+
Rigid hinge	-/-	-/-	-/-	-

+ Unrestricted mobility; - restricted mobility

Despite the agreements on many aspects of total knee design, there is an impressive number of knee implants currently on the market. This reflects not only commercial interests but also design controversies. For decades there has been an ongoing discussion as to whether stability should be provided by the soft tissues in conjunction with low conforming prosthetic surfaces, by only the posterior cruciate ligament (PCL) in conjunction with shallow or moderately conforming (curved, dished) surfaces, by ultra-conforming surfaces without the cruciate ligaments, or by conforming surfaces augmented by an intercondylar stabilizing arrangement or even a hinge.

A brief historical review reveals that total knee prostheses first appeared in the 1950s, in the shape of simple hinges. These implants failed to account for the complexities of knee motion and suffered high failure rates due to aseptic loosening. They were also associated with unacceptably high rates of postoperative infection. In 1971, Gunston recognized that the knee does not rotate on a single axis like a hinge; rather, the femoral condyles roll and glide on the tibia with multiple, momentary centers of rotation [1]. His polycentric knee endoprosthesis enjoyed early successes with its improved kinematics but ultimately failed because of inadequate alignment and fixation to the bone. The highly conforming and constrained Geomedic knee arthroplasty introduced in 1973 ignored Gunston's principles, giving rise to the kinematic conflict. Other designs followed, either following Gunston's principle in attempting to reproduce normal knee kinematics or allowing a conforming articulation to govern knee motion. Hinged implants are still used today, though largely in special cases or as revision components. If an artificial knee is hinged it is described as being maximally constrained. Due to the problems of constrained components, new designs were introduced that were semi-constrained or even unconstrained. For such knees to be effective, the soft-tissue envelope had to be functionally intact. Stability following the knee arthroplasty was provided by the patient's own ligaments, rather than by the intrinsic stability of the implant itself.

Each of the various design concepts proved more or less successful in the past, and each has its individual strengths and limitations. Thus we started from the published data and our own experiences and developed an implant concept for primary knee joint replacement, which will be discussed below. At our hospital, we use, in descending order, implants retaining the PCL (~70%), implants replacing the PCL (~20%), implants with intercondylar stabilization (~7%), and hinged implants (~3%). Before we describe the indications for these implant types we will give a brief overview of the experiences published to date on different design variants with various levels of constraint. The results reported in the literature and our own experience formed the basis for our implant concept, which we present in this chapter.

Experiences with Different Implant Designs with Various Levels of Constraint

When considering the issue of implant constraints one has to take into account some fundamental principles. One approach to enable free, multiaxial mobility, as far as possible, is to reduce the intrinsic constraint of the artificial joint by using flat tibial glide surfaces and to ensure the stability of the joint by preserving the soft-tissue envelope. Such implants are characterized by the attributes of "low congruency, low constraint, high mobility, high contact stress". High contact stresses as a consequence of non-conforming surfaces may lead to increased wear of the polyethylene component in these implants [2, 3]. Theoretically, polyethylene damage can be reduced by using highly congruent bearing surfaces with significantly larger contact areas. However, this increases the intrinsic constraint of the implant. Consequently, the mobility of the implant is reduced, which gives rise to increased internal constraint forces with the risk of damage to the implant-bone fixation. The design principle in this case can be summarized as "high congruency, high constraint, low mobility, low contact stress". A compromise is achieved in designs with components providing sufficient relative mobility to minimize the risk of loosening through constraint forces on the one hand. On the other hand, the contact areas of the conforming bearings are large enough to reduce contact stresses and thus polyethylene wear. These designs also offer adequate intrinsic stability to withstand external forces in conjunction with the extrinsic soft-tissue stabilizers. There are numerous designs that have successfully applied this compromise. The biomechanically promising functional principle, "high congruency, low constraint, high mobility, low contact stress", can be realized by mobile bearings. Depending on the degrees of freedom of the mobile platform, internal constraint forces can be avoided, to a large extent, while high mobility is maintained. At the same time, wear in the femorotibial articulation is minimized by using highly congruent bearing surfaces. Although congruency of the bearings is maximum in these designs, their intrinsic stability is low due to the mobility of the bearings. For this reason, implants with mobile bearings require a stable and perfectly balanced soft-tissue apparatus to function properly. Therefore, an advanced operating technique, especially with regard to the soft-tissue and gap-balancing procedures, is a prerequisite for the success of mobile-bearing designs.

The most common examples of the implant concepts cited above with exclusive focus on the aspect of insufficient constraint will be discussed below. First we present an overview of the problems that can arise when using implants offering insufficient constraint, and of the arguments for using implants with higher constraint in certain situations. Other important arguments for or against certain implant types are treated in other chapters of this book. At this point, we ought to highlight again our fundamental principle, "as little constraint as possible (i.e., posterior cruciate-retaining or -substituting implants as first choice, if sufficient extrinsic stability can be provided by the soft tissues), as much constraint as necessary (i.e., intercondylar stabilized or hinged implants in special cases)", in order to counteract the impression that using high-constraint implants were the preferable solution for reasons of principle.

Posterior Cruciate-retaining (PR) Designs and Cruciate-substituting (PS) Designs

Posterior cruciate-retaining (PR) designs, which are used in the majority of cases, are characterized by relatively low intrinsic stability. Their longevity depends on the presence of a functionally intact soft-tissue envelope, more specifically of a well-balanced posterior cruciate ligament. To fulfill its kinematically important functions in TKA, the functionality of the posterior cruciate ligament needs to be restored during surgery, if necessary by release, which can present a major technical challenge [4]. Consequently, critics of the cruciate-retaining designs argue that the precise balancing of the PCL, which is usually pathologically deformed in patients suffering from osteoarthritis or rheumatoid arthritis, is technically difficult or even impossible [5, 6]. In a cadaver study, Mahoney showed that retaining the correct length of the PCL when implanting a PCL-preserving joint is problematic and that the ligament tension changes significantly even if the thickness of the tibia component is changed only very slightly [7]. A posterior cruciate ligament that is too tight narrows the flexion gap and can thus result in a painful restriction of flexion and in increased wear of the polyethylene component. In contrast, excessive laxity of the PCL can lead to clinically apparent flexion instability [8,9]. Waslewski reported instabilities suffered by patients with PCL-retaining designs, caused by the early occurrence of PCL insufficiencies. His advice was to remember this problem in cases of clinical instability complaints but normal radiological findings. In a prospective randomized study Straw found no differences, either in the function score or in the range of movement, between cruciate-sacrificing, cruciate-substituting, and cruciate-retaining designs after an average follow-up of 3.5 years. In the same study, significantly worse outcomes were found only with patients whose posterior cruciate ligaments required balancing by release [10]. Hence, advocates of cruciate substitution point out that this procedure is technically more forgiving, more reproducible, and therefore less fraught with complications. Gait analyses generally produced unphysiological findings in patients with TKA compared with healthy volunteers. Several authors proved a kinematic advantage in favor of cruciate retention, although these studies used cruciate-sacrificing implants without substitution as the control group, for which lack of femoral roll-back must be expected [11-13]. However, kinematic studies by Dennis and Stiehl have shown that femoral roll-back failure will also occur with cruciate-retaining designs. Instead, in many such cases a paradoxical, discontinuous anterior femur movement is observed [14-16]. This anterior slip is thought to be the cause for increased polyethylene damage, as well as for reduced effectiveness of the extension apparatus, e.g., when climbing stairs [17]. In contrast, cruciate-substituting implants help to achieve more reproducible kinematics, at least, which comes closer to the physiological situation, even if no implant can exactly reproduce the natural kinematics of the native knee joint [7, 14-16]. Despite good clinical results with cruciate-retaining implants, the use of these designs is questionable, at least in the presence of severe deformities in the frontal and sagittal planes, because achieving adequate extrinsic stability, i.e., a balance between intrinsic and extrinsic stability of the joint, with a pathologically changed soft-tissue apparatus (severely contracted and overstretched structures) can be extremely difficult. As reported by Scott, even with careful soft-tissue release a contracted posterior cruciate can hamper the mediolateral balance (gap symmetry) [18]. In addition to this, balancing of the extension and flexion gaps (gap congruency) can also be more difficult in such a case. In a study by Laskin, patients with significant varus deformities of more than 15° profited more from cruciate-substituting designs, in the long run, at least if flat inlays were used in the cruciate-retaining variants and if the PCL was not recessed regularly [19]. For patients with rheumatoid arthritis, too, a cruciate-retaining joint replacement should be considered with caution. Laskin found an increased revision rate in such cases, due to flexion instabilities and secondary genu recurvatum [20]. In the same way, secondary cruciate ruptures must be taken into account in the context of the arthritic condition. In conclusion, in the presence of severe deformities in the frontal (varus, valgus) and sagittal (flexion contracture, genu recurvatum) planes, in cases of global instability and in the presence of inflammatory joint diseases, the use of cruciate-retaining implants is questionable, to say the least. Conventional cruciate-retaining and cruciate-substituting implants have in common that they cannot ensure any intrinsic varus-valgus stability, and can provide only little, if any, rotational stability. Whiteside showed in an in vitro study that adequate varus-valgus stability in the frontal plane, achieved by correct balancing of the collateral ligaments, automatically resulted in sufficient rotational stability, making additional intrinsic rotational stability of the implant unnecessary [21].

Implants with Intercondylar Stabilizing (ICS) Arrangements

Implants with intercondylar stabilizing arrangements provide a significant degree of rotational and varus-valgus stability due to their central cam-post design. However, Auley pointed out that it appears questionable whether these implants can provide sufficient long-term stability in the frontal plane without any ligament support. Hence, there is a risk of recurring instabilities [22]. Nevertheless, the post can provide short-term support for healing collateral structures or in association with collateral reconstruction. Severe flexion instability is another limitation for intercondylar stabilized implants. Despite the taller post, the implant can still dislocate posteriorly in case of a severe laxity in flexion. Other authors reported good clinical results with low complication rates (peroneal nerve palsy, flexion instability) in the medium- to long-term outcome for the primary implantation of the intercondylar stabilized CCK knee (Zimmer) in older, low-demand patients with severe valgus deformity. The authors consider intercondylar stabilized implants for such cases as a suitable therapy option in primary knee arthroplasty, which helps to avoid instability problems due to insufficient implant constraint [23].

Implants with Mobile Components

Implants with mobile components represent a special category. With them, the principle of "high congruency, low constraint, high mobility, low contact stress" can be realized in order to improve kinematics, reduce polyethylene wear, and allow implant self-alignment. However, as a large part of the forces in the knee have to be carried off through soft-tissue stabilizers (i.e.; extrinsically), this clearly requires particularly precise reconstruction of the soft-tissue balance, putting high demands on the skills and experience of the surgeon. Critics of mobile components point to polyethylene wear arising from the additional articulation at the underside of the mobile polyethylene components. A recent knee simulator study by Bourne, in particular, caused some concern. The worst gravimetric polyethylene wear was found with mobile components that enable rotation and translation, followed by reduced wear in pure rotation components and the lowest wear in fixed bearings (Genesis II, Smith and Nephew) [24]. This is attributed to the additional articulating surface of mobile components. Comparative wear tests under standard (ISO) conditions are required to gain further insights into these aspects. Dislocations of mobile components are rare and caused mostly by mistakes made during implantation [25]. However, incongruence of the extension and flexion gaps, especially, can lead to an increased incidence of component dislocations, too

[26]. Dislocations of rotating platforms following primary implantation are even rarer in comparison to the meniscal bearings, although their incidence is generally higher after revision operations.

Hinged Implants

The limited mobility of hinged implants, which should be employed only for certain indications, gives rise to internal constraint forces, which must be transferred though appropriate anchoring elements to the load-bearing bone in order to avoid implant fixation failure. This leads to decisive drawbacks of such implants (larger primary bone loss, secondary bone loss due to stress shielding, risk of infections with primarily diaphyseal involvement, risk of periprosthetic fractures, and increased stress for the extension apparatus due to lack of femoral roll-back). Still, the hinged systems offer the advantage that the load-transferring surfaces can be completely congruent, which reduces wear. Another advantage is that these systems do not require any technically demanding soft-tissue balancing procedures and thus help to avoid potential faults that can lead to clinically manifest complications [27]. When marked deformities in the frontal and sagittal planes require correcting, the contracted soft-tissue parts can be sacrificed without risking any instability. Even if the collateral ligaments are completely insufficient, or in cases of neuropathic joints, these systems can be implanted successfully. More recent designs with rotating hinges generally have produced more encouraging clinical and radiographic outcomes than the earlier uniaxially hinged designs [28, 29].

Choosing the Correct Implant Constraint According to the Classification of the Knee Joint Deformities

Ultimately; every implant design can be only a more or less successful compromise regarding the sometimes mutually exclusive biomechanical requirements, resulting in advantages in some respects and disadvantages in others. There is no such thing as the ideal implant that meets the requirements of every patient and every situation. Therefore, to reduce trouble caused by insufficient constraint, it is important to arrive at a patient-adapted decision for a certain implant in every individual case. When the surgical technique and the implant design are decided on, the extent of the deformity with its osseous and soft-tissue components is of crucial importance, in our opinion. The bone inventory, the soft-tissue situation, and the implant constraint must be assessed as interdeterminative components of a complex system. Therefore, we use a systematic classification system for knee joint

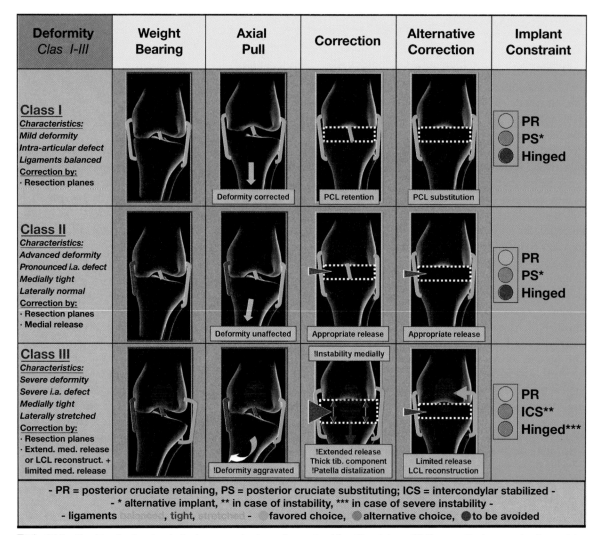

Deformity *Clas I-III*	Weight Bearing	Axial Pull	Correction	Alternative Correction	Implant Constraint
Class I *Characteristics:* *Mild deformity* *Intra-articular defect* *Ligaments balanced* *Correction by:* *· Resection planes*		Deformity corrected	PCL retention	PCL substitution	○ PR ◐ PS* ● Hinged
Class II *Characteristics:* *Advanced deformity* *Pronounced i.a. defect* *Medially tight* *Laterally normal* *Correction by:* *· Resection planes* *· Medial release*		Deformity unaffected	Appropriate release	Appropriate release	○ PR ◐ PS* ● Hinged
Class III *Characteristics:* *Severe deformity* *Severe i.a. defect* *Medially tight* *Laterally stretched* *Correction by:* *· Resection planes* *· Extend. med. release* *or LCL reconstruct. +* *limited med. release*		!Deformity aggravated	!Instability medially !Extended release Thick tib. component !Patella distalization	Limited release LCL reconstruction	○ PR ◐ ICS** ◐ Hinged***

- PR = posterior cruciate retaining, PS = posterior cruciate substituting; ICS = intercondylar stabilized -
- * alternative implant, ** in case of instability, *** in case of severe instability -
- ligaments balanced, tight, stretched - ◐ favored choice, ◐ alternative choice, ● to be avoided

Fig. 12-1a. Algorithm for choosing the implant constraint depending on the deformities of classes I-III, illustrated by the example of varus deformities.

Table 12-2. Catalog of measures for balancing the extrinsic soft-tissue stabilizers for a fixed varus deformity

When?	What?
During approach	Medial meniscectomy Excision of the meniscotibial ligament Removal of medial osteophytes Intra-articular subperiostal shifting-off of the medial and posteromedial capsule from the tibia
After the bone resections at the distal femur and proximal tibia	Extensive subperiostal exposure of the medial proximal tibia Release of the anterior portion of the medial collateral ligament at the tibia Release of the posterior portion of the medial collateral ligament at the proximal tibia Detaching the semimembranosus insertion at the tibia Release of the posteromedial capsule and the gastrocnemius insertion at the femur Release of the pes anserinus at the tibia Reconstruction of the lateral collateral ligament
Change of implant type, i.e. increasing the level of constraint	Substitution of the posterior cruciate ligament (PS) Intercondylar stabilized implant (ICS) Hinged implant

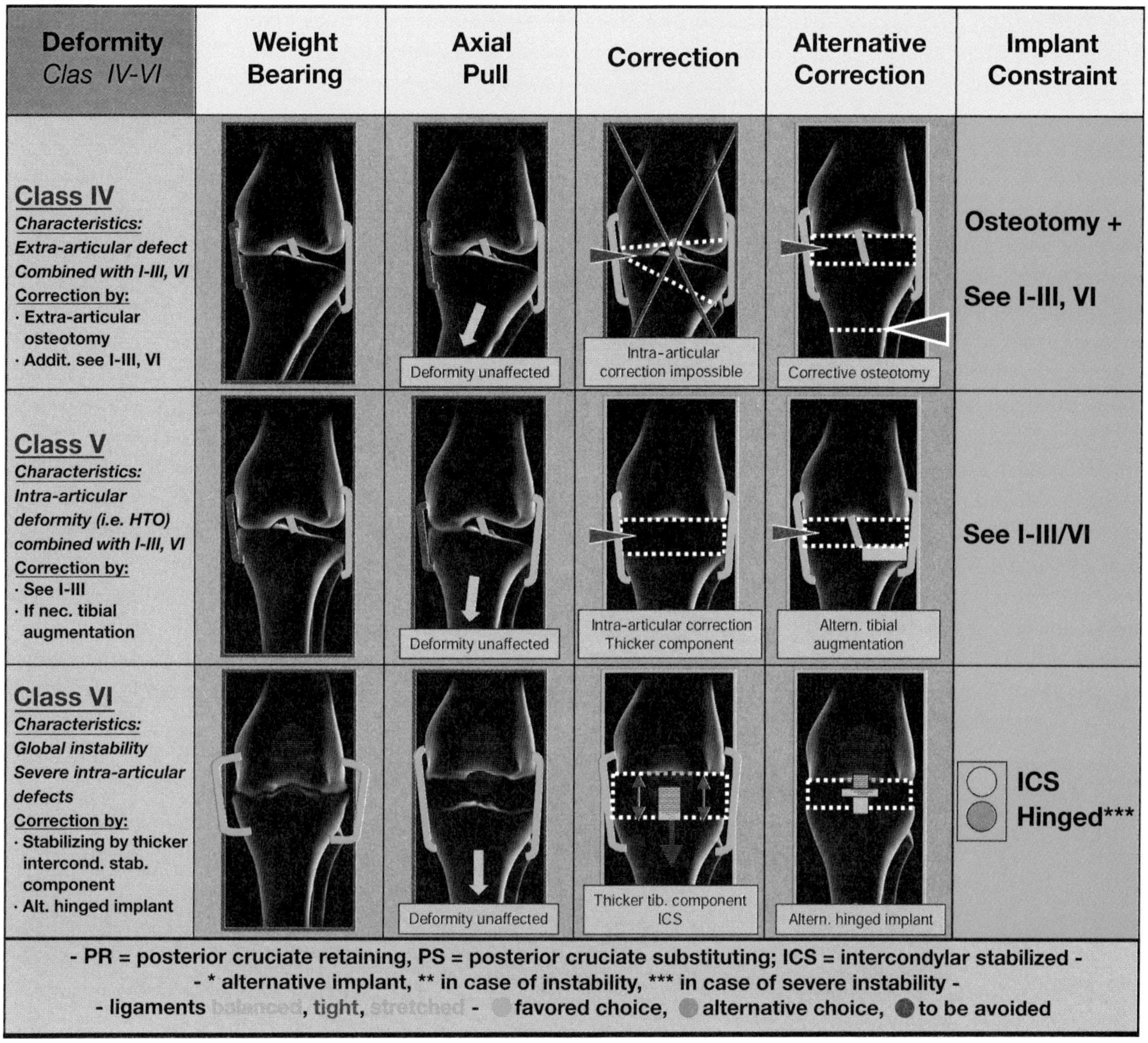

Deformity Clas IV-VI	Weight Bearing	Axial Pull	Correction	Alternative Correction	Implant Constraint
Class IV Characteristics: Extra-articular defect Combined with I-III, VI Correction by: · Extra-articular osteotomy · Addit. see I-III, VI	Deformity unaffected	Deformity unaffected	Intra-articular correction impossible	Corrective osteotomy	Osteotomy + See I-III, VI
Class V Characteristics: Intra-articular deformity (i.e. HTO) combined with I-III, VI Correction by: · See I-III · If nec. tibial augmentation		Deformity unaffected	Intra-articular correction Thicker component	Altern. tibial augmentation	See I-III/VI
Class VI Characteristics: Global instability Severe intra-articular defects Correction by: · Stabilizing by thicker intercond. stab. component · Alt. hinged implant		Deformity unaffected	Thicker tib. component ICS	Altern. hinged implant	○ ICS ○ Hinged***

- PR = posterior cruciate retaining, PS = posterior cruciate substituting; ICS = intercondylar stabilized -
- * alternative implant, ** in case of instability, *** in case of severe instability -
- ligaments balanced, tight, stretched - ● favored choice, ● alternative choice, ● to be avoided

Fig. 12-1b. Algorithm for choosing the implant constraint depending on the deformities of classes IV-VI, illustrated by the example of varus deformities

Table 12-3. Catalog of measures for balancing the extrinsic soft-tissue stabilizers in case of a fixed valgus deformity

When?	What?
During approach	Lateral approach if necessary Lateral meniscectomy Removal of lateral osteophytes Circumferential shift-off of the capsule from the posterolateral tibia
After the bone resections at the distal femur and proximal tibia	Lateral retinaculum release Detaching the popliteus tendon from the femoral insertion Successive detachment of the lateral collateral ligament at the femur or recessing it Release of the posterolateral capsule and the gastrocnemius insertion at the femur Detaching the iliotibial band from Gerdi's tubercle or recessing it Reconstruction of the medial collateral ligament
Change of implant type, i.e., increasing the level of constraint	Substitution of the posterior cruciate ligament (PS) Intercondylar stabilized implant (ICS) Hinged implant

deformities, from which one can derive an algorithm that facilitates the decision for a certain implant constraint and the appropriate soft-tissue treatment (Fig. 12-1a, b).

The required soft-tissue release must be carried out in a dosed manner, adjusted to the individual situation, to prevent excessive release and the resulting instability and to avert the necessity of using an implant with a higher degree of constraint. Hence, the soft-tissue balancing procedures listed in Tables 12-2 and 12-3 are meant as suggestions, which can be varied, e.g., regarding their sequential order and timing. The principles involved in soft-tissue balancing are illustrated by means of a strongly simplified model (Fig. 12-2).

The stabilizers represented by symbols in this model (medial and lateral collateral stabilizers, posterior cruciate ligament, and posterior capsule) can be either contracted or lax. As a rule, contracted structures are released until a balanced situation is obtained; lax structures can be tightened and reconstructed in certain situations. The medial and lateral structures determine stability in both flexion and extension, or in flexion or extension only (Table 12-4). The posterior capsule is tight only in ex-

tension and thus defines among other stabilizers the width of the extension gap. The tension of the posterior cruciate ligament controls mainly the flexion gap.

Following our principle of "as little constraint as possible," and as the final decision about the actual procedure is made intraoperatively, according to the individual situation, an implant of the next higher constraint level than that determined preoperatively on the basis of certain deformities should at least be available during the operation. In this way the risk of insufficient constraint can be minimized. Therefore, at our hospital we have modular systems available which allow us to choose between cruciate-retaining, cruciate-substituting, and intercondylar stabilized components, depending on the pre- and intraoperative decision. For certain cases hinged implants are considered, too. However, such implants are not kept on hand permanently, but are made available according to preoperative planning. Especially when using implants with low constraint (for example, mobile-bearing designs) a stable and balanced soft-tissue situation is crucial along with optimum component alignment. Since 1999 we have been gaining experience with the comput-

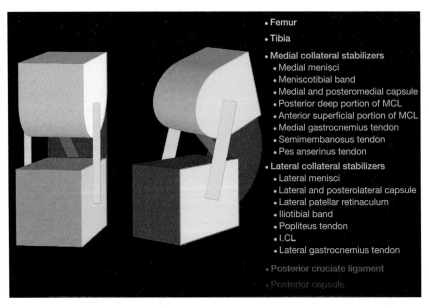

- Femur
- Tibia
- Medial collateral stabilizers
  - Medial menisci
  - Meniscotibial band
  - Medial and posteromedial capsule
  - Posterior deep portion of MCL
  - Anterior superficial portion of MCL
  - Medial gastrocnemius tendon
  - Semimembanosus tendon
  - Pes anserinus tendon
- Lateral collateral stabilizers
  - Lateral menisci
  - Lateral and posterolateral capsule
  - Lateral patellar retinaculum
  - Iliotibial band
  - Popliteus tendon
  - LCL
  - Lateral gastrocnemius tendon
- Posterior cruciate ligament
- Posterior capsule

Fig. 12-2. Simplified knee model showing the soft-tissue stabilizers (extrinsic stabilizers) relevant for soft-tissue balancing

Table 12-4. Soft-tissue structures and their contribution to stability in flexion and extension

Medial stabilizers	Pes anserinus	Semi-membranosus	Gastrocnemius	Posterior capsule	MCL, anterior part	MCL, posterior part
Flexion	-	-	-	-	+	(+)
Extension	+	+	+	+	(+)	+

Lateral stabilizers	Iliotibial band	Popliteus	Gastrocnemius	Posterior capsule	LCL	Postero-lateral corner
Flexion	-	+	-	-	+	(+)
Extension	+	(+)	+	+	+	+

er-navigated implantation (OrthoPilot navigation system, B. Braun Aesculap) of knee endoprostheses. The latest OrthoPilot Version 4.0 allows not only navigated component positioning but navigated soft-tissue and gap balancing as well, in order to achieve perfect gap symmetry and congruency. In our view, computer-navigation presents a very promising tool to reduce requirements concerning intrinsic implant stability and constraint by optimizing component alignment and soft-tissue balancing. This might help to avoid failures due to insufficient implant constraint in the future.

In the following we introduce the different deformity classes (based on the classification of Kenneth A. Krackow) and their consequences for soft-tissue treatment and the choice of an implant type. Please note that, in clinical reality, the boundaries between the individual classes cannot always be clear-cut, and that combinations of classes are possible.

Deformity Class I. This category is characterized by mild-to-medium varus or valgus deformity with corresponding intra-articular substance loss (cartilage and bone defects). The soft tissues are still balanced (i.e., not contracted on the concave side and not overstretched on the convex side). This deformity can be corrected by appropriate bone resection without relevant soft-tissue release and treated with a low-constraint implant (PR or PS).

Deformity Class II (◘ Fig. 12-3a). This category is typified by a higher-degree varus or valgus deformity with corresponding intra-articular substance loss (cartilage and bone defects). The soft tissues are not balanced (i.e., contracted on the concave side, but not yet significantly overstretched on the convex side). This deformity can usually be corrected through appropriate bone resection combined with adjusted soft-tissue release and treated with a low-constraint implant (PR or PS).

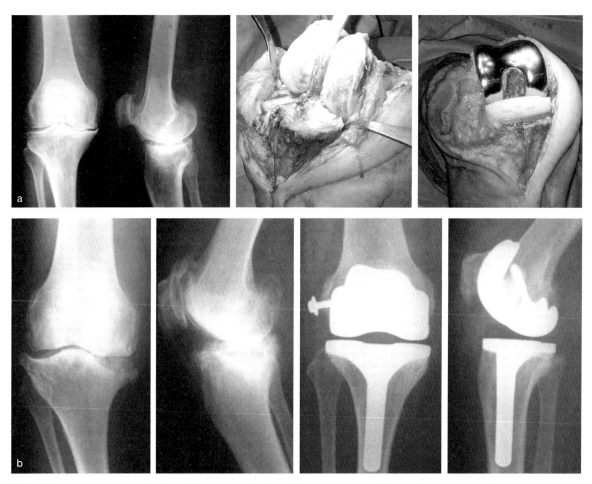

◘ **Fig. 12-3a, b.** *a* Management of a class-II deformity. Correctly aligned bone resections were followed by extensive medial release (see *intraoperative site, left*) until mediolateral soft-tissue balance is attained (gap symmetry). Following that, a slightly thicker polyethylene plateau (12 mm) was inserted to achieve adequate ligament tension. In this way the correction of the deformity was achieved using a low-constraint implant, retaining the posterior cruciate ligament (see *intraoperative site, right*). *b* Management of a class-III deformity. Correctly aligned bone resections were followed by medial release. To limit the extent of the release, and thus the risk of overcorrection and the emergence of large gaps necessitating the use of a thick polyethylene component with resulting patella distalization, the lateral collateral ligament was reconstructed. This was done by centralizing the osseous femoral insertion on the epicondyle and fixing it with a screw. This made possible the use of a low-constraint implant (PR) even with this degree of deformity. Due to the tibial defect situation, a tibial stem was inserted.

12

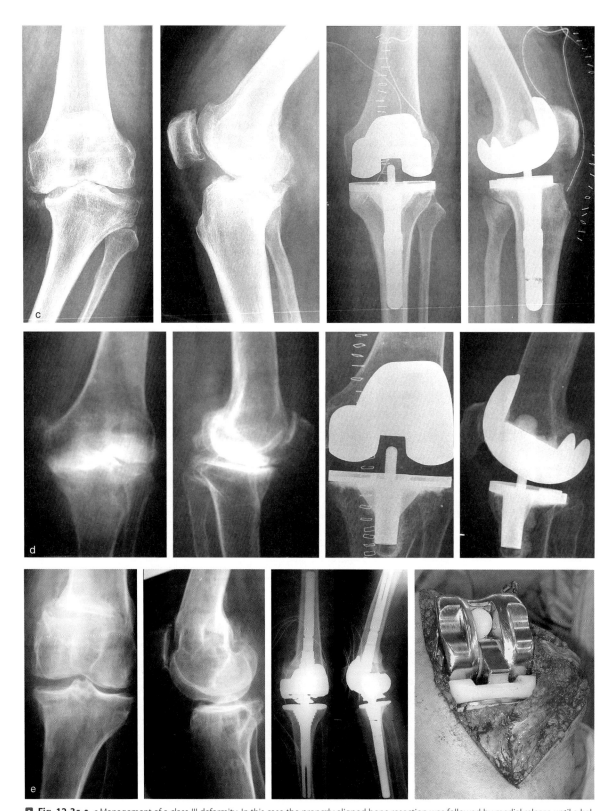

◘ **Fig. 12-3c-e.** *c* Management of a class-III deformity. In this case the properly aligned bone resection was followed by medial release until a balanced mediolateral ligament tension was achieved. The knee was replaced with an intercondylar stabilized implant. Due to the tibial defect situation, a tibial stem was inserted. *d* Management of a class-VI deformity. Following bone resections, the joint was stabilized using a thicker polyethylene component with intercondylar support. In this way the implantation of a hinged prosthesis could be avoided, even in this situation of a severe osseous defect. *e* Management of a class-V/VI deformity. In this case an unstable joint after tibial and femoral correction osteotomy was present in a patient suffering from general muscle insufficiency. Due to the neuropathically insufficient muscle envelope a maximum-constraint implant (hinged prosthesis with rotating platform) was used here in order to ensure long-term joint stability

Deformity Class III (◘ Fig. 12-3b, c). This category shows considerable varus or valgus deformity with significant intra-articular substance loss (cartilage and bone defects). The soft tissues are significantly out of balance (i.e., contracted on the concave side and markedly overstretched on the convex side). This deformity can be corrected through appropriate bone resection with extensive soft-tissue release on the concave side. This extensive soft-tissue release has the disadvantage that it involves the risk of instability caused by overcorrection, and of gap widening, necessitating the use of thicker polyethylene components and resulting in distalization of the patella. In cases of valgus deformity there is the additional risk of peroneal nerve palsy. These factors may necessitate alternative ligamentous reconstruction on the convex side, combined with a limited release on the concave side, though this is technically demanding and must be taken into account in postoperative rehabilitation. With adequate soft-tissue balancing, this condition can be treated with an implant with relatively low constraint (PS) in certain cases. However, the option of using the next higher constraint level (intercondylar stabilized or hinged) should be available intraoperatively, especially if very extensive soft-tissue release or reconstruction was carried out.

Deformity Class IV. This category is characterized by an extra-articular deformity (e.g., post-traumatic) combined with an intra-articular deformity according to deformity classes I-III or VI. This deformity cannot be corrected by intra-articular bone resection alone. In these cases, an extra-articular corrective osteotomy needs to be carried out. This can be done simultaneously with the TKA or at a different time, prior to the TKA. The knee endoprosthesis is implanted according to the criteria for the intra-articular deformity of class I, II, III, or VI.

Deformity Class V (◘ Fig. 12-3e). This category is typified by the presence of an intra-articular bone deformity, e.g., following a high tibial osteotomy. The other components of the deformity conform to deformity classes I-III or VI. This deformity can be controlled as described under deformity classes I, II, III, or VI, but if the resection of larger amounts of bone substance becomes necessary to compensate for an osseous defect, the defect should be augmented appropriately (autogenous bone, metal blocks or wedges, cement).

Deformity Class VI (◘ Fig. 12-3d, e). This category shows marked defects with global instability. The situation can be controlled by correctly aligned bone resections and stabilization of the overstretched soft tissues using an intercondylar stabilized implant with a polyethylene component of adequate thickness or, alternatively, using a hinged implant. Application of an excessively thick polyethylene component leads to corresponding patella distalization and frontal impingements [30].

References

1. Gunston FH et al (1971) Polycentric knee arthroplasty. Prosthetic simulation of normal knee movement. J Bone Joint Surg [Br] 53:272-277
2. Blunn GW, Walker PS, Joshi A, Hardinge K (1991) The dominance of cyclic sliding in producing wear in total knee replacements. Clin Orthop 273:253-260
3. Swany MR, Scott RD (1993) Posterior polyethylene wear in posterior cruciate ligament-retaining total knee arthroplasty. A case study. J Arthroplasty 8:439-446
4. Ritter MA, Faris PM, Keating EM (1988) Posterior cruciate ligament balancing during total knee arthroplasty. J Arthroplasty 3:323-326
5. Hirsch HS, Lotke PA, Morrison LD (1994) The posterior cruciate ligament in total knee surgery. Save, sacrifice, or substitute? Clin Orthop 309:64-68
6. Incavo SJ, Johnson CC, Beynnon BD, Howe JG (1994) Posterior cruciate ligament strain biomechanics in total knee arthroplasty. Clin Orthop 309:88-93
7. Mahoney OM, Noble PC, Rhoads DD, Alexander JW, Tullos HS (1994) Posterior cruciate function following total knee arthroplasty. A biomechanical study. J Arthroplasty 9:569-578
8. Pagnano MW, Hanssen AD, Lewallen DG, Stuart MJ (1998) Flexion instability after primary posterior cruciate retaining total knee arthroplasty. Clin Orthop 356:39-46
9. Waslewski GL, Marson BM, Benjamin JB (1998) Early, incapacitating instability of posterior cruciate ligament-retaining total knee arthroplasty. J Arthroplasty 13:763-767
10. Straw R, Kulkarni S, Attfield S, Wilton TJ (2003) Posterior cruciate ligament at total knee replacement. Essential, beneficial or a hindrance? J Bone Joint Surg [Br] 85:671-674
11. Andriacchi TP, Galante JO, Fermier RW (1982) The influence of total knee-replacement design on walking and stair-climbing. J Bone Joint Surg [Am] 64:1328-1335
12. Dorr LD, Ochsner JL, Gronley J, Perry J (1998) Functional comparison of posterior cruciate-retained versus cruciate-sacrificed total knee arthroplasty. Clin Orthop 236:36-43
13. Kelman GJ, Biden EN, Wyatt MP, Ritter MA, Colwell CW Jr (1989) Gait laboratory analysis of a posterior cruciate-sparing total knee arthroplasty in stair ascent and descent. Clin Orthop 248:21-26
14. Dennis DA, Komistek RD, Hoff WA, Gabriel SM (1996) In vivo knee kinematics derived using an inverse perspective technique. Clin Orthop 331:107-117
15. Dennis DA, Komistek RD, Colwell CE Jr, Ranawat CS, Scott RD, Thornhill TS, Lapp MA (1998) In vivo anteroposterior femorotibial translation of total knee arthroplasty: a multicenter analysis. Clin Orthop 356:47-57
16. Stiehl JB, Komistek RD, Dennis DA, Paxson RD, Hoff WA (1995) Fluoroscopic analysis of kinematics after posterior-cruciate-retaining knee arthroplasty. J Bone Joint Surg [Br] 77:884-889
17. Blunn GW, Walker PS, Joshi A, Hardinge K (1991) The dominance of cyclic sliding in producing wear in total knee replacements. Review. Clin Orthop 273:253-260
18. Scott RD, Volatile TB (1986) Twelve years' experience with posterior cruciate-retaining total knee arthroplasty. Clin Orthop 205:100-107
19. Laskin RS (1996) The Insall Award. Total knee replacement with posterior cruciate ligament retention in patients with a fixed varus deformity. Clin Orthop 331:29-34
20. Laskin RS (1997) The Insall Award. Total knee replacement with posterior cruciate ligament retention in rheumatoid arthritis. Problems and complications. Clin Orthop 345:24-28
21. Whiteside LA, Amador DD (1989) Rotational stability of a posterior stabilized total knee arthroplasty. Clin Orthop 242:241-246
22. McAuley JP, Engh GA (2003) Constraint in total knee arthroplasty: when and what? J Arthroplasty 18:51-54
23. Easley ME, Insall JN, Scuderi GR, Bullek DD (2000) Primary constrained condylar knee arthroplasty for the arthritic valgus knee. Clin Orthop 380:58-64

24. Bourne RB, Masonis J, Anthony M (2003) An analysis of rotating-platform total knee replacements. Clin Orthop 410:173-180

25. Weaver JK, Derkash RS, Greenwald AS (1993) Difficulties with bearing dislocation and breakage using a movable bearing total knee replacement system. Clin Orthop 290:244-252

26. Bert JM (1990) Dislocation/subluxation of meniscal bearing elements after New Jersey low-contact stress total knee arthroplasty. Clin Orthop 254:211-215

27. Fehring TK, Valadie AL (1994) Knee instability after total knee arthroplasty. Clin Orthop 299:157-162

28. Westrich GH, Mollano AV, Sculco TP, Buly RL, Laskin RS, Windsor R (2000) Rotating hinge total knee arthroplasty in severly affected knees. Clin Orthop 379:195-208

29. Barrack RL et al (2001) Evolution of the rotating hinge for complex total knee arthroplasty. Clin Orthop 392:292-299

30. Verborgt O, Victor J (2004) Post impingement in posterior stabilised total knee arthroplasty. Acta Orthop Belg 70:46-50

12

13   Surface Damage and Wear in Fixed, Modular Tibial Inserts: The Effects of Conformity and Constraint

J. D. Haman, M. A. Wimmer, J. O. Galante

Summary

The degree of conformity and constraint are thought to play an important role in the severity of wear damage of the polyethylene insert of total knee replacement (TKR). Wear is thought to diminish as a function of increasing conformity and hence increased surface areas and thus diminished contact stresses. However, a study of retrieved polyethylene components of less conforming CR prostheses (MG2) and more conforming PS and CCK devices (IBII) showed more severe wear damage (delamination and pitting) on the articulating surfaces of the more conforming design. In addition, the IB2 post showed substantial wear-related damage, implicating it as an important source of particulate debris. Wear in TKR is a complex phenomenon influenced by many variables beyond the simple relationship between conformity and surface area.

Introduction

Clinical results reported to date with contemporary total knee replacements (TKR) indicate high survivorship coupled with satisfactory functional performance. There are, however, a number of controversies that relate to long-term function and the potential for late failure. One such controversy centers on the geometric characteristics of the articular surfaces, specifically, the degree of conformity and constraint of the polyethylene (PE) inserts and the subsequent effect on wear and damage. The classic assumption that a direct relationship exists between contact stress and the severity of wear has had major implications in prosthetic design. Proponents of highly conforming (i.e., large contact area) articular surfaces base their design criteria on this assumption, thus predicting an overall decrease in wear of the polyethylene insert. Consequently, it is perceived that so-called flat-on-flat (less-conforming) geometries, while allowing a greater degree of tibiofemoral rotation and translation, may result in decreased tibiofemoral contact areas, increased predicted contact stresses, and, thus, increased polyethylene wear.

By virtue of the geometric and motion requirements of the human knee, conformity is most frequently attached to varying degrees of constraint. Posterior cruciate-substituting prostheses and constrained condylar designs take the constraint one step further and include a central post for added stability. This design feature can become an additional source of wear debris.

Taking the direct relationship between contact stress and wear to its ultimate implications, a mobile-bearing design or a rotating platform can substantially increase the available contact areas and provide the greatest degree of conformity, not only on the frontal plane but in the sagittal plane as well.

The alternative, minimally constrained articulating surfaces, requires less conforming designs, with a flat or nearly flat surface on the coronal plane on the tibia and varying degrees of curvature on the femur. This is a design requirement in posterior cruciate ligament-sparing devices or in unicompartmental prostheses where unconstrained relative motion of the articulating surfaces is needed to allow for the necessary kinematics.

This chapter will focus on observations from retrieved specimens that allow a comparison of wear and damage from surfaces with different degrees of conformity and constraint. The ultimate purpose of these and future studies is to relate these findings to the mechanism of polyethylene wear in total knees and associated principles of prosthetic design.

Wear

Although a source of concern in long-term follow-up, wear is not at the present time a major cause of failure in TKR [1]. The clinical consequences of wear include the possibility of mechanical failure due to the major loss of integrity of the polyethylene insert; more commonly of synovitis secondary to an inflammatory response to the presence of polyethylene particles; and less frequently of osteolysis.

While osteolysis can result in catastrophic failure of the arthroplasty with major bone loss, it has not had (in total knees) the overall major clinical impact that it has exhibited in total hip arthroplasty [2]. The incidence of osteolysis is variable and related to a number of factors including the quality and manufacturing process of the polyethylene insert, the design of the implant, the presence and quality of modular junctions, and the method of fixation.

Osteolysis is most frequently related to the motion between the polyethylene insert and the underlying tibial plate (i.e., the stability of the modular junction between tibial plate and insert). The generated backside wear can produce very small particles with high osteolytic potential. Osteolysis is probably more common in cementless designs. Granulomas seem to be associated with the presence of screw holes that act as pathways for polyethylene particle migration to the peripheral tissues.

The average diameter of polyethylene particles originating from TKR is larger than that found in total hip replacements. Their biological activity is thus less pronounced than those produced as a result of wear in total hips. This size difference is most probably a reflection of the prevalent mechanism of wear.

In total hips adhesive wear is the predominant mechanism. Adhesion is capable of producing very small particles in the micron and submicron range, which are easily phagocytosed. Thus, these particles are capable of inducing the phenomenon of cell activation eventually leading to granuloma formation and, subsequently, to osteolysis. By contrast, in total knees the predominant mechanism of wear is associated with surface fatigue, a phenomenon that leads to the generation of larger, less biologically active particles.

Wear Appearances and Related Mechanisms

Characteristic wear appearances of three major wear mechanisms, adhesion, abrasion, and surface fatigue, have been observed on the articulating surfaces of total knee prostheses and are documented in an extensive body of literature. Typical wear appearances for the tibial polyethylene plateau [3] include: polishing (or burnishing), scratching, abrasion, surface deformation, embedded debris, pitting, and delamination. In the following paragraphs we will tie these "damage modes" with the wear mechanisms that produce them. In several references surface deformation, creep, or cold flow is listed as a damage mode; however, this type of surface change does not create particles and is therefore, strictly speaking, not wear damage.

Surface fatigue is the most common wear mechanism seen in TKR. It is typically associated with repetitive loading as it occurs during sliding, rolling motion. Its wear appearance such as pitting and delamination is often

reported for the polyethylene liner. Third-bodies such as cement debris, bone fragments, or polyethylene particles, which repeatedly slide or roll within the wear track, may also initiate this type of wear.

Abrasion is an often-reported mechanism because scratches and grooves are always obvious. Abrasion may be induced by many sources from outside and inside the system. System-inherent abrasive bodies are compacted wear debris, or large flakes generated as a consequence of adhesion. External abrasive bodies may originate from bone cement or the bone itself.

A polished appearance of the tibial polyethylene plateau is linked to adhesion. Microscopic welding between tibial plateau and femoral condyle generates fibrils on the surface of the polymeric material. These fibrils may be torn off and pulled away, resulting in elongated particles.

Factors in Polyethylene Wear at the Tibial Articulation

In addition to the shape of the articulating surfaces and the resulting kinematics, there are numerous factors that contribute to polyethylene wear, including those that are intrinsic or extrinsic to the material properties of the polyethylene itself.

Intrinsic factors that have been shown to affect the wear performance of UHMWPE include the presence of fusion defects or inclusions, the stiffness of the polyethylene, the nature of the base resin, the molecular weight, the method of fabrication (machined versus molded), the presence of residual free radicals in the matrix, and the degree of cross-linking.

Factors unrelated to the material properties of the polyethylene (extrinsic factors) include the thickness of the polyethylene, the counterface material, the counterface roughness, the presence or absence of metal backing, the presence and stability of modular connections, and the presence of any third bodies.

As previously stated, TKRs are more likely to produce larger particulate as a result of surface fatigue and third-body wear. The intrinsic factors that contribute most to surface fatigue are resin type [4] and consolidation method [5], while the use of additives is thought to be a cause of third-body wear [6] and surface fatigue [7]. We found these factors to be important in a study comparing retrievals of two flat-on-flat designs (MG1 and MG2, successive generations of a prosthetic design) [8].

Compression-molded inserts manufactured from H1900 resin without calcium stearate (MG1), were compared with machined, ram-extruded inserts manufactured from GUR 4150 with calcium stearate (MG2). The compression-molded inserts had significantly longer service lifetimes than did the ram-extruded inserts with

Chapter 13 · Surface Damage and Wear in Fixed, Modular Tibial Inserts – J. D. Haman et al.

87   **13**

respect to delamination (a surface-fatigue damage mode). Pitting, also associated with third-body wear, was not different between the two designs. Pitting was seen to increase for those implants that were cemented, indicating a potential effect from retained cement particles.

One of the significant conclusions from this study was that, in spite of articular surfaces that were virtually identical in shape and thus had virtually identical kinematics, there were major differences in wear behavior between the two implants. These differences were related solely to the different intrinsic properties of the polyethylene used in each design. The effect of these properties must be taken into account when evaluating wear in retrieved components, as it can easily obscure the influence of other variables such as conformity and constraint.

The Effect of Conformity and Constraint

The amount of constraint in the prosthesis can markedly affect the contact mechanics of the joint. Banks et al. [9] found significant differences in the contact kinematics between cruciate-retaining (less conforming) and posterior-stabilized (more conforming) designs. Guan Li et al. [10, 11] outlined that only cruciate-retaining knees may achieve displacement patterns similar to those of natural knees. It has been suggested that limited anteroposterior movement of the femur on the tibia influences function during daily activities [12]. While it is generally accepted that stresses resulting from compressive forces inside the bulk polyethylene are reduced with higher conformity [13], limited freedom of motion can increase tangential (constraint) forces on the tibial plateau, thus confounding and compounding the severity of the wear produced.

To ascertain the effect of conformity on the severity of wear, we examined retrieved polyethylene tibial inserts of two designs from the same manufacturer [14]. The retrieval collection consisted of 85 tibial inserts. Forty-five inserts came from a total knee design with conforming, moderately constrained articulating surfaces (IBII). Of those, 20 were posterior stabilized (PS) with a standard

tibial cam, and 25 were constrained condylar implants (CCK) with an elevated tibial cam. The mean implantation time was 20.9 months (range 1-84). There were 40 inserts retrieved from a total knee design with less conforming, unconstrained, tibiofemoral geometry (MG2, Zimmer). These components were fully conforming in the coronal plane and non-conforming in the sagittal plane. The mean implantation time was 29.3 months (range 1-85). All implants were manufactured by one company (Zimmer Inc., Warsaw, IN) applying the same processing technique and identical resin (ram extrusion and subsequent machining from GUR 415). There was no significant demographic difference between any of the designs with respect to age, implantation time, or gender.

Wear damage to the articulating and post surfaces of the inserts was inspected visually and, where necessary, at 5-7 x magnification. Delamination, pitting, creep, and polishing were scored for all surfaces by three independent investigators. In addition to simple frequency counts, severity was rated on a 0-3 scale and multiplied by extent of damage (rated on a 0-4 scale) to give a total wear score. All four investigated damage modes were present in both retrieved designs, MG2 and IBII. Surprisingly, there were more implants in the more conforming design group with fatigue-type wear than in the less conforming design group. Pitting and delamination occurred with a higher frequency in the IBII retrievals (◻ Fig. 13-1). Conforming articular surfaces had significantly greater wear scores than non-conforming articular surfaces with the exception of medial pitting and lateral delamination. However, the non-conforming surfaces were more likely to undergo polishing, and the associated wear score was significantly greater than for conforming surfaces. Finally, edge loading was noted almost exclusively for the conforming inserts, with only one incident (on the posterior portion of the lateral compartment) reported for the non-conforming inserts.

In addition to the changes seen in the articulating surfaces, the post itself may be regarded as a source of polyethylene wear. All surfaces of the post of the IBII components were damaged in some way, with at least 84% of all the inserts showing damage [15]. Separating the data

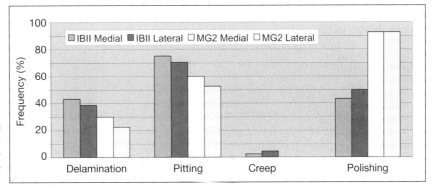

◻ **Fig. 13-1.** Frequency of observed damage modes in IBII and MG2 implants. Data are categorized with respect to medial and lateral compartments

by design (CCK vs. PS) showed that the incidence of delamination and pitting – severe damage modes – was low for most surfaces of both post designs. For most surfaces, polishing was the damage mode most likely to occur, followed by creep. When wear scores were compared, only pitting was found to significantly differ ($p=0.005$) for the PS and CCK designs, with the CCK design having the greater damage. However, the major source of particulate expected from these results would be secondary to the rather severe polishing damage. Thus the particulate would be smaller and more likely to be an osteolytic instigator.

Interestingly, when the relationships between post and articular surface damage were examined, there appeared to be some correlation between these two phenomena. This may implicate the post in the production of third-body particulate and thus significant, severe articular damage.

Discussion

The characterization of the wear behavior of PE through both retrieval analyses and laboratory knee wear simulation is fraught with a number of difficulties. This explains the lack of complete understanding of the wear behavior of total knees and the controversies that surround issues of prosthetic design. For instance, the vast majority of inserts available in retrieval collections are a result of revision surgery, and are therefore considered to be failures. By far, the most valuable information is obtained from autopsy specimens, as the wear patterns are not likely to be affected by complications such as malalignment, instability, loosening, infection, or pain, which may alter the pattern of motion and joint loading.

Less obvious difficulties, but more onerous, are those associated with the method used to qualify or quantify the wear damage itself. Both photomicrographs or direct visual inspection present difficulties in quantifying accurately the severity of wear such as the number of pits present, the average size of the damaged area, etc., and thus the results can be brought into question.

Knee wear simulators designed to mimic the motions and loads of the knee joint are widely used to evaluate polyethylene wear. However, the wear scars and patterns observed in simulators do not always reflect the kind of patterns seen in retrieved specimens, and thus some of the conclusions derived from knee simulators may not be valid.

The impact of the cruciate-retaining versus -substituting design issues on tibial component wear and clinical outcome is still unclear and the subject of much debate. Low conformity (as seen in cruciate-retaining designs) was found to produce more wear and less clinical success in the studies of Collier et al. [16] and Feng et al. [17]. This was not observed by Blunn et al. [18] and Ritter et al. [19], who were in agreement with our findings described above. Ritter promoted low conformity as a primary reason for success: The cylinder-on-flat design allows freedom of rotation and translation, which reduces constraint forces and thus surface damage. An additional source of concern is the damage observed in posts in both PS and CCK designs. This damage is the result, to some extent, of adhesive wear and is capable of generating a large volume of particles with considerable biological activity.

Most in vitro and modeling studies indicate that more conformity would lead to lower stresses in the PE due to greater contact areas. However, supporting our findings, a recent in vitro study by Mazzucco and Spector indicates that within the range of normal loading, wear rate increases linearly with contact area and is not affected by contact stress. The authors suggested that more conformity/constraint, i.e., more contact area, in TKR would lead to greater volumetric wear [20].

An important issue of biological significance relates to the predominant mechanism of wear. Under conditions of increasing conformity it is expected that adhesive wear will eventually predominate. Thus, in the extreme of total conformity, such as in a meniscal-bearing design, adhesive wear conditions could be operating at both mobile interfaces. The result would be the generation of small particles with the capacity to induce cell activation and eventually lead to osteolysis.

In summary, recent retrieval and in vitro studies by our group and others indicate that wear damage is not necessarily reduced in conforming implants in vivo; on the contrary, it appears to be increased. Ultimately, the results of these and various other studies indicate that the problem of wear in TKRs is much more complex than can be explained by conformity alone.

References

1. Sharkey PF et al (2002) Insall Award paper. Why are total knee arthroplasties failing today? Clin Orthop 404:7-13
2. Huang CH et al (2002) Osteolysis in failed total knee arthroplasty: a comparison of mobile-bearing and fixed-bearing knees. J Bone Joint Surg [Am] 84:2224-2229
3. Hood RW et al (1983) Retrieval analysis of total knee prostheses: a method and its application to 48 total condylar prostheses. J Biomed Mater Res 17:829-842
4. Eyerer P (1986) Kunststoffe in der Gelenkendoprothetik. Z Werkstofftechnik 17:284
5. Furman B et al (1997) Effect of resin type and manufacturing method on UHMWPE oxidation and quality at long aging and implant times. Trans of 43rd Annual Meeting of the Orthopaedic Research Society
6. Lewis G (1997) Polyethylene wear in total hip and knee arthroplasties. J Biomed Mater Res 38:55-75
7. Schmidt MB, Hamilton JV (1996) The effects of calcium stearate on the properties of UHMWPE. Trans of 42nd Annual Meeting of the Orthopedic Research Society 21:239

Chapter 13 · Surface Damage and Wear in Fixed, Modular Tibial Inserts – J. D. Haman et al.

89   **13**

8. Berzins A et al (2002) Surface damage in machined ram-extruded and net-shape molded retrieved polyethylene tibial inserts of total knee replacements. J Bone Joint Surg [Am] 84:1534-1540

9. Banks SA et al (1997) Total knee replacement mechanics during gait. Trans of 43rd Annual Meeting of the Orthopedic Research Society 22:263

10. Bertin KC et al (2002) In vivo determination of posterior femoral rollback for subjects having a NexGen posterior cruciate-retaining total knee arthroplasty. J Arthroplasty 17:1040-1048

11. Li G et al (2001) Cruciate-retaining and cruciate-substituting total knee arthroplasty: an in vitro comparison of the kinematics under muscle loads. J Arthroplasty 16 [Suppl 1]:150-156

12. Andriacchi TP, Galante JO (1988) Retention of the posterior cruciate in total knee arthroplasty. J Arthroplasty 3 [Suppl]:S13-19

13. Bartel DL et al (1995) Stresses in polyethylene components of contemporary total knee replacements. Clin Orthop 317:76-82

14. Haman JD, Wimmer MA (2003) Tibial plateau damage in retrieved conforming and non-conforming TKAs. Proc Annual Meeting of Society for Biomaterials 25:383

15. Haman JD, Wimmer MA (2003) Tibial post damage in TKAs is associated with tibial plateau damage. Trans of 49th Annual Meeting of the Orthopedic Research Society 28:6

16. Collier JP et al (1991) Analysis of the failure of 122 polyethylene inserts from uncemented tibial knee components. Clin Orthop 273:232-242

17. Feng EL et al (1994) Progressive subluxation and polyethylene wear in total knee replacements with flat articular surfaces. Clin Orthop 299:60-71

18. Blunn GW et al (1992) Polyethylene wear in unicondylar knee prostheses. 106 retrieved Marmor, PCA, and St. Georg tibial components compared. Acta Orthop Scand 63:247-255

19. Ritter MA et al (1995) Flat-on-flat, nonconstrained, compression molded polyethylene total knee replacement. Clin Orthop 321:79-85

20. Mazzucco D, Spector M (2003) Effect of contact area on the wear of ultrahigh molecular weight polyethylene in bidirectional pin-on-flat articulation. Trans of 49th Annual Meeting of the Orthopedic Research Society 28:1

14 Failure in Cam-Post in Total Knee Arthroplasty

R. B. Bourne, J. V. Baré

Summary

Ideally, a total knee arthroplasty would mimic normal knee motion. Fluoroscopic studies have suggested a need for "guided motion" to provide a better approximation of normal knee kinematics. The development of the post-cam mechanism in posterior cruciate ligament-sacrificing designs of total knee arthroplasty is an attempt in this direction. Analysis has revealed that all post-cam mechanisms are not the same and that substantial differences exist from one implant type to another. Mikulak et al. have suggested that a substantial number of post-cam implants do not engage as designed. They have also raised the concept of rotational constraint leading to tibial post wear and the transmission of tibial rotational stresses to the modular interfaces (resulting in backside wear) and to the bone-implant interfaces (potentially resulting in loosening). The Puloski et al. study has also emphasized that post-cam mechanisms might result in increased wear debris and hence in negative outcomes such as osteolysis, aseptic loosening, and reactive synovitis. This group found more wear with varus/valgus constrained implants and advised caution with this design. They also described two tibial polyethylene posts that either fractured or were worn away, resulting in an unstable knee that required revision. This indicates that a post-cam mechanism cannot substitute for proper implant alignment and soft-tissue balancing. As we look into the future, the designers of future knee replacements that rely on a post-cam mechanism for guided motion within a total knee replacement must be aware of the surgical and design factors necessary to make this mechanism function properly.

Introduction

Whether or not to sacrifice the posterior cruciate ligament (PCL) during primary total knee replacement remains a subject of controversy. Excellent long-term clinical outcomes have been achieved with both PCL-retaining and -sacrificing total knee arthroplasties [2-6, 9, 12-14]. Many surgeons prefer PCL-sacrificing devices when treating patients with deformities greater than 15°, with inflammatory rheumatoid arthritis, with a prior high tibial valgus osteotomy, or with a prior patellectomy. Recent fluoroscopic studies have also played a role in encouraging an increasing number of surgeons to consider PCL sacrifice during total knee arthroplasty [15]. These fluoroscopic studies have suggested a rather haphazard tibiofemoral contact pattern with PCL-retaining implants and a more guided motion pattern with PCL-sacrificing devices.

Should the surgeon select a PCL-sacrificing total knee arthroplasty, options to prevent anteroposterior instability are limited to the use of a posterior-stabilized design with a tibial post and femoral cam or a dished polyethylene insert with a raised anterior lip. A short-term, randomized clinical trial comparing these two devices has shown comparable short-term clinical outcomes [7]. The deep-dished, PCL-sacrificing design has the advantage of not relying on a small post to control anteroposterior stability, but the disadvantage of not allowing roll-back during knee flexion, which might limit knee range of motion and the mechanical advantage of various muscles about the knee joint.

Wear of the polyethylene insert is the primary limiting factor in the longevity of current total knee arthroplasties [1, 2, 10, 11, 16]. Recently, increased attention has been directed towards the post-and-cam type of PCL-sacrificing knee arthroplasties as a potential source of polyethylene damage and wear debris. The purpose of this chapter is to alert the orthopedic surgeon to the fact that cam-post PCL-sacrificing devices can be an additional source of polyethylene wear debris and that there is variability in the wear patterns observed among different PCL-sacrificing designs due to differences in the cam-post mechanics, post location, and post geometry. The surgeon should be aware that the cam-post interface is not an innocuous articulation.

Retrieval Studies

Puloski et al. retrieved and analyzed 23 post-cam, PCL-sacrificing tibial inserts over a 2-year period (1996-1998) from the practices of four orthopedic surgeons operating at his center [11]. The retrieved implants had been inserted over a period of 17 years (1981-1998) and had an average implantation duration of 36 months (2-107 months). Seven inserts had been implanted as primary components and 16 had been inserted during revision knee arthroplasties. The tibial inserts collected were parts of modular cemented systems from four different manufacturers. There were four Genesis I and three Genesis II inserts (Smith & Nephew, Inc., Memphis, Tennessee), one Kinematic I, one Kinematic II, and five Kinemax inserts (Stryker Osteonics Howmedica, East Rutherford, N.J.), two AMK and five Coordinate inserts (Johnson & Johnson, Depuy, Warsaw, IN), and one Insall-Burstein II and one CCK insert (Zimmer, Warsaw, IN). Eighteen inserts were manufactured from standard ultra-high-molecular-weight polyethylene (UHMWPE) and five were manufactured from Hylamer (Johnson and Johnston DePuy, Warsaw IN). Five of the Kinematic/Kinemax components were heat-pressed. The polyethylene sterilization procedure was identified for 21 inserts (gamma irradiation in air - 13, ethylene oxide - 6, and gas plasma - 2). Regarding the revision implants, six were revised for aseptic loosening, one for osteolysis, seven for infection, two for pain, five for instability, and one for stiffness.

All 23 inserts were examined for wear on the stabilizing post, using stereomicroscopy and digital image analyses. A wear score was applied to each post to calculate a "wear grade" and "surface area" affected (◘ Table 14-1).

Initial examination of all 23 retrieved implants revealed evidence of wear in varying degrees over some portion of the post surface. All three mechanisms of wear occurred and the morphology of damage included pitting, delamination, scratching, abrasions, burnishing, and surface deformation. There was no notable evidence of embedded cement debris. The mean prevalence of all wear as a percentage of the posts' total surface area was 39.9% (range, 18.5%-60%). The most predominant mechanism observed was adhesive wear or "burnishing", occurring on 21 of the 23 implants (93%) and covering 24% (range, 0-48%) of the entire post surface. Fatigue

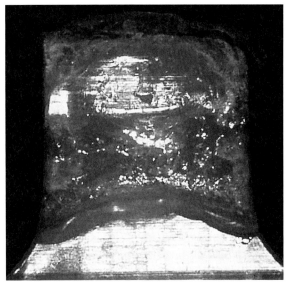

◘ **Fig. 14-1.** Posterior surface of post from Kinematic (Howmedica, Rutherford, NJ) implant. Delamination covers over 60% of the surface. The implant was revised for aseptic loosening after 107 months

wear representing mainly delamination was evident on eight implants (36%), covering 11% (range, 0-64%) of the overall surface area. Abrasive damage involving primarily "scratching" was evident on 12 implants (55%), covering a surface area of 4% (range, 0-19%).

Severe post wear, involving gross loss of polyethylene was apparent in seven of the 23 inserts (30%), primarily in the form of delamination (◘ Fig. 14-1). Three of these seven inserts had been heat-pressed. The structural integrity of the post and capacity to prevent posterior subluxation was impaired in two implants. One of these implants, a revision Genesis I (Smith & Nephew, Memphis, TN) removed for instability after 35 months, had a fractured post that had completely dissociated from the tibial insert (◘ Fig. 14-2).

A Kinemax (Howmedica, Rutherford, NJ) insert, also revised for instability, had complete disintegration of 4.1 mm, or 33% of the superior apex of the post (◘ Fig. 14-3). Al-

◘ **Table 14-1.** Wear grading system

Wear mechanism	Damage mode	Score	Severity	Add	Overall grade
Adhesive wear	Burnishing	1	Mild- surface finish altered	0	1
			Mod – complete loss of machining grain	1	2
			Severe – palpable step around affected region	2	3
Abrasive wear	Scratching	2	Mild – damage density <1/3 surface	0	2
	Abrasions		Mod – damage density <2/3 surface	1	3
	Embedded debris		Severe – damage density >2/3 surface	2	4
Fatigue wear	Delamination, pitting	3	Mild – subsurface changes, surface intact	0	3
			Mod – surface removed, subsurface exposed	1	4
			Severe – notable wear over exposed subsurface	2	5

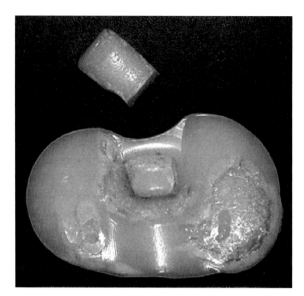

◘ **Fig. 14-2.** Genesis (Smith & Nephew, Memphis, TN) tibial insert revised for instability after 35 months. The stabilizing bar was found to be fractured at the time of revision

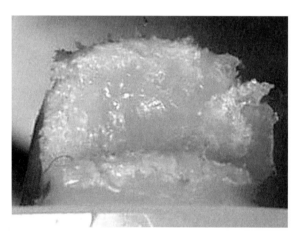

◘ **Fig. 14-3.** Anterior surface of stabilizing post from Kinematic (Howmedica Rutherford, NJ) tibial insert. This implant exhibited catastrophic wear with severe loss of polyethylene. Over 30% of superior apex of the post is worn away. This implant was revised after 77 months due to instability

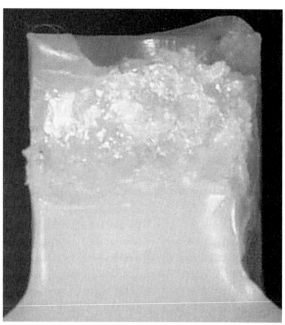

◘ **Fig. 14-4.** Anterior surface of stabilizing post from AMK (DePuy, Warsaw, IN) insert. Significant post wear with minimal condylar surface wear was observed in this component. The implant was revised after 45 months for pain from a chronic synovitis

Post wear scores (PWS) from 22 of the 23 retrieved inserts were determined. Wear analysis from one component was inapplicable, as iatrogenic damage during removal was too extensive for accurate quantitative assessment. A mean total wear score of 3.56 (±3.18, 0.7-12.4) was calculated for all components with an average implantation period of 35.7 months (range, 2.3-107). PWS, period of implantation, and revision diagnosis for all implants are shown in ◘ Table 14-2.

The Pearson product-moment correlation coefficient comparing period of implantation with PWS was 0.61, suggesting an increasing wear score with duration (◘ Fig. 14-5). With the numbers available, no significant differences in normalized wear scores were noted be-

though formal grade analysis was not completed on the articular surfaces of the tibial inserts in this study, severe wear of the tibial post did appear to coincide with appreciable wear over the articular surface. Certainly, delamination occurring over the post surface seemed to correspond with similar damage over the articular surface in five of the seven severely damaged inserts. Interestingly, a single AMK insert, revised for pain after 45 months duration, exhibited severe wear over a portion of the anterior and posterior post surface without evidence of similar articular surface wear (◘ Fig. 14-4). Intra-operative records made during explantation of this component describe an inflammatory cyst and generalized reactive synovitis with appreciable evidence of polyethylene debris.

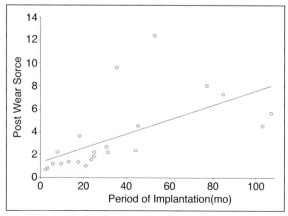

◘ **Fig. 14-5.** Post wear score and period of implantation for all implants. Pearson product-moment correlation coefficient, r=0.61

◻ **Table 14-2.** Implant demographics and tibial post wear scores

Implant	Model	Manufacturer	Material	Sterilization	Period (months)	Revision diagnosis	Post wear score (PWS)
1	Kinemax	Howmedica	UHMWPE	Gamma	33.6	Aseptic loosening	N/A
2	Kinemax	Howmedica	UHMWPE	Gamma	5.8	Instability	1.2
3	Kinemax	Howmedica	UHMWPE	Gamma	25.0	Infection	2.1
4	Kinemax	Howmedica	UHMWPE	Gamma	107.2	Aseptic loosening	5.6
5	Kinemax	Howmedica	UHMWPE	Gamma	77.1	Instability	8.0
6	Kinematic II	Howmedica	UHMWPE	Gamma	53.0	Osteolysis	12.4
7	Kinematic I	Howmedica	UHMWPE	Gamma	103.3	Aseptic loosening	4.5
8	CCK	Zimmer	UHMWPE	N/A	18.4	Aseptic loosening	3.6
9	IB II	Zimmer	UHMWPE	N/A	17.7	Infection	1.4
10	Genesis II	Smith & Nephew	UHMWPE	ETO	3.5	Stiffness	0.8
11	Genesis II	Smith & Nephew	UHMWPE	ETO	23.6	Pain	1.6
12	Genesis II	Smith & Nephew	UHMWPE	ETO	2.3	Infection	0.7
13	Genesis	Smith & Nephew	UHMWPE	ETO	31.3	Infection	2.2
14	Genesis	Smith & Nephew	UHMWPE	Gamma	84.8	Recurrent effusion	7.3
15	Genesis	Smith & Nephew	UHMWPE	Gamma	35.4	Instability	9.6
16	Genesis	Smith & Nephew	UHMWPE	ETO	30.7	Aseptic loosening	2.7
17	AMK	Depuy	UHMWPE	Gas plasma	9.8	Infection	1.2
18	AMK	Depuy	UHMWPE	Gamma	45.3	Pain	4.5
19	Coordinate	Depuy	Hylamer	Gas plasma	21.2	Infection	1.0
20	Coordinate	Depuy	Hylamer	Gamma	8.0	Infection	2.2
21	Coordinate	Depuy	Hylamer	Gamma	24.7	Aseptic loosening	1.9
22	Coordinate	Depuy	Hylamer	Gamma	13.1	Instability	1.4
23	Coordinate	Depuy	Hylamer	Gamma	44.1	Instability	2.4

tween design types. Similarly, no significant differences in normalized post wear scores were noted when comparing inserts manufactured from Hylamer or standard UHMWPE, or between sterilization procedures. The normalized PWS for heat-pressed inserts were appreciably higher than the non-heat-pressed inserts, but with the small numbers available, no significance was determined.

Average wear score and period of implantation in components revised for infection was 1.56 (±0.65), aseptic loosening was 3.7 (±1.48), osteolysis was 12.4; pain was 2.29 (±1.96), instability was 4.5 (±3.98), and recurrent effusions was 7.2. With the small sample size and absence of complete tibial surface analysis, significance of testing of post-wear score and revision diagnosis would be irrelevant. It was noted, however, that implants revised for sepsis did exhibit normalized wear scores and wear patterns similar to those of the rest of the cohort. Fatigue wear was not observed over the post in any of the implants revised for infection, but the average duration was relatively short; 16.5 (range, 2.3-31.3).

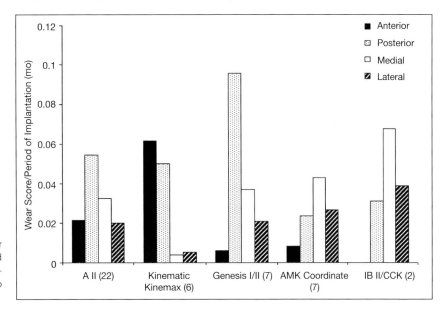

◻ **Fig. 14-6.** Mean normalized wear scores by surface location combined for all implants and for individual designs. Number of implants per group in parentheses

Wear occurred over all four surfaces of the post and the prevalence varied between implant designs (◘ Fig. 14-6). The most predominant location of wear and highest wear scores occurred over the posterior surface, prevalent in all 22 (100%) of the inserts with a mean wear score of 1.86 (±1.53). The incidence of anterior wear was not insignificant, occurring in eight (36%) of the implants with a mean wear score of 0.93 (±1.56). The overall extent of anterior wear was skewed by the high incidence and severity of wear in the group of Kinematic/Kinemax (Howmedica, Rutherford, NJ) inserts. All six of these inserts (100%) had evidence of anterior wear and exhibited significantly ($p<0.05$) higher normalized wear scores over the anterior surface when compared with the other designs.

With the numbers available, no significant difference between medial and lateral post wear was identified. The predominant morphology of wear over the medial and lateral surfaces was burnishing, with minimal evidence of fatigue. Posts with a relatively wider medial-lateral dimension had increased evidence of damage over these surfaces. This was evident in six implants, five Co-ordinate (DePuy, Warsaw, IN) and one CCK (Zimmer, Warsaw, IN), which had ultra-constraining posts used to resist varus-valgus deformity and to limit tibial rotation to a few degrees. Normalized wear scores were substantially higher over the medial and lateral surfaces of these constrained posts when compared with wear scores over the same regions from implants of a similar model type (◘ Fig. 14-7). This is evident in the relatively high mean scores in the two groups containing these implants (see Fig. 14-6). In two cases, significant wear of either the medial or lateral articular surface appeared to have caused a mild varus-valgus deformity, which appeared to accelerate wear over the opposite surface of the post.

Wear occurred over all four surfaces of the post, but the prevalence varied among implant designs. The most predominant location of wear was the posterior surface, and this was found to be worn in all 22 inserts. Anterior wear was noted in 36% (eight of the 22 implants). Medial-lateral wear of the post was common; the predominant morphology was burnishing. Medial-lateral wear was worse in the six varus/valgus constrained implants.

We can conclude that PCL-sacrificing post-cam devices may contribute to the production of additional wear debris and be associated with negative outcomes such as reactive synovitis, aseptic loosening, and osteolysis. The surgeon should be aware that the cam-post interface is not an innocuous articulation. Manufacturers should strive to limit wear and damage to these components. Finally, highly congruent varus/valgus designs demonstrate increased wear and should be used with caution.

Clinical Studies

Mikulak et al. analyzed 557 consecutive press-fit condylar modular knee prostheses with a PCL-substituting design (PFC, Johnson & Johnson Orthopaedics, Raynham, MA) implanted by a single surgeon between July 20, 1989 and October 14, 1994 [10]. All knees were inserted according to a standard protocol. At a mean of 56 months (37-89 months) postoperatively, 22 (3.9%) of the 557 primary knee arthroplasties had been revised. Four (0.7%) were revised because of infection, two (0.4%) because of a supracondylar fracture, and 16 (2.9%) because of aseptic loosening and osteolysis.

The authors went on to provide a detailed description of the 16 knee replacements (15 patients) which had been revised because of aseptic loosening. The study population of failed total knee arthroplasties was made up of eight women and seven men with a mean age of 65 years (46-80 years). All patients were doing well at 1 year, with Knee Society clinical and functional scores of 95 and 86 points, respectively. These scores declined to 48 and 45 points, respectively, prior to revision. Six patients had isolated loosening of the femoral component with osteolysis, six had loosening of both the femoral and tibial components with osteolysis, and two had isolated loosening of the tibial component with osteolysis. At retrieval, the machine marks on the posterior aspect of the polyethylene post were preserved in six of the 12 retrieved polyethylene inserts, indicating a lack of substantial repetitive contact between the tibial post and the femoral cam of the components. All 12 inserts had burnishing on both the medial and lateral aspects of the tibial post. In ten of the 12 knees, grooves of variable depth associated with burnishing and delamination were found at the anteromedial and anterolateral edges of the post. A horizontal burnished groove across the anteroinferior aspect of the polyethylene post was seen in nine of the 12 inserts. With as little as a 1-mm reduction in the thickness of the tibial condylar polyethylene, the top of the tibial post impinged on the roof of the femoral box housing. An

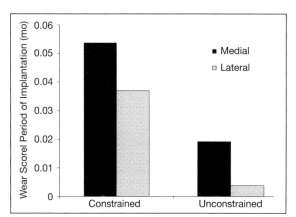

◘ **Fig. 14-7.** Normalized mean wear scores from medial and lateral surfaces of *constrained* (CCK, Co-ordinate) and *unconstrained* (AMK, Insall-Burstein II) inserts of same manufacturer and similar modular design

asymmetric loss of polyethylene from the top of the post reflected this impingement. Overall, patient activity, younger age, and greater height were correlated with increased wear on the medial side of the tibial insert. So-called backside wear was seen on all 12 of the tibial polyethylene inserts.

In summary, this clinical study made several interesting observations with regard to the post-cam mechanism in this particular PCL-substituting total knee arthroplasty. Six of the 12 retrieved tibial components demonstrated little evidence of cam-post engagement, despite a good range of motion. When the cam-post mechanism did engage, as suggested by wear on the posterior aspect of the tibial polyethylene post, none of these patients revealed any type of surface damage on the articulating or back sides of the tibial insert, suggesting that when the cam-post mechanism works, the vector sum of the tibial femoral forces and the cam-post forces are compression into the tibia. The authors also found evidence of surface damage to the medial and lateral sides and base of all posts retrieved. With the design of total knee replacements studied, the authors concluded that rotational forces generated by impingement of the side walls of the intracondylar box on the polyethylene post produced surface damage. The authors also demonstrated that the top of the polyethylene post could impinge in the roof of the box in the femoral component if even minimal wear occurred in the polyethylene insert. The authors ended this study by implicating rotational constraint in post-cam types of PCL-substituting total knee arthroplasties as a cause of post wear and the transmission of rotational stresses to the modular interfaces resulting in wear into the bone-implant interfaces, potentially resulting in loosening.

References

1. Blunn GW, Joshi AB, Minns RJ., Lidgren L, Lilley P, Ryd L, Engelbrecht E, Walker PS (1997) Wear in retrieved condylar knee arthroplasties. A comparison of wear in different designs of 280 retrieved condylar knee prostheses. J Arthroplasty 12:281-290
2. Colizza WA, Insall JN, Scuderi GR (1995) The posterior stabilized total knee prosthesis. Assessment of polyethylene damage and osteolysis after a ten-year minimum follow-up. J Bone Joint Surg [Am] 77:1713-1720
3. Diduch DR, Insall JN, Scott WN, Scuderi GR, Font-Rodriguez D (1997) Total knee replacement in young, active patients. Long-term follow-up and functional outcomes. J Bone Joint Surg [Am] 79:575-582
4. Font-Rodriguez DE, Scuderi GR, Insall JN (1997) Survivorship of cemented total knee arthroplasty. Clin Orthop 345:79-86
5. Hirsch HS, Lotke PA, Morrison LD (1994) The posterior cruciate ligament in total knee surgery. Save, sacrifice, or substitute? Clin Orthop 309:64-68
6. Insall JN, Lachiewicz PF, Burstein AH (1982) The posterior stabilized condylar prosthesis: a modification of the total condylar design. Two to four year clinical experience. J Bone Joint Surg [Am] 64:1317-1323
7. Laskin RS, Maruyama Y, Villaneuva M, Bourne RB (2000) Deep-dish congruent tibial component use in total knee arthroplasty. A randomized prospective study. Clin Orthop 38:36-44
8. Lewis P, Rorabeck CH, Bourne RB, Devane P (1994) Posteriomedial tibial polyethylene failure in total knee replacements. Clin Orthop 299:11-17
9. Martin SD, McManus JL, Scott RD, Thornhill TS (1997) Press-fit condylar total knee arthroplasty: 5- to 9-year follow-up evaluation. J Arthroplasty 12:603-614
10. Mikulak SA, Mahoney OM, Dela Rosa MA, Schmalzreid TP (2001) Loosening and osteolysis with the press-fit condylar posterior-cruciate substituting total knee replacement. J Bone Joint Surg [Am] 83:398-403
11. Puloski SKT, McCalden RW, MacDonald SJ, Rorabeck CH, Bourne RB (2001) Tibial post wear in posterior stabilized total knee arthroplasty. An unrecognized source of polyethylene debris. J Bone Joint Surg [Am] 83:390-397
12. Ranawat CS, Luessenhop CP, Rodriguez JA (1997) The press-fit condylar modular total knee system. Four to six year results with a posterior-cruciate-substituting design. J Bone Joint Surg [Am] 79:342-348
13. Ritter MA, Campbell E, Faris PM, Keating EM (1989) Long-term survivor analysis of the posterior cruciate condylar total knee arthroplasty. A 10-year evaluation. J Arthroplasty 4:293-296
14. Schai PA, Thornhill TS, Scott RD (1998) Total knee arthroplasty with the PFC system. Results at a minimum of ten years and survivorship analysis. J Bone Joint Surg [Br] 80:850-858
15. Stiehl JB, Dennis DA, Komistek RD, Crane HS (1999) In vivo determination of condylar lift-off and screw-home in a mobile-bearing total knee arthroplasty. J Arthroplasty 14:293-299
16. Wright TM, Bartel DL (1986) The problem of surface damage in polyethylene total knee components. Clin Orthop 205:67-74

15 Flexion Instability

J. Bellemans

Summary

Mid-flexion instability is an issue that has only recently gained the attention of knee arthroplasty surgeons. It is a not uncommon problem which has been overlooked in the past, and which has probably been responsible for a relatively large number of patients with poor outcome after TKA surgery. Despite the former belief that mid-flexion instability was a rather vague and poorly defined concept, recent advances in knowledge about the function of the normal and the prosthetic knee have clarified this problem, with regard not only to its diagnosis, but also to the appropriate treatment and prevention.

Introduction

Flexion instability can be defined as: "The presence of excessive laxity in flexion after TKA. Such laxity can be present in the anteroposterior direction, the mediolateral direction, or both. Normal stability is noted in extension. Depending on the degree of flexion at which excessive laxity is noted, the instability is defined as early-flexion instability (at 30°-60°) or mid-flexion instability (90°)".

Flexion instability can be caused by many factors. In most cases, however, it is either the consequence of an important mismatch between the flexion and extension space or the result of PCL insufficiency. It is therefore important to carefully assess the directions of the instability, since a flexion-extension gap mismatch will provoke not only anteroposterior but also mediolateral laxity, while in the case of PCL insufficiency only anteroposterior laxity will be seen.

Causal Factors

Inadequate flexion and extension gap balancing is probably the most frequent cause of mid-flexion instability. Most surgeons today realize that one of the most important issues in the surgical TKA technique is adequate creation of the flexion and extension spaces. These spaces are defined as the opening of the knee joint space after completion of the bone cuts, while the knee is held in extension (extension space) or flexion (flexion space). These spaces are subsequently filled up by the prosthetic components, and their size is therefore critical since too large a space may lead to underfilling by the prosthetic components, with insufficient soft-tissue tension and instability as the result.

Since most contemporary knee arthroplasty designs have an identical thickness of metal on their extension and flexion regions, the creation of the flexion and extension spaces should therefore be equal in size. Despite the fact that the amount of bone resection is controlled by the surgeon, reality shows that unequal flexion and extension spaces are not seldom obtained during TKA surgery.

In the specific case where the flexion space is left much larger than the extension space, the surgeon does not have the option of filling up the flexion space with a thicker insert, since this will prevent the knee from extending. Instead, he will tend to use the appropriate insert thickness for extension, with the consequence of underfilling the flexion space and flexion instability (◻ Fig. 15-1).

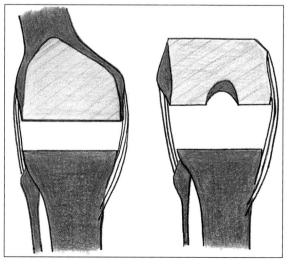

◻ **Fig. 15-1.** Flexion space too large compared with extension space

□ Table 15-1. Causal factors in mid-flexion instability

— Flexion space > extension space
  – Insufficient resection of distal femur
  – Undersized femoral component (anterior referenced)
  – Anteriorization of femoral component
  – Femoral component positioned in extension
  – Excessive tibial slope
  – Insufficient posterior condylar offset
— PCL insufficiency

Several factors can contribute to the intraoperative creation of an excessive flexion space (□ Table 15-1). For example, insufficient distal femoral bone resection will lead to a relatively small extension space, unless more proximal tibia is resected. The latter will not reduce the imbalance with the flexion space, however.

Excessive resection of the posterior condylar bone should also be avoided, since this increases the flexion space while the extension space is unaltered. Such over-resection occurs relatively frequently when an anterior referencing technique is used, since most surgical technical guides suggest the use of the smaller femoral component when in between two sizes.

Anterior or extension placement of the femoral component has the same effect of enlarging the flexion space, while the extension space remains unaltered (see Fig. 15-6). In this regard, we have previously described the so-called posterior condylar offset as an important parameter [1-3].

Posterior Condylar Offset

The posterior condylar offset is defined as the maximal thickness of the posterior condyle, projected posteriorly to the tangential of the posterior cortex of the femoral shaft, and it can be measured easily on a lateral radiograph (□ Fig. 15-2). It is obviously an important factor with regard to the flexion space.

Decreasing the posterior condylar offset excessively during TKA surgery may lead to a loose flexion space and flexion instability. In the same way, decreasing the posterior condylar offset will slacken the PCL, with relative PCL insufficiency as a consequence. This mechanism is responsible for the so-called paradoxical roll-forward of the femur that is noted in the majority of contemporary PCL-retaining TKAs. The slackened PCL is indeed, in this situation, not capable of provoking the normal roll-back of the femur, which instead will slide forward during flexion (□ Fig. 15-3).

A last causal factor is excessive down-sloping of the tibial component. The reason why extra sloping of the tibial component may lead to flexion instability is three-fold. First, down-sloping leads to extra space in the pos-

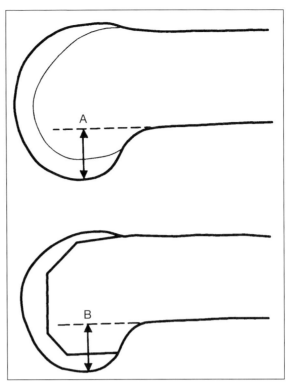

□ Fig. 15-2. Measurement of posterior condylar offset (*A*) before and (*B*) after operation. (Reprinted, with permission, from [3])

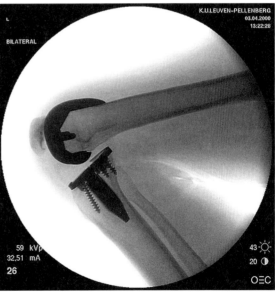

□ Fig. 15-3. Paradoxical roll-forward of the femur due to relative PCL insufficiency (Reprinted, with permission, from [3])

terior aspect of the joint, which is where the femorotibial contact points will be during flexion. In extension the contact points are located anterior. Down-sloping the tibia therefore tends to loosen the knee in flexion, without influencing the knee in extension.

Second, excessive slope on the tibial bone cut will damage the proximal insertion of the PCL fibers on the tibia, which weakens the PCL. Third, sloping the tibia leads to an increased overall anteroposterior laxity. This has been substantiated by M. Bonnin, who determined that for every degree of tibial slope, an extra 0.6 mm of anteroposterior laxity is induced [4].

Diagnosis

Although the diagnosis of flexion instability may be obvious in severe cases, it is important to realize that some patients will present somewhere in the continuum between normal laxity and excessive instability (◘ Table 15-2). In more subtle cases the diagnosis may be less obvious, but fortunately, these patients can usually accept their situation and seldom require revision surgery.

In more serious cases the symptoms are usually such that the patient will seek further help. Typically, the patient will complain of a rather poorly specified feeling of general discomfort or pain in the knee, sometimes together with a feeling of instability or lack of confidence in the replaced knee. Usually, there are also signs of synovial inflammation, such as recurrent effusions and periarticular soft-tissue swelling. Load-bearing activities in flexion are usually difficult, for example descending stairs or rising from a chair.

On clinical examination a marked anteroposterior laxity is present during the anteroposterior drawer test with the knee in 90° of flexion. When varus and valgus stress testing in flexion demonstrates excessive laxity as well, the mid-flexion instability is the consequence of an

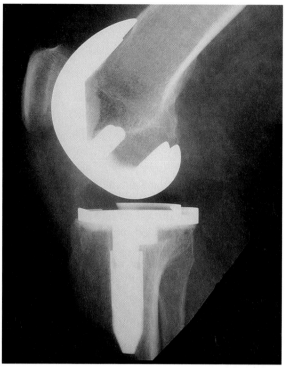

◘ **Fig. 15-4.** Weight-bearing radiograph of a patient with early-flexion instability: Paradoxical slide-forward of the femoral component is already present in early flexion

◘ **Table 15-2.** Diagnostic characteristics of the patient with mid-flexion instability

- Symptoms
  - Discomfort or pain
  - Lack of confidence in knee
  - Recurrent effusions and soft-tissue swelling
  - Problematic stair descent/ascent and chair rise
- Clinical examination
  - Excessive laxity on AP drawer test (90° flexion)
  - Excessive laxity on varus/valgus stress in flexion, not in extension
  - Effusion
- Radiographic signs
  - Paradoxical slide-forward of femoral component on weight-bearing X-rays (0° and 90° flexion)
  - Radiographic evidence of causal factors:
    - undersized femoral component
    - anterior position of femoral component
    - extension position of femoral component
    - decreased posterior condylar offset
    - excessive tibial slope
    - PCL-retaining implant
- Other technical investigations (joint fluid/blood sample/scintigraphy)
  - Negative

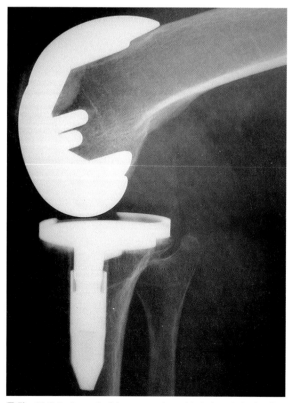

◘ **Fig. 15-5.** Radiograph of the same patient with the knee in further flexion, showing even more paradoxical slide-forward of the femoral component

15

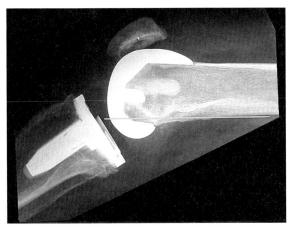

Fig. 15-6. Poor restoration of posterior condylar offset, with extension positioning of femoral component

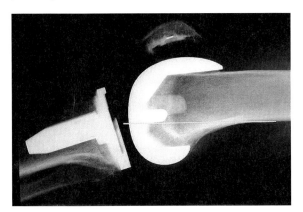

Fig. 15-7. Adequate restoration of posterior condylar offset

◘ **Table 15-3.** Intra-operative correction of mid-flexion instability during primary TKA

In case of combined AP and varus/valgus laxity:
– Use larger femoral component (anterior referenced)
– Flex the femoral component (max. 5°)
– Resect more distal femur and use thicker insert
In case of isolated AP laxity (stable on varus/valgus stress):
– Use posterior-stabilized implant
– Reduce tibial slope

reduced, while the arthrotomy is temporarily closed with the help of two towel clamps.

At the same time, varus and valgus stress testing should be performed in flexion, and joint line opening should be assessed. Any anteroposterior play greater than 10 mm should not be accepted, while medial and lateral joint line opening should not exceed 5 mm. Asymmetrical opening on either the medial or the lateral side greater than 5 mm is frequently not a major problem, but when both sides open more than 5 mm the patient is at very high risk of developing mid-flexion instability.

From a strategic standpoint it is important to assess both anteroposterior and varus/valgus laxity. For example, if both AP and varus/valgus laxity are present an excessive flexion space is the problem, and the surgeon should therefore aim to reduce the flexion space or to increase the extension space. This can be achieved by several methods. Choosing a larger femoral component is one of the easiest options, but care should be taken to avoid mediolateral component overhang, since this may cause pain by irritating the retinacular structures.

Flexing the femoral component is another was of reducing the flexion space and can be performed without adverse effects as long as one stays within 5° of flexion with reference to the intramedullary axis. Resecting more distal femur will also be helpful, since this increases the extension space and allows the use of a thicker tibial insert.

If the joint is stable on varus/valgus testing in flexion but shows excessive anteroposterior laxity on the drawer test, insufficiency of the PCL is the problem. The surgeon should therefore switch to a posterior-stabilized implant to compensate for the PCL insufficiency. Reducing the tibial slope will thereby be of further help, since this will additionally reduce the anterior laxity.

excessive flexion space problem. When such varus/valgus stress testing is normal while the anteroposterior drawer test is markedly positive, PCL insufficiency is responsible for the flexion instability. Standard weight-bearing radiographs in extension and at 30°, 60°, and 90° of flexion will demonstrate a paradoxical anterior translation of the femoral component, together with one or more of the causal factors that were described above (◘ Figs. 15-4 and 15-5).

Typically, an important reduction in posterior condylar offset will be noted (◘ Figs. 15-6 and 15-7). Further technical investigations such as joint fluid analysis, CRP, and sedimentation rate, but also bone scintigraphy, will be normal.

Intra-operative Strategy

The presence of mid-flexion laxity can usually be detected during the primary TKA surgery when the surgeon is aware of this potential problem (◘ Table 15-3). It is sufficient to perform a standard AP drawer test in 90° of flexion, once the trial implants are inserted and the patella is

Revision for Mid-flexion Instability

The same principles can be applied when revising a knee with mid-flexion instability (◘ Table 15-4). Most often the primary knee will be a PCL-retaining design, although occasionally a posterior stabilized implant may require re-intervention for mid-flexion instability.

☐ **Table 15-4.** Revision for mid-flexion instability

In case of combined AP and varus/valgus laxity:
– Start revising femoral component
– Restore posterior condylar offset
  – upsize femoral component
  – position femoral component in slight flexion (max. 5°)
– Slightly proximalize new femoral component (occurs almost automatically)
– Consider additional tibial revision with:
  – switch to posterior-stabilized insert
  – less down-slope
– Consider constraint implant if the above is not sufficient (CCK/rotating hinge)
In case of isolated AP laxity (stable on varus/valgus stress):
– Exchange insert to posterior-stabilized (cam-post or deep dished)
– Reduce tibial slope

Again, one should differentiate between (a) excessive laxity in AP direction and varus/valgus laxity - which means that an excessive flexion space is the problem, or (b) isolated AP laxity with normal varus/valgus stability - which means that PCL insufficiency is the problem. In the first situation (AP + varus/valgus laxity) revision of only the femoral component with restoration of the posterior condylar offset may be sufficient in less severe cases. This again can be achieved by upsizing the femoral component and inserting it with a little flexion. When this is done, some beneficial proximalization of the distal femoral cut is usually automatically achieved, which will open the extension space and allow the use of a thicker insert.

If the tibial base plate allows, a posterior-stabilized insert can be inserted to improve the anteroposterior laxity. If this is not the case, revision of the tibial component may be necessary, while the revision tibial implant is inserted with less down-slope. In extreme cases, where the above-mentioned steps have proven to be insufficient, a constrained-type insert (CCK) or rotating hinge should be considered.

In the second situation (isolated AP laxity), exchanging the tibial polyethylene insert for a posterior-stabilized insert is almost always sufficient. This can be achieved by using a standard cam-post or deeply dished design. When this requires changing the tibial base plate, one should again attempt to reduce the slope.

Conclusion

Mid-flexion instability is a not uncommon problem after TKA. The knee arthroplasty surgeon should be familiar with this entity and should be able to recognize and adequately address it during the primary procedure. In this chapter we have described the diagnostic and strategic principles that can be used as guidelines when faced with this problem.

References

1. Banks S et al (2003) Knee motions during maximum flexion in fixed and mobile bearing arthroplasties. Clin Orthop Rel Res 410:131-138
2. Banks et al (2003) Making sense of knee arthroplasty kinematics: news you can use. J Bone Joint Surg [Am] 85:64-72
3. Bellemans J et al (2002) Fluoroscopic analysis of the kinematics of deep flexion in total knee arthroplasty. The influence of posterior condylar offset. J Bone Joint Surg [Br] 84:50-53
4. Bonnin M (1990) La subluxation tibial antérieure en appui monopodal dans les ruptures du ligaments croisés antérieure. Etude clinique et bioméchanique. Thèse Med. Lyon, n° 180

15

16 Lessons Learned from Cementless Fixation

G. L. Rasmussen

Summary

For any implant system, evaluating the causes of past failure is the best way to determine necessary improvements for future success. Even though cemented fixation of total knee arthroplasties has become the standard for comparison, the plateau of success for this form of fixation has been reached. Cementless fixation has the potential to reach higher levels of success. This chapter, by reviewing the causes of past failures, addresses ways of achieving higher levels of success with cementless fixation of total knee arthroplasties.

Introduction

Cemented fixation of total knee arthroplasties has become the standard to which all other forms of fixation must be compared. Cemented fixation has produced consistent reliable results and – on a percentage basis – better knee rating scores and better longevity than cementless fixation [1-3]. However, when factors of "ideal fixation" of total knee arthroplasty (TKA) are taken into account, such as osseointegration (biocompatibility), risk of infection, longevity with high-demand activities [4], less invasive surgery, skeletal augmentation, and ease of revision without significant bone loss, cemented fixation falls short. Therefore, these problems will most likely be solved in the future through cementless fixation. This chapter reviews: (a) an abridged history of cementless TKA including lessons learned, (b) the author's experience, and (c) new technology which should lead to better success rates.

History

Assisted by Boyd, Campbell developed and implanted Vitallium (cobalt chromium alloy, CoCr) femoral interposition-mold arthroplasty plates. He reported the preliminary results in 1940 [5]. Smith-Petersen also developed and implanted femoral Vitallium-mold arthroplasties [6]. The Massachusetts General Hospital (MGH) femoral mold arthroplasty was reported in 1967 [7]. In 1952, Mc-Keever and Elliot [8] developed a tibial plateau prosthesis consisting of unicompartmental metal (Vitallium) spacers with a short truncated T-shaped keel which fixed into slots made in the tibial condyle. The MacIntosh hemiarthroplasty 1954 [9] consisted first of acrylic and later of CoCr metal discs inserted between the femur and the tibia. In 1953, Townley [10] designed a tibial metal articular plate hemiarthroplasty fixed with screws. While an improvement for the time, these designs all had a high percentage of suboptimal results and failures.

Cementless-hinge total knee arthroplasty was popularized by Walldius. The first joints he implanted in 1951 were made of acrylic. By 1958 he had converted to stemmed metal (first stainless steel and later CoCr) hinge joints [11]. Subsequently, several other surgeons developed modifications of the Walldius hinge design. Hinge knee arthroplasties have had a high incidence of loosening because the increased constraint causes greater implant bone-interface forces.

The first cementless condylar total knee arthroplasties were the Kodama-Yamamoto [12], the Imperial College London Hospital (ICLH) in 1977 (Freeman) [13], the "Ring" prosthesis also in 1977 [14], the Low Contact Stress (LCS) in 1978 (Buechel and Pappas) [15] (DePuy, Warsaw, IN), the Porous Coated Anatomic (PCA) in 1980 (Hungerford, Kenna, and Krackow) [16] (Howmedica, Rutherford, NJ), the Anatomic Total Knee (ATK) in 1980 (Townley) [10], the Ortholoc I in 1982 (Whiteside) [17] (Wright Medical Technology, Arlington, TN), the Tricon-M (Smith & Nephew, Memphis, TN) in 1983 (Laskin) [18], the Miller-Galante (MG-I) in 1984 [19] (Zimmer, Warsaw, IN), the Anatomic Graduated Component (AGC) in 1984 (Ritter, Keating and Faris) [20] (Biomet, Warsaw, IN), the Press Fit Condylar (PFC) in 1985 (Scott and Thornhill) [21] (Depuy, Warsaw, IN), the Natural-Knee in 1985 (Hofmann) [22] (Zimmer, Warsaw, IN), and the Genesis I in 1988 (Smith & Nephew, Memphis, TN).

Most failures of cementless TKA have been the result of either suboptimally designed metal-backed patellar components or loosening and wear of the tibial base. Many of the patellar components had an endoskeleton of metal with thin polyethylene. Early wear of the polyethylene down to metal or dissociation of the polyethylene from the metal backing resulted in a high revision rate. Tibial component loosening was primarily the result of failure to achieve both primary and secondary fixation. Loosening and wear have often led to significant osteolysis. The patellar problem can be solved by not resurfacing the patella, by cementing an all-polyethylene patella, or by using a metal-backed design with thicker polyethylene and without an endoskeleton of metal. Hence, tibial component fixation is, in the author's opinion, the primary challenge to achieving success with cementless TKA. Therefore, cementless tibial component fixation will be the emphasis of this chapter. It is important to note that cementless TKA implants vary widely in both materials and design. Generalizations about this broad category are not always appropriate. If one cementless TKA design has a high failure rate, similar designs and materials may also have the same results. However, this does not mean all cementless TKA designs will have a high failure rate.

Lessons Learned from Early Cementless TKA Designs

The ICLH Knee used finned polyethylene pegs for fixation. This knee was a roller in a trough design. The knee was subsequently modified to the Freeman-Samuelson Knee (FS), a condylar design with a patellar groove, which also used finned polyethylene pegs for fixation. The patella was resurfaced with an all polyethylene finned peg component. The tibial component was initially all polyethylene with finned pegs. Over time it became apparent that the polyethylene-bone interface was not ideal. Therefore, the tibial component was later modified to a metal-backed component. It is noteworthy that the finned peg polyethylene patellar component has had a better survival rate than many metal-backed patellar components. Subsequently, a stem was added to the tibial metal base. The metal base and stem did not have a porous ingrowth surface. The CoCr femoral component, which also did not have a porous ingrowth surface, used two polyethylene pegs for fixation. These knees had a higher incidence of loosening and lower knee rating scores than comparable cemented condylar knees.

The Tricon-M Knee developed in the early 1980s also used finned polyethylene pegs for primary fixation. This knee had metal-backed tibial and patellar components. In addition to the finned polyethylene pegs, the femoral, tibial, and patellar components of the Tricon-M knee had a porous bead ingrowth surface for secondary fixation. This knee seemed to do better than the cementless ICLH or FS, presumably because of the secondary fixation of the porous beads.

The cementless LCS knee has had a better survival rate than most [23]. This is likely due to a tibial component with a central stem or keel that was porous coated, which was different from most other early cementless knees. Reduced bone-implant interface forces due to the meniscal-bearing or rotating-platform design may also have contributed to the low incidence of loosening. Controversy still exists regarding which are better: mobile or fixed bearings. Dislocating mobile bearings and mobile bearing wear have been an issue.

The PCA knee used CoCr femoral, tibial, and patellar components with pegs. The bone-interface surfaces and pegs were coated with porous beads for bone ingrowth. The tibial base did not have a stem/keel. The early results were promising; however, pain scores were slower to improve and subsequently, compared with cemented condylar knees, a higher loosening rate of the patellar and tibial components occurred. The femoral component compared favorably with cemented femoral components [24].

The Miller-Galante Knee used titanium alloy (Ti) femoral, tibial, and patellar components with titanium fiber metal mesh for bone ingrowth. The tibial base did not have a stem/keel. As with the PCA, pain scores were slower to improve and a higher loosening rate was seen. However, also as with the PCA, a suboptimal patellar component design led to a high incidence of patellar failures. The incidence of patellar failure was higher than tibial component failure, which was higher than femoral component failure [25].

The Ortholoc I Knee made of CoCr used smooth pegs and a stem for early fixation and a porous tibial base undersurface for secondary fixation. In the Ortholoc II, tibial component fixation was enhanced with four peripheral screws [17]. Long-term follow-up results of the Ortholoc Knee implanted without a metal-backed patella have been good [26].

The cementless AGC Knee tibial component was CoCr with a central smooth I-beam stem/keel press fit without screws. The undersurface of the tibial base was porous coated [20]. Early and apparently late postoperative results suggest knee scores to be much lower than the scores for the cemented prosthesis [27].

The cementless PFC Knee titanium tibial base had a smooth central finned stem/keel and a porous undersurface. The early results were equivalent to those with the cemented knee, but with time a significantly higher revision rate was found in the uncemented knees [28].

The early design of the Natural Knee was a titanium metal femoral component, with Ti metal-backed patellar and tibial components. The tibial component was fixed with four peripheral spikes and two screws. The bone interface surfaces were coated with cancellous structured titanium [22]. Later, the tibia was modified with the addition of a smooth central finned stem/keel. The long-term follow-up of the later design has been good [29].

Author's Experience

My experience with cementless TKA began with the Freeman-Samuelson Knee (FS). The first two TKAs I performed in private practice, in 1985, were fully cementless in a patient with RA. These knees are doing well and still surviving nearly 20 years later (◘ Fig. 16-1). However, due to overall suboptimal pain and function scores, in 1988 I changed to the cementless Genesis I Knee (Smith & Nephew, Memphis, TN). This ponons-coated knee was made of "state-of-the-art" materials (CoCr femoral component and titanium tibial component) and had a metal-backed patellar component that was a better design than most. There was no endoskeleton of metal with thin polyethylene. This knee worked better, with knee scores that were improved over the FS; however, the knee scores were not as good as a comparable series of cemented Genesis I knees. Radiographs of the cementless Genesis I knees showed a significant incidence of radiolucent lines around the smooth tibial stem (◘ Fig. 16-2).

The bone-prosthesis interface around the central stem/keel is a good indicator of the fixation of the component. I took part in an IDE study comparing the Genesis I tibial base with and without hydroxyapatite (HA) coating. The HA-coated knees did better than the non-HA-coated knees. Radiographs showed no lucent lines around the tibial stem. In fact, the HA-coated knees scored as well as the cemented Genesis I knees (◘ Fig. 16-3).

In 1995 we evaluated knee fixation in the Biomechanics Research Institute at our hospital (The Orthopedic Specialty Hospital, TOSH). The best cementless fixation of a tibial base to cadaver bone was achieved with a component that had a central stem/keel, peripheral pegs or spikes, and four screws. The Advantim Knee

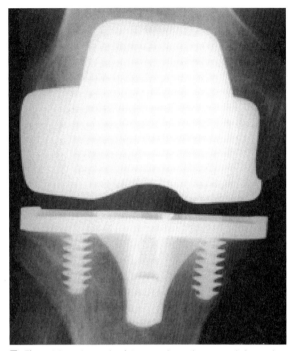

◘ **Fig. 16-2.** Radiograph of Genesis I knee showing radiolucent line around the tibial stem

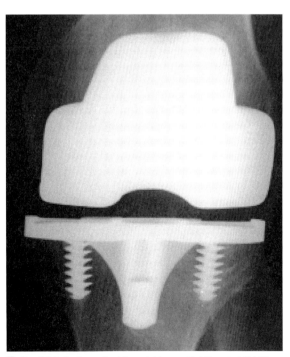

◘ **Fig. 16-3.** Radiograph of Genesis I knee with HA-coated tibial base plate. No radiolucent line is present around the tibial stem

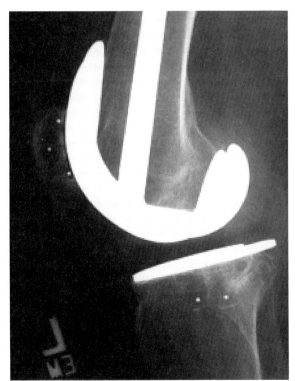

◘ **Fig. 16-1.** Radiograph of cementless FS knee implanted for nearly 20 years

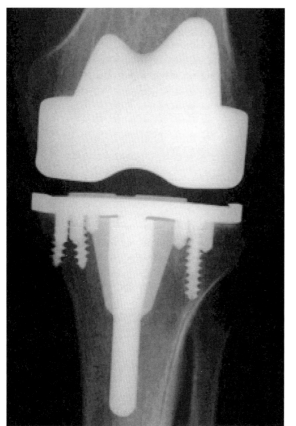

Fig. 16-4. Radiograph of cementless Advantim knee

formed with PMMA cement (incidence of infection less than 0.3% compared with 1%).

Rationale for Currrent Designs

Experience with cementless implants has shown that bone prefers rough surfaces to smooth for ongrowth or ingrowth. In 1997, I implanted a series of ProFix Knees (Smith & Nephew Memphis, TN). The ProFix Ti tibial base has a central corundum blasted stem with peripheral spikes and four screws for fixation (Fig. 16-5).

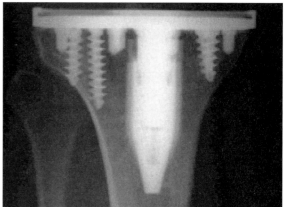

Fig. 16-5. Radiograph of Profix knee showing no radiolucent line around the tibial stem

(Wright Medical Arlington, TN), met these design criteria (Fig. 16-4). The other knee that met these design criteria at the time was the Natural Knee. Clinical experience correlated with the biomechanical studies. The knee scores of the Advantim knee proved to be better than those of the cementless non-HA-coated Genesis I knee, but not as good as those of the cemented Genesis I series. Also, radiographs of the Advantim knees show a lower, but still a significant incidence of lucent lines around the smooth central tibial stem.

The author's experience with infection rates in cemented versus cementless TKA is as follows. In 1981, as part of a fixation study, I implanted bilateral TKAs in ten dogs. One knee was implanted with cement and the contralateral knee was implanted without cement. Nine of ten cemented knees became infected, but only one cementless knee became infected. The one cementless knee that became infected did so only after the contralateral cemented knee had first developed an infection. These results correlate with Petty's finding that methylmethacrylate (PMMA) bone cement has a negative immunological effect [30, 31]. Infection rates are difficult to evaluate but, the infection rate at TOSH, where most TKAs are performed without PMMA cement, have been lower than at other hospitals in the area where most TKAs are per-

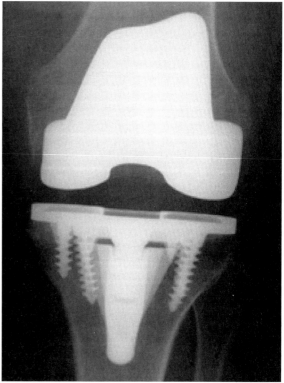

Fig. 16-6. Radiograph of Genesis II knee showing no radiolucent line around the tibial stem

The results of this cementless clinical series were the best to date. No lucent lines have been observed around the central stem. The solution seems to lie in having an aggressive stem/keel with a rough surface. This finding may explain the good results obtained with the cementless LCS knee.

Since 1999 I have implanted a series of Genesis II (Smith & Nephew Memphis, TN) cementless knees (◘ Fig. 16-6) and a series of Advance Medial-Pivot (Wright Medical Arlington, TN) cementless knees (◘ Fig. 16-7).

Both designs, like the ProFix knee, have a corundum blasted, roughened, central finned stem/keel with peripheral spikes and four screws. The early clinical and radiographic results of all three of these knees (Profix, Genesis II, and Advance Medial-Pivot) have been excellent. The clinical results correlate well with the cadaver tibial implant fixation studies. I believe, we are on the right course for the future success of cementless TKA (◘ Fig. 16-8).

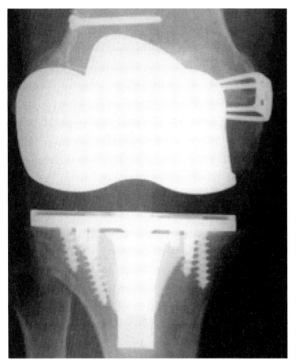

◘ **Fig. 16-7.** Radiograph of Advance Medial-Pivot knee showing no radiolucent line around the tibial stem

New Technology

New technology which should improve cementless TKA success includes alloys with improved bone ingrowth qualities and structure such as tantalum (Ta) trabecular metal (Zimmer, Warsaw, IN), new Ti-alloy structures, and zirconium (Zr) alloys with oxidized surfaces (oxinium, Smith & Nephew, Memphis, TN) which could reduce polyethylene wear. Other factors which either have been shown to or could enhance cementless fixation (in order of apparent effectiveness) are growth factors, bone morphogenic protein, autogenous bone graft, ultrasound, fresh-frozen allogeneic bone graft, factor VIII, calcium phosphate coatings (hydroxyapatite HA), prostaglandin, electrical stimulation, calcium phosphate granules, freeze-dried allogeneic bone graft, fibrin glue, and demineralized bone matrix.

The future of cementless TKA appears bright. Reduced infection rates, improved biomechanical fixation, and better materials and bone ingrowth surfaces, along with bone growth-enhancing agents, should lead to high-demand knees with longevity.

References

1. Insall JN, Ranawat CS, Scott WN, Walker P (1976) Total condylar knee replacement: preliminary report. Clin Orthop 120:149-154
2. Font-Rodriguez DE, Scuderi GR, Insall IN (1997) Survivorship of cemented total knee arthroplasty. Clin Orthop 345:79-86
3. Rodriguez JA, Bhende H, Ranawat CS (2001) Total condylar knee replacement: a 20-year follow-up study. Clin Orthop 388:10-17
4. Diduch DR, InsallJN, Scott WN, et al (1997) Total knee replacement in young, active patients: long-term follow-up and functional outcome. J Bone Joint Surg 79A: 575-582
5. Campbell WC (1940) Interposition of Vitallium plates in arthroplasty of the knee: preliminary report. Am J Surg 47:639

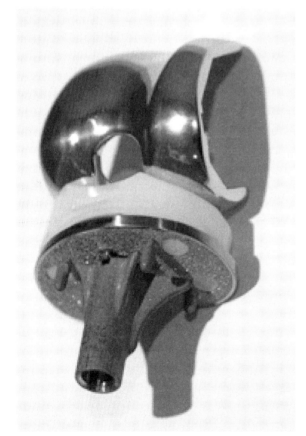

◘ **Fig. 16-8.** Photograph of Advance Medial-Pivot knee showing the corundum blasted finned tibial stem, peripheral spikes, screw holes, and porous coating on the undersurface of the tibial base. The Profix and Genesis II knees have similar design features

6. Riley LH Jr (1976) The evolution of total knee arthroplasy. Clin Orthop 120:7-10
7. Jones WN, Aufranc OE, Kermont WL (1967) Mold arthroplasy of the knee. J Bone Joint Surg [Am] 49:1022
8. McKeever DC, Elliott RB (1960) Tibial plateau prosthesis. Clin Orthop 18:86-95
9. MacIntosh DL (1958) Hemiarthroplasty of the knee using a space occupying prosthesis for painful varus and valgus deformities. J Bone Joint Surg [Am] 40:1431
10. Townley CO (1985) The anatomic total knee resurfacing arthroplasty. Clin Orthop 192:82
11. Walldius B (1960) Arthroplasty of the knee joint using endoprosthesis. Acta Orthop Scand 30:137
12. Yamamoto S (1979) Total knee replacement with the Kodama-Yamamoto knee prothesis. Clin Orthop 145:60
13. Freeman MA, McLeod HC, Levai JP (1983) Cementless fixation of prosthetic components in total arthroplasty of the knee and hip. Clin Orthop 176:88-94
14. Ring PA (1980) Uncemented surface replacement of the knee joint. Clin Orthop 148:106-111
15. Buechel FF, Pappas MJ (1989) New Jersey low contact stress knee replacement system, ten year evaluation of meniscal bearings. Orthop Clin North Am 20:147-177
16. Hungerford DS, Kenna RV, Krackow KA (1982) The porous-coated anatomic total knee. Orthop Clin North Am 13:103
17. Whiteside LA (1989) Clinical results of Whiteside Ortholoc total knee replacement. Orthop Clin North Am 20:113-124
18. Laskin RS (1988) Tricon-M uncemented total knee arthroplasty. A review of 96 knees followed for longer than 2 years. J Arthroplasty 3:27-38
19. Landon GC, Galante JO, Maley MM (1986) Noncemented total knee arthlroplasty. Clin Orthop 205:49-57
20. Ritter MA, Keating EM, Faris PM (1989) Design features and clinical results of the anatomic graduated components (AGC) total knee replacement. Clin Orthop 19:641
21. Scott RD, Thornhill TS (1994) Posterior cruciate supplementing total knee replacements using conforming inserts and cruciate recession: effect on range of motion and radiolucent lines. Clin Orthop 309:146
22. Hofmann AA, Wyatt RW, Beck SW, Alpert J (1991) Cementless total knee arthroplasty in patients over 65 years old. Clin Orthop 271:28-34
23. Buechel FF Sr, Buechel FF Jr, Pappas MJ, D'Alessio JD (2001) Twenty-year evaluation of meniscal bearing and rotating platform knee replacements. Clin Orthop 388:41-50
24. Collins DN, Heim SA, Nelson CL, Smith P III (1991) Porous-coated anatomic total knee arthroplasty. A prospective analysis comparing cemented and cementless fixation. Clin Orthop 267:128-136
25. Berger RA, Lyon JH, Jacobs JJ, Barden RM, Berkson EM, Sheinkop MB, Rosenberg AG, Galante JO (2001) Problems with cementless total knee arthroplasty at 11 years follow-up. Clin Orthop 392:196-207
26. Whiteside LA (2001) Long-term follow-up of the bone-ingrowth Ortholoc knee system without a metal-backed patella. Clin Orthop 388:77-84
27. Ritter MA, Berend ME, Meding JB, Keating EM, Faris PM, Crites BM (2001) Long-term follow-up of anatomic graduated components posterior cruciate-retaining total knee replacement. Clin Orthop 388:51-57
28. Duffy GP, Berry DJ, Rand JA (1998) Cement versus cementless fixation in total knee arthroplasty. Clin Orthop 356:66-72
29. Hofmann AA, Evanich JD, Ferguson RP, Camargo MP (2001) Ten- to 14-year clinical follow-up of the cementless natural knee system. Clin Orthop 388:85-94
30. Petty W (1978) The effect of methylmethacrylate on bacterial phagocytosis and killing by human polymorphonuclear leukocytes. J Bone Joint Surg [Am] 60:752
31. Petty W (1983) Influence of skeletal implant materials on infection. Trans Orthop Res Soc 8:137

16

17 Lessons Learned from Mobile-Bearing Knees

J. V. Baré, R. B. Bourne

Summary

With the issues over the surgical treatment of the young osteoarthritic knee far from being resolved, the intellectual concepts associated with a mobile-bearing prosthesis are indeed attractive. The current challenges in knee prosthetic design are centered around attempting to produce normal kinematics, reducing wear and hence achieving greater longevity. Initially, it was hoped that mobile-bearing designs might go a long way toward achieving these aims. These hopes have yet to be borne out in practice.

Introduction

Fixed-bearing knee prostheses have been shown to have excellent long-term survival and good to excellent clinical results [4, 5]; however, with concerns regarding polyethylene debris, implant fixation, and function in younger, more active patients, the mobile-bearing total knee arthroplasty (MBKA) was designed as an attractive alternative. By increasing conformity between the tibial and femoral bearing surfaces and thus increasing the contact area without the associated constraints that conformity produces in fixed-bearing implants, the dual-surface articulation was intended to reduce wear at the bearing surfaces and the consequent osteolytic effects of wear debris. It was also designed to reduce stress at the bone-implant interface, thus improving longevity of the implant. Subsequently, other characteristics have been attributed to MBKAs. These include improved stability, range of movement, and kinematics which should then translate into a more physiologically functioning knee. To date, however, none of these intended benefits have been clearly documented in a clinical setting.

Mobile-Bearing Designs

There are currently many different designs of MBKA on the market. Basic design types based on bearing move-

ments have been classified by Walker and Sathasivam [19]. These include:

1. Pure rotation around a centrally located post
2. Rotation around a medially located post to better simulate the medial pivot kinematics of a "normal" knee
3. Rotation and AP translation (including meniscal-bearing TKA)
4. Guided motion which allows rotation, as in type 1, but with translation guided by cams or guide surfaces

Each prosthetic design has its own characteristics with regard to the conformity of the tibiofemoral component, mobility of the insert, and kinematics of the knee.

The mobile-bearing TKA with the longest clinical follow-up is the New Jersey Low Contact Stress (LCS) (DePuy, Warsaw, IN) [1]. This was originally designed as both a posterior cruciate-retaining, meniscal-bearing prosthesis which allowed AP translation and some rotation and a cruciate-sacrificing rotating platform prosthesis. The Oxford Unicompartmental Knee Replacement (Biomet Ltd., Bridgend, UK), which was originally designed as a bicompartmental replacement, has an unconstrained meniscal bearing, and the Self-aligning (SAL) TKA (Zimmer, Warsaw, IN) combines both rotation and AP translation in its bearing movement. Additional issues with these and other mobile-bearing designs include: cruciate ligament retention or sacrifice; type of congruence between bearing surfaces; type of restraint used to prevent bearing dislocation; and the addition of stops to prevent excessive AP translation or rotation. These stops have been associated with increased polyethylene wear [13, 19].

A gait-congruous TKA such as the LCS rotating platform has a dual radius of curvature of the femoral component in the sagittal plane. A larger radius anteriorly allows congruence during the stance phase of gait, while a smaller radius posteriorly allows reduced conformity with knee flexion and hence the possibility of normal femoral roll-back and increased flexion (Fig. 17-1).

Other MBKAs, such as the SAL, which is congruent up to 90° of flexion (Fig. 17-2a) and the Oxford, which is designed with the same single radius of curvature of the femoral component and articulating surface of the polyethylene bearing (see Fig. 17-2b), allow greater con-

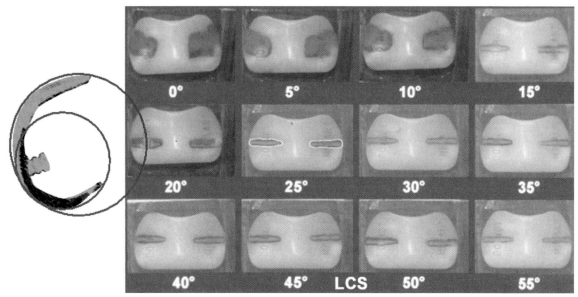

Fig. 17-1. The New Jersey Low Contact Stress (LCS) (DePuy, Warsaw, IN). This shows the dual radius of curvature and the tibio-femoral contact area through a range of flexion. Note the concept of "gait congruence" with a greater contact area (congruence) in extension than flexion

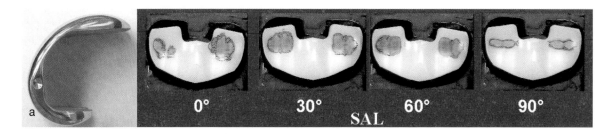

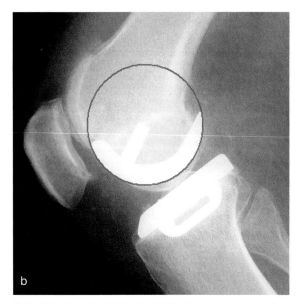

Fig. 17-2a, b. *a* The Self-Aligning (SAL) TKA (Zimmer, Warsaw, IN) with its bearing contact area showing tibiofemoral congruity up to 90° of flexion. *b* The Oxford Unicompartmental Knee Replacement (Biomet Ltd., Bridgend,UK), demonstrating a single radius of curvature of the femoral component. This articulates with the concave upper surface of the polyethylene bearing which has the same radius of curvature, enabling congruency through a full range of motion

gruity. This keeps bearing surfaces congruous up to 90° in the case of the SAL, and through a full range of motion in the case of the Oxford. Congruous bearings allow sliding but no rolling, and femoral roll-back is therefore addressed by allowing AP translation at the underside of the polyethylene bearing. The issue of gait congruence or full congruency has implications for knee kinematics and polyethylene wear patterns.

Polyethylene Wear

Wear of the polyethylene insert in TKA remains a significant problem and one of the main reasons behind the design and development of MBKA. The generation of particulate debris arises from both the bearing surface and the "backside" or metallic tibial tray-polyethylene interface. The amount and type of debris produced will influence its biological activity and may eventually affect the implant longevity through osteolysis or premature polyethylene failure (Fig. 17-3).

It is not possible to generalize the effect that a mobile bearing has on polyethylene wear, as different prosthesis designs have different degrees of conformity, mobility,

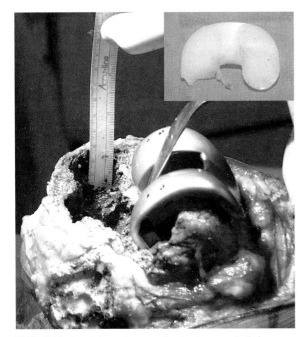

Fig. 17-3. Aseptic loosening secondary to advance polyethylene wear and osteolysis

imens of the Oxford Medial Unicompartmental Knee Arthroplasty. This is an unconstrained meniscal-bearing device which is congruent through a full range of motion due to the spherical nature of both femoral and polyethylene bearing surfaces in sagittal and coronal planes. Murray [13] reported linear wear rates as low as 0.001 mm/year in these specimens. Interestingly, he also noted that this wear rate increased to 0.003 mm/year if there was any impingement and, unlike fixed-bearing devices, the wear rate was not correlated to the thickness of the bearing.

Motion in congruent bearings tends to be predominantly sliding with low contact stresses, while that in an incongruent bearing is a combination of rolling and sliding with much higher contact forces and subsurface stresses. This results in the production of more UHMW-PE particulate debris of larger size than a congruent bearing. Subsurface stresses above 6.9 MPa result in increased wear and those above 9 MPa result in failure with pitting and delamination [16]. Despite the fact that the congruent bearing produces less linear or fatigue wear, it produces more volumetric wear in the form of granular debris [18]. With a knee simulator study comparing wear in a fully congruent, multidirectional UHMWPE platform and a fixed-bearing device over 10 million cycles, Jones et al. [11] showed that the MBKA exhibited less linear wear but approximately 30% more volumetric wear. This granular debris has been associated with more osteolysis than the particulate debris. Huang et al. [8, 9] reviewed a series of failed primary mobile-bearing (LCS) and fixed-bearing TKAs that had undergone revision surgery. They found that although there was evidence of advanced polyethylene wear in both groups, the prevalence of osteolysis was significantly higher in the mobile-bearing group. Histological specimens showed smaller particulate debris and more granular debris in the mobile-bearing knees.

and constraint. In addition, polyethylene wear is also influenced by articular kinematics and the polyethylene quality, including its processing, sterilization, and shelf-life. However, in general it is assumed that the wear rates in TKAs are reduced as the contact area increases. Sathasivam et al. [17] confirmed this theory with an in vitro study analyzing wear rates and particle size production with differing contact areas of ultra-high-molecular-weight polyethylene (UHMWPE) on polished metal surfaces. There was a significant (inverse) relationship between the size of the contact area and the production of polyethylene debris. There was also a trend noticed with a smaller particle size production in the larger contact area. This work is supported clinically with retrieval spec-

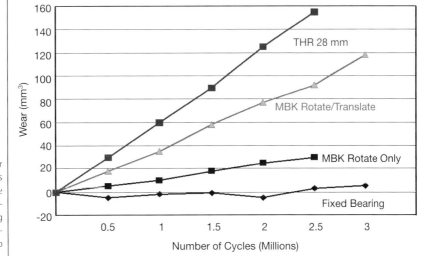

Fig. 17-4. Knee simulator wear studies showing the relative amounts of volumetric wear produced by three different designs of total knee arthroplasty [fixed bearing, mobile bearing (rotate only) and mobile bearing (rotate and translate] and a total hip arthroplasty

It is worth noting that the volumetric wear of any MBK is significantly less than the volumetric wear produced by a total hip arthroplasty containing a standard 28-mm metal head on UHMWPE acetabulum. In addition, mobile-bearing designs that rotate and translate show more volumetric wear than those that rotate only (see ◘ Fig. 17-4). In the hip, the amount of volumetric wear can be substantially reduced with the use of cross-linked polyethylene instead of UHMWPE. This may have design implications on TKA as cross-linked polyethylene displays its best wear characteristics with "sliding" type movements (as in a hip arthroplasty) and therefore may be used only with fully congruent bearing surfaces.

Survival

Despite concerns regarding the increased potential for osteolysis in mobile-bearing prostheses, this has not been reflected clinically in long-term survival figures. Buechel [1] and Callaghan [3] have each reported excellent long-term results of the LCS. Ninety-five to 100% 10- to 20-year survival figures are reported for the rotating platform. The meniscal-bearing design has survival figures of 97.4% at 10 years and 83% at 16 years. Similar 5- to 8-year results have been reported on the SAL TKA [2] and the Oxford bicompartmental replacement (ACL intact) [6]. These results are comparable to results of conventional fixed-bearing TKA. Investigators have consistently reported 95% good to excellent results and greater than 94% survival rates at 10-15 years [4, 5].

Kinematics and Function

From the evidence presented so far, it would seem that the amount and type of polyethylene debris produced in a mobile-bearing TKA do not positively or adversely affect the long-term survival of the prosthesis. Does, then, a mobile bearing impart some kinematic advantage which would improve function in TKAs? In order to answer this question, we must first be able to understand normal knee kinematics; second, we require an accurate, reproducible way of measuring these kinematics both in the normal and in the prosthetic knee. Iwaki et al. [10], Hill et al. [7], and Nakagawa et al. [14] attempted to define normal knee kinematics with a series of MRI studies on cadaveric and living knees. As an oversimplification of these complex tests, they showed femoral "roll-back" with flexion, much greater on the lateral side than on the medial side. This roll-back was minimal before 90° of flexion and then increased to full flexion to the point of subluxing the lateral femoral condyle off the posterior lateral tibial plateau. The lateral contact point

moved an average of 28 mm posteriorly with full flexion (162°), while the medial femoral condyle moved an average of only 4.5 mm posteriorly.

Ideally, the design features of a mobile-bearing knee prosthesis would incorporate full conformity with the ability to translate posteriorly and externally rotate the femur with flexion. Because of the absence of functioning cruciate ligaments in TKA, this rotation and translation would somehow need to driven by a design feature that did not interfere with congruency. Clearly, all of these features do not exist in any currently available prosthesis.

How, then, do the kinematics of available MBKAs compare with those of normal knees and those of fixed-bearing knees? The most common method used to make this comparison is video fluoroscopy. When compared with normal knees, fixed-bearing TKA tends to exhibit paradoxical anterior femoral sliding with flexion. This is seen more in posterior cruciate-retaining prostheses, but also in posterior-stabilized implants, as the post does not usually engage the cam until beyond the flexion range of most functional activities [2]. Dennis et al. [2] reported on the fluoroscopic results of MBKA. They showed that meniscal-bearing TKAs tended to have a posterior contact point in full extension and then, with flexion, displayed the same paradoxical movement as cruciate-retaining fixed-bearing TKA. The posterior cruciate-sacrificing, rotating platform MBKA (LCS) showed minimal AP movement with the normal gait cycle, but with knee flexion to 90°, the lateral femoral condyle contact point moved posteriorly an average of 3.3 mm. However, in 40% of these cases some anterior paradoxical movement was noted. In patients managed with a posterior-stabilized rotating platform (LCS), again little AP movement was seen in the normal gait pattern; however, with flexion to 90° an average of 5.9 mm posterior movement was seen on the lateral side while very little movement was seen on the medial side.

This same group of patients were also tested for knee range of movement. The greatest range was seen with a fixed-bearing posteriorly stabilized TKA (127°) and the smallest range with the posterior cruciate-sacrificing rotating platform (108°) [2].

Normal knee kinematics does not exist in any TKA. While the congruent bearings of some MBKAs seem to impart a relatively consistent pattern of movement in a fashion which comes closer to resembling that of a normal knee than non-congruent bearings do, this comes at the expense of reducing the flexion range. It appears that the potential to achieve more normal kinematics would involve a prosthetic design which incorporated congruency with guided motion.

To date, there are few comparative data available on the effects of MBKA on the patellofemoral joint. Intuitively, one would assume that by designing a tibiofemoral joint that is more consistent in its movement and reduces the amount of paradoxical anterior femoral movement, the patellofemoral forces would be minimized and the quadriceps mechanism could function more efficiently; however, this remains to be proven.

Although we have long-term clinical results on case series involving both fixed-bearing and mobile-bearing knees, there are no long-term controlled trials available to compare these two groups. Price et al. [15] recently reported on the short-term follow-up of 40 patients involved in a randomized controlled trial. These patients each underwent sequential bilateral TKA while under one anesthetic. On one side a well-established posterior cruciate-retaining TKA was inserted (AGC; Biomet, Bridgend, UK); on the other a new MBKA (Total Meniscal Knee (TMK); Biomet, Bridgend, UK) was inserted. This MBKA is a fully congruent TKA with a mobile bearing that rotates and translates around a central peg. Results were reported at 1 year. They included American Knee Society Scores, Oxford Knee Scores, and pain scores. There was a small but significant difference between the groups in favor of the mobile-bearing knee. No difference was noted in the range of motion. Interestingly, the only revision procedure was required for a dislocated bearing. Longer-term follow-up is required to see if this initial benefit is maintained.

Problems Associated with MBKA

So far we have seen little evidence to suggest that any clinical benefit exists of a mobile-bearing knee arthroplasty over a fixed-bearing arthroplasty. In addition, there are problems which may be isolated to the mobile-bearing prosthesis. Bearing dislocation and breakage have been reported with different designs of MBKA [12]. Dislocation is probably the result of failing to accurately balance flexion and extension gaps. A reduced margin of error with regard to soft-tissue balancing may make this surgery more technically demanding, which carries with it the problems of a steep learning curve and the complications that accompany this learning curve. Even without dislocation, an excessively mobile bearing can cause problems with subluxation or even soft-tissue impingement. Because of these concerns, difficulty balancing a knee at the time of surgery should be a contraindication to inserting a mobile-bearing prosthesis. One theoretical surgical benefit of the MBKA is that because of its self-aligning properties it has the potential to correct a malrotated tibial component. However, there may be evidence to suggest that a malrotated tibial component is associated with increased backside wear [2].

Despite the much lower linear wear rates reported in MBKA, a mobile bearing does not give a knee immunity from such problems. Many examples of catastrophic polyethylene wear and subsequent failure have been reported (◘ Fig. 17-5).

Conclusion

In over 25 years of experience with mobile-bearing knee arthroplasties, many lessons have been learned. We now know that, compared with a fixed-bearing TKA, a constrained mobile-bearing arthroplasty will produce less linear wear but more volumetric wear. Video fluoroscopy has shown that the kinematics of some MBKAs more closely resembles that of a normal knee, especially when guided motion is involved; however, there is no total knee arthroplasty that has normal knee kinematics. And finally, we have seen complications occurring in MBKA that do not occur in the fixed-bearing device.

Despite these documented differences, what remains to be shown is a practical difference in terms of clinical outcome. Clinical case series have shown that there are some mobile-bearing prostheses available with long-term clinical results equal to those of the best fixed-bearing TKAs [1]. Unfortunately, due to the lack of controlled comparative clinical studies, the question of whether any true long-term benefit exists with mobile-bearing total knee arthroplasty over fixed-bearing arthroplasty remains unanswered. In addition, with an ever-increasing array of mobile-bearing designs, a comparison between them may prove to be just as complex as the comparison between mobile- and fixed-bearing designs.

Bearing mobility forms only part of the complex picture surrounding future potential for TKA design. Issues such as congruency, bearing surface materials, and guided motion need careful detailed evaluation. Challenges for the future will involve establishing how best to use the lessons that we have learned from mobile-bearing prostheses to design an implant that will better serve the younger, more active patient with knee osteoarthritis.

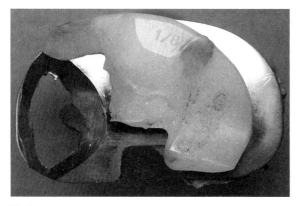

◘ **Fig. 17-5.** Retrieval specimen at 8 years post implantation showing advanced polyethylene wear in a mobile bearing knee arthroplasty

References

1. Buechel FF Sr (2002) Long-term follow-up after mobile-bearing total knee replacement. Clin Orthop 404:40-50
2. Callaghan JJ, Insall JN, Greenwald AS, Dennis DA, Komistek RD, Murray DW, Bourne RB, Rorabeck CH, Dorr LD (2001) Mobile-bearing knee replacement: concepts and results. Instr Course Lect 50:431-449
3. Callaghan JJ, Squire MW, Goetz DD, Sullivan PM, Johnston RC (2000) Cemented rotating-platform total knee replacement. A nine to twelve-year follow-up study. J Bone Joint Surg [Am] 82:705-711
4. Colizza WA, Insall JN, Scuderi GR (1995) The posterior stabilized total knee prosthesis. Assessment of polyethylene damage and osteolysis after a ten-year minimum follow-up. J Bone Joint Surg [Am] 77:1713-1720
5. Gill GS, Joshi AB, Mills DM (1999) Total condylar knee arthroplasty: 16- to 21-year results. Clin Orthop 367:210-215
6. Goodfellow JW, O'Connor J (1986) Clinical results of the Oxford knee. Surface arthroplasty of the tibiofemoral joint with a meniscal bearing prosthesis. Clin Orthop 205:21-42
7. Hill PF, Vedi V, Williams A, Iwaki H, Pinskerova V, Freeman MA (2000) Tibiofemoral movement 2: the loaded and unloaded living knee studied by MRI. J Bone Joint Surg [Br] 82:1196-1198
8. Huang CH, Ho FY, Ma HM, Yang CT, Liau JJ, Kao HC, Young TH, Cheng CK (2002) Particle size and morphology of UHMWPE wear debris in failed total knee arthroplasties – a comparison between mobile bearing and fixed bearing knees. J Orthop Res 20:1038-1041
9. Huang CH, Ma HM, Liau JJ, Ho FY, Cheng CK (2002) Osteolysis in failed total knee arthroplasty: a comparison of mobile-bearing and fixed-bearing knees. J Bone Joint Surg [Am] 8412:2224-2229
10. Iwaki H, Pinskerova V, Freeman MA (2000) Tibiofemoral movement. 1: the shapes and relative movements of the femur and tibia in the unloaded cadaver knee. J Bone Joint Surg [Br] 82:1189-1195
11. Jones VC, Barton DC, Fitzpatrick DP, Auger DD, Stone MH, Fisher J (1999) An experimental model of tibial counterface polyethylene wear in mobile bearing knees: the influence of design and kinematics. Biomed Mater Eng 9:189-196
12. Jordan LR, Olivo JL, Voorhorst PE (1997) Survivorship analysis of cementless meniscal bearing total knee arthroplasty. Clin Orthop 338:119-123
13. Murray DW, Goodfellow JW, O'Connor JJ (1998) The Oxford medial unicompartmental arthroplasty: a ten-year survival study. J Bone Joint Surg [Br] 80:983-989
14. Nakagawa S, Kadoya Y, Todo S, Kobayashi A, Sakamoto H, Freeman MA, Yamano Y (2000) Tibiofemoral movement. 3: full flexion in the living knee studied by MRI. J Bone Joint Surg [Br] 82:1199-1200
15. Price AJ et al (2003) A mobile-bearing total knee prosthesis compared with a fixed-bearing prosthesis. A multicentre single-blind randomised controlled trial. J Bone Joint Surg [Br] 85:62-67
16. Rostoker W, Galante JO (1979) Contact pressure dependence of wear rates of ultra high molecular weight polyethylene. J Biomed Mater Res 13:957-964
17. Sathasivam S, Walker PS, Campbell PA, Rayner K (2001) The effect of contact area on wear in relation to fixed bearing and mobile bearing knee replacements. J Biomed Mater Res 58:282-290
18. Vertullo CJ, Easley ME, Scott WN, Insall JN (2001) Mobile bearings in primary knee arthroplasty. J Am Acad Orthop Surg 9:355-364
19. Walker PS, Sathasivam S (2000) Design forms of total knee replacement. Proc Inst Mech Eng [H] 214:101-119

17

III Kinematics

18 Understanding and Interpreting In Vivo Kinematic Studies

S. A. Banks

Summary

Radiographic imaging and shape-matching techniques have been used since the late 1980s to quantify the motions of knee replacements in vivo. These studies have shown how knee implants move in vivo, how implant design affects knee kinematics, and how different surgical and design factors influence knee mechanics and patient function. In general, knee implants that definitively control the anteroposterior position of the femur with respect to the tibia achieve greater weight-bearing flexion and exhibit kinematics that are more likely to result in better patient function and implant longevity.

Three-dimensional Kinematics from Two-dimensional Images

By the late 1980s, total knee arthroplasty (TKA) had become a fairly routine procedure for the treatment of severe knee arthritis. A wide variety of implant designs were being utilized with predictable success and reasonable durability. The focus of designers was shifting from basic knee function and implant fixation to improving knee performance and implant longevity. In part, what was needed to continue evolving knee replacements was more precise information on how knee replacements moved once implanted. Unfortunately, the gait laboratories and CT scanners of the day were not able to provide accurate three-dimensional (3D) kinematic information about knee replacement motion during weight-bearing dynamic activities.

In 1988 I was given the mandate to develop a better method for measuring knee kinematics for my doctoral dissertation. Having failed to use the gait laboratory motion capture system to accurately measure implant motion, W. Andrew Hodge suggested we should directly image the joint with X-ray fluoroscopy and develop an image-based motion measurement technique. This "shape-matching" approach proved to work well [1, 2], and this technique and its evolved forms have been used since to provide a better understanding of knee replacement function.

The details of shape-matching-based motion measurement are beyond the scope of this volume, but the process follows several logical steps: Radiographic images are produced when X-rays pass through space and are attenuated by the patient's anatomy before striking a sensitive medium to cause a chemical or electrical reaction. The X-ray beam emanates from a point source, with rays diverging in all directions, creating a central or perspective projection of the object - in essence a shadow (◘ Fig. 18-1). The location of the X-ray source with respect to the image plane can be measured so that the same optics can be reproduced on a computer. Computer-aided design (CAD) information is available for the knee implant components, and bone surfaces can be reconstructed from CT or MR (◘ Fig. 18-2), making it a simple process to synthesize on the computer images of implants at any possi-

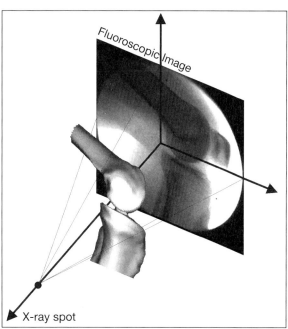

◘ **Fig. 18-1.** Fluoroscopic and radiographic projections are created by a spot source of rays so that the image is a "perspective" projection, or shadow, that is a three-dimensional function of the projection geometry and the position and orientation of the bones. This geometry allows three-dimensional kinematics to be derived from sequences of two-dimensional radiographic images

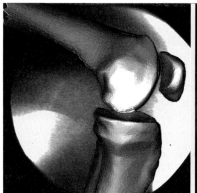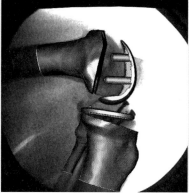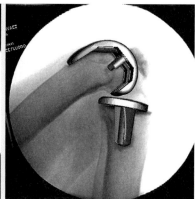

Fig. 18-2. Three-dimensional measurement of dynamic knee motion using fluoroscopy and shape-matching techniques has been performed for natural knees (*left*), knees with partial arthroplasty (*middle*), and knees with total arthroplasty (*right*). The bone surface models can be created from CT and MR scans and the implant models are obtained from the manufacturer or 3D laser scans

ble position. These synthetic views can be iteratively modified until they match the views obtained from patients. Once matched, the positions and orientations of the models represent the physical position and orientation of the patient's implants that created the radiographic projection.

Many groups the world over have used shape-matching techniques for determining implant motion from single-plane radiographic views, studying a range of activities including gait [3], stair-climbing [4], and deep knee bends [5]. Although the details of the methods vary, measurement precision for each moving segment is typically 0.5-1.0 mm for implant motions parallel to the image plane and 0.5°-1.0° for rotations. Importantly, this is monocular vision, not stereo or binocular, and all of these techniques have much reduced accuracy for translations perpendicular to the image plane, where precisions are typically 3.0-6.0 mm. If these measurement errors are extended to the articular surfaces, one can typically expect measurement uncertainties of greater than 1.2 mm for single observations of condylar contact or separation.

Positional Findings

Findings from image-based TKA studies can be organized into positional and dynamic observations. The positional observations relate closely to how implant design and surgical alignment influence articular contact and knee function at the extreme ranges of motion.

Knee implants typically are designed to maximize tibiofemoral contact area with the knee in extension and to accommodate 10°-15° of hyperextension. Implant wear testing is performed such that the implants reach 0° relative flexion at simulated early stance. Yet neither context takes account of the fact that surgical alignment may place the implants in positions which differ from 0° relative flexion. Femoral components implanted using in-

tramedullary rods or extramedullary techniques seek alignment orthogonal to the distal femur. The anterior bow of the femoral shaft results in the femoral implant component being flexed forward in the sagittal plane by 5°-7°. Similarly, tibial implant techniques range from alignment perpendicular to the long axis of the tibia to an alignment matching the normal posterior slope of the tibial plateau. The net result of typical surgical placement is that the implants are in 5°-12° of relative hyperextension. Simultaneous measures of skeletal flexion, using goniometry or motion capture (**Fig. 18-3**), and of implant flexion using fluoroscopy have shown an average 9.5° of implant hyperextension compared with the skeletal flexion angle [6].

There are at least three important ramifications of this simple and intuitive observation. First, implants that have hyperextension stops will likely experience much greater contact and possible wear than the designers anticipated [6, 7]. Posterior stabilized designs with tibial

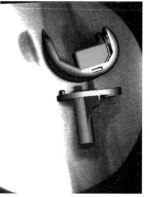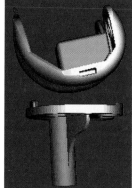

Fig. 18-3. Knees with well-aligned implants commonly show implant hyperextension. Anterior bow of the femur and posterior slope of the tibial plateau bias implant alignment by an average of 10° hyperextension. Thus, when the knee is fully extended at toe-off during gait (*left*), the implants are in hyperextension (*right*)

posts and some PCL-retaining designs accommodate limited hyperextension, often 5°-15°. With the implants routinely placed in almost 10° of hyperextension at 0° of knee flexion, many of these designs will experience anterior impingement during routine activity. Second, standard evaluations of TKA designs, whether by computer or by machine, do not account for implant alignment. The evaluations assume that the straight leg corresponds to 0° of implant flexion. Given that many designs have surfaces with changing curvatures in early flexion, it is possible that these tests will predict performance differing from the clinical experience. Third, implant features designed to guide implant motions at particular flexion angles will engage later in the flexion arc. Post and cam mechanisms in posterior stabilized knees will engage at approximately 10° greater anatomical flexion than anticipated by the design. In very deep flexion, there is some concern that the proximal "edge" of the femoral condyles (where the articular and bone-cut surfaces meet) will dig into the tibial articular surface. Normal implant alignment means this phenomenon will occur 10° later in the flexion arc, if at all.

Fluoroscopic evaluations have elucidated the mechanics of total knee arthroplasties in deeply flexed postures. It has long been assumed that greater posterior femoral translation on the tibia permits greater knee flexion [8]. In a study of 16 different TKA designs in patients with excellent clinical outcomes, a significant linear relationship was seen between the amount of posterior femoral translation and maximum weight-bearing flexion [9]. This relationship, 1.4° greater flexion for each additional millimeter of posterior femoral translation, held true for all types of TKA design (◘ Fig. 18-4). Implant designs that definitively controlled tibiofemoral position in flexion achieved greater femoral "roll-back", and demon-

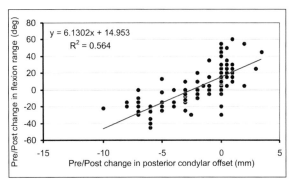

◘ **Fig. 18-5.** Correlation of restoration of posterior condylar offset (postoperative minus preoperative) with postoperative flexion gain(+)/loss(-) for 150 consecutive knees. Overlapping points are not shown. (Reprinted from [7])

strated greater weight-bearing flexion than designs that required the soft tissue and muscles to control tibiofemoral position. These findings suggest that the flexion space, particularly in PCL-retaining TKA, ought not to be made too loose, as additional laxity may allow unwanted anterior translation of the femur and a concomitant decrease in maximum weight-bearing flexion.

Similar analyses have shown the importance of posterior condylar geometry on knee flexion range. Bellemans et al. [10] showed a significant linear relationship between changes in the posterior condylar offset, the maximum AP distance from the femoral shaft to the most posterior point on the condyles, and changes in the passive ROM. They found that reducing the posterior condylar offset by 1 mm from its anatomical value decreased the passive ROM by 6° (◘ Fig. 18-5). This finding is particularly relevant for surgeons using anterior referencing instrumentation: When a knee measures in-between component sizes, common practice argues for selecting the smaller component. This will typically reduce the anatomical posterior condylar offset by several millimeters, potentially reducing the flexion range by 10° or more! Using the larger femoral component, when possible, or adjusting the position of the smaller femoral component can reduce the effect on the posterior condylar offset and provide the patient with the best possible range of motion.

Dynamic Characteristics

Early fluoroscopic studies of TKA kinematics showed that dynamic motions could differ markedly from those of the normal knee [11]. These and subsequent studies showed that, lacking the anterior cruciate ligament and menisci, there is a tendency for the femur to slide forward on the tibia with flexion and backward with extension. However, tibial rotations were normal with the tibia rotating inward with flexion. A simple method to quantify these

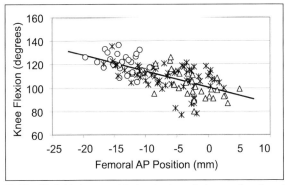

◘ **Fig. 18-4.** Maximum weight-bearing knee flexion as a function of femoral AP position for 121 knees. Femoral posterior positions are *negative*, anterior is *positive*, and *zero* represents the AP midpoint of the tibial component. *Circles* represent posterior-stabilized knees, *asterisks* represent posterior cruciate-retaining fixed bearing knees, and *triangles* represent the mobile-bearing knees. The *solid line* shows the linear regression with a slope of 1.4° more flexion per millimeter femoral posterior translation (R=0.64, *p*<0.001). (Reprinted from [6]).

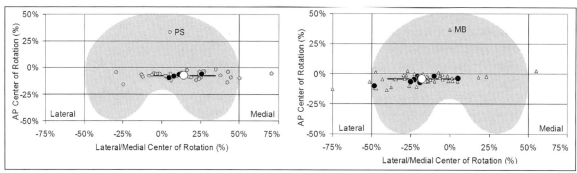

Fig. 18-6. The average center of rotation is strongly influenced by the intrinsic constraints of the implant design for stair-step activities. Posterior-stabilized knees, which force the femur posterior on the tibia with flexion, mostly show medial centers of rotation (*left*). Gait-congruent mobile-bearing knee designs allow relatively free AP translation of the femur in flexion, with most knees showing a lateral center of rotation (*right*). Each *open symbol* (○,△) represents the center of rotation in one knee; the *filled black circles* represent the average center of rotation for a specific implant design, and the *large white circle* represents the average center of rotation for all knees of that type. (Reprinted from [9])

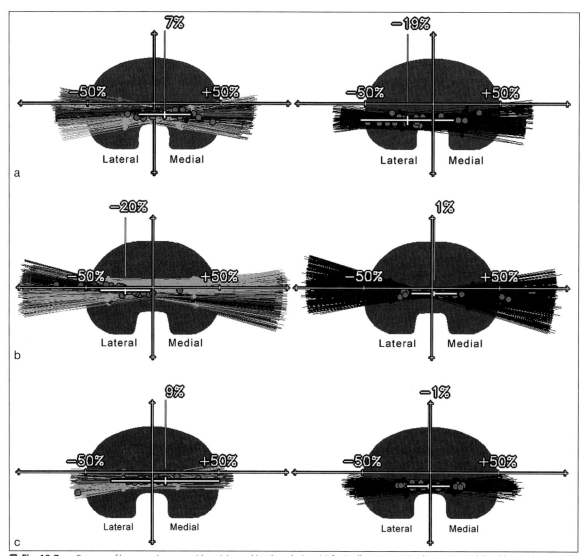

Fig. 18-7a-c. Patterns of knee motion vary with activity and implant design. (*a*) Sagittally unconstrained posterior-stabilized knees show medial center of rotation during stair-climbing activities, but greater femoral sliding and a lateral center of rotation during the stance phase of gait. (*b*) Gait-congruent rotating-platform mobile-bearing knees show anterior slding of the femur in flexion during stair activities and a lateral center of rotation, but are constrained to pure internal/external tibial rotation with flexion during the stance phase of gait. (*c*) Knees that maintain similar conformity over the flexion range show more similar knee motion patterns for the gait and stair activities. Each line represents the location and orientation of the femoral condyles with respect to the tibial plateau for all frames of data for a group of subjects. The *gray dots* indicate the average center of rotation for a single motion trial, and the *white cross* indicates the mean and standard deviation for the group average center of rotation. (Graphs reprinted from [10])

translations and rotations is to consider the average center of rotation: In the healthy knee posterior translation of the femur and internal rotation of the tibia with flexion result in a medial center of rotation. The lateral condyle moves posterior with flexion about a relatively stationary medial condylar position. In unconstrained TKA, the medial condyle is observed to slide forward with flexion about a relatively stationary lateral condylar position. Thus, a lateral center of rotation has been observed in unconstrained TKA designs. In an analysis of stair-climbing motions in 25 different TKA designs a significant relationship was found between the intrinsic constraints of the implant and the average center of rotation (◘ Fig 18-6): Designs with greater intrinsic control had central or medial centers of rotation, while up to 86% of unconstrained devices showed lateral centers of rotation [12]. This analysis included only patients with high satisfaction and excellent clinical scores, showing that a wide range of knee motion patterns are compatible with good clinical results. This suggests that implant designers and surgeons have wide latitude to modulate knee motion patterns to achieve further improvements in patient strength, range of motion, and implant longevity.

Fluoroscopic studies of TKA kinematics comparing different activities have shown that TKA motions can vary dramatically, depending on the activity and the implant design [13]. Many implant designs have articular surfaces with varying curvatures or mechanisms that engage at different parts of the flexion arc. Intuitively, these changing constraints might result in different kinematic patterns depending on the flexion range of the activity. Conversely, implant designs with consistent intrinsic constraint over the flexion arc might be expected to show similar motion patterns across the range of activities. Comparison of TKA motions during the stance phase of gait and during stair activities confirms these concepts (◘ Fig. 18-7). For example, posterior stabilized fixed-bearing TKA designs consistently showed more medial centers of rotation during stair activities than during gait (Fig.18-7a). During stair-climbing, the post-cam mechanism controls motion and forces posterior femoral translation with flexion. During gait, the post-cam mechanism is not engaged and the femur tends to slide posterior with extension, more so on the medial side. The opposite situation is observed in rotating platform mobile-bearing knees with gait-congruent articulations (Fig.18-7b). During gait the tibiofemoral articulation is fully conforming and allows only axial rotation with flexion/extension. Stair-climbing flexes the knee beyond the range of tibiofemoral congruency and the femur slides forward on the tibia with flexion, more on the medial side. Implants having condyles with the same sagittal radius from 0° to 75° of flexion, and correspondingly consistent tibiofemoral constraint, did exhibit similar motions for the gait and stair activities (Fig. 18-7c).

Other Applications for In Vivo Data

In vivo kinematic data are unquestionably useful for understanding the interplay of implant design and surgical factors in TKA performance. In addition, these data provide important corroboration or guidance for other studies. For example, interpretations of wear patterns on retrieved tibial inserts are greatly enhanced with knowledge of that particular implant's in vivo kinematics [14]. In vivo kinematics can be used to implement increasingly realistic and more powerfully predictive mechanical wear tests. With advanced computer codes, it is now possible to input in vivo kinematics and make reasonably accurate predictions of an implant"s wear performance over its service life [15].

Conclusion

Fluoroscopy has provided a unique window for direct observation and measurement of dynamic knee replacement motions. Shape-matching-based measurements have provided a powerful tool for accurately quantifying knee motions and providing informative characterizations of implant design and surgical factors influencing patient outcomes. In addition to providing an enhanced understanding of implant design and surgical issues, these in vivo data provide a useful complement to retrieval studies, gait laboratory analyses, and computer simulations.

References

1. Banks SA (1992) Model-based 3D kinematic estimation from 2D perspective silhouettes: application with total knee prostheses. Doctoral dissertation, Massachusetts Institute of Technology, Cambridge, MA
2. Banks SA, Hodge WA (1996) Accurate measurement of three-dimensional knee replacement kinematics using single-plane fluoroscopy. IEEE Trans Biomed Eng 43/6:638-649
3. Dennis DA et al (2003) In vivo fluoroscopic analysis of fixed-bearing total knee replacements. Clin Orthop 410:114-130
4. Fantozzi S et al (2003) Fluoroscopic and gait analysis of the functional performance in stair ascent of two total knee replacement designs. Gait Posture 17:225-234
5. Kanekasu K et al (2004) Fluoroscopic analysis of knee arthroplasty kinematics during deep flexion kneeling. J Arthroplasty 19:998-1003
6. Banks SA et al (2002) The mechanism of anterior impingement damage in TKR. J Bone Joint Surg [Am] 84 [Suppl 2]:37-42
7. Callaghan JJ et al (2002) Tibial post impingement in posterior-stabilized total knee arthroplasty. Clin Orthop 404:83-88
8. Walker PS, Garg A (1991) Range of motion in total knee arthroplasty. A computer analysis. Clin Orthop 262:227-235
9. Banks SA et al (2003) Tibio-femoral translation and maximum weight-bearing flexion in fixed and mobile bearing knee arthroplasties. Clin Orthop Rel Res 410:131-138
10. Bellemans J et al (2002) Fluoroscopic analysis of the kinematics of deep flexion in total knee arthroplasty. Influence of posterior condylar offset. J Bone Joint Surg [Br] 84:50-53
11. Banks SA et al (1991) In vivo bearing motion with meniscal bearing TKR. Orthop Trans 15:544

12. Banks SA, Hodge WA (2004) Implant design affects knee arthroplasty kinematics during stair-stepping. Clin Orthop Rel Res 426:187-193

13. Banks SA, Hodge WA (2004) Design and activity dependence of kinematics in fixed and mobile bearing knee arthroplasties - The Hap Paul Award Paper. J Arthroplasty 19:809-816

14. Harman MK et al (2001) Polyethylene damage and knee kinematics after total knee arthroplasty. Clin Orthop Rel Res 392:383-393

15. Fregly BJ, Sawyer WG, Harman MK, Banks SA (2005) Computational wear prediction of a total knee replacement from in vivo kinematics. J Biomech 38(2): 305-14

19   The Importance of the ACL for the Function of the Knee: Relevance to Future Developments in Total Knee Arthroplasty

A. M. Chaudhari, C. O. Dyrby, T. P. Andriacchi

Summary

This chapter discusses the importance of the anterior cruciate ligament (ACL) for the function of the knee by examining the functional role of the cruciate ligaments in healthy knee joints and the functional results of different total knee designs. The cruciate ligaments influence the motion of the knee in multiple planes, restraining AP translations as well as axial rotations to varying degrees, based on the angle of flexion. Functional analyses of knee arthroplasty designs that retain no cruciate ligaments, the PCL only, and both ligaments show differences, with unicompartmental knee arthroplasties retaining function that is the closest to normal function. After total knee arthroplasties, even asymptomatic patients showed gait abnormalities such as quadriceps avoidance that could lead to reduced functional ability to perform activities of daily living over time. These results and continuing positive short- and long-term follow-up of patients who have received ACL-retaining prostheses should increase enthusiasm for these procedures in the future.

Introduction

Over the past 40 years, total knee arthroplasties (TKA) have become the standard of care for end-stage knee arthritis, with excellent long-term clinical outcomes for patients. The most common TKA procedures involve removal of the anterior cruciate ligament (ACL), and often of the posterior cruciate ligament (PCL) as well. While these procedures do result in positive overall results for patients, they also result in changes in functional abilities, such as quadriceps avoidance [3] and changed upper-body mechanics during stair-climbing and rising from a chair [5]. Several authors have also reported postero-medial wear of the tibial component following TKA [10, 13, 15].

Alternatives to the standard ACL-sacrificing TKA are not nearly as common, but they have been shown to also have excellent long-term results in patients. The Cloutier prosthesis, which retains both cruciate ligaments, has been shown to have good or excellent results in 97% of patients after 9-11 years, with no evidence of the postero-medial wear on the tibial component observed in ACL-sacrificing TKA [9]. Unicompartmental knee arthroplasties (UKA) have also shown excellent clinical results, in both the short and the long term [7]. Furthermore, compared with total knee arthroplasty, the cost saving from the prosthesis, length of stay, and reduced blood products make UKA an even more attractive alternative. Thus, interest in unicompartmental arthroplasty is resurging.

In most patients, UKA has potential advantages over both proximal tibial osteotomy and total knee arthroplasty. Compared with total knee arthroplasties, UKA is a preserving procedure. First, the bone stock is preserved. Second, with UKA the patellofemoral joint, the ACL and PCL, and the meniscus with the articular surface of the opposite compartment are preserved. Finally, if necessary, a UKA can be easily revised to a total knee arthroplasty.

Differences in the patterns of motion when the cruciate ligaments are retained versus when they are sacrificed may also result in differences in the wear characteristics of the metal and polyethylene components. These differences may affect the longevity of the prosthesis, which is especially relevant today as knee arthroplasties are considered for younger, more active populations.

Functional Role of the Cruciate Ligaments

The cruciate ligaments appear crossed when viewed in the sagittal plane and their function has often been related to the mechanics of a four-bar linkage. However, the cruciate ligaments are actually crossed in three-dimensional space, resulting in behavior that is more closely associated with elastic cables that provide an envelope of stability and motion. For example, at any angle of knee flexion there is a range of possible anterior-posterior translations that are possible. It has been shown that in a neutral position the passive knee joint will move within a certain range without noticeable resistance to applied loads. This region can be considered as a region of extremely low stiffness or high mobility of the knee joint. This envelope of stiffness or flexibility varies with the angle of knee flexion. At full extension the envelope of motion is quite small and the knee remains quite stable, with the ACL completely tensed. As the knee flexes from full extension, the ACL relaxes. The PCL does not begin to tighten until the knee flexes beyond 40° of flexion. Thus, as the knee flexes from full extension the envelope (anterior-posterior motion) increases. At approximately 20° of flexion there is a minimum of restraint to anterior-posterior motion of the knee. As the knee flexes past 40° to deep flexion, the PCL tightens to reduce the envelope of motion again. This changing envelope of stability at the knee is important from a functional viewpoint. At full extension, the knee is passively stable, allowing for standing posture with a minimal amount of muscular demand. During dynamic activities such as walking (where the knee typically flexes to approximately 20° during mid-stance), the ligaments are relatively relaxed; and dynamic stability is provided by large muscle forces generated by muscle contraction.

The interaction between the orientation of the cruciate ligaments and the cam-like shape of the femoral condyles are the primary determinants of how the knee changes its passive stability with flexion. ◘ Figure 19-1 illustrates the interaction between the cam-shaped geometry of the femoral condyles and the orientation of the cruciate ligaments. In full extension the sagittal plane orientation of the ACL is at its greatest angle with respect to the joint line, while the PCL is at its closest to horizontal. As the knee flexes to 90°, the ACL becomes horizontal and the PCL becomes perpendicular to the joint line. Thus,

when the knee is flexed the posterior cruciate provides distraction stability to the knee. This function is likely important for activities involving deep flexion such as squatting, where knee flexion can exceed 130° of flexion.

The cruciate ligaments influence stability and motion in planes other than the sagittal plane. The attachment of the ACL on the medial portion of the lateral femoral condyle relative to its tibial attachment, and the attachment of the PCL on the lateral portion of the medial femoral condyle relative to its tibial attachment orient the ligaments obliquely in the frontal plane (◘ Fig. 19-2). This oblique orientation of the cruciate ligaments is compatible with the asymmetry in the geometry of the distal femoral condyles. As previously described (Fig. 19-1), the femur rolls posteriorly during flexion from full extension. Since the distal curvature of the lateral femoral condyle is larger, the lateral femoral condyle will move posteriorly a greater distance than the medial femoral condyle. As a re-

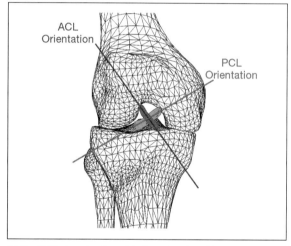

◘ **Fig. 19-2.** Anterior view of the knee showing oblique orientation of anterior cruciate ligament (red) and posterior cruciate ligament (green)

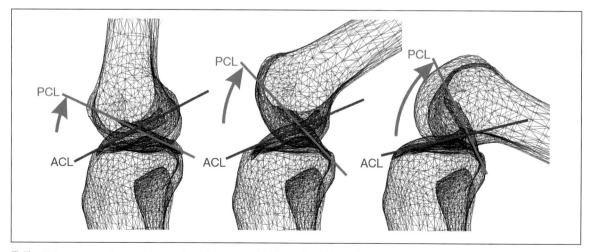

◘ **Fig. 19-1.** Interaction between the cam-shaped geometry of the femoral condyles and the orientation of the cruciate ligaments

Chapter 19 · The Importance of the ACL for the Function of the Knee – A.M. Chaudhari et al.

123   **19**

sult, the femur will rotate externally with flexion relative to the tibia. With extension, the femur will rotate internally relative to the tibia, a motion commonly referred to as "screw-home" motion. The cruciate ligaments act as fulcrums to further guide and constrain the motion, creating a balance between rolling and sliding motions and maintaining the normal tension in these ligaments throughout the range of motion.

When one or both of these ligaments are missing, this envelope of motion becomes disrupted. ACL-deficient patients experience reduced internal femoral rotation and reduced anterior tibial translation throughout the gait cycle during walking [1]. The geometric interaction between the anatomy of the cruciate ligaments and the geometry of the distal femoral condyles is likely an important consideration in the design of knee arthroplasties where retention of the cruciate ligaments is considered. Clearly, the interaction with the femoral condyles and the orientation of the cruciate ligament play a fundamental role in the function of the knee joint.

Functional Analyses of Knee Arthroplasty Designs

In a study of the influence of TKA design on walking and stair-climbing [3], it was found that after TKA, even asymptomatic patients with excellent clinical results had a gait abnormality. The feature of the abnormality consisted of shorter stride length, reduced mid-stance knee flexion, and abnormal patterns of external flexion-extension moment. Furthermore, patients with less constrained designs which retain both cruciate ligaments, such as the Cloutier and Gunston prostheses, seemed to have a more normal gait during stair-climbing than patients with more constrained cruciate-sacrificing designs.

In this analysis the Cloutier prosthesis retained the most of the native structure of the knee; both cruciate ligaments, an unconstrained articulation, and the native patellofemoral joint. This prosthesis, which anatomically most simulated the native knee functionally, performed most closely to the native knee. Furthermore, this prosthesis most closely simulated a unicompartmental knee arthroplasty.

Chassin et al. reported on the functional analysis of patients with medial unicompartmental knee arthroplasties [8]. The study found that 70% of the ten patients with unicompartmental knee arthroplasties maintained the normal biphasic pattern of flexion/extension moments about the knee during gait. Throughout the stance phase, this normal moment pattern oscillates between an initial flexion moment, then an extension moment, and once again to a flexion moment. Two of the patients exhibited quadriceps avoidance patterns that had pre-

Table 19-1. Percentage prevalence of biphasic, quadriceps avoidance, and quadriceps overuse in the normal, UKA, and TKA groups. (Reproduced from [8])

	Normal (n=29)	Group UKA (n=10)	TKA (n=35)
Biphasic	79	70	23
Quadriceps avoidance	16	20	46
Quadriceps overuse	5	10	31

dominantly extensional patterns, where the moment remained extensional throughout stance phase. The other patient with an abnormal pattern exhibited a quadriceps overuse pattern. This pattern had a predominantly flexional moment pattern, where the moment remained flexional throughout stance phase.

The distribution of gait patterns was compared with those of a previously published group of normal control subjects [2] and a previously published group of TKA subjects [3]. In the normal group, 79% exhibited a normal flexion/extension pattern. Using a Fisher's exact test, there was no difference in distribution of flexion/extension moment patterns between the unicompartmental knee arthroplasties and the normal knees. However, there was a significant difference between the total knee arthroplasties and the normal knees. Finally, there was a difference between the UKA and the TKA groups. The distribution of the moment patterns for normal knees, unicompartmental knee arthroplasties, and total knee arthroplasties is summarized in ◻ Table 19-1. Since 16% have a quadriceps avoidance pattern and 5% have a quadriceps overuse pattern in the normal population [2], the 20% quadriceps avoidance and 10% quadriceps overuse patterns in the UKA patients appear to be a reflection of the variability normally found in the flexion/extension moments about the knee.

The retention of the ACL in the unicompartmental knee arthroplasty population provides a possible explanation for the functional difference between the UKA and TKA populations. Sacrifice of the ACL removes a constraint to the anterior displacement of the tibia produced by quadriceps contraction near full extension. Patients with ACL deficiency developed a quadriceps avoidance type of gait [4], suggesting that the similar quadriceps avoidance pattern of gait found in the total knee arthroplasty patients is at least in part the result of sacrifice of the ACL during the procedure. Prostheses which retain the ACL, such as the Cloutier prosthesis or a UKA, have a low prevalence of the quadriceps avoidance pattern and therefore function more closely to the normal knee. This normal knee function affects not only the knee, but also the kinematics of the entire body.

Proper knee function is crucial to ascending stairs and rising from a chair. The stresses on the lower body joints during these activities are more than those that occur during gait. It has been shown by other investigators that TKA patients neither ascend stairs nor rise from a chair normally [5]. Furthermore, it has been shown that for comparing lower extremity performance in contrasting subject groups, ascending stairs and particularly rising from a chair are superior to gait analysis in reproducibility and in controlling incremental alterations in mechanical demands on the subject [6].

Berger et al. reported functional performance differences between seven unicompartmental knee arthroplasties and six PCL-sparing total knee arthroplasties [5]. Twelve healthy women with no musculoskeletal complaints were used as a control group. Participants rose from four chair heights: 115%, 100%, 80%, and 65% of each participant's knee height. The participants also ascended a standard staircase.

When rising from a chair, both knee arthroplasty groups experienced lower knee flexion moments than the normal group, although the UKA group averaged only 17% lower peak moments while the TKA group averaged 26% lower peak moments. The peak knee flexion moment is attained just as the subject lifts off the chair. At this point in the motion, the knee flexion angle is greatest and the participant's weight is furthest from the knee joint. The mechanical demands on the body increase as chair height is diminished. Normal subjects are able to increase their knee moment as chair height is diminished. Not only do both unicompartmental and total knee arthroplasty groups develop a smaller knee moment at every chair height than normal; they also demonstrate less ability to meet increasing knee extensor demands, resulting in larger and larger differences from the normal group as the chair height is decreased. However, compared with TKA patients, UKA patients are able to produce a more normal knee moment at every chair height. Total knee arthroplasty patients demonstrate a flat plateau from 80% to 65%, indicating a limit of ability to generate a knee moment. Unicompartmental knee arthroplasty patients show less of the plateau effect, although their knee moment response is not as much as the normal response [5].

Berger et al. also examined the difference in upper body velocity between groups when rising from a chair. Upper body velocity is attained just prior to lift off and is a measure of the upper body's momentum. This momentum is then harnessed to aid the lower body in rising [14]. For each successive reduction in chair height, normals produce incrementally more upper body velocity. All three groups initially attained approximately the same upper body velocity at the highest, least demanding chair height. Unlike the normal and the UKA groups, the TKA group generated significantly more upper body velocity as the mechanical demands of rising increased with de-creasing chair height. The UKA group attained only slightly more upper body velocity than the normal group even at the highest chair height [5]. Since the effects on the knee were less extreme in the UKA group, they were not required to make as extreme compensations when performing this very common and necessary activity of daily living. Making these compensations may cause other secondary problems to these patients, such as excess muscle strain in the arms or back.

Moreover, it has been reported that elderly subjects often are near the limits of their knee extensor strength when rising from a chair [12]. In this study, Hughes et al. found that this population required 97% of their available strength when rising from the lowest chair height from which they could successfully rise. Since it is well known that in the elderly, disuse leads to muscle wasting and continued use is necessary to muscle maintenance [11], the quadriceps disuse that occurs as a result of the quadriceps avoidance gait observed most often in TKA patients may reduce their functional ability to perform activities of daily living such as rising from a chair and ascending stairs.

Conclusions

The cruciate ligaments perform several important functions in the healthy knee, from controlling the allowable envelope of anterior-posterior motion in the knee to controlling motion in other planes as well. The anterior cruciate ligament in particular affects the function of the knee extensor mechanism as an antagonist to the action of the patellar ligament at low flexion angles. The functional effects of sacrificing the ACL have been shown in several studies of walking, ascending stairs, and rising from a chair. While all knee arthroplasties do cause changes in the knee motion as well as in the total body response during these activities, ACL-retaining arthroplasties such as the Cloutier prosthesis and unicompartmental knee arthroplasties appear to retain function that is closer to normal. In addition, these knee arthroplasties offer long-term results similar to those with other total knee arthroplasty designs. Unicompartmental knee arthroplasties have the added advantages of replacing only the degenerated portion of the joint, retaining more of the bone stock, and requiring shorter hospital stays and fewer blood products. Continued positive short- and long-term follow-up of patients who have received these alternative, ACL-retaining procedures should increase enthusiasm among clinicians in the future and improve both clinical and functional outcomes for patients even further.

19

Chapter 19 · The Importance of the ACL for the Function of the Knee – A.M. Chaudhari et al.

125   **19**

References

1. Andriacchi TP et al (2004) Interactions between kinematics and loading during walking for the normal and ACL-deficient knee. J Biomech (in press)
2. Andriacchi TP, Strickland AB (1985) Biomechanics of normal and pathological human articulating joints. Proceedings of the NATO Advanced Study Institute. 93/83, Martinus Nijhoff, Dordrecht
3. Andriacchi TP, et al (1982) The influence of total knee-replacement design on walking and stair-climbing. J Bone Joint Surg [Am] 64:1328-1335
4. Berchuck M, et al (1990) Gait adaptations by patients who have a deficient anterior cruciate ligament. J Bone Joint Surg [Am] 72:871-877
5. Berger RA, et al (1990) Functional differences following unicompartmental and total knee replacements. Trans 36th Annu Meeting Orthopedic Research Society 15/1:282, American Association of Orthopedic Surgeons, Rosemont, IL
6. Berger RA, et al (1989) Advantages of rising from a chair to quantitate human performance, Trans 35th Annu Meeting Orthopedic Research Society 14/91, American Association of Orthopedic Surgeons, Rosemont, IL
7. Berger RA, et al (1999) Unicompartmental knee arthroplasty. Clinical experience at 6- to 10-year follow-up. Clin Orthop Rel Res 367:50-60
8. Chassin EP et al (1996) Functional analysis of cemented medial unicompartmental knee arthroplasty. J Arthroplasty 11:553-559
9. Cloutier JM, et al (1999) Total knee arthroplasty with retention of both cruciate ligaments. A nine to eleven-year follow-up study. J Bone Joint Surg [Am] 81:697-702
10. Feng EL, et al (1994) Progressive subluxation and polyethylene wear in total knee replacements with flat articular surfaces. Clin Orthop Rel Res 299:60-71
11. Hopp JF (1993) Effects of age and resistance training on skeletal muscle - a review, Phys Ther 73:361-373
12. Hughes MA et al (1996) The role of strength in rising from a chair in the functionally impaired elderly. J Biomech 29:1509-1513
13. Lewis P et al (1994) Posteromedial tibial polyethylene failure in total knee replacements. Clin Orthop Rel Res 299:11-17
14. Schenkman M et al (1990) Whole-body movements during rising to standing from sitting. Phys Ther 70:638-651
15. Wasielewski RC et al (1994) Wear patterns on retrieved polyethylene tibial inserts and their relationship to technical considerations during total knee arthroplasty. Clin Orthop Rel Res 299:31-43

20 Kinematics of Mobile Bearing Total Knee Arthroplasty

D. A. Dennis, R. D. Komistek

Summary

Review of the kinematic patterns of fixed- vs. mobile-bearing TKA has not demonstrated major differences, with the following exceptions. Less (minimal) anteroposterior translation of both the medial and lateral femoral condyles was observed during gait in patients who received mobile-bearing designs than in those implanted with fixed-bearing TKA. This is likely secondary to the increased sagittal femorotibial conformity present in most mobile-bearing designs. This reduces polyethylene shear stresses and should result in lower polyethylene wear rates in mobile-bearing TKA.

In rotating-platform mobile-bearing designs, axial rotation occurs primarily on the inferior surface of the polyethylene bearing, as compared with primarily on the superior surface in fixed-bearing TKA. This should reduce shear forces on the superior aspect of the polyethylene bearing, thereby lessening wear. Additionally, while average axial rotational values following TKA were limited (<10°), a significant number of subjects exhibited higher magnitudes (>20°) of rotation which exceed the rotational limits of most fixed bearing TKA designs. This may be an advantage of rotating-platform mobile-bearing TKA designs which can accommodate a wider range of axial rotation without creation of excessive polyethylene stresses.

Introduction

Various methods have been utilized to analyze kinematics of the normal knee and the knee after implantation of total knee arthroplasty (TKA) [1, 11-13, 15, 26-29, 33-36, 40, 41, 46, 49, 50, 59-66]. These have included in vitro cadaveric evaluations [19, 21, 30, 43, 45, 51, 53], gait laboratory motion analysis systems [1-3, 19, 40, 47, 68], roentgen stereophotogrammetric analyses (RSA) [34-36, 49, 50], quasi-dynamic MRI testing [27, 33], and in vivo video fluoroscopy [11-13, 15, 26, 28, 29, 41, 57, 61]. Unfortunately, cadaveric studies often do not simulate in vivo conditions since the actuators utilized to apply joint loads are often unable to accurately reproduce in vivo motions. RSA analyses have often been performed under non-weight-

bearing conditions and are quasi-dynamic [34-36, 49, 50]. Error analyses of gait laboratory evaluations have suggested that these systems can induce significant out-of-plane rotational and translational error due to motion between skin markers and underlying osseous structures [40, 46]. Murphy [46, 47] determined that the out-of-plane rotational error could be as high as 18° for internal-external knee rotation, quite unacceptable for analyses of TKA rotation, which is often less than 5° degrees during certain activities [18].

More recently, video fluoroscopy has been utilized to assess kinematics of both non-implanted and implanted knees [11-13, 15, 26, 28, 29, 41, 59-66]. This method has the advantage of testing under in vivo, weight-bearing, and fully dynamic conditions, while subjects perform various activities. Development of automated model-fitting methods allow for three-dimensional (3D) analyses to be conducted from two-dimensional (2D) fluoroscopic images with minimal in-plane or out-of-plane error [29, 41]. Three-dimensional evaluation of sequential fluoroscopic images can then be performed to accurately determine knee kinematic patterns.

The objective of the following report is to summarize our various in vivo kinematic analyses of multiple groups of patients implanted with various designs of mobile-bearing TKA and to compare their in vivo knee kinematic patterns with those found in studies of fixed-bearing TKA and the normal knee.

Methods

In vivo knee kinematics (anteroposterior translation, axial rotation, femoral condylar liftoff, and range-of-motion) have been determined in several studies following implantation of multiple designs of fixed- and mobile-bearing TKA [4, 7, 11-13, 24, 28, 29, 39, 52, 55, 59, 60, 61, 63, 67]. The material presented is a summation analysis of over 90 individual studies performed in our research facility over the past 10 years.

All subjects were analyzed under fluoroscopic surveillance, either during the stance-phase of gait from heel-strike to toe-off or during a deep knee bend maneuver from full extension through 90° of flexion. For gait analysis, individual fluoroscopic videoframes at heel-strike, 33% of stance phase, 66% of stance phase, and at toe-off were digitized, whereas videoframes at 0°, 30°, 60°, and 90° flexion were digitized for deep knee bend analyses. Knees analyzed included those considered normal (nonimplanted) or those implanted with 33 different designs of fixed- and mobile-bearing TKA. All knee replacement subjects analyzed were judged clinically successful (Hospital for Special Surgery Knee Scores [31] rated excellent) without any significant ligamentous laxity or functionally limiting pain.

Fluoroscopic images were captured and downloaded to a workstation computer for analysis. Three-dimensional kinematics for each knee were recovered from the 2D fluoroscopic images using a previously described automated model-fitting technique that determines the in vivo orientation of the femoral component relative to the tibial component and, subsequently, the contact positions between the femoral and tibial components [57]. Extensive error analyses of the 3D model fitting technique have shown a translational 3D error of less than 0.5° [29, 41]. Sequential fluoroscopic videoframes were then analyzed to determine kinematic patterns. A femorotibial contact position anterior to the midline was denoted as positive and a posterior position was denoted as negative. The magnitudes of anteroposterior translation were then determined for six individual increments of gait and six flexion increments of a deep knee bend (☐ Table 20-1).

The measurements of anteroposterior (AP) translation represented either pure AP linear motion or rotation of the femoral component relative to the tibial component, or a combination of both. The reported measurements comprised the amount of motion each condyle moves along the AP axis fixed on the tibia plateau. If pure linear translation occurred, both condyles moved in the same direction along this axis. If rotation occurred, one condyle moved anteriorly, whereas the other condyle moved in the posterior direction.

After completion of the AP femorotibial translation kinematic evaluations, axial rotation patterns were determined. To accomplish this, a line was created from the medial condylar contact point to the lateral condylar contact point. A second line was then constructed, bisecting the center of the tibial plateau in the coronal plane. The angle created between these two lines was measured and denoted as the axial rotation angle. If the lateral condylar contact position was more anterior than the medial condylar contact position, then the axial rotation angle was denoted as negative. If the medial condylar contact point was more anterior than the lateral condylar contact point, the axial rotation angle was denoted as positive.

The magnitudes of axial rotation were then determined for the same six individual increments of gait and six flexion increments of a deep knee bend, as had been done in the evaluation of AP translation (☐ Table 20-1). This was accomplished by subtracting the axial rotation angle at the beginning of the increment to be analyzed from the axial rotation angle at the end of the analyzed increment. If the change in rotation was positive, then it was denoted as a positive (normal) magnitude of axial rotation (☐ Fig. 20-1) and a negative change was considered a negative magnitude of axial rotation (or reverse axial rotation; ☐ Fig. 20-2). In the normal knee, the axial rotation angle is negative at full extension (lateral condylar contact position more anterior than the medial contact

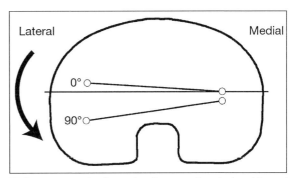

☐ **Fig. 20-1.** Example of normal axial rotation where the lateral femoral condyle rotates more posteriorly than the medial condyle (i.e., internal tibial rotation) as flexion increases

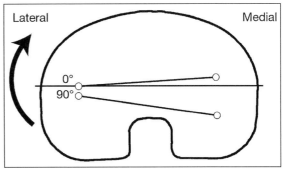

☐ **Fig. 20-2.** Example of a reverse axial rotational pattern where the medial femoral condyle rotates more posteriorly than the lateral condyle (i.e., external tibial rotation) as flexion increases

☐ **Table 20-1.** Individual increments analyzed during gait and a deep knee bend

Stance phase of gait	Deep knee bend
Heel-strike to 33% of stance phase	Full extension to 30° of knee flexion
Heel-strike to 66% of stance phase	Full extension to 60° of knee flexion
Heel-strike to toe-off	Full extension to 90° of knee flexion
33%-66% of stance phase	30°-60° of knee flexion
33% of stance phase to toe-off	30°-90° of knee flexion
66% of stance phase to toe-off	60°-90° of knee flexion

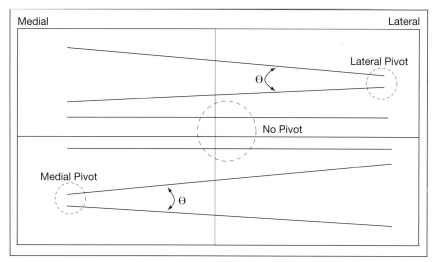

Fig. 20-3. The location of the pivot position was determined from the convergence angle between the lines connecting the medial and lateral condyle contact positions at full extension and at 90° of knee flexion. If the angle between these lines (Θ) converged on the medial half of the tibial insert a medial pivot point was denoted, and if this angle converged on the lateral half, a lateral pivot point was denoted. If this angle did not have a definite convergence and tended towards infinity, no pivot position was denoted

position) and in deeper flexion, the axial rotation angle is positive (medial contact position more anterior than lateral). Therefore, a positive axial rotation pattern occurred when the tibia internally rotated with increasing knee flexion (positive screw-home rotational pattern), and a negative axial rotation pattern (reverse screw-home rotational pattern) occurred when the tibia externally rotated with increasing knee flexion.

Next, the condylar pivot position was determined by analysis of medial and lateral condylar contact positions at full extension and 90° flexion. Two lines were constructed between the medial and lateral condylar contact positions at full extension and also at 90° of flexion (Fig. 20-3). An angle (Θ) was then determined between these two lines. If the full extension and 90° flexion lines converged on the medial half of the tibia in the coronal plane (apex of angle Θ), it denoted that a medial pivot location occurred. If the lines converged on the lateral half of the tibial insert, it denoted that a lateral pivot location had occurred. If these lines remained parallel to each other and the angle appeared to approach infinity, no convergence was found and it denoted that there was no pivot location.

Upon completion of the sagittal plane kinematic analyses, the grouped implants were rotated to a frontal view to assess for femoral condylar liftoff. This was determined by measuring the distances from the medial and lateral femoral condyles to the tibial tray (Fig. 20-4). If the difference in the medial vs. lateral condylar distance was greater than our error value of 0.75 mm (3.0 standard deviations from our true error value of 0.25 mm), it was determined that femoral condylar liftoff had occurred [42].

Range of motion was determined under weight-bearing conditions by measuring the femorotibial angle in maximum extension and by analyzing the angle at the maximum flexion videoframe. Finally, the existing model-fitting methodology for 3D kinematic analyses of TKA was adapted to determine the 3D kinematics of the normal femorotibial joint [29, 38, 57]. Ten normal knees were evaluated using this methodology. An initial advantage of analyzing TKA kinematics was that the required computer-assisted design (CAD) models could be created from manufacturer blueprints. However, because the skeletal geometry is variable for every person, computer-generated 3D models of the normal femur, tibia, and fibula had to be created for each specific subject. To determine normal knee kinematics, the 3D models of each subject's femur, tibia, and fibula were registered precisely to the 2D fluoroscopic images using an optimization algorithm that automatically adjusts the pose of the model at various knee flexion angles [38]. For each activity, the femorotibial contact patterns of normal knees were determined for the medial and lateral condyles and plotted with respect to knee flexion angle.

Results and Discussion

Anterior-Posterior Translation in Gait

In a multicenter analysis [16], AP translation patterns (i.e., posterior femoral roll-back vs. anterior femoral trans-

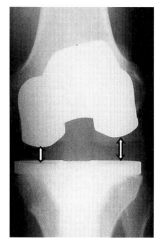

Fig. 20-4. Method of determination of femoral condylar liftoff in which the distances between the femoral condyles and the tibial tray (*arrows*) are determined and compared

lation) of 261 knees during gait were analyzed: 251 had been implanted with a TKA and ten were judged to be normal knees. Fifteen of the implanted knees were ACL-retaining fixed-bearing TKAs. Eighty-three knees had been implanted with a PCL-retaining fixed-bearing TKA, 74 knees received a posterior-stabilized fixed-bearing TKA, ten knees received a PCL-retaining mobile-bearing TKA, 35 knees received a posterior-stabilized mobile-bearing TKA, and 34 knees received a posterior cruciate-sacrificing mobile-bearing TKA.

From heel-strike to toe-off, nine of ten subjects (90%) with a normal knee experienced posterior motion of their lateral femoral condyle, whereas the medial condyle translated posteriorly in five of the ten knees (50%; □ Fig. 20-5). The average total lateral condyle motion from heel-strike (0% of stance phase) to toe-off (100% of stance phase) was -5.8 mm (4.3 to -23.1 mm; SD=8.1), whereas the medial condylar motion was less, averaging only -0.4 mm

(10.6 to -19.5 mm; SD=6.6). As the direction of knee flexion angle changed from extension to flexion, the lateral condyle translated in the posterior direction. When the angle changed from flexion into extension, the lateral condyle translated anteriorly.

The *average* magnitudes of AP translation observed during gait were minimal (typically <2 mm) both medially and laterally for all fixed- and mobile-bearing TKA subjects when compared with normal knees (□ Fig. 20-6). Similar patterns were observed in both PCL-retaining and PCL-substituting TKA subjects. This has been attributed to the fact that the cam-and-post mechanism of most PCL-substituting TKA designs does not engage during lesser flexion activities such as gait.

While the *average* magnitudes of AP translation of fixed- versus mobile-bearing TKA designs of similar type (i.e., fixed-bearing PCL-retaining versus mobile-bearing PCL-retaining, etc.) were not statistically different, analy-

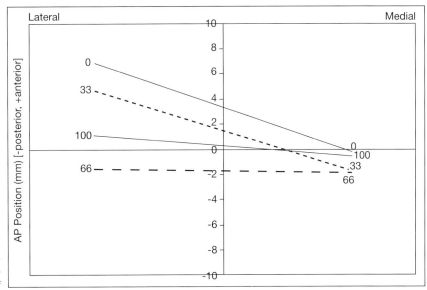

□ **Fig. 20-5.** Average medial and lateral condylar contact positions for the normal knee from heel-strike to toe-off

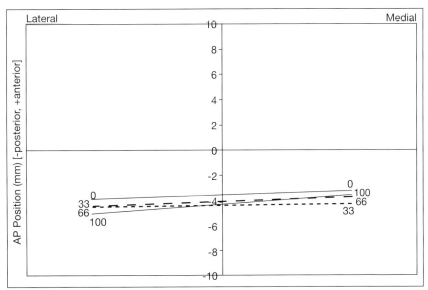

□ **Fig. 20-6.** Average medial and lateral condyle contact positions for a fixed-bearing posterior cruciate-retaining total knee arthroplasty from heel-strike to toe-off

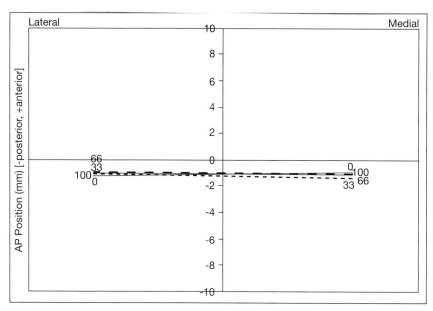

Fig. 20-7. Average medial and lateral condylar contact positions for a rotating-platform posterior cruciate-sacrificing total knee arthroplasty from heel-strike to toe-off

sis of interval segments of the stance phase of gait demonstrated higher magnitudes of AP translation in fixed-bearing than in mobile-bearing designs (p<0.05). Additionally, much greater variability in contact position (anterior versus midline versus posterior) on the tibial component was seen in fixed-bearing TKA designs. Typically, minimal AP motion of both the medial and lateral femoral condyles was observed during gait in patients who received mobile-bearing TKAs (■ Fig. 20-7). This phenomenon is likely related to the higher sagittal femorotibial conformity present in most mobile-bearing designs. They also demonstrated less paradoxical anterior femoral sliding during the flexion segments of the stance phase of gait. This results in reduced polyethylene shear stresses and may account, at least in part, for the low polyethylene wear rates reported with long-term clinical use of mobile-bearing TKA [8, 48].

Anterior-Posterior Translation in a Deep Knee Bend

In the same multicenter study [16], 550 knees were analyzed during a deep knee bend maneuver. Ten were normal knees and ten had been implanted with an ACL-retaining fixed-bearing TKA. Of the remainder, 136 knees had received a PCL-retaining fixed-bearing TKA, 163 knees had a posterior-stabilized fixed-bearing TKA, 69 knees had a PCL-retaining mobile-bearing TKA, 103 knees had a posterior-stabilized mobile-bearing TKA, and 59 knees had been implanted with a posterior cruciate-sacrificing mobile-bearing TKA.

The magnitudes of AP translation were substantially higher in deep flexion in normal knees and in all TKA groups tested than in a lesser flexion activity such as gait.

All ten (100%) subjects with a normal knee experienced posterior motion (i.e., posterior femoral roll-back) of the lateral femoral condyle from full extension to 90° of knee flexion, whereas nine of ten (90%) subjects experienced posterior motion of the medial condyle (■ Fig. 20-8). On average, posterior motion of the lateral femoral condyle was -19.2 mm (-5.8 to -31.6 mm; SD=8.4) and medial condylar motion was -3.4 mm (3.3 to -11.8 mm; SD=4.6) in the posterior direction. All subjects experienced posterior motion of both condyles from full extension to maximum flexion, but three of ten (30%) subjects had greater than 3 mm of medial condyle anterior translation during at least one analyzed increment of flexion. All lateral femoral condyles experienced only posterior motion. Only one of ten (10%) subjects experienced a lateral pivot motion, eight of ten (80%) had a medial pivot motion, and one of ten (10%) did not experience a pivot motion.

Similar to the subjects with a normal knee, all ten (100%) patients with an ACL-retaining fixed-bearing TKA experienced posterior motion of their lateral condyle, and nine of ten (90%) patients had posterior motion of their medial condyle (■ Fig. 20-9). The average amount of posterior motion of the lateral condyle was -13.6 mm (-10.0 to -20.3 mm; SD=3.7) and the medial condylar motion was -6.1 mm (5.6 to -15.0 mm; SD=6.3), posteriorly. One of ten (10%) patients experienced paradoxical anterior femoral motion of the medial condyle greater than 3 mm from full extension to 90° of knee flexion and six of ten (60%) patients experienced greater than 3 mm of medial condyle anterior translation during any increment of knee flexion. Similar to the normal knee, all lateral femoral condyles had only posterior motion; only one of ten (10%) patients experienced a lateral pivot motion, seven of ten (70%) had a medial pivot mo-

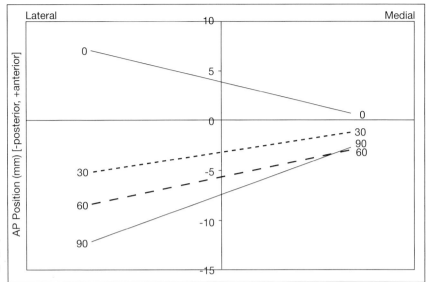

Fig. 20-8. Average medial and lateral condyle contact positions during a deep knee bend for the normal knee (0°-90° flexion)

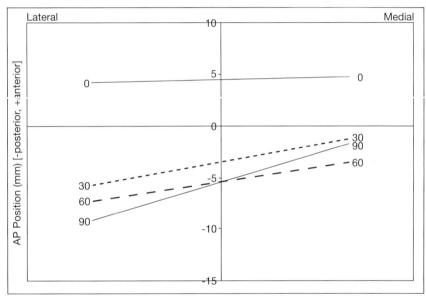

Fig. 20-9. Average medial and lateral condyle contact positions during a deep knee bend for a fixed-bearing anterior cruciate-retaining total knee arthroplasty (0°-90° flexion)

tion, and two of ten (20%) did not experience a pivot motion pattern.

Analysis of all remaining fixed- and mobile-bearing TKA groups demonstrated reduced magnitudes and percentages of posterior motion of both the medial and lateral femoral condyles, a higher incidence of paradoxical anterior femoral translation, and a reduced percentage of subjects exhibiting a medial pivot pattern (□ Table 20-2). No statistical differences in amounts of posterior translation during flexion were observed between fixed- and mobile-bearing posterior-stabilized TKAs or between fixed- and mobile-bearing PCL-retaining TKAs (p>0.2). However, subjects with both fixed- and mobile-bearing posterior-stabilized TKA designs exhibited higher magnitudes of posterior femoral translation than either fixed- or mobile-bearing designs that lacked a cam-and-post mechanism (p<0.01). The magnitudes of posterior trans-

lation presented in Table 20-2 may underestimate the maximum amounts of posterior femoral translation occurring during extreme flexion in posterior stabilized TKA designs since analysis was performed only to a maximum of 90° of flexion. Many posterior-stabilized implants are designed to have late cam-post engagement (>70° of knee flexion), which may result in additional posterior translation at flexion increments greater than 90°.

In the current study, patients with either a fixed- or a mobile-bearing PCL-retaining TKA experienced the highest incidence and magnitude of paradoxical anterior femoral translation of either femoral condyle. During a deep knee bend, 72% of patients with a PCL-retaining fixed-bearing TKA and 60% of patients with a PCL-retaining mobile-bearing TKA experienced greater than 3 mm of paradoxical femoral translation during knee

◻ Table 20-2. Average for all groups during a deep knee bend from full extension to 90° flexion

Implant type	No. of subjects	Percent with posterior motion		Average motion 0°-90° (mm)		> 30 mm 0°-90° (%)[a]	<30 mm any time (%)[b]	Maximum motion (mm)	Standard deviation		Pivot position		
		L	M	L	M	M or L	M or L		L	M	LP	MP	NP
Normal	10	100	90	-19.2	-3.4	0	30	5	8.4	4.6	10.0	80.0	10.0
ACL-retaining	10	100	90	-13.6	-6.1	10	60	8.1	3.7	6.3	10.0	70.0	20.0
PCL-retaining	136	64	34.6	-1.6	1.0	28	72	8.4	3.4	3.5	41.2	52.9	7.4
Posterior stabilized	163	83.4	60.1	-3.7	-1.0	4	43	6.3	3.3	2.7	22.7	68.7	8.6
PCL retaining mobile-bearing	69	68.1	46.4	-1.3	0.4	25	60	11.7	3.5	3.8	43.5	40.6	15.9
Posterior-stabilized mobile-bearing	103	84.5	49.5	-3.9	-0.8	7	34	6.2	2.9	2.8	32.0	63.1	4.9
PCL-sacrificing mobile-bearing	59	84.7	37.3	-2.1	0.4	18	54	6.8	2,7	2.6	45.8	49.2	5.1
Average		76.9	45.6	-2.5	0.0	17	52	7.9	3.1	3.1	37.0	54.9	8.4

L lateral condyle, *M* medial condyle, *LP* percent of subjects exhibiting a lateral pivot position, *MP* percent of subjects exhibiting a medial pivot position, *NP* percent of subjects exhibiting no pivot position
[a] >3.0 mm anterior motion for either condyle, measuring difference between full extension and 90° flexion positions
[b] >3.0 mm anterior motion for either condyle, occurring at any time during a deep knee bend

flexion. Predominantly during anterior femoral translation, both condyles shift anteriorly. Patients who had either a fixed- or mobile-bearing posterior-stabilized TKA also experienced anterior femoral motion, but it occurred primarily on the medial side after the cam and post had engaged (flexion >60°). At cam-post engagement, the medial condyle experiences the greatest shear forces and translates anteriorly as the lateral femoral condyle levers posteriorly. This finding was determined by analyzing the data in flexion increments greater than 60°. After a patient achieves 60° of knee flexion, the medial femoral condyle typically shifts anteriorly to a similar extent as the lateral condyle translates posteriorly.

The anterior translation of the femur on the tibia observed in our investigation has numerous potential negative consequences. First, anterior femoral translation results in a more anterior axis of flexion, lessening maximum knee flexion [11, 14]. Second, the quadriceps moment arm is decreased, resulting in reduced quadriceps efficiency. Third, anterior sliding of the femoral component on the tibial polyethylene surface risks accelerated polyethylene wear. In a laboratory evaluation of polyethylene wear, Blunn et al. [7] reported dramatically increased wear with cyclic sliding as compared with compression or rolling, because of increased subsurface shear stresses.

While the majority of normal knees demonstrated a medial pivot pattern during a deep knee bend activity, this was much less common in both fixed- and mobile-bearing TKA groups. Overall, during a deep knee bend maneuver, 313 of 540 subjects (58%) with a TKA had a medial pivot pattern, 184 of 540 TKA patients (34%) had a lateral pivot pattern, and 43 of 540 subjects (8%) with a TKA did not exhibit a pivot pattern.

When the effects of surgeon variability on AP motion patterns of subjects who received the same TKA design were investigated, no statistical differences among surgeons were noted in mobile-bearing TKA groups (p>0.2). In contrast, statistically significant differences among differing surgeons were observed in subjects who received fixed-bearing TKA devices of the same type (p<0.05). This may be attributed, at least in part, to the increased sagittal conformity commonly present in mobile-bearing TKA implants, which provides enhanced control of kinematic patterns, therefore lessening the affect of variances in technique among surgeons.

There also was great variability among TKA types within each group (posterior-stabilized fixed-bearing,

20

PCL-retaining fixed-bearing, etc.). For example, patients with a PCL-retaining fixed-bearing TKA with asymmetric femoral condyles experienced more than twice the amount of posterior femoral motion and substantially less paradoxical anterior femoral translation when compared with patients who had a PCL-retaining fixed-bearing TKA with symmetric femoral condyles [6]. Although it has often been assumed that all posterior-stabilized fixed-bearing TKA designs have similar kinematic patterns, the opposite is actually true. Differing incidences and magnitudes of posterior femoral roll-back typically were seen when comparing differing fixed-bearing posterior-stabilized TKA designs. One such design, for example, showed an excessively posterior contact position throughout the flexion range, thereby never achieving cam-post engagement.

Axial Rotation in Gait

In a multicenter evaluation of axial rotation during gait, 267 knees were analyzed [18]. Of these, 252 had been implanted with a TKA, ten were judged to be normal knees, and five were non-implanted, ACL-deficient knees. Fifteen of the implanted knees were ACL-retaining (ACR) fixed-bearing TKAs. Eighty-three knees had been implanted with a PCL-retaining (PCR) fixed-bearing TKA, 74 with a posterior-stabilized (PS) fixed-bearing TKA, ten with a PCL-retaining mobile bearing TKA, 35 with a PS mobile-bearing TKA, and 35 with a posterior cruciate-sacrificing (PCS) mobile-bearing TKA.

From heel-strike to toe-off, eight of ten subjects (80%) with a normal knee experienced normal axial rotation (tibia internally rotating with increasing knee flexion) and eight of ten subjects (80%) experienced reverse rotation during at least one analyzed increment of the stance phase of gait.

The normal knee did not experience progressive increasing axial rotation during stance-phase of gait, rather demonstrating a variable pattern that involves extension, flexion, extension and then flexion before toe-off. It would therefore be expected that subjects experience some reverse rotation during gait. The average amount of axial rotation from heel-strike to toe-off for normal knees was 5.7° and the average maximum axial rotation at any increment during stance-phase increased to 11.1°. The maximum amount of normal rotation observed for any individual normal knee at any analyzed increment was 24.0° (tibia internal rotation) and the maximum reverse rotation observed was -10.1° (tibia external rotation). Nine of ten subjects (90%) achieved at least 5.0° of normal rotation, five of ten (50%) greater than 10.0°, and five of ten (50%) demonstrated greater than -5.0° of reverse rotation.

Analysis of all fixed- and mobile-bearing TKA groups demonstrated reduced average rotational values (average 1.2°) and a reduced incidence of normal axial rotation patterns when compared with the normal knee during gait (Table 20-3). The axial rotation patterns for the fixed- and mobile-bearing PS TKA groups were similar, as were the axial rotation patterns for the fixed- and mobile-bearing PCL-retaining TKA groups. Although most subjects with a PCL-sacrificing mobile-bearing TKA did experience axial rotation, the *average* rotation for this group was 0°. Only 146 of 252 knees (58%) experienced a normal axial rotational pattern during the stance phase of gait; this was a decrease from the normal knees, which experienced 80% normal rotation, but was not statistically different ($p=0.15$). Also, only 86 of the 252 TKAs (34%) experienced greater than 5.0° of axial rotation at any analyzed increment, a significant decrease from that observed in normal knees (90%; $p<0.05$). This trend continued for knees experiencing greater than 10.0° of axial rotation. Only 15 of 252 (6%) TKAs experienced greater than 10.0° of axial rotation, compared with 50% of the normal knee group ($p=0.01$).

Axial Rotation in a Deep Knee Bend

In the same multicenter evaluation of axial rotation [18], 760 knees were analyzed during a deep knee bend. Ten were normal knees, five were ACL-deficient knees and ten were ACL-retaining fixed bearing TKAs. There were 183 knees that had been implanted with a PCL-retaining fixed-bearing TKA (163 with a functional PCL and 20 with the PCL sacrificed), 212 knees with a PS fixed-bearing TKA, 107 knees with a PCL-retaining mobile bearing TKA, 157 knees with a PS mobile-bearing TKA, and 76 knees with a PCL-sacrificing mobile-bearing TKA.

Increased axial rotation occurred more during deep flexion than during gait in all study groups. From full extension to 90° of knee flexion, all ten normal knees experienced normal axial rotation (tibia internally rotating with increasing knee flexion), and only four of ten subjects (40%) demonstrated reverse rotation during at least one analyzed flexion increment of a deep knee bend.

The average amount of axial rotation for normal knees from full extension to 90° of knee flexion was 16.5° and the average maximum amount of axial rotation at any flexion increment was 17.3°. The maximum amounts of normal and reverse rotation of any normal knee at any flexion increment were 27.7° and -7.3°. All ten knees achieved at least 5.0° of normal rotation, nine of ten (90%) greater than 10.0°, and only one of ten (10%) greater than -5.0° of reverse rotation.

Patients who received an ACL-retaining fixed-bearing TKA also achieved excellent axial rotation patterns, while those with an ACL-deficient knee experienced more variable rotational patterns (Table 20-4). Seven of ten knees (70%) implanted with an ACL-retaining fixed-bearing

Table 20-3. Summation analysis of axial rotation of all knee types during gait

Implant type	No. of knees	Normal rotation[a] HS-TO (%)	Reverse rotation[b] HS-TO (%)	Normal rotation all increments[c] (%)	Reverse rotation any increments[d] (%)	Average rotation HS-TO (degrees)	Average max. rot. all increments[f] (degrees)	Average max. rev. all increments[g] (degrees)	Maximum norm. rot. all increments[h] (degrees)	Maximum rev. rot. all increments[i] (degrees)	Normal rot.[j] >5.0° (%)	Normal rot.[k] >10.0° (%)	Reverse rot.[l] >-5.0° (%)
Normal	10	80	20	20	80	5.7	11.1	-4.1	24.0	-10.1	90	50	50
Fixed-bearing ACR	15	33	67	27	73	2	3.5	-1.6	12	-5.4	13		
ACL deficient	5	60	40	0	100	2	10.4	-7.4	17.5	-19.3	80	40	40
Fixed-bearing PCR (+PCL)	83	69	31	8	92	2.1	5.3	-3.1	9.6	-7.6	40	10	22
Fixed-bearing PS	74	53	46	12	88	1.4	4.3	-2.9	8.2	-7.0	31	3	19
Mobile-bearing PCR	10	60	40	20	80	0.1	5.1	-5	9.9	-26.6	40	0	40
Mobile-bearing PS	35	60	37	9	91	2.2	4.7	-2.6	12.0	-5.9	37	14	11
Mobile-bearing PCS	35	51	49	11	86	0.0	3.0	-3.2	7.3	-10.1	31	0	14
Average of all knees		59	40	17	83	1.9	5.9	-3.7	12.6	-11.5	37	9	20
Average of all TKA		58	41	12	88	1.2	4.5	-3.3	9.4	-11.4	34	6	18

a Percentage of knees experiencing normal rotation from heel-strike to toe-off.
b Percentage of knees experiencing reverse rotation from heel-strike to toe-off.
c Percentage of knees experiencing normal rotation during all increments of stance phase of gait.
d Percentage of knees experiencing reverse rotation during at least one increment of stance phase of gait.
e Average rotation from heel-strike to toe-off.
f Average maximum normal rotation each knee experienced at any increment of stance phase of
g Average maximum reverse rotation each knee experienced at any increment of stance phase of gait.
h Maximum normal rotation each knee achieved at any increment of stance phase of gait.
i Maximum reverse rotation each knee achieved at any increment of stance phase of gait.
j Percentage of knees experiencing at least 5.0° of normal axial rotation at any increment of stance phase of gait.
k Percentage of knees experiencing at least 10.0° of normal axial rotation at any increment of stance phase of gait.
l Percentage of knees experiencing at least -5.0° of reverse axial rotation at any increment of stance phase of

20

■ Table 20-4. Summation analysis of axial rotation of all knee types during a deep knee bend

Implant type	No. of knees	Normal rotation[a] (90-0, in %)	Reverse rotation[b] (90-0, in %)	Normal rotation all increments[c] (%)	Reverse rotation any increments[d] (%)	Average rotation (90-0[e], in degrees)	Average max. rot. all increments[f] (degrees)	Average max. rev. all increments[g] (degrees)	Maximum norm. rot. all increments[h] (degrees)	Maximum rev. rot. all increments[i] (degrees)	Normal rot.[j] >5.0° (%)	Normal rot.[k] >10.0° (%)	Reverse rot.[l] >-5.0° (%)
Normal	10	100	0	60	40	16.5	17.3	-0.3	27.7	-7.3	100	90	10
Fixed-bearing ACR	10	70	20	40	60	8.1	11.8	-3.3	20.9	-14.1	90	40	60
ACL deficient	5	60	40	20	80	9.8	13.3	-4.3	21.2	-9.8	80	60	40
Fixed-bearing PCR (+PCL)	163	79	21	20	80	3.7	6.5	-2.7	13.0	-9.7	66	13	20
Fixed-bearing PCR (-PCL)	20	40	60	5	95	-1	2.7	-3.4	5.8	-9.5	5	0	25
Fixed-bearing PS	212	76	23	24	75	3.1	5.5	-2.1	11.5	-7.6	52	15	12
Mobile-bearing PCR	107	69	28	20	80	3.9	7.3	-4.1	15.6	-11.4	64	25	27
Mobile-bearing PS	157	80	19	31	69	3.9	6.5	-2.5	12.5	-8.9	58	21	15
Mobile-bearing PCS	76	63	33	18	80	3.3	5.5	-2.1	11.4	-5.9	51	12	16
Average all knees		74	24	27	69	5.7	8.5	-2.8	15.5	-9.4	58	18	18
Average all TKA		74	24	23	76	2.8	5.7	-2.8	11.6	-8.9	57	17	18

a Percentage of knees experiencing normal rotation from 0° to 90° of knee flexion.
b Percentage of knees experiencing reverse rotation from 0° to 90° of knee flexion.
c Percentage of knees experiencing normal rotation during all increments of knee flexion.
d Percentage of knees experiencing reverse rotation during at least one increment of knee flexion.
e Average rotation from 0° to 90° of knee flexion.
f Average maximum normal rotation each knee experienced at any increment of knee flexion.
g Average maximum reverse rotation each knee experienced at any increment of knee flexion.
h Maximum normal rotation each knee achieved at any increment of knee flexion.
i Maximum reverse rotation each knee achieved at any increment of knee flexion.
j Percentage of knees experiencing at least 5.0° of normal axial rotation at any increment of knee flexion.
k Percentage of knees experiencing at least 10.0° of normal axial rotation at any increment of knee flexion.
l Percentage of knees experiencing at least -5.0° of reverse axial rotation at any increment of knee flexion.

TKA experienced normal rotation from full extension to 90° of knee flexion, and six of ten (60%) experienced reverse rotation during at least one flexion increment. The average amount of axial rotation from full extension to 90° of knee flexion was 8.1° and the average maximum amount at any increment of a deep knee bend increased to 11.8°. The maximum amounts of normal and reverse rotation in any ACL-retaining TKA at any flexion increment were 20.9° and -14.1°. Nine of ten (90%) knees achieved at least 5.0° of normal rotation, four of ten (40%) greater than 10.0°, and six of ten (60%) greater than -5.0° of reverse rotation.

Both the percentage of subjects experiencing normal rotational patterns and the magnitudes of axial rotation decreased in all remaining fixed- and mobile-bearing TKA groups compared with normal knee subjects during a deep knee bend maneuver ($p<0.01$; Table 20-4). The axial rotation patterns for the fixed- and mobile-bearing posterior-stabilized TKA groups were similar, as were the axial rotation patterns for the fixed- and mobile-bearing PCL-retaining TKA groups. No statistically significant difference in average amount of axial rotation was noted between PCL-retaining and posterior-stabilized knee groups ($p>0.2$). As with posterior femoral translation, however, the present data may underestimate the maximum magnitudes of axial rotation occurring during extreme flexion in posterior-stabilized TKA designs, since analysis was performed only to a maximum of 90° of flexion. Since many posterior-stabilized implants have late cam-post engagement (>70° of knee flexion), additional axial rotation at flexion increments greater than 90° may occur.

Increased axial rotation was present in deep flexion if the ACL was intact. Average values in normal and ACL-retaining TKA subjects (16.5° and 8.1°) were significantly higher than in TKA study groups in which the ACL was absent (<4.0°; $p<0.01$).

High variability in axial rotation patterns and magnitudes was found among differing TKA categories, between differing implant designs within the same implant category, and among identical designs implanted by different surgeons. This suggests that axial rotation is determined by many factors, including implant design, individual patient anatomical variances, and the surgical technique of TKA. For example, the range of average axial rotation was -1.0°–10.4° for the posterior-stabilized fixed-bearing TKA group. Similarly, the maximum amount of normal rotation ranged from 7.0° to 35.9° and from 9.5° to 22.4° for subjects in the PCL-retaining and posterior-stabilized mobile-bearing TKA groups, respectively.

Considering all TKAs during a deep knee bend, only 551 of 745 knees (74%) experienced a normal axial rotational pattern; this was a significant decrease from the normal knee group, in which 100% (ten of ten) demonstrated a normal axial rotational pattern ($p=0.001$). Also,

only 425 of 745 TKAs (57%) experienced greater than 5.0° of axial rotation at any flexion increment, a significant decrease from the normal knee group (100%, ten of ten; $p=0.001$). This trend continued for the number of knees experiencing greater than 10.0° of axial rotation. Only 127 of 745 (17%) subjects with a TKA experienced greater than 10.0° of axial rotation compared with 90% (nine of ten) of normal knees ($p=0.001$).

While average magnitudes of axial rotation in fixed- vs. mobile-bearing TKA groups were similar, additional analysis suggests the site of rotation differs. Two in vivo, video fluoroscopic analyses of two different designs of rotating-platform TKA have been performed to assess polyethylene bearing mobility [25, 39]. Tantalum beads were embedded within the mobile polyethylene bearings to determine the amount of polyethylene-bearing mobility during a deep knee bend. In both studies it was found that the polyethylene bearing typically rotated in conjunction with the femoral component, confirming the presence of bearing mobility. Similar findings were observed by D'Lima et al. [10] in a cadaveric analysis of axial rotation following mobile-bearing TKA. Therefore, in rotating-platform TKA designs, axial rotation typically occurs on the inferior surface of the polyethylene bearing, whereas rotation obviously occurs on the superior surface in fixed-bearing TKA. This may play a role in reduction of polyethylene wear following mobile-bearing TKA. Bearing mobility should reduce shear forces on the superior aspect of the polyethylene bearing, thereby lessening wear. Otto et al. [54] have demonstrated that low contact stresses (≤8 MPa) are present on the inferior surface of rotating-platform polyethylene bearings when articulating against a highly polished cobalt-chromium surface, which should minimize polyethylene wear during activities requiring axial rotation.

Reverse axial rotational patterns during individual increments of a deep knee bend were common in all fixed- and mobile-bearing study groups. It was uncommon for subjects in any TKA group to demonstrate a progressive normal rotational pattern (i.e., internal tibial rotation) throughout all increments of deep flexion. Typically, alternating patterns of internal and external tibial rotation were observed as flexion increased. Reverse axial rotation is undesirable, risking patellofemoral instability due to lateralization of the tibial tubercle during deep flexion, as well as lessening maximum knee flexion due to reduced posterior femoral roll-back of the lateral femoral condyle.

Finally, while average axial rotational values following TKA were limited, a review of individual TKA subjects revealed a substantial number with high magnitudes (>20°) of both normal and reverse axial rotation, which exceeds the rotational limits of most fixed-bearing TKA designs. This may be an advantage for rotating-platform mobile-bearing TKA designs, which can accommodate a wider range of axial rotation without creation of excessive polyethylene stresses.

Femoral Condylar Liftoff

The incidence and magnitude of femoral condylar liftoff has been evaluated in numerous studies of both fixed- and mobile-bearing TKA [15, 24, 55, 61]. Initially, a series of 20 fixed-bearing PCL-retaining and 20-fixed bearing PCL-substituting TKA were analyzed during a deep knee bend maneuver [15]. All analyzed knees were judged clinically excellent, with no measurable ligamentous laxity or functionally limiting pain. The incidence of femoral condylar liftoff was similar in both fixed-bearing TKA groups, occurring in 70% (14 of 20) of PCL-retaining knees and 80% (16 of 20) of PCL-substituting knees. It occurred with similar frequency medially and laterally in subjects implanted with PCL-substituting knees, but was observed predominantly on the lateral side in those with PCL-retaining knees. Femoral condylar liftoff was most commonly observed between 60° and 90° of flexion in both groups. The average magnitudes of liftoff observed were small (< 2.0 mm) in these well-functioning knees. Since initial studies to assess for condylar liftoff, additional analyses have produced higher magnitudes of femoral condylar liftoff (as high as 8.0 mm; ◘ Fig. 20-10), particularly in subjects with suboptimal clinical results.

A similar incidence (45%-100%) and magnitude (0.78-3.53 mm) of femoral condylar liftoff during both gait and a deep knee bend has been observed in various designs of mobile-bearing TKA [24, 55, 61]. Femoral condylar liftoff was again observed more commonly on the lateral side of the joint, particularly if the posterior cruciate ligament was preserved, and has been attributed to an adduction moment occurring during the mid-stance phase of gait [15]. It was most commonly observed

between 60° and 90° of flexion during a deep knee bend activity and during the mid-stance phase of the gait cycle.

In summary, femoral condylar liftoff is a frequent phenomenon which occurs in many TKA types and does not appear to be affected by the presence of bearing mobility. It occurs most commonly on the lateral side of the joint during the deep flexion phase of a deep knee bend activity and during the mid-stance phase of gait. Lift-off occurred both medially and laterally in subjects implanted with fixed- and mobile-bearing TKA designs in which both cruciate ligaments were sacrificed, but was observed predominantly on the lateral side in those with PCL-retaining TKA. This may be related, at least in part, to the presence or absence of the cruciate ligaments. In the knee with intact cruciate ligaments, the ACL originates at the lateral femoral condyle while the femoral attachment of the PCL is medial. We theorize, therefore, that the ACL acts as a checkrein, limiting lateral femoral liftoff, with the PCL similarly resisting femoral liftoff medially. In knees with both cruciate ligaments resected, the incidence of femoral condylar liftoff was similar both medially and laterally; whereas in TKA subjects with the PCL preserved, femoral condylar liftoff occurred predominantly laterally, possibly due to the intact PCL resisting liftoff medially.

These findings support the importance of coronal femorotibial curvature and conformity in TKA design. In a laboratory analysis, Miller et al. [44] evaluated peak tibial polyethylene stresses under eccentric loading conditions in both flat-on-flat and more coronally curved femorotibial implant geometries. They observed substantially higher polyethylene stresses in flat-on-flat designs, often exceeding the yield strength of polyethylene, whereas designs with increased coronal curvature and conformity proved less sensitive to eccentric loading conditions with lesser peak polyethylene stresses.

Additionally, these studies support the use of metal-backed tibial components with central stems to reduce peak subchondral cancellous bone loads, should femoral condylar liftoff occur. Bartel et al.[5] conducted a finite element analysis of the effect of metal backing on peak subchondral cancellous stresses. They reported reductions in peak cancellous stresses of 16%-39% with metal-backed versus all-polyethylene tibial components when evaluated under eccentric loading conditions. This analysis is supported by clinical studies. Ritter et al. [56] evaluated 2001 cases of a metal-backed PCL-retaining TKA with a flat-on-flat coronal plane geometry (Anatomical Graduated Components; Biomet Corporation, Warsaw, IN). A 98% implant survival rate was observed at 10 years. Faris et al. [20] reviewed 536 cases of the same prosthetic design, with the exception that an all-polyethylene tibial component was utilized. At an average follow-up of 10 years, survival of only 68.11% was found. Fifty-eight (73.4%) of the 79 failures observed occurred in association with loosening or collapse of the bone beneath the

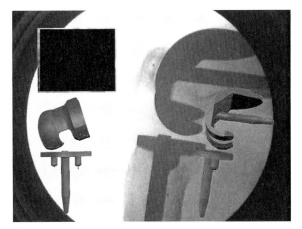

◘ **Fig. 20-10.** Fluoroscopic image and computer-assisted design overlay of a TKA, demonstrating marked femoral condylar liftoff

medial tibial plateau. We postulate that lateral femoral condylar liftoff may have played a role in the premature failure of these all-polyethylene, flat-on-flat tibial components. If lateral liftoff occurs, excessive medial loads are created. In the absence of tibial component metal backing, these high loads become transmitted to the underlying medial subchondral bone, resulting in osseous collapse and eventual tibial component loosening.

Range of Motion

Numerous analyses have been performed to assess magnitudes of range of motion of various designs of TKA [14, 52, 60, 63]. On average, subjects with a normal knee experienced 139° and 135° of knee flexion under passive, non-weight-bearing and weight-bearing conditions, respectively [14]. Under passive conditions, subjects with fixed-bearing PCL-retaining (123°) or -substituting TKAs (127°) experienced similar magnitudes of knee flexion. When tested under weight-bearing conditions, however, subjects with a PCL-substituting TKA experienced statistically more flexion (113°) than those implanted with a PCL-retaining TKA (103°; $p<0.024$). The reduction of motion observed under weight-bearing conditions in the PCL-retaining TKA group is likely related to paradoxical anterior femoral translation during progressive knee flexion, which is commonly noted in these designs. This kinematic abnormality may limit maximum flexion due to anteriorization of the axis of flexion, earlier impingement of the posterior soft-tissue structures, and tightening of the extensor mechanism (from anterior femoral displacement). Alternatively, patients implanted with PCL-substituting TKAs routinely demonstrate posterior femoral roll-back, dictated by interaction of the femoral cam and tibial post mechanism of the PCL-substituting design, regardless of weight-bearing status [11].

Similar studies have subsequently been completed to assess whether bearing mobility influences range of motion [52, 60, 63]. These are summarized in ❑ Table 20-5.

In summary, when tested under weight-bearing conditions, subjects implanted with mobile-bearing TKA did not have superior range of motion compared with those who had fixed-bearing designs (range, 99°-119°). In most mobile-bearing TKA designs, a reduced range of motion was observed. This may be related to the increased sagittal conformity typically seen in most mobile-bearing designs, which limits posterior femoral roll-back due to the increased prominence of the posterior lip of mobile polyethylene bearings. Additionally, the sagittal dwell point (the point where the polyethylene is the thinnest) of the mobile-bearing TKA designs tested is positioned more anteriorly than in most fixed-bearing TKA designs [14]. This may position the axis of flexion more anteriorly and limit maximum flexion. In summary, knee range of mo-

❑ **Table 20-5.** Average range of motion for various types of TKA

Knee type	Passive (degrees)	Weight-bearing (degrees)
Normal [14]	139	135
Fixed-bearing TKA		
PFC PS [14]	127	113
PFC PCR [14]	123	103
PFC Sigma PS [9]	127	113
Mobile-bearing TKA		
LCS RP [63]	108	99
LCS MBª [60]	123	103
LCS RP PS [22]	121	104
LCS AP Glide [52]	129	119
PFC Sigma PS RP [17]	124	114

ª Meniscal bearing

tion is determined more by implant condylar geometry than by bearing mobility.

References

1. Andriacchi TP, Stanwyck TS, Galante JO (1986) Knee biomechanics and total knee replacement. J Arthroplasty 1:211-219
2. Andriacchi TP (1993) Functional analysis of pre- and post-knee surgery. Total knee arthroplasty and ACL reconstruction. J Biomech Eng 115:575-581
3. Andriacchi TP, Galante JO, Fermier RS (1994) Patient outcomes following tricompartmental total knee replacement. JAMA 271:1349
4. Argenson JN, Komistek RD, Aubaniac JM, Dennis DA, Northcut EJ, Anderson DT, Agostini S (2002) In vivo determination of knee kinematics for subjects implanted with a unicompartmental arthroplasty. J Arthroplasty 17:1048-1054
5. Bartel DL, Burstein AH, Santavicca EA, Insall JN (1982) Performance of the tibial component in total knee replacement. J Bone Joint Surg [Am] 64:1026-1033
6. Bertin KC, Komistek RD, Dennis, DA, Hoff WA, Anderson DT, Langer T (2002) In vivo determination of posterior femoral rollback for subjects having a NexGen posterior cruciate retaining total knee arthroplasty. J Arthroplasty 17:1040-1048
7. Blunn GW, Walker PS, Joshi A, Hardinge K (1991) The dominance of cyclic sliding in producing wear in total knee replacements. Clin Orthop 273:253-260
8. Buechel FF, Buechel FF, Pappas MJ, Dalessio J (2002) Twenty-year evaluation of the New Jersey LCS rotating platform knee replacement. J Knee Surg 15:84-89
9. Callaghan JJ, Insall JN, Greenwald AS, Dennis DA, Komistek RD, et al (2000) Mobile bearing knee replacement. J Bone Joint Surg [Am] 82:1020-1041
10. D'Lima DD, Trice M, Urquhart AG, Colwell CW Jr (2001) Tibiofemoral conformity and kinematics of rotating-bearing knee prostheses. Clin Orthop 386:235-242
11. Dennis DA, Komistek RD, Hoff WA, Gabriel SM (1996) In vivo knee kinematics derived using an inverse perspective technique. Clin Orthop 331:107-117
12. Dennis DA, Komistek RD, Cheal EJ, Stiehl JB, Walker SA (1997) In vivo femoral condylar lift-off in total knee arthroplasty. Orthop Trans 21:1112
13. Dennis DA, Komistek RD, Colwell CE, Ranawat SC, Scott RD, Thornhill TS, Lapp MA (1998) In vivo anteroposterior femorotibial translation of total knee arthroplasty: a multicenter analysis. Clin Orthop 356:47-57
14. Dennis DA, Komistek RD, Stiehl JB, Walker SA, Dennis K (1998) Range of motion following total knee arthroplasty: The effect of implant design and weight-bearing conditions. J Arthroplasty 13:748-752

20

15. Dennis DA, Komistek RD, Cheal EJ, Walker SA, Stiehl JB (2001) Femoral condylar liftoff in vivo in total knee arthroplasty. J Bone Joint Surg [Br] 83:33-39

16. Dennis DA, Komistek RD, Mahfouz MR, Haas BD, Stiehl JB (2003) Multi-center determination of in vivo kinematics after total knee arthroplasty. Clin Orthop 416:37-57

17. Dennis DA, Komistek RD (2003) Evaluation of range of motion after PFC Sigma posterior stabilized rotating platform total knee arthroplasty. Internal Report at the Rocky Mountain Musculoskeletal Research Laboratory

18. Dennis DA, Komistek RD, Mahfouz MR, Walker SA, Tucker A (2004) A multicenter analysis of axial femorotibial rotation after total knee arthroplasty. Clin Orthop 428:180-189

19. Draganich LF, Andriacchi T, Andersson GBJ (1987) Interaction between intrinsic knee mechanics and the knee extensor mechanism. J Orthop Res 5:539-547

20. Faris, PM, Ritter MA, Keating EM, Meding JB, Harty LD (2003) The AGC all-polyethylene tibial component: a ten-year clinical evaluation. J Bone Joint Surg [Am] 85:489-493

21. Fukubayashi T, Torzilli PA, Sherman MF, Warren RF (1982) An in vitro biomechanical evaluation of anterior-posterior motion of the knee. Tibial displacement, rotation, and torque. J. Bone Joint Surg [Am] 64:258-264

22. Haas BD, Dennis DA, Komistek RD, Brumley JT, Hammill C (2001) Range of motion of posterior-cruciate-substituting total knee replacements: the effect of bearing mobility. J Bone Joint Surg [Am] 83 [Suppl 2]:51-55

23. Haas BD, Komistek RD, Dennis DA (2002) In vivo kinematics of the low contact stress rotating platform total knee. Orthopedics 25 [Suppl 2]: 219-26

24. Haas BD, Komistek RD, Stiehl JB, Anderson DT, Northcut EJ (2002) Kinematic comparison of posterior cruciate sacrifice versus substitution in a mobile bearing total knee arthroplasty. J Arthroplasty 17:685-692

25. Haas BD, Komistek RD, Kilgus D, Smith A, Hammill C, Walker SA (2005) Polyethylene bearing motion relative to the tibia and the femur in mobile bearing total knee arthroplasty. J Arthroplasty (submitted for publication)

26. Haas B, Komistek RD, Dennis DA (1999) In vivo kinematic comparison of posterior cruciate sacrificing and stabilized mobile total bearing knee arthroplasty. (Unpublished data, Rocky Mountain Musculoskeletal Research Laboratory; Denver, CO)

27. Hill PF, Williams VV, Iwaki H, Pinskerova V, Freeman MAR (2000) Tibiofemoral movement. 2: The loaded and unloaded living knee studied by MRI. J Bone Joint Surg [Br] 82:1196-1200

28. Hoff WA, Komistek RD, Dennis DA, Walker SA, Northcut EJ, Spargo K (1996) Pose estimation of artificial knee implants in fluoroscopy images using a template matching technique. Proc. 3rd Workshop on Applications of Computer Vision, IEEE, Sarasota, FL, Dec. 2-4, pp 181-186

29. Hoff WA, Komistek RD, Dennis DA, Gabriel SA, Walker SA (1998) A three-dimensional determination of femorotibial contact positions under in vivo conditions using fluoroscopy. J Clin Biomech 13:455-470

30. Hsieh HH, Walker PS (1976) Stabilizing mechanisms of the loaded and unloaded knee joint. J. Bone Joint Surg [Am] 58:87-93

31. Insall JN, Hood RW, Flawn LB, Sullivan DJ (1983) Total condylar knee prosthesis in gonarthrosis: a five- to nine-year follow-up of the first one hundred consecutive replacements. J Bone Joint Surg [Am] 65:619-628

32. Insall JN, Scuderi GR, Komistek RD, Math K, Dennis DA, Anderson DT (2002) Correlation between condoylar lift-off and femoral component alignment. Clin Orthop 403:143-152

33. Iwaki H, Pinskerova V, Freeman MAR (2000) Tibiofemoral movement. 1: The shapes and relative movements of the femur and tibia in unloaded cadaver knee. J Bone Joint Surg [Br] 82:1189-1195

34. Jonsson J, Karrholm J, Elmquist LG (1989) Kinematics of active knee extension after tear of the anterior cruciate ligament. Am J Sports Med 17:796-802

35. Karrholm J, Jonsson H, Nilsson KG, Soderqvisy I (1994) Kinematics of successful knee prosthesis during weight-bearing: three dimensional movements and positions of screw axes in the Tricon-M and Miller-Galante designs. Knee Surg Sports Traumatol Arthrosc 2:50-59

36. Karrholm J, Brandsson S, Freeman MAR (2000) Tibiofemoral movement. 4: Changes of axial tibial rotation caused by forced rotation at the weight-bearing knee studied by RSA. J Bone Joint Surg [Br] 82:1201-1203

37. Komistek RD, Scott RD, Dennis DA, Yasgur D, Anderson DT, Hajner ME (2002) In vivo comparison of femorotibial contact positions for press-fit posterior stabilized and posterior cruciate-retaining total knee arthroplasties. J Arthroplasty 17:209-216

38. Komistek RD, Dennis DA, Mahfouz MR (2003) In vivo fluoroscopic analysis of the normal knee. Clin Orthop 410:69-81

39. Komistek RD, Dennis DA, Mahfouz MR, Walker SA, Outten J (2004) In vivo polyethylene mobility is maintained in posterior stabilized total knee arthroplasty. Clin Orthop 428:207-213

40. Lafortune M, Cavanagh P, Sommer I III, Kalenak A (1992) A three-dimensional kinematics of the human knee during walking. J Biomech 25:347-357

41. Mahfouz MR (2001) In vivo estimation of six degrees of freedom position and orientation for non-implanted human joints from single plane fluoroscopy. PhD Dissertation, Colorado School of Mines, Engineering, Golden, CO

42. Mahfouz MR, Hoff WA, Komistek, RD, Dennis DA (2003) A robust method for registration of three-dimensional knee implant models to two-dimensional fluoroscopy images. IEEE Trans Med Imaging 22:1561-1574

43. Mahoney OM, Nobel PC, Rhoads DD, Alexander JW, Tullos HS (1994) Posterior cruciate function following total knee arthroplasty: a biomechanical study. J Arthroplasty 9:569

44. Miller GJ, Perry W, Goll C (1995) Congruency and varus/valgus loading effect on prosthetic knee contact stress. Combined Orthopedic Research Society (English Speaking World), San Diego, CA, Nov 6-8

45. Muller W (1983) The knee. Form, function and ligament reconstruction: kinematics. Springer-Verlag, Berlin Heidelberg New York, pp 8-17

46. Murphy M (1990) Geometry and the kinematics of the normal human knee. Ph.D. thesis, Dept of Mechanical Engineering, Massachusetts Institute of Technology

47. Murphy MC, Zarins B, Jasty M, Mann RW (1995) In vivo measurement of the three-dimensional skeletal motion at the normal knee. Trans Orthop Res Soc, p 142

48. Murray DW, Goodfellow JW, O'Connor JJ (1998) The Oxford medial unicompartmental arthroplasty: a ten-year survival study. J Bone Joint Surg [Br] 80:983-989

49. Nilsson KG, Karrholm J, Ekelund L (1990) Knee motion in total knee arthroplasty. A roentgen stereophotogrammetric analysis of the kinematics of the Tricon-M knee prosthesis. Clin Orthop 256:147-161

50. Nilsson KG, Karrholm J, Gadegaard P (1991) Abnormal kinematics of the artificial knee. Roentgen stereophotogrammetric analysis of 10 Miller-Galante and five New Jersey LCS knees. Acta Orthop Scand 62:440-446

51. O'Connor J, Shercliff T, Fitzpatrick D, Biden E, Goodfellow J (1990) Mechanics of the knee, In: Daniel DM, Akeson WH, O'Connor JJ (eds) Knee ligaments: structures, function, injury and repair. Raven, New York, pp 201-237

52. Oakshott R, Komistek RD, Anderson DT, Haas BD, Dennis DA (2000) In vivo passive vs weight-bearing knee kinematics for subjects implanted with a mobile bearing that can freely translate and rotate. Internal report at Rocky Mountain Musculoskeletal Research Laboratory

53. Oishi CS, Kaufman KR, Irby SE, Colwell CW Jr (1996) Effects of patellar thickness on compression and shear forces in total knee arthroplasty. Clin Orthop 331:283-290

54. Otto JK, Callaghan, JJ, Brown TD (2001) Mobility and contact mechanics of a rotating platform total knee replacement. Clin Orthop 392:24-37

55. Ranawat CS, Komistek RD, Rodriguez JA, Dennis DA, Anderle M (2004) In vivo kinematics for fixed and mobile-bearing posterior stabilized knee prostheses. Clin Orthop 419:1-7

56. Ritter MA, Worland R, Saliski J, Helphenstine JV, Edmondson KL, Keating EM, Faris PM, Meding JB (1995) Flat-on-flat, nonconstrained, compression-molded polyethylene total knee replacement. Clin Orthop 321:79-85

57. Sarojak ME (1998) Model-fit: an interactive pose-determining system. Engineering thesis, Colorado School of Mines, Golden, CO

58. Scuderi GR, Komistek RD, Dennis DA, Insall JN (2003) The impact of femoral component rotational alignment on condoylar liftoff. Clin Orthop 410:148-54

59. Stiehl JB, Komistek RD, Dennis DA, Paxson RD (1995) Fluoroscopic analysis of kinematics after posterior-cruciate-retaining knee arthroplasty. J Bone Joint Surg [Br] 77:884-889

60. Stiehl JB, Dennis DA, Komistek RD, Keblish PA (1997) In vivo kinematic analysis of a mobile-bearing total knee prosthesis. Clin Orthop 345:60-66

61. Stiehl JB, Dennis DA, Komistek RD, Crane H (1999) In vivo determination of condylar liftoff and screw home in a mobile bearing total knee arthroplasty. J Arthroplasty 14:293-299

62. Stiehl JB, Komistek RD, Dennis DA (1999) Detrimental kinematics of a flat-on-flat total condoylar knee arthroplasty. Clin Orthop 365:139-148

63. Stiehl JB, Dennis DA, Komistek RD, Keblish P (2000) In vivo comparison of posterior cruciate retaining and sacrificing mobile bearing total knee arthroplasty. Am J Knee Surg 13:13-18

64. Stiehl JB, Komistek RD, Cloutier JM, Dennis DA (2000) The cruciate ligaments in total knee arthroplasty: a kinematic analysis of 2 total knee arthroplasties. J Arthroplasty 15:545-550

65. Stiehl JB, Komistek RD, Dennis DA (2001) A novel approach to knee kinematics. Am J Orthop 30:287-293

66. Stiehl JB, Komistek RD, Haas BD, Dennis DA (2001) Frontal plane kinematics after mobile-bearing total knee arthroplasty. Clin Orthop 392:56-61

67. Walker PS, Komistek RD, Barrett DS, Anderson D, Dennis DA, Sampson M (2002) Motion of a mobile bearing knee allowing translation and rotation. J Arthroplasty 17:11-19

68. Wilson SA, McCann PD, Gotlin RS, Ramakrishnan HK, Wootten ME, Insall JN (1996) Comprehensive gait analysis in posterior-stabilized knee arthroplasty. J Arthroplasty 11:359

21 Cruciate Deficiency in the Replaced Knee

J. Victor

Summary

At least one of the cruciate ligaments is sacrificed in most total knee arthroplasties. This can lead to important functional changes in the joint. In severe cases, instability causes early failure and revision of the implant. In a less extreme form, the cruciate deficiency leads to abnormal kinematics, affecting activities of daily life and reducing functional capacity of the knee joint. Technological advances opened the potential for studying the in vivo characteristics of the replaced knee. Significant differences in kinematics between the normal and the replaced knee have been reported in the literature. Many of these differences can be attributed to either anterior or posterior cruciate ligament deficiency following total knee arthroplasty.

Introduction

In the normal human knee, passive stability is provided by the ligaments, the menisci, and the congruency of the joint surfaces. The cruciate ligaments play an important role as stabilizers in the sagittal plane. The anterior cruciate ligament (ACL) is the primary restraint against anterior translation of the tibia relative to the femur. The posterior cruciate ligament (PCL) is the primary restraint against posterior translation of the tibia relative to the femur. In the horizontal plane both cruciate ligaments resist excessive internal rotation of the tibia relative to the femur. In the coronal plane, the PCL is a secondary restraint against valgus angulation of the tibia, relative to the femur. In addition to their stabilizing and proprioceptive function, the cruciate ligaments also play a crucial role in guiding the kinematics of the knee during the arc of motion, as their location, length, and insertion are closely related to the geometrical characteristics of the distal femur and the proximal tibia [21, 32].

When a total knee arthroplasty is inserted, much of this delicate mechanical system is altered. Today's resurfacing-type knee prostheses mimic the condylar shape of the knee but are far from being truly anatomical. In addition, in most total knee arthroplasties the ACL is resect-

ed. Many types of total knees also require resection of the PCL. It is clear that this will alter the stability and the kinematics of the replaced knee in comparison to a healthy normal knee joint. Historically, the loss of primary and secondary stabilizers (cruciate ligaments and menisci) was recognized at an early stage by the designers of the total condylar knee. They attempted to restore the sagittal stability of the knee joint by creating a concave tibial surface that accommodated the femoral condyles. Later on, this design was converted to the posterior stabilized knee to avoid the posterior kinematic conflict and still maintain sufficient stability [23].

Design Solutions for Obtaining Stability in the Sagittal Plane

There are basically two options for improving sagittal stability in the replaced knee without completely constraining the joint as in a hinged design. One option is to alter the surface congruity, the other is to include a type of cam-and-post mechanism. Altering the surface congruity is often misinterpreted, as the terminology is misleading.

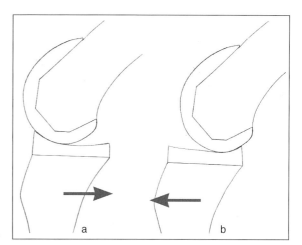

◩ Fig. 21-1a, b. *a* An anterior build-up of the polyethylene insert provides resistance against posterior translation of the tibia with respect to the femur and is a substitute for PCL function. *b* A posterior lip on the polyethylene insert provides resistance against anterior translation of the tibia with respect to the femur and is a substitute for ACL function

21

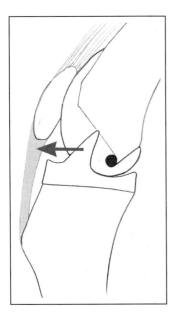

Fig. 21-2. Near full extension the extensor mechanism exerts an anterior pull on the tibia. This can lead to anterior subluxation of the tibia and disengagement of the cam-post mechanism. The point at which the cam and post engage during the flexion cycle depends upon the thickness of the patella-button complex, the geometry of the femoral component, the surface geometry of the tibial polyethylene, the position of the post and the cam, and the surgical positioning of the components. In some knees, contact between the cam and the post never occurs during the flexion cycle

An 'anterior build-up' of the polyethylene provides a buffer towards *posterior* translation of the tibia relative to the femur, whereas a 'posterior lip' provides a buffer towards *anterior* translation of the tibia relative to the femur. In terms of sagittal stability, the 'anterior build-up' is an attempt to copy the PCL function (Fig. 21-1a). The 'posterior lip', on the other hand, is an attempt to copy ACL function (Fig. 21-1b).

The cam-and-post mechanism can provide a mechanical buttress against posterior translation of the tibia with respect to the femur. It should be understood, however, that this cam-and-post mechanism is without function as long as there is no contact between the two components. More specifically, if there is increased anterior laxity of the tibia with respect to the femur (deficient ACL function), the initial anterior-directed force vector of the extensor mechanism can pull the tibia forward [33] and disengage the cam-and-post mechanism (Fig. 21-2).

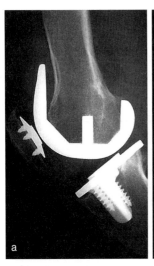
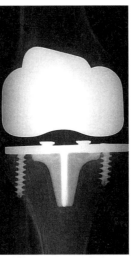
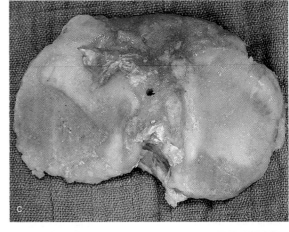
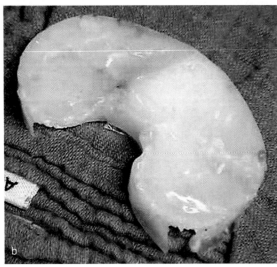
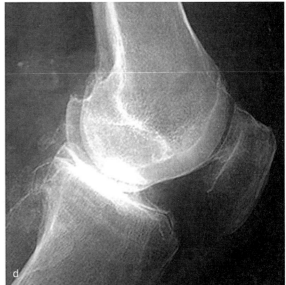

Fig. 21-3a-d. Sagittal instability leading to polyethylene wear with anterior subluxation of the tibia (*a*). The synovial hypertrophy is conspicuous as a soft-tissue shadow on the lateral X-ray. The retrieved specimen (*b*) shows a wear pattern that is strikingly similar to the arthritic wear pattern (*c*) of the chronic ACL-deficient knee (*d*), suggesting that the mechanism of failure (sagittal instability) is similar

In other words, in the absence of normal ACL function, the traditional cam-and-post mechanism can only prevent nonphysiological posterior translation, starting from a given position and in a given direction, and is not able to provide gradual stabilization of the joint during the full range of motion.

Instability as a Clinical Entity

Sagittal instability has been described as a clinical complication after TKA. The above-described mechanisms to improve functional sagittal stability can function only when the collateral ligaments provide sufficient stability during flexion. Their incapacity to do so is referred to as „flexion gap" instability. This can lead to clinical symptoms such as reduced range of motion, pain, and giving way [7]. If the instability is significant, dislocation of the knee can occur, depending upon the design of the cam-and-post mechanism [26]. The most notorious complication of sagittal instability is early polyethylene wear (◘ Fig. 21-3).

Sharkey et al. [35] recently investigated the causes for revision total knee arthroplasty. Instability was the reason for early revision in 21% of cases and the reason for late revisions in 22%. The biomechanical explanation for the detrimental effect of repetitive sliding on the polyethylene was described by Blunn et al. [9]. There is further clinical evidence from outcome studies that looked at the results of polyethylene exchange for wear. Babis et al. [3] reported a re-revision rate of these polyethylene exchanges of 25% at a mean of 3 years. These findings were confirmed by Brooks et al. [11], who found a re-revision rate of 29% at less than 5 years. These data strongly suggest that the cause of failure is not intrinsic to the polyethylene but is related to the instability of the replaced knee.

Another potential consequence of sagittal instability is anterior knee pain. Excessive posterior laxity of the tibia increases the patellofemoral joint reaction force. The use of a posterior-stabilized knee arthroplasty has been advocated in case of prior patellectomy.

The Relation Between Sagittal Instability and Kinematic Characteristics

All in vivo studies using fluoroscopy as a tool to investigate the kinematics of the knee after implantation of a total knee arthroplasty report abnormal kinematics as compared with the normal knee [2, 4, 5, 8, 13-16, 20, 22, 27, 31, 37-41, 44, 45]. These differences include less posterior lateral femoral roll-back as the knee moves from extension to flexion, abnormal axial rotation between the femur and the tibia, a different center of rotation of the knee in the horizontal plane, and condylar liftoff. The reported results for the posterior cruciate ligament-retaining (CR) knees are consistently more variable than for the posterior-stabilized (PS) knees. Non-physiological roll-forward of the medial femoral condyle during flexion is a common finding. Roll-back on the lateral side during flexion is noted to a greater extent in the PS than in the CR devices. Overall, PS knees display greater roll-back and have a better range of motion [5, 6, 15, 20, 44, 45].

The role of the posterior cruciate ligament in total knee arthroplasty (TKA) has been discussed at large in the orthopedic literature. Arguments of theoretical order [19], functional order [1, 17, 36], and survivorship [18, 34, 46] have been used to prove the advantage of retention over substitution and vice versa. Other papers focused on the degree of deformity [28, 36] or the underlying cause of arthritis [29] as indications for resecting the PCL and using a PS design. Numerous authors are capable of producing good clinical outcome results with either technique, CR or PS [10, 17, 30, 34, 42, 44, 45]. A recent paper by Straw [42] shows equal results for patients with PCL-retaining total knee arthroplasty and PS knees. Significantly worse results are reported for patients with a CR knee replacement where a tight PCL has been released.

The ambition to reproduce normal knee kinematics after the implantation of a TKA has been questioned [16]. Others consider the reproduction of normal kinematic patterns the best option to preserve stability and range of motion [43]. As most modern knee prostheses are surface replacements that mimic the anatomical form of the human knee, this seems a logical assumption to us. Normal knee kinematics under loaded conditions (deep knee bend) have recently been studied by dynamic MRI [21], biplanar image-matching of X-rays [2], and fluoroscopy [25, 31]. It has been shown that the posterior part of the medial femoral condyle has a single radius of curvature, acting like a ball-in-socket up from 20° to 110° of flexion, allowing the lateral condyle to pivot around it [21, 24]. This mechanism positions the lateral femorotibial contact point in deep flexion extremely posterior on the tibia. Asano et al. [2] used a biplanar image-matching technique to describe the kinematic behavior of the normal human knee. They found a medial center of rotation in the horizontal plane as the knee moved from full extension to 120° of flexion. The mean axial rotation of the femur relative to the tibia was 22° at a flexion angle of 90° and 23.8° at a flexion angle of 120°. The medial contact point moved backward by 6.9 mm and the lateral contact point moved backward by 27.4 mm at 120° of flexion. The differences between these fluoroscopic findings and the dynamic MRI data with respect to the kinematics on the medial side of the knee can be attributed to the different description of the kinematic characteristics of the knee. Depending upon the use of the tibiofemoral contact area or the center of rotation in describing the movement of

21

the knee, the kinematics of the medial side are different [21, 24]. The reported in vivo kinematic studies and the present study use the tibiofemoral contact area.

Mahfouz et al. [31] used fluoroscopy to study and to compare normal knee kinematics with kinematics of the anterior cruciate-deficient knee during a loaded deep knee bend. All ten normal knees displayed femoral roll-back as the knee moved into flexion. At 120° of flexion the mean posterior translation of the medial condyle was 1.9 mm; the mean posterior translation of the lateral condyle was 21 mm; and the mean axial rotation of the femur relative to the tibia was 23.7°. In the anterior cruciate-deficient knee, reduced magnitudes of anteroposterior translation and increased variability in kinematic patterns were observed (reversed axial rotation between 30° and 45° of flexion).

These reported kinematic patterns are difficult to reproduce in patients with TKA. Several authors compared the kinematic behavior of CR implants with those of PS implants. These results are summarized in ◘ Table 21-1. Udomkiat et al. [44] found a mean value of femoral roll-forward during flexion on the medial side of 2.7 mm and

a mean roll-back of -2.2 mm on the lateral side for CR knees. In the PS design, the mean value was 0 mm on the medial side and -1.3 mm on the lateral side. Dennis et al. [15] compared the findings of CR and PS implants from their multicenter data. They reported better lateral roll-back for the PS group as compared with the CR group. Forward sliding of the medial femoral condyle during flexion was present in 50% of the CR patients and in 70% of the PS patients. Bertin et al. [8] claimed to have found better kinematic behavior for a CR implant. Of 20 subjects who had undergone a CR NexGen TKA, 13 experienced femoral roll-back on the medial side and 19 on the lateral side. The mean values were -3.1 on the medial side and -3.9 on the lateral side. Although forward sliding of the medial femoral condyle during flexion was far less frequently present than in previous reports [5, 6, 16, 20, 22, 44], the absolute value on the lateral side of -3.1 mm is still far from the normal mean value ranging from 21 to 27 mm [2, 31]. Despite the differences in the implants that were used, a clear trend appears from these papers. Axial rotation is less pronounced in the replaced knee than in the human knee, forward sliding of the medial femoral

◘ **Table 21-1.** The author's data compared with a summary of reported kinematics in papers that describe normal human knees or compare posterior-stabilized versus cruciate-retaining total knee prostheses. The first two papers describe the normal knee and serve as a reference baseline. The other papers compare CR with PS. The data all refer to a loaded deep knee bend

	No of knees tested	Knee type	Range of motion	Medial femoral roll-back	Lateral femoral roll-back	Axial rotation	% Paradoxical motion, medial	% Paradoxical motion, lateral	Maximum flexion	Method of measuring maximum flexion
Asano et al [2]	6	Normal	0°-120°	-6.9	-27.4	23.8°				
Mahfouz et al [31]	10	Normal	0°-120°	-1.9	-21	23.7°				
Udomkiat et al [43]	10	CR Apollo	0°-90°	2.7	-2.2	not listed	not listed	not listed	119	Clinical NWB
Udomkiat et al [43]	10	PS Apollo	0°-90°	0	-1.3	not listed	not listed	not listed	118	Clinical NWB
Dennis et al [15]	20	CR Multi-center	0°-90°	-0.1	-1.7	-0.1°	50	40	103	Fluoroscopy WB
Dennis et al [15]	20	PS Multi-center	0°-90°	0.9	-7.1	10.4°	70	0	113	Fluoroscopy WB
Banks et al [5]	6	CR AMK	0°-90°	0.4	-5.7	9.6°	not listed	not listed	107	Fluoroscopy WB
Banks et al [5]	5	PS Osteonics	0°-90°	0.2	-1.5	4.9°	not listed	not listed	110	Fluoroscopy WB
Haas et al [20]	5	CR LCS	0°-90°	0.1	-2.4	-1.4°	not listed	not listed	not	
Haas et al [20]	5	PS LCS	0°-90°	-2	-5.9	5.3°	not listed	not listed	not	
Victor et al [44]	8	CR Genesis II	0°-115°	-2.7	-11.9	6.3°	not listed	not listed	114	Fluoroscopy WB
Victor et al [44]	7	PS Genesis II	0°-115°	-11.9	-15.5	5.1°	not listed	not listed	117	Fluoroscopy WB

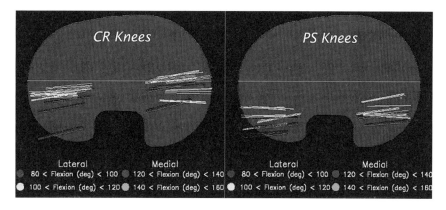

Fig. 21-4. Kinematic behavior of the replaced knee, comparing a cruciate-retaining (CR) against a posterior-stabilized (PS) knee in deep knee bend. The *colored lines* represent the tibiofemoral contact positions at different angles of flexion. The contact lines are normalized for a size-five tibial component. The PS knees display a more posterior contact position than the CR knees

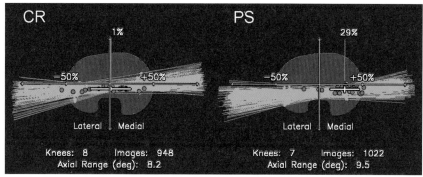

Fig. 21-5. Kinematic comparison of cruciate-retaining (CR) and posterior-stabilized (PS) knee between 50° and 90° of flexion during stair-stepping. The forward sliding of the medial condyle in the CR group is apparent. The *gray dots* represent the centers of rotation. In the PS knees they tend to cluster on the medial side, whereas the CR group shows a more scattered pattern

condyle during flexion on the medial side is present for all CR types of knees, and lateral femoral roll-back is better for the PS than for the CR devices. Maximum flexion tends to be better in the PS than in the CR groups.

In a study performed by the author [45], the difference in maximum flexion during lunge between CR and PS patients was not significant, although the gain in flexion relative to the preoperative status was greater in the PS (14°) than in the CR (5°) group. The better flexion in the PS group correlates with earlier findings [15, 42]. The explanation for this better flexion probably lies in the greater posterior translation of the femur on the tibia [6]. The PS group displayed on average a more posterior contact area in flexion than the CR group (Figs. 21-4 and 21-5). This posterior position of the femoral component clears the back of the knee and helps to avoid impingement between polyethylene and the posterior cortex of the femur (Fig. 21-6). This phenomenon is synergistic with the posterior condylar offset as described by Bellemans et al. as a determinant for maximum flexion [7].

The forward sliding of the medial femoral condyle in CR knees during flexion can be explained as follows: The initial force vector of the patellar tendon keeps the tibia anterior ('the quadriceps active test') [12], but with increasing flexion, the direction of pull switches to a more vertical position. The gastrocnemius and hamstring muscles now exert a posterior pull on the tibia, leading to posterior tibial subluxation in case of an insufficient PCL. This phenomenon can be partially compensated in PS

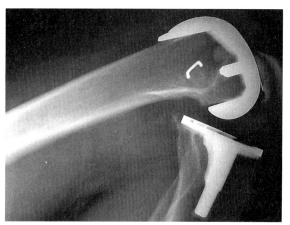

Fig. 21-6. Anterior sliding of the femur during flexion causes impingement between the polyethylene and the posterior cortex of the femur. This mechanism can limit maximum flexion

knees, as the cam-post mechanism acts as a buttress against posterior subluxation of the tibia relative to the femur (see Fig. 21-5; Fig. 21-7).

The fact that it still partially occurs with PS knees can be explained by the absence of the stabilizing function of the anterior cruciate ligament. In early flexion, the patellar tendon force vector can translate the tibia anteriorly (see Fig. 21-2). This positions the femur relatively posterior with respect to the tibia. Reduction of this position to the midline causes anterior sliding of the femur on the tibia, which is stopped eventually when the cam-post

21

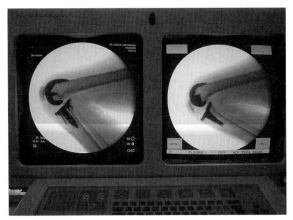

7. Bellemans J et al (2002) Fluoroscopic analysis of the kinematics of deep flexion in total knee arthroplasty. Influence of posterior condylar offset. J Bone Joint Surg [Br] 84:50-53
8. Bertin KC et al (2002) In vivo determination of posterior femoral rollback for subjects having a NexGen posterior cruciate retaining total knee arthroplasty. J Arthroplasty 17:1040-1048
9. Blunn GW et al (1991) The dominance of cyclic sliding in producing wear in total knee replacements. Clin Orthop 273:253-260
10. Bolanos AA et al (1998) A comparison of isokinetic strength testing and gait analysis in patients with posterior cruciate-retaining and substituting knee arthroplasties. J Arthroplasty 13:906-915
11. Brooks DH et al (2002) Polyethylene exchange only for prosthetic instability. Clin Orthop 405:182-188
12. Daniel DM et al (1988) The use of the quadriceps active test to diagnose posterior cruciate ligament disruption and measure posterior laxity of the knee. J Bone Joint Surg [Am] 70:386-391
13. Dennis DA et al (1998) Range of motion after total knee arthroplasty: the effect of implant design and weight bearing conditions. J Arthroplasty 13:748-752
14. Dennis DA et al (2001) Femoral condylar lift-off in vivo in total knee arthroplasty. J Bone Joint Surg [Br] 83:33-39
15. Dennis DA et al (2003) In vivo fluoroscopic analysis of fixed-bearing total knee replacements. Clin Orthop 410:114-130
16. Dennis DA et al (2003) Multicenter determination of in vivo kinematics after total knee arthroplasty. Clin Orthop 416:37-57
17. Dorr LD et al (1988) Functional comparison of posterior cruciate retained versus sacrificed total knee arthroplasty. Clin Orthop 236:36-43
18. Font-Rodriguez DE et al (1997) Survivorship of cemented total knee arthroplasty. Clin Orthop 345:79-86
19. Freeman MAR et al (1988) Should the posterior cruciate ligament be retained or resected in condylar knee arthroplasty: the case for resection. J Arthroplasty 3:3-12
20. Haas BD et al (2002) Kinematic comparison of posterior cruciate sacrifice versus substitution in a mobile bearing total knee arthroplasty. J Arthroplasty 17:685-692
21. Hill PF et al (2000) Tibiofemoral movement. 2: The loaded and unloaded living knee studied by MRI. J Bone Joint Surg [BR] 82:1196-1200
22. Hoff WA et al (1998) A three dimensional determination of femorotibial contact positions under in vivo condtitions using fluoroscopy. J Clin Biomech 13:455-470
23. Insall JN (1993) Historical development, classification, and characteristics of knee prosthesis. In: Insall JN (ed) Surgery of the knee. Churchill Livingstone, New York
24. Iwaki H et al (2000) Tibiofemoral movement. 1: The shapes and relative movements of the femur and the tibia in unloaded cadaver knee. J Bone Joint Surg [Br] 82:1189-1195
25. Kanisawa I et al (2003) Weight bearing knee kinematics in subjects with two types of anterior cruciate ligament reconstructions. Knee Surg Sports Traumatol Arthrosc 11:16-22
26. Kocmond JH et al (1995) Stability and range of motion of Insall-Burstein condylar prostheses. J Arthroplasty 10:383-388
27. Komistek RD et al (2002) In vivo kinematics for subjects with and without an anterior cruciate ligament. Clin Orthop 404:315-325
28. Laskin RS (1996) Total knee replacement with posterior cruciate ligament retention in patients with a fixed varus deformity. Clin Orthop 331:29-34
29. Laskin RS et al (1997) Total knee replacement with posterior cruciate ligament retention in rheumatoid arthritis. Problems and complications. Clin Orthop 345:24-28
30. Lombardi AV et al (2001) An algorithm for the posterior cruciate ligament in total knee arthroplasty. Clin Orthop 392:75-87
31. Mahfouz M et al (2004) In vivo determination of normal and anterior cruciate ligament deficient knee kinematics. Scientific Exhibit at AAOS 71sr Annual Meeting, San Francisco
32. Müller W (1983) The knee: form, function and ligament reconstruction. Springer-Verlag Berlin Heidelberg New York
33. O'Connor J et al (1990) Geometry of the knee. In: Dale D et al (eds) Knee ligaments, structure, function, injury and repair. Raven, New York
34. Ritter MA et al (1995) Flat-on-flat, nonconstrained, compression molded polyethylene total knee replacement. Clin Orthop 321:79-85

Fig. 21-7. Fluoroscopic image of two different knees. The total knee arthroplasty on the *left* (cruciate-retaining) has significantly more anterior sliding of the femur with respect to the tibia during flexion than the knee on the *right* (posterior-stabilized). Flexion is limited in the unstable cruciate-retaining knee because impingement between the posterior polyethylene and the posterior cortex occurs

mechanism engages. This is supported by the work of Komistek et al. [27]. They compared the in vivo kinematics of an ACL-sparing knee prosthesis with those of a classical PS (ACL-sacrificing) prosthesis and related a posterior tibiofemoral contact position near full extension to an ACL that was 'not functioning properly' or absent (PS group). Further confirmation of this hypothesis is found in papers dealing with kinematics following TKA implantation [16, 40], where the authors reported the highest posterior translation in ACL-sparing total knee designs.

Conclusion

Abnormal kinematics and sagittal instability have been reported after implantation of a total knee prosthesis. These abnormalities are related to deficient ACL and PCL function. Surface congruity and cam-post mechanisms can partially compensate for the sacrificed ligaments if the „flexion gap" is accurately sized.

References

1. Andriacchi TP et al (1988) Retention of the posterior cruciate in total knee arthroplasty. J Arthroplasty 3:13-19
2. Asano T et al (2001) In vivo three dimensional knee kinematics using a biplanar image-matching technique. Clin Orthop 388:157-166
3. Babis GC et al (2002) The effectiveness of isolated tibial insert exchange in revision total knee arthroplasty. J Bone Joint Surg [Am] 84:64-68
4. Banks SA, Hodge WA (1996) Accurate measurement of three-dimensional knee replacement kinematics using single-plane fluoroscopy. IEEE Trans Biomed Eng 43/ 6, June
5. Banks SA et al (1997) In vivo kinematics of cruciate retaining and substituting knee replacements. J Arthroplasty 3:297-304
6. Banks S et al (2003) Knee motions during maximum flexion in fixed and mobile bearing arthroplasties. Clin Orthop 410:131-138

35. Sharkey PF et al (2002) Why are total knee arthroplasties failing today? Clin Orthop 404:7-13

36. Simmons S et al (1996) Proprioception following total knee arthroplasty with and without the posterior cruciate ligament. J. Arthroplasty 11:763-768

37. Stiehl JB et al (1995) Fluoroscopic analysis of kinematics after posterior-cruciate-retaining knee arthroplasty. J Bone Joint Surg [Br] 77:884-889

38. Stiehl JB et al (1997) In vivo kinematic analysis of a mobile bearing total knee prosthesis. Clin Orthop 345:60-66

39. Stiehl JB et al (2000) In vivo kinematic comparison of posterior cruciate ligament retention or sacrifice with a mobile bearing total knee arthroplasty. Am J Knee Surg 13:13-18

40. Stiehl JB et al (2000) The cruciate ligaments in total knee arthroplasty. J Arthroplasty 15:545-550

41. Stiehl J (2001) Femoral roll back is obtainable and beneficial (not sure). In: Laskin RS (ed) Controversies in total knee replacement. Oxford University Press, Oxford, pp 118-131

42. Straw R et al (2003) Posterior cruciate ligament at total knee replacement. J Bone Joint Surg [Br] 85:671-674

43. Sultan PG et al (2003) Optimizing flexion after total knee arthroplasty. Clin Orthop 416:167-173

44. Udomkiat P et al (2000) Functional comparison of posterior cruciate retention and substitution knee replacement. Clin Orthop 378:192-201

45. Victor J et al (2005) Posterior stabilised knee replacements have more natural kinematics than cruciate retaining knee replacements. J Bone Joint Surg [Br] (in press)

46. Windsor R et al (1989) Mechanisms of failure of the femoral and tibial components in total knee arthroplasty. Clin Orthop Rel Res 248:15-20

22 Kinematic Characteristics of the Unicompartmental Knee

J. N. Argenson, R. D. Komistek, D. A. Dennis

Summary

Knee kinematics were analyzed in subjects with unicompartmental knee arthroplasty (UKA) during deep knee bend (DKB) and stance phase of gait, using video fluoroscopy. Femorotibial contact positions were determined using a computer-automated model-fitting technique. During DKB, subjects with medial UKA experienced on average -0.8 mm of posterior femoral roll-back (PFR), those with lateral UKA -2.5 mm. During stance phase of gait, subjects with medial UKA experienced on average 0.8 mm of PFR, those with lateral UKA -0.4 mm. During DKB normal axial rotation was found for two thirds of subjects (average = 3.3° and 11.2°, respectively, for medial and lateral UKA) and during stance phase of gait for half of the subjects with medial UKA and one quarter with lateral UKA (average of 0.9° and -6.0°, respectively). On average, subjects with UKA experienced kinematic patterns similar to those of the normal knee. The kinematic variability for some subjects suggests progressive laxity of the anterior cruciate ligament, which confirms its role for maintaining satisfactory knee kinematics in UKA.

Introduction

Since the introduction of unicompartmental knee arthroplasty (UKA), many improvements have been made in patient selection, preoperative planning, and surgical instrumentation [1-3], while recently, due to the technical evolution in the field of minimally invasive surgery, a renewed interest in UKA has been noted among knee surgeons [4].

The main failure mode for UKA has been polyethylene wear [5, 6]. More recently, failures secondary to catastrophic polyethylene wear have been observed, attributed to less conforming articular geometries, polyethylene sterilization methods, or disturbed knee kinematics. A better understanding of knee joint kinematics is important to explain the premature polyethylene wear failures observed and serves as the purpose of this investigation.

To date, most experimental studies of knee kinematics have involved cadaveric in vitro analyses or have not tested the knee in a weight-bearing mode [7]. Previously, we determined the in vivo femorotibial and patellofemoral motions of various types of TKA using video fluoroscopy, demonstrating numerous kinematic variances compared with the normal knee, such as paradoxical anterior femoral translation and femoral condylar liftoff [8, 9]. The purpose of the present study was to analyze the kinematics of UKA in which the ACL was intact at the time of the operative procedure, under in vivo weight-bearing conditions, during a deep knee bend, and during stance phase of gait.

Material and Methods

All subjects evaluated received the same UKA (M/G Unicompartmental Arthroplasty, Zimmer, Warsaw, IN, USA) and were operated on in the same department of orthopedic surgery in Marseille, France. For the deep knee bend (DKB) study, 20 knees were evaluated, 17 implanted with a medial UKA and three with a lateral UKA. For the gait analysis study, 19 knees were evaluated, 15 implanted with a medial UKA and four with a lateral UKA. All UKAs were judged as clinically successful (HSS scores >90), without substantial ligamentous laxity or pain, and the ACL was considered to be functionally present in all cases.

Under fluoroscopic surveillance, each subject was asked to perform successive weight-bearing deep knee bend maneuvers up to maximum flexion, while the knee kinematic patterns were assessed at full extension and at 15°, 30°, 45°, 60°, 75°, and 90° of knee flexion. Likewise, each subject was asked to perform the normal stance phase of gait, while the kinematics were analyzed at heel-strike, at 33% and 66% of stance phase, and at toe-off.

The contact position between the medial femoral condyle (medial UKA) or the lateral femoral condyle (lateral UKA) and the tibia was determined using a three-dimensional (3D) model-fitting technique [10]. The 3D computer-aided design (CAD) solid models of the femoral and tibial components were overlaid and fit onto the two-dimensional (2D) fluoroscopic perspective view images (◘ Fig. 22-1).

Chapter 22 · Kinematic Characteristics of the Unicompartmental Knee – J. N. Argenson et al.

149   **22**

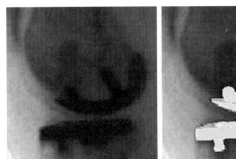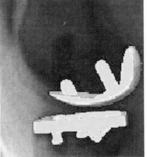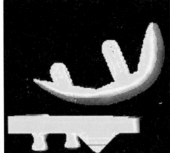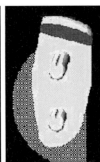

Fig. 22-1. Example of the 3D model-fitting process showing a fluoroscopic image (*far left*), 3D overlay (*center left*), pure sagittal view (*center right*), and top view (*far right*)

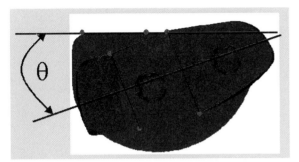

Fig. 22-2. Technique used to determine the axial rotation of the UKA

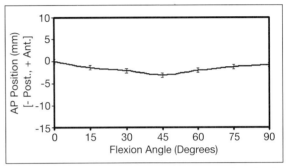

Fig. 22-3. Average anteroposterior contact position, evaluated on the sagittal view, for subjects with a medial UKA, during deep knee bend

A contact position anterior to the midline of the tibia was denoted as positive, and a position posterior was denoted as negative. For rotation, the angle between the longitudinal axis of the femoral component on the coronal view and the fixed axis passing through the tibial component was measured either medially or laterally (■ Fig. 22-2).

Error analyses for this 3D model-fitting technique have been conducted previously and demonstrated translational errors less of than 0.5 mm, and rotational errors of less than 0.5° [10].

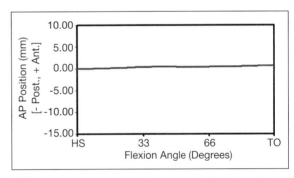

Fig. 22-4. Average anteroposterior contact position, evaluated on the sagittal view, for subjects with a medial UKA, during stance phase of gait, from heel-strike (*HS*) to toe-off (*TO*)

Results

Anteroposterior Translation

Medial UKA

On average, during DKB the femoral component moved 3.1 mm posteriorly from 0° to 45° and then 2.3 mm anteriorly from 45° to 90° (■ Fig. 22-3). Thus from 0° to 90° the femoral components moved an average of 0.8 mm posteriorly. Eight knees (47 %) displayed anterior tibiofemoral contact at 0°. In the remaining nine knees the inital contact was more posterior.

At heel-strike, the average contact position for subjects with a medial UA was -0.2 mm (6.1 to -7.2), moving an average of 0.3 mm in the anterior direction to an average contact position of 0.3 mm (6.6 to -7.2) at 33% of gait stance phase (■ Fig. 22-4). The subjects with a medial UKA

remained in a similar position at 66% of stance phase with a contact position of 0.4 mm (7.7 to -6.0). From 66% of stance phase to toe-off, these subjects experienced an average anterior motion, having a contact position of 0.6 mm (7.2 to -8.0) at toe-off. Eleven of the 15 subjects experienced less than 2.0 mm of medial UKA motion (anterior or posterior), which is similar to the medial condyle for the normal knee during gait.

Lateral UKA

During DKB, two knees exhibited minimal anteroposterior motion of the femoral component from 0° to 90°, and one exhibited posterior motion of 7.6 mm. Between 0°

22

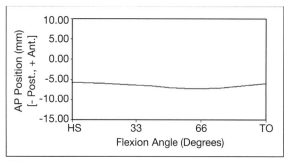

Fig. 22-5. Average anteroposterior contact position, evaluated on the sagittal view, for subjects with a lateral UKA, during stance phase of gait, from heel-strike (*HS*) to toe-off (*TO*)

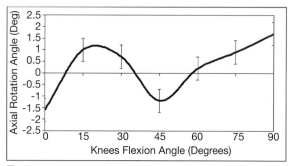

Fig. 22-6. Average axial rotation pattern for subjects having a medial UKA, during deep knee bend

and 90°, all three knees exhibited both anterior and posterior motion at different points in the arc.

On average, during stance phase of gait, subjects with a lateral UA experienced -0.4 mm of posterior motion from heel-strike to toe-off (Fig. 22-5).

At heel-strike, the average contact position for subjects with a lateral UA was -5.7 mm (-3.9 to -83.9), at 33% of stance phase the average was -6.4 mm (-5.7 to -7.6), at 66% of stance phase the average was -7.3 mm (-2.4 to -9.9), and at toe-off the average contact position was -6.1 mm (-4.3 to -8.0). On average, the greatest amount of posterior motion occurred from heel-strike to 66% of stance phase (-1.6 mm), while an anterior slide of 1.2 mm occurred from 66% of stance phase to toe-off. Overall, all four subjects experienced less than 2.1 mm of motion, whether the motion occurred in the anterior or the posterior direction.

Axial Tibiofemoral Rotation

Medial UKA

On average, during DKB the 17 knees displayed 3.3° of internal tibial rotation between the two components of the

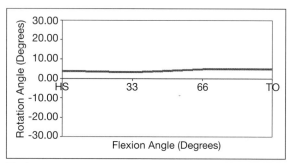

Fig. 22-7. Average axial rotation pattern for subjects with a medial UKA, during stance phase of gait, from heel-strike (HS) to toe-off (TO)

prosthesis between 0° and 90° flexion (Fig. 22-6). Three knees displayed external tibial rotation, two displayed negligible (<1.0°) rotation, and the remainder rotated internally with a mean of 10.1° (range 1.2°-17.3°).

On average, during stance phase of gait, subjects with a medial UA experienced 0.94° of normal axial rotation from heel-strike to toe-off (Fig. 22-7). Eight of 15 (53.3%) subjects with a medial UKA experienced normal axial rotation from heel-strike to toe-off (Fig. 22-8).

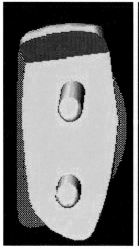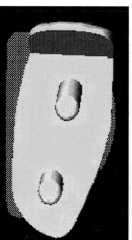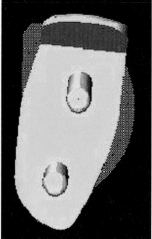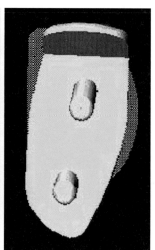

Fig. 22-8. Top view of a subject with a medial UKA, depicting normal axial rotation during gait

Chapter 22 · Kinematic Characteristics of the Unicompartmental Knee – J. N. Argenson et al.

151   **22**

Lateral UKA

During DKB, it was found that in two knees the tibia rotated internally with flexion, but in one knee the tibia rotated externally. As with AP motion, the direction of axial rotation in an individual knee changed from point to point over the range from 0° to 90°.

During stance phase of gait, and contrary to those with a medial UKA, subjects with a lateral UKA experienced on average -6.0° of opposite axial rotation from heel-strike to toe-off. Two of four subjects with a lateral UKA experienced greater than 10° of opposite axial rotation.

Discussion

Kinematic evaluations of the normal knee have demonstrated anterior femorotibial contact in full extension and 14.2 mm of posterior roll-back of the lateral femoral condyle (PFR) with progressive flexion, while during stance phase of gait minimal motion (1.0-2.0 mm) of the medial condyle and approximately 4.0 mm of posterior roll-back of the lateral condyle is seen, leading to the normal axial rotation of the femur relative to the tibia [10].

The present study has determined that on average subjects with a medial UKA experienced a normal AP kinematic pattern, but less pronounced in magnitude than in the normal knee, with the medial condyle remaining in a similar contact position throughout a deep knee bend and during stance phase of gait. On average, subjects with a medial UKA experienced only 0.8 mm of average motion during stance phase of gait and 11 of 15 subjects experienced either 2.0 mm or less motion, similar to the range for the normal knee. The results for the few lateral UKAs showed more variability, with the lateral condyle either moving in the posterior direction or demonstrating minimal motion. During gait, subjects with a medial UKA experienced more normal axial rotation patterns than subjects with a lateral UKA, with 0.9° of normal axial rotation for medial UKA (compared with 4.0° for the normal knee) from heel-strike to toe-off, while subjects with a lateral UA experienced -6.0° of opposite axial rotation.

The results of this study may suggest that for some subjects progressive laxity of the ACL may occur over time [11]. This finding was very similar to what was reported based on fluoroscopic evaluations of PCL-retaining TKA in which the ACL is absent [9]. The functional role of the ACL for maintaining satisfactory knee kinematics has been previously demonstrated both in cadaveric and clinical studies [12, 13]. The deficient ACL function found in these UKA patients may be related to various factors such as unrecognized tears at the time of operation, or chronic attenuation occurring after implantation secondary to minor traumata, or by abrasion caused by persistent notch osteophytes. The clinical adverse consequence could be a potentially higher risk for accelerated tibial polyethylene wear as demonstrated during laboratory evaluation [14]. Therefore, one of the reasons for premature failure observed in some studies of UKA may be related, at least in part, to kinematic abnormalities secondary to disturbed ACL function.

In conclusion, this study has shown that during weight-bearing activities, such as when performing a deep knee bend or during walking, certain subjects exhibited normal knee motion patterns after implantation of UKA, but the amount of motion was less than the magnitudes reported for the normal knee. For some subjects abnormal kinematic patterns were found, possibly related to progressive dysfunction of the ACL over time. The subjects in this study who exhibited normal kinematic patterns demonstrated PFR and internal tibial rotation with progressive flexion, similar to the normal knee.

References

1. Berger RA, Nedeff DD, Barden RM, Sheinkop MM, Jacobs JJ, Rosenberg AG, Galante JO (1999) Unicompartmental knee arthroplasty. Clinical experience at 6- to 10-year follow-up. Clin Orthop 367:50-60
2. Cartier P, Sanouiller JL, Grelsamer RP (1996) Unicompartmental knee arthroplasty surgery. 10-year minimum follow-up period. J Arthroplasty 11:782-788
3. Argenson JN et al (2002) Modern cemented metal-backed unicompartmental knee arthroplasty. A 3- to 10-year follow-up study. J Bone Joint Surg [Am] 84:2235-2239
4. Price AJ, Webb J, Topf H, Dodd CAF, Goodfellow JW, Murray DW (2001) Rapid recovery after Oxford unicompartmental knee arthroplasty through a short incision. J Arthroplasty 16:970-976
5. Palmer SH, Morrison PJ, Ross AC (1998) Early catastrophic tibial component wear after unicompartmental knee arthroplasty. Clin Orthop 350:143-148
6. Argenson JN, O'Connor JJ (1992) Polyethylene wear in meniscal knee replacement. A one- to nine-year retrieval analysis of the Oxford knee. J Bone Joint Surg [Br] 74:228-232
7. Lafortune MA et al (1992) Three-dimensional kinematics of the human knee during walking. J Biomech 25:347-357
8. Dennis D et al (1998) In vivo anteroposterior femorotibial translation: a multicenter analysis. Clin Orthop 356:47-57
9. Komistek R et al (2000) An in vivo determination of patellofemoral contact positions. Clin Biomech 15:29-36
10. Dennis DA et al (1996) In vivo knee kinematics derived using an inverse perspective technique. Clin Orthop 331:107-117
11. Argenson JN et al (2002) In vivo determination of knee kinematics for subjects implanted with a unicompartmental arthroplasty. J Arthroplasty 17:1049-1054
12. Deschamps G, Lapeyre B (1987) Rupture of the anterior cruciate ligament: a frequently unrecognized cause of failure of unicompartmental knee prostheses. Rev Chir Orthop 73:544-551
13. Moller JT et al (1985) Unicompartmental arthroplasty of the knee. Cadaver study of the importance of the anterior cruciate ligament. Acta Orthop Scand 56:120-123
14. Blunn GW, Walker PS, Joshi A, Hardinge K (1991) The dominance of cyclic sliding in producing wear in total knee replacements. Clin Orthop 273:253-260

23 In Vitro Kinematics of the Replaced Knee

S. Incavo, B. Beynnon, K. Coughlin

Summary

Important information on knee kinematics can be obtained using in vitro methods. Specifically, mounting a cadaver lower extremity on an "Oxford" knee jig allows loading of the knee joint and makes it possible to observe physiological motion. This approach can provide a detailed description of the displacements and rotations of the patella, femur, and tibia, and direct measurement of load at both the patellofemoral and tibiofemoral articulations. Using this approach, the "two-axis" description of tibiofemoral kinematics has been advanced. Another application of this method describes lower patellofemoral contact forces when a more posterior femorotibial contact point is present after total knee arthroplasty. This kinematic information is useful when considering new designs in knee arthroplasty.

Introduction

Although it is clear that the forces and moments transmitted across the patellofemoral and tibiofemoral joints affect metabolism of articular cartilage in the normal knee, and wear of joint replacements, very little is known about the magnitude and direction of these forces in vivo. In part, this is because the tools that are currently available permit only accurate measurement of displacements and rotations in vivo; they do not permit quantification of the forces and moments. Indeed, a great deal is known about the displacement biomechanics of normal and especially prosthetic joints in vivo, while very little is known about the forces and moments transmitted across these joints. In an effort to gain insight into the loads and moments transmitted across the knee, many in vitro studies have used a knee-loading fixture, commonly referred to as an "Oxford" knee jig. These loading fixtures have been developed to recreate common activities such as squatting by attempting to simulate muscle contraction and weight bearing. The quadriceps are the most common muscle group that has been simulated, because contraction of these muscles is important during daily activity, and because the orientation of the quadriceps, patella,

and patellar tendon makes it readily accessible to produce a realistic muscle action simply by pulling on the quadriceps tendon. Two approaches have been used to apply body weight to the knee. Either the ankle joint is held stationary and the hip is allowed to translate in a vertical direction, or the hip joint remains stationary and the ankle joint translates in a vertical direction. Both approaches permit 6° of freedom at the knee, such that flexion-extension movement of the knee is constrained by articular contact and the soft tissues that span this joint, and not the loading fixture. With these techniques, the knee is loaded such that a flexion moment is created, and stability is obtained by applying a tensile load to the quadriceps tendon through a load sensor. Compressive loads can be applied about the hip to simulate body weight, and using this feature, activities such as stair-climbing or squatting are simulated.

A tensile load applied to the quadriceps results in a compressive load at the knee joint. Ideally, an additional load is applied to the hamstrings and gastrocnemius muscles. Because the loading jig allows completely unrestrained knee joint motion, very accurate kinematic measurements can be made during physiological knee motion. While kinematic measurements can be made using different techniques, we have utilized electromagnetic position sensors rigidly fixed to the femur, tibia, and patella. Additionally, load sensors can be used to measure joint forces during physiological knee motion (◘ Fig. 23-1). Thus, this in vitro approach allows detailed description of the displacements and rotations of the patella, femur, and tibia, and direct measurement of load at the patellofemoral and tibiofemoral interfaces.

There are, however, several limitations associated with using cadaver models to simulate the in vivo condition. First, the actual magnitude of muscle contraction involved during squatting is unknown, and thus it can only be estimated, through analytic prediction. An alternative approach is to recreate the load of body weight and then apply a force to the extensor mechanism such that equilibrium is established or flexion-extension motion is created. Second, when using a cadaver model to simulate squatting, body-weight loads are typically applied through the center of the hip and ankle joints throughout

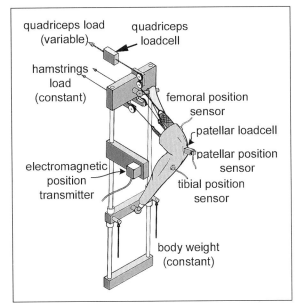

Fig. 23-1. Oxford loading jig. Hip and ankle joints provide all rotational degrees of freedom. Tibiofemoral kinematics are measured by electromagnetic position sensors. Constant body-weight and hamstring loads are applied, while flexion cycles are activated by varying the quadriceps load

and recent studies challenge conventional understanding of the instantaneous center of rotation model. Several controversial aspects of knee arthroplasty are addressed by in vitro study, such as the role of the PCL and the kinematic behavior of various knee designs. Another area in which in vitro studies have provided new information involves patellar forces associated with knee arthroplasty. These topics will be discussed separately.

Kinematics of The Normal Knee

It is somewhat surprising that the kinematic behavior of the normal human knee has been variously described in apparently contradictory ways. These descriptions include the instantaneous center of rotation model, the helical-axis model, and the two-axis model. A brief description of the first two is included, and is followed by a more detailed description of the two-axis theory, which is supported by more recent in vitro studies.

Instantaneous Center of Rotation

The motion of the knee in the sagittal plane has traditionally been modeled as a four-bar linkage [9]. One of the bars represents the ACL, one represents the PCL, and the two remaining bars connect the tibial ACL and PCL attachments and the femoral ACL and PCL attachments. At a given knee flexion angle the intersection of the ACL and PCL is termed the "instantaneous center of rotation". At different knee flexion angles, the intersection between the ACL and the PCL changes. Moving from extension to flexion, the instantaneous center of rotation follows a semicircular pathway (referred to as the "J" curve), which produces a changing roll-glide ratio with the tibia relative to the femur. That is, the femur does not roll posteriorly off the tibia, but also slides on the tibia during increasing flexion.

The model has been used to explain the posterior translation of the femur relative to the tibia during flexion, and it has been used to explain resistance to posterior drawer motion. The model is useful in showing that the center of rotation of the knee is not rigidly fixed to the femur or the tibia.

The four bar linkage model has proven to be useful in enhancing our understanding of the motions of the knee, although the model assumptions have limitations. The cruciate ligaments are modeled as rigid bars, when, in reality, the ligaments elongate during knee motion. In addition, the knee is modeled in two dimensions (flexion-extension in the sagittal plane) only, and the model is not applicable if rotation of 15° or more exists in the other planes [17]. In fact, out-of-plane rotation will lead to errors of up to 20 mm, which is too large to accurately describe knee kinematics [3].

the entire flexion-extension motion of the knee. In contrast, when squatting in vivo, the force produced by body weight acts through the center of gravity of the trunk, which is located anterior to the hip, while the force produced by the ground reaction acts through the forefoot, which is located anterior to the ankle joint. Thus, the extension moment arm may be smaller in vivo than in vitro, and the corresponding muscle forces required to extend the leg or maintain a fixed flexion angle would be much less. For these reasons, the quadriceps force applied to flex and extend a cadaver lower extremity with a fixed body-weight load may be greater than the quadriceps forces that occur in vivo. A third concern associated with the use of a cadaver model to recreate knee biomechanics is that few studies have simulated contraction of the extensor and flexor muscle groups, specifically the combined contraction of the hamstring and gastrocnemius muscles. Clearly, contraction of these muscles has an effect on the biomechanical behavior of the knee, and studies including these combined contractions should be more meaningful than earlier studies.

Another in vitro approach utilizes a robotic system [15]. The robotic testing system serves as both a position-control device and a force-moment sensor. When a knee specimen is mounted and moved through a range of motion, the specimen's motion pattern is "learned" and then repeated after the specimen has been modified.

Even with these limitations, in vitro studies have provided important insights into several areas of knee kinematics and biomechanics. Specifically, the kinematic behavior of the normal knee is not universally agreed upon,

Helical Axes of Rotation

It is well known that motions of the knee are coupled. Thus, the functional axis of rotation of the knee is not parallel to the frontal or the coronal planes. Modeling knee motions using the helical axis of rotation accounts for the oblique angle of the functional axis relative to commonly referenced anatomical axes. The helical-axis model describes rotations about, and translations along, a fixed axis. Blankevoort showed that patterns of the helical axes are reproducible and consistent when care is taken to ensure that the motion pathways are consistent [2]. The helical-axis technique has been used in vivo combined with roentgen stereophotogrammetric analysis [13,14,18] and in vitro [1].

The helical axis is not dependent on the choice of the anatomical coordinate system. When the instantaneous helical-axis model is used, the center of rotation is not necessarily the intersection of the ACL and the PCL, suggesting that the colateral ligaments and the articular geometry of the knee are also responsible for the location of the helical axis.

Although the helical-axis theory models the knee in three dimensions, there are several drawbacks. The data from the helical-axis model are not unique; they are dependent on the particular motion pathway. Obtaining the model data requires accurate measurement techniques. Position and direction parameters of the helical axes are highly susceptible to measurement errors when the rotations are small [19]. Finally, it is difficult to discuss the helical axis in clinically meaningful terms and anatomical planes.

Two-Axis Model

As mentioned above, descriptions of knee kinematics based on the instantaneous center of rotation method or helical-axis method have been called into question. Because of this, investigators began to look for a more straightforward approach to describing knee kinematics. This was based, in part, on the recognition that the posterior femoral condyles can be described as circular. Prior to this recognition, the femur – when viewed from that anatomical lateral – view was thought to be elliptical in the posterior aspect. Based on this circular profile, a single fixed knee flexion axis passing through the condylar centers has been postulated [8]. Building on this concept, Hollister et al. described knee kinematics based on motions about two fixed axes: a flexion axis located in the femur and a rotational axis in the tibia [10].

To more fully evaluate knee kinematics and expand on these findings, a mathematical modeling technique was applied to cadavers in an Oxford-loaded knee rig by Churchill et al. [3]. The modeling technique identifies

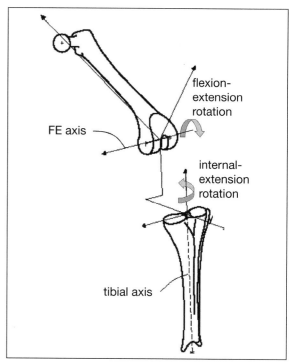

Fig. 23-2. The "two-axis" theory of knee kinematics, with the femoral epicondylar axis as the flexion axis and the tibial axis as the internal-external rotational axis

both the optimal knee flexion axis and the longitudinal rotational axis. Once the flexion axis is identified, it can be compared to the femoral epicondylar axis and the longitudinal rotational axis can be compared to the tibial axis.

Two significant findings of this work were noted. First, optimal flexion and longitudinal rotation axes were accurately identified for each specimen from 5° to 90° of flexion. Second, the location of the axes was identified. The flexion axis very closely aligned with the femoral epicondylar axis (±3 mm, 3°), and the longitudinal rotational axis was found to intersect the tibial plateau in the region of the medial tibial plateau sulcus. This verifies earlier studies which showed that the knee has two bony-fixed primary axes. This model has been described as a "compound hinge model" but is better termed the "two-axis theory" of knee kinematics (Fig. 23-2).

At both extremes of the flexion cycle, the two-axis theory does not necessarily apply, however. Noncircular portions of the femoral condyles come into contact with the tibia and menisci in terminal extension (screw-home mechanism) and in flexion beyond 90° (roll-back mechanism). Nonetheless, this theory represents a subtle, but important distinction in the understanding of knee kinematics, especially throughout the most functional range of knee motion.

Upon first inspection, the two-axis theory appears to contradict the accepted phenomenon of femoral roll-back. However, this is explained by the fact that the longitudinal rotational axis is located in the medial tibial plateau. With tibial rotation, more lateral tibial plateau motion occurs than medial plateau motion. Because of this, even though the longitudinal rotational axis does not move posteriorly with respect to the femoral epicondylar axis (roll-back), the femur appears to roll back with knee flexion. This phenomenon can be referred to as "apparent roll-back." Churchill et al. reported that no true femoral roll-back occurs during much of the flexion cycle (0°-75°). However, true roll-back does occur for flexion angles generally greater than 75°. Stated differently, "apparent roll-back" occurs from 0° to 75°, and true roll-back occurs over 75° [3].

Once the femoral epicondylar axis is considered to be the flexion axis of the knee, it is logical to examine the tibial and patellar axes in relation to the femoral epicondylar axis. A follow-up in vitro study supports this logic [5]. When the femoral epicondylar axis was used to reference the tibial axis, the tibial shaft axis was found to be perpendicular to the femoral epicondylar axis (average 90.5° from 5° to 90° of knee flexion(Fig. 23-3).

Tibial rotation was observed to be 5°-15° throughout the flexion cycle. However, nearly all rotation occurred near terminal extension. With flexion greater than 10°-15°, virtually no tibial rotation occurs.

The two-axis theory of knee kinematics has favorable implications for knee arthroplasty. When using a "classical" (perpendicular) tibial cut, rotationally aligning the femoral component along the femoral epicondylar axis should result in a rectangular flexion gap because of the perpendicular relationship of the epicondylar and tibial axes. Furthermore, a femoral component with a circular sagittal profile can yield constant colateral ligament tensioning throughout the functional knee motion. Con-

cerning tibial rotations, several aspects of arthroplasty component design should be noted. If the terminal tibial external rotation is excluded (as likely happens after total knee arthroplasty), then the neutral tibial rotational position is more externally rotated than traditionally considered. This externally rotated tibial base-plate position is also supported by a recent MRI study [12]. If the femoral epicondylar axis is selected for femoral component rotation, the mid portion (rather than the medial one third) of the tibial tubercle may be a preferable rotational landmark for the tibial base plate.

It is important to mention that while the two-axis model is an excellent description of femoral and tibial motions, it represents a simplification of knee kinematics. For example, the tibial axis is not always perpendicular to the epicondylar axis, but ranges from 85° to 94° throughout the flexion cycle. Nonetheless, one angle must be selected for placement of the tibial component in TKA, and the average experimentally observed angle of 90° to the tibial shaft axis (a classical tibial cut) reflects both biomechanical and clinical logic.

The two-axis theory is directly applicable to a rotating-platform (mobile-bearing) TKA design. For a rotating tibial design, the rotational center can be located either centrally or off-center, but most rotating-bearing designs utilize a central rotation point.

In vitro studies are particularly suitable to examine options for a given prosthetic design: for example, PCL retention vs. substitution and fixed vs. mobile-bearing articulations. Multiple in vitro studies have examined the role of the PCL in knee arthroplasty [4,11]. Agreement exists that in a PCL-retaining design, anterior positioning of the femur on the tibia (paradoxical roll-back) occurs and is worsened if the PCL is deficient. For knee kinematics to be restored even partially, either an intact PCL or a cam-spine mechanism is necessary.

Several in vitro studies have compared fixed-bearing and mobile-bearing design options for the same knee arthroplasty system [7,16]. In general, little tibial insert rotation occurs, and increasing conformity or rotational constraint in mobile-bearing designs does not adversely affect knee kinematics.

Three-Axis Model

To extend the two-axis model to include the patellofemoral joint we have examined patellar tracking in vitro and referenced this to the femoral epicondylar axis. In a plane perpendicular to the epicondylar axis the patellar axis can be described as a circle with the center approximately 10 mm anterior and 10 mm proximal to the epicondylar axis (Fig. 23-4). Minimal medial-lateral movement (4 mm) is observed along the epicondylar axis (Fig. 23-5). This biomechanical finding supports the

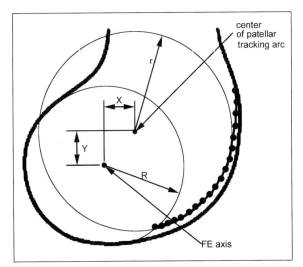

 Fig. 23-3. Average tibial varus-valgus angulation throughout the knee flexion cycle. The tibial shaft axis was found to be perpendicular to the femoral epicondylar axis (average 90.5° (1.9°) from 5° to 90° of knee flexion. (From [5])

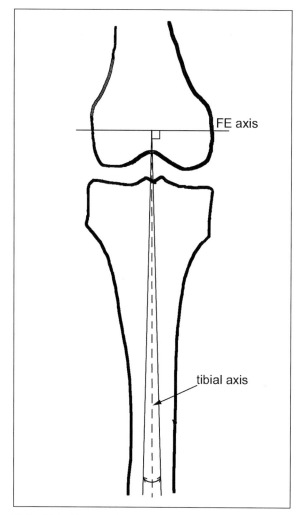

Fig. 23-4. Schematic of a distal femur (*dark line*) and the path of the patellar tracking from full extension to 90° flexion (*right*). The center of the arc describing the patellar path is located at a distance (approximately 10 mm anteriorly and 10 mm proximally) from the FE axis [3]. *R* Radius of the epicondylar circle, *r* radius of the arc describing the patellar tracking

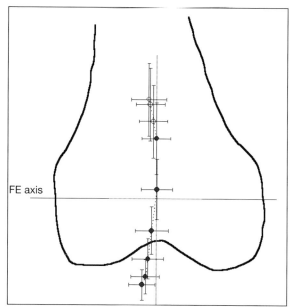

Fig. 23-5. The average patella shift in the frontal plane along the FE axis is 4.3 mm. *Open circles* represent the patellar position at flexion angles between 0° and 15°; *solid circles* represent the patellar position at flexion angles between 20° and 90°. (From [5])

clinical observation that external rotation of the femoral component aids patellar tracking in TKA.

Patellar Component Forces

Patellar tracking and patellar component failure are important aspects of total knee arthroplasty. While fluoroscopic in vivo studies provide data regarding tibiofemoral kinematics, they do not show the effect of tibiofemoral kinematics on the patellofemoral articulation. In vitro studies can provide helpful information on patellar kinematics and patellar loading by including a patellar force transducer while measuring kinematics. In one study, the anterior-posterior position of the femur on the tibia was examined and direct comparisons were made based on the status of the PCL [4]. The specific conditions that were studied included the intact PCL, the loose PCL, and a PCL-substituting design. Additionally, the post position was varied from 2 mm more anterior to 4 mm more posterior. These implant conditions were shown to directly affect the anterior-posterior position of the femur on the tibia (◘ Fig. 23-6a). Simultaneous measurement of patellofemoral contact forces demonstrated about 20% lower forces for the most posterior femoral position (◘ Fig. 23-6b).

Another in vitro study by D'Lima et al. also supports these findings that a more posterior femoral position (roll-back) significantly decreases patellar compressive forces [6]. This occurs in a normal knee with an intact PCL or with a posterior-stabilized implant but is less likely in a PCL-retaining design, especially when the PCL is loose or deficient.

In vitro setups have also been used to study patellar preparation in TKA [20]. Comparisons were made for different patellar prosthesis designs (resurfacing vs. inset). When measuring anterior patellar bone strain, it was concluded that a patellar resurfacing design is superior (less alteration to strain) to an inset design and that the osteotomy for patellar resurfacing is more tolerant to error by excess cutting than is the reaming technique required for an inset design. Another finding of the study was that if the ideal depth of the cut or reaming is surpassed (making the patella too thin), attempts to recreate the original patellar thickness by using a thicker prosthesis are mechanically detrimental.

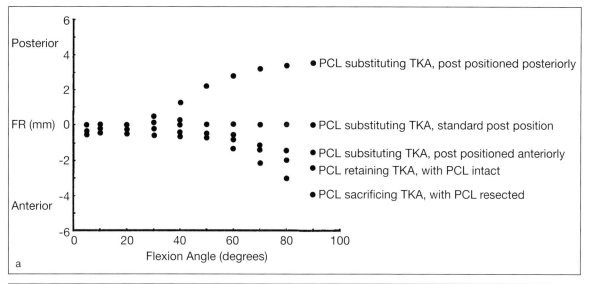

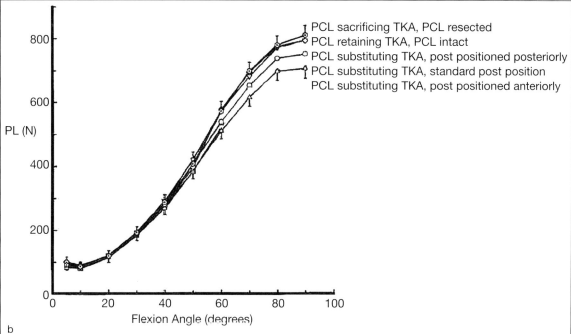

☐ **Fig. 23-6a, b.** *a* Average difference in the femoral roll-back (☐ FR) versus flexion. ☐ FR is the difference in femoral roll-back between the treatment of interest and the reference (standard post position) treatment. *b* Average patellofemoral contact load (*PL*) versus flexion. (From [4])

Conclusions

Knee kinematics and TKA design have been successfully studied using in vitro methods and represent useful complements to in vivo studies. In particular, in vivo studies can examine individual cases, while in vitro studies are most useful to study the same specimen with a variety of different treatment options.

References

1. Blaha JD et al (2003) Kinematics of the human knee using an open chain cadaver model. Clin Orthop 410:25-34
2. Blankevoort L et al (1990) Helical axes of passive knee joint motions. J Biomech 23:1219-1229
3. Churchill DL et al (1998) The transepicondylar axis approximates the optimal flexion axis of the knee. Clin Orthop 356:111-118
4. Churchill DL et al (2001) The influence of femoral roll-back on patellofemoral contact loads in total knee arthroplasty. J Arthroplasty 16:909-918
5. Coughlin KM et al (2003) Tibial axis and patellar position relative to the femoral epicondylar axis during squatting. J Arthroplasty 18:1048-1055

23

6. D'Lima DD et al (2003) Impact of patellofemoral design on patellofemoral forces and polyethylene stresses. J Bone Joint Surg [Am] 85 [Suppl 4]: 85-93

7. D'Lima DD et al (2000) Comparison between the kinematics of fixed and rotating bearing knee prostheses. Clin Orthop 380:151-157

8. Elias S et al (1990) A correlative study of the geometry and anatomy of the distal femur. Clin Orthop 260:98-103

9. Frankel V (1971) Biomechanics of the knee. Orthop Clin North Am 2:175-190

10. Hollister AM et al (1993) The axes of rotation of the knee. Clin Orthop 290:259-268

11. Incavo SJ et al (1997) Knee kinematics in genesis total knee arthroplasty. A comparison of different tibial designs with and without posterior cruciate substitution in cadaveric specimens. Am J Knee Surg 10:209-215

12. Incavo SJ et al (2003) Anatomic rotational relationships of the proximal tibia, distal femur, and patella: implications for rotational alignment in total knee arthroplasty. J Arthroplasty 18:643-648

13. Jonsson H et al (1994) Three-dimensional knee joint movements during a step-up: evaluation after anterior cruciate ligament rupture. J Orthop Res 12:769-779

14. Karrholm J et al (1994) Kinematics of successful knee prostheses during weight-bearing: three-dimensional movements and positions of screw axes in the Tricon-M and Miller-Galante designs. Knee Surg Sports Traumatol Arthrosc 2:50-59

15. Li G et al (2001) Cruciate-retaining and cruciate-substituting total knee arthroplasty: an in vitro comparison of the kinematics under muscle loads. J Arthroplasty 16 [Suppl 1]:150-156

16. Most E et al. (2003) The kinematics of fixed- and mobile-bearing total knee arthroplasty. Clin Orthop 416:197-207

17. Nordin M, Frankel VH (2001) Biomechanics of the knee. In: Nordin M, Frankel VH (eds) Basic biomechanics of the musculoskeletal system. Lippencott Williams and Wilkins, Philadelphia

18. Weidenhielm L et al (1993) Knee motion after tibial osteotomy for arthhrosis. Acta Orthop Scand 64:317-319

19. Woltring H et al (1985) Finite centroid and helical axis estimation from noisy landmark measurements in the study of human joint kinematics. J Biomech 18:379-389

20. Wulff W, Incavo SJ (2000) The effect of patella preparation for total knee arthroplasty on patellar strain: a comparison of resurfacing versus inset implants. J Arthroplasty 15:778-782

24 The Virtual Knee

B. W. McKinnon, J. K. Otto, S. McGuan

Summary

The Virtual Knee is a 3-D, dynamic, physics-based software that simulates in vivo functional activities for the purpose of evaluating the kinematic and kinetic performance of TKR designs. Implant models are virtually implanted onto a lower-leg purdue-like knee simulator that is driven through activities including gait and deep knee bend using active quadriceps and hamstring actuators. The surrounding soft tissues, including LCL, MCL, and capsule, are modeled. By varying parameters such as implant geometry, ligament tensions, component positioning, and patient anthropometrics, this complex system can be understood, which allows the design of better-performing implants.

Introduction

The typical engineering design process for most complex mechanical systems is illustrated in ◧ Fig. 24-1. This process is followed by many industries including the aerospace, the automotive, and of course the orthopedic industry. In this process, virtual testing and physical testing design-iteration loops are employed, both of which arc important methods for arriving at a final design that meets the design inputs.

The virtual testing loop uses computational methods to evaluate performance before physical components are ever made. Although virtual methods cannot perfectly model the physical world, the advantages of this method are that many design iterations can be evaluated quickly and cheaply. Moreover, all variables are controlled, and quality measurements can be extracted for nearly everything modeled in the system. Virtual testing is a powerful method for characterizing the system and understanding how specifically varied parameters affect the results. With the exception of finite element analysis, the orthopedic industry has generally been without a robust, dynamic analytical testing method. Consequently, total knee replacement design has relied heavily on physical testing methods.

Although the physical testing loop measures real-world performance, it is time consuming and expensive.

Drawings must be prepared and tooling and gaging must all be designed and manufactured just to produce a high-fidelity prototype implant. The physical testing machines for TKR performance evaluation include servohydraulic machines (e.g., MTS and Instron), wear simulators [1, 2], and Oxford/Purdue-type knee simulators [3, 4]. But these machines have their shortcomings. They often generate insufficient data because inline force transducers provide only force magnitude and not direction, multi-degree of freedom transducers are large and expensive, and multiple transducers add complexity. Some testing machines oversimplify the real-world conditions. Often derived resultant forces are applied to the implants, leaving out major stability-contributing tissues (e.g., quadriceps, hamstrings, collateral ligaments, and capsule). Also, the nonlinear properties of these tissues are hard to replicate and

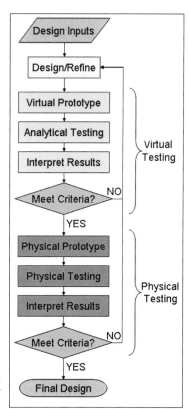

◧ **Fig. 24-1.** Engineering design process for complex systems

they are difficult to attach to testing fixtures. The simulations are generally limited to less demanding activities like walking, stair climbing, and deep knee bend because of inertia, fixture interference, and limited actuator stroke. More demanding activities (e.g., running, tennis, and skiing) are too challenging to replicate. When cadavers are used, they are variable in size, shape, and location of anatomical landmarks. In addition, great care must be taken to minimize implantation alignment errors.

Because of high cost and long lead times, the number of physical design iterations is severely limited. In addition, the confounding factors of the physical testing machines make it difficult to interpret the results and make educated decisions about design changes. As a result, TKR design has evolved slowly, and the kinematic and kinetic performance has not been optimized. Recently, an analytical tool called the Virtual Knee (Biomechanics Research Group, San Clemente, Calif., USA) has been used to address the shortcomings of the physical testing phase, and it has the potential to greatly advance TKR design.

Materials and Methods

The Virtual Knee is a 3-D, dynamic, physics-based software that simulates in vivo functional activities for the purpose of evaluating the kinematic and kinetic performance of TKR designs. Every parameter during the simulation is controlled and can be kept identical between trials. By comparing the results between design iterations, changes in kinematics and kinetics can be directly attributed to changes in the articular geometry, allowing designers to more easily meet performance design goals.

The Virtual Knee models a lower limb mounted to a Purdue-like knee testing rig (Fig. 24-2). Anatomically accurate 3-D bone models of the femur, tibia, and patella with the desired anthropometrics are mounted to the rig and serve as reference for implant placement, joint line position, scale, and ligament/muscle attachment.

The constraints imparted on the simulation include the hip and ankle joint, passive soft tissues, intrinsic geometric contact constraint, and active muscle elements. The hip joint is modeled as a revolute joint, parallel to the flexion axis of the knee, and is allowed to slide vertically. The ankle joint is modeled as a combination of several joints that combine to allow free translation in the ML direction and free rotation in flexion, axial, and varus/valgus directions. Passive tissue constraints are modeled as spring/damper elements and are attached to the virtual bones at their respective anatomical locations [5]. The mechanical properties of the tissues were obtained from Woo [6]. The LCL is simulated with a single constraint element, and the MCL is modeled with two separate constraint elements to simulate the anterior and posterior

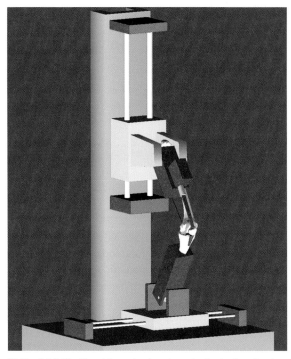

Fig. 24-2. The Virtual Knee simulates lower leg in vivo functional activities for the purpose of evaluating the kinematic and kinetic performance of TKR designs

fibers (Fig. 24-3). For posterior cruciate-retaining knees, a PCL element is added and attached at the respective anatomical locations. The final soft-tissue constraint is the general capsule force, which simulates the general soft-tissue reactions of the knee capsule. This force is directed such that it draws the femur and tibia together in a similar manner to the capsular tissues in the actual knee.

Intrinsic geometric constraints are imparted by the conformity of the TKR models, which includes stick/slip friction and stiffness characteristics. A contact algorithm models the articular surfaces, which are discretized into quadrilateral elements, as a bed of springs with the stiffness characteristics of polyethylene. The method allows for intermittent contact, contact pressure, and center of pressure determination. This algorithm is used to model contact of the patellofemoral joint, the tibiofemoral joint, between the cam and post, and between the quadriceps tendon and femoral component.

The active, driving elements in the model are the quadriceps and hamstrings muscle forces. The quadriceps muscle attaches to the quadriceps tendon and is discretized into six components which conform to the distal head of the femur or anterior flange of the femoral component, permitting proper force transmission to the femur and patella. The patella is attached to the tibial tubercle through the patellar ligament, which conforms to the polyethylene insert component. The simulation is driven by a controlled actuator arrangement similar to the

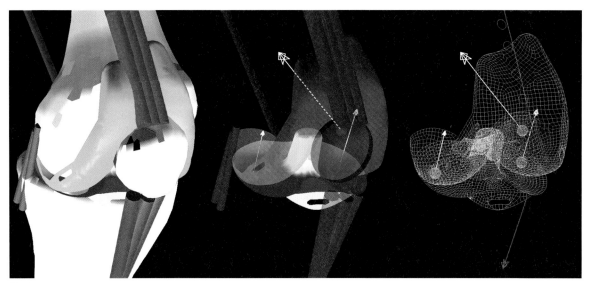

☐ **Fig. 24-3.** Bones, passive soft tissues, active muscles, and component contact are modeled

physical machine. A closed-loop controller is used to apply tension to the quadriceps and hamstring muscles to match a prescribed knee flexion vs. time profile. No large antagonistic forces are modeled. Ground reaction forces are applied as varus/valgus forces and internal/external torques during the cycle using time history data derived from force plate experiments [7]. Two main activities are simulated, a complete cycle gait, and a 0°-160°-0°-160° double deep knee bend cycle. The double cycle is performed so as to capture the inertial loading conditions at full extension (the second 0°).

Three different reference frames are utilized for the reporting of data. These reference frames are rigidly attached to the femur, tibia, and patella at the respective interfaces where the implant models meet the bone models, so as to easily resolve the interface forces and moments. In the simulation, most kinematic and kinetic data are reported relative to the reference frame fixed in the tibia. Kinematic and kinetic data for the patella are also reported with respect to the femur. Component orientation is reported using a three-cylindric model of knee motion similar to Grood and Suntay [8].

Data are reported via graphical animations and numerical results. The graphical animations serve as a powerful communicative tool to design teams and surgeons. Bones, muscles, soft tissues, and implants can all be selectively displayed during the animations. The center-of-pressures for articular contact are displayed as spheres, and all contact forces and tissue forces are displayed as scaled force vectors (Fig. 24-3). Currently, 84 data time-histories are reported for each simulation. These include patellofemoral and tibiofemoral kinematics, soft-tissue forces and locations, actuator forces and locations, contact forces and center-of-pressure locations, contact area, interface forces and locations, and all externally applied forces and locations. All the data are post-processed in a custom in-house spreadsheet, allowing graphical comparative analysis between trials.

The Virtual Knee has been validated in a variety of ways including mechanical, cadaver, and live subject tests. Mechanical tests have been used to tune the performance of the contact force algorithm for both the shear component (friction/stiction) of the force and the normal component of the force. The shear component of the contact force was tuned by comparing the Instron test machine results for the ASTM 1223 component laxity test with a virtual model of the laxity test. The normal component of the forces was tuned by comparing the resulting contact area of virtual compression tests with the contact areas reported from Instron-Fuji film tests. With the current set of contact parameters, the contact algorithm has consistently delivered results within 10% of mechanical tests [9]. Cadaver tests have been used to tune the soft tissues (attachment locations and mechanical properties) and the system controller function comparing the virtual rig results with physical machine results. Human tests have been used to compare kinematic trends between the virtual simulation and in vivo data derived from fluoroscopy [10].

Discussion

Analytical functional simulation tools like the Virtual Knee provide key information that engineers and surgeons need to enable the use of several other powerful analytical tools and methods to design advanced TKR systems. These tools include statistical methods such as sensitivity analysis, response surface methodology, and design of experiments (widely used today to study, control, and optimize manufacturing systems). Through functional simulation, designers can now define, isolate,

24

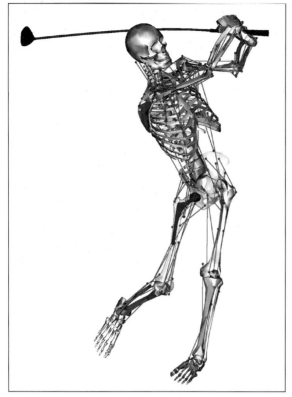

and control the factors affecting the TKR system, analyze the factors using these statistical tools, and subsequently understand how to manipulate the factors to optimize performance.

Factors of particular interest to surgeons are those that affect stability and performance (and which can be variably controlled during simulation) including ligament tension, muscle strength, component alignment, surgical technique, patient anthropometric variability, implant selection, size mismatch, and material selection.

Future analytical functional simulation of TKR systems could involve the use of full-body muscle-driven simulations (◻ Fig. 24-4) rather than the single-leg simulation of the Virtual Knee. In these simulations, motion capture data drive the skeletal model in displacement control, and the muscles are "trained" to perform the activity. After applying forward dynamics analysis, the muscles then drive the motion, and implant performance is evaluated. These simulations are not limited to the standard gait, stair climbing, and deep knee bend movements, but instead allow for more demanding activities.

With the addition of other active and passive tissues, normal knee kinematics and kinetics could be compared with those of the replaced knee for various functional activities, possibly defining new TKR performance testing methods and measures that are more closely correlated to in vivo performance. Furthermore, the Virtual Knee does

not have to be limited to TKR design. Patellofemoral and unicondylar designs could all benefit. In addition, awareness of implantation alignment sensitivities can also drive improved instrument design.

The current state of the art in computer modeling, analytical simulation, and statistical analysis offers exciting opportunities for the designing surgeon and engineer. All of the key ingredients now exist to enable a revolution in TKR design. Parametric 3-D CAD models of implants can now be precisely controlled and quickly manipulated in a manner that allows for optimization of the geometry. Reverse-engineered CT and MRI knee scans can provide the geometry required to optimize implant shape, fit, and size. Analytical tools such as the Virtual Knee can accurately model knee function, provide critical measures not possible with physical testing, and reduce cost and lead times. The resulting kinematics measured from the Virtual Knee can be used to drive dynamic finite element analyses [11], providing an enhanced picture of polyethylene stresses, which may be used as a predictor of in vivo wear performance [12]. Finally, proven statistical methods can be used to effectively consider the many factors affecting TKR performance, allowing optimization of those factors to create the desired performance envelope. In the end, the patient will benefit the most by receiving thoroughly tested and optimized knee replacements implanted by surgeons who are more aware of the factors that most affect the desired results.

References

1. Walker PS et al (1997) A knee simulating machine for performance evaluation of total knee replacements. J Biomech 30:83-89
2. Burgess IC et al (1997) Development of a six-station knee wear simulator and preliminary wear results. Proc Inst Mech Eng [H] 211:37-47
3. Biden E, O'Connor J (1990) Knee ligaments: structure, function, injury, and repair. Raven, New York
4. Zachman NJ (1977) Design of a load simulator for the dynamic evaluation of prosthetic knee joints. MS Thesis. Mechanical Engineering, Purdue University, West Lafayette, IN
5. Blankevoort L, Huiskes R (1991) Ligament-bone interaction in a three-dimensional model of the knee. J Biomech Eng 113:263-269
6. Woo SL et al (1991) Tensile properties of the human femur-anterior cruciate ligament-tibia complex. The effects of specimen age and orientation. Am J Sports Med 19:217-225
7. Winter D (1990) Biomechanics and motor control of human movement. Wiley-Interscience, New York
8. Grood ES, Suntay WJ (1983) A joint coordinate system for the clinical description of three-dimensional motions: application to the knee. J Biomech Eng 105:136-144
9. Masson M et al (1996) Computer modeling of articular contact for assessing total knee replacement constraint criteria. 10th Conference of the European Society of Biomechanics, Leuven
10. Banks SA et al (1997) The mechanics of knee replacements during gait. In vivo fluoroscopic analysis of two designs. Am J Knee Surg 10:261-267
11. Godest AC et al (2002) Simulation of a knee joint replacement during a gait cycle using explicit finite element analysis. J Biomech 35:267-275
12. Fregly BJ et al (2003) Computational prediction of in vivo wear in total knee replacements. Proc 2003 Summer Bioengineering Conference, American Society of Mechanical Engineers, New York

IV Surgical Technique

25 Optimizing Alignment

M. A. Rauh, W. M. Mihalko, K. A. Krackow

Summary

Optimizing alignment in total knee arthroplasty requires an understanding of the assumptions of a chosen instrumentation system. This understanding involves knowing the possible alignment errors of a system and knowing how the particular system leads the surgeon through the various steps of component placement. Current intramedullary and extramedullary instrumentation can assist in component placement; however, the surgeon must be aware of situations such as extra-articular deformities that can affect the final alignment. Additionally, computer-assisted knee navigation is available for routine use. These systems allow for more accurate positioning of jigs, the ability to correctly establish femoral component rotation, instantaneous feedback on overall alignment, and the ability to prevent implantation of malpositioned components. Overall, computer assistance results in decreased variability and the elimination of outliers. An armamentarium of alternative techniques must be kept in mind for use as secondary checks on the primary technique and in situations of distorted or absent anatomical landmarks.

Introduction

Optimizing total knee arthroplasty alignment requires an understanding of the assumptions of a chosen instrumentation system. This understanding involves knowing the possible alignment errors of a system and knowing how the particular system leads the surgeon through the various steps of component placement. Current intramedullary and extramedullary instrumentation can assist in component placement; however, the surgeon must be aware of situations such as extra-articular deformities that can affect the final alignment. An armamentarium of alternative techniques must be kept in mind for use as secondary checks on the primary technique and in situations of distorted or absent anatomical landmarks.

The History of Optimal Alignment

A consensus exists on most aspects of "normal" knee alignment. Such normal alignment involves issues of the proper mechanical axis and joint line orientation. More specifically, proper alignment at the knee can be characterized by two independent conditions:

1. The normal or prosthetic knee joint should be centered on the mechanical axis of the lower extremity.
2. "Proper" orientation of the joint line should exist. Few dispute that the single most important element to successful and long-lasting total knee arthroplasty is accurate alignment of the implants [1-7]

Historically, instrumentation systems have been grouped under two headings, referred to here as classical alignment and anatomical alignment [8]. In the classical, most common variety, the theoretically correct goal is the establishment of a joint line perpendicular to the reconstituted mechanical axis. As a result, the proximal tibial cut is perpendicular to the overall tibial shaft axis; and since the distal femoral cut is perpendicular to the femoral portion of the mechanical axis, it is oriented at an angle β, approximately 6° relative to the femoral shaft axis (◘ Fig. 25-1).

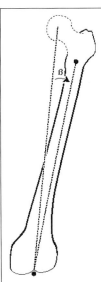

◘ **Fig. 25-1.** Variation in alignment from the mechanical to the anatomical axes of the femur

This angle β typically ranges between 5° and 7° of valgus [9-11]. Understanding these angles and having drawn them accurately on preoperative radiographs is helpful when it is necessary to judge the accuracy of instrument placement intraoperatively. Regardless of the ultimate depth or thickness of the distal femoral or proximal tibial cut, the angular orientation selected by the instrumentation system should lead to a bone resection situation that resembles what was drawn and was predicted on the planning films.

Historically, instrumented approaches to establishing proper varus or valgus orientation of the distal femoral cut involved several different techniques: (a) intramedullary alignment rods, (b) extramedullary alignment rods that are meant to parallel the femoral shaft, and (c) extramedullary alignment that is intended to point toward the femoral head. The first two are obviously directed toward referencing the anatomical femoral shaft axis, and the third references the mechanical femoral axis. Whichever axis one decides to reference, theoretically the same angular orientation of cuts should be determined by any one of the three techniques [8].

Each of these three approaches has its sources of error, which should be understood along with their magnitudes. One type of error relates to incorrect mediolateral positioning of an alignment instrument, either in the region of the knee or at the hip. Simple high school trigonometric calculations indicate that 1-in mediolateral placement errors in location of a femoral head will lead to a 3°-4.5° error in the orientation of the cut. At the hip, medial displacement leads to valgus change, whereas lateral displacement leads to varus change.

At the knee itself, the possibility also exists for mediolateral error, either at the entry point for an intramedullary rod drill hole or as other types of instruments are applied to the end of the femur. Whether the alignment guide points to the femoral head or is directed up the femoral shaft, mediolateral error in placement of the instrument at the knee leads to a similar varus or valgus error. At the distal femur, lateral displacement leads to valgus change and medial displacement to varus positioning. Mediolateral displacement distally has been minimized as a source of error. However, even at 1° or 2° it is still a possible source that can add to other causes. Sagittal plane alignment must also be considered with intramedullary femoral instrumentation. Minimal displacement can lead to malalignment of femoral components, and proper orientation of the femoral starting hole can influence the flexion of the ultimate component [12].

Intramedullary femoral instrumentation for establishing the varus and valgus orientation of the femoral cut is clearly the most popular. With the use of an intramedullary alignment rod, it may be argued that uncertainty about the position of the proximal tip of the rod is minimized. This is certainly true as long as (a) the rod readily achieves a position in the neighborhood of the femoral isthmus and (b) the rod does not bend. However, as the resting point of the proximal tip of the rod comes to be more distal, closer to the knee, i.e., if the rod does not pass easily up the shaft, then the potential for error is significant. The possibility of problems from a flexible rod has to be considered a source of very significant, essentially uncontrollable error.

Originally, nearly all proximal tibial resections were performed perpendicular to the tibial shaft axis, and a relatively short cutting instrument was used on the anterior tibial crest. An obvious source of error was the potential of a proximal bow of the tibial cortex. It was hoped this would be offset, however, by a tendency to hold the overall axis of the tibia in a vertical position and to use this overall orientation to keep the cuts perpendicular.

More specific tibial alignment guides have been introduced. Two available types focus on (a) extramedullary alignment from the center of the knee to the ankle and (b) an intramedullary system. Just as with the femoral case, one is specifically cautioned concerning the accuracy of mediolateral placement of any such guides. Erroneous lateral positioning at the ankle moves the instrument toward a varus error, as would inappropriate medial positioning at the proximal surface of the tibia. The magnitude of errors for a given amount of mediolateral displacement is similar in the tibia – actually slightly higher, because the bone is usually shorter.

One must also be careful with the use of intramedullary rods at the tibia. The obvious shortcomings of intramedullary instrumentation can be even more frequent and less obvious on the tibial side. Intramedullary alignment instrumentation will clearly direct proper placement when a non-flexible rod traverses the entire length of the tibia. It is not uncommon, however, for a medial convexity not only to block the full transverse of the IM rod but also to lead the tip into a medial direction which directs a fixed cutting jig into valgus.

Another factor interfering with full placement of the rod is the generally narrower tibial canal. The tibial intramedullary diameter seems to be approximately 2 mm less than that of the femur. However, one must resist the temptation to address this problem by simply using a smaller tibial alignment rod, as any flexibility of the rod will be equally problematic.

Accurate placement of tibial alignment instruments is also a concern. The specific cutting guides themselves need to be placed in the proper position. However, play in the instruments, and especially inadvertent movement of fixation pins, can lead to very realistic errors of 1°-4°. If you consider this statement along with the similar one from the femoral section earlier, it is possible to see how surgeons using even sophisticated; modern total knee arthroplasty instruments can make overall varus or valgus alignment errors exceeding 5°.

Whenever one talks about 1° and 2° alignment or jig placement errors a typical comment arises: "But how accurately can we perform cuts or make any of these placements anyway?" The implication is that we do not need to worry about sources of error which are on the order of 1°-2°. This line of reasoning or casualness is fallacious. We have multiple steps and multiple sites or sources of 1°-2°, even 3°-4° possible errors. The combination of several sources of error all "lining up" in the same direction may be quite rare. Nonetheless, who wants to have even 1-100 cases with 5°-7° of varus or valgus error? A total knee replacement with a tibiofemoral angulation of 11° instead of 6° is quite obviously crooked. A varus error of 5°-6° may not be cosmetically obvious; mechanically, however, it may be even worse.

The topic of femoral component rotation introduces yet another aspect of knee arthroplasty that must be considered in the quest for optimal alignment. However, prior to focusing on the mechanics of establishing rotational alignment with total knee instruments, the surgeon should keep foremost in mind the patient's preoperative rotational characteristics. How do the patient's clinical, anatomical landmarks appear preoperatively in a standing position, during gait, and especially on the examining or operating table? In particular, does the knee appear, in general, to be internally or externally rotated? What is the preoperative position of the tibial tubercle, the intermalleolar axis, and the long axis of the foot? Ideally, the surgeon ought to know how these all line up before disrupting the bony and soft-tissue relationships with surgery.

The crude instrumentation of the early 1970s made no clear-cut provision for femoral rotation, and, historically, surgeons generally aligned the cutting instrument with the "horizon of the room." Later attempts involved orienting the anterior and posterior femoral cuts in a rotational sense so that the flexion space created was approximately rectangular. Preferred techniques developed which involved specific referencing from particular aspects of the bony architecture of the distal femur. Here, in general terms, an attempt is made to reconstruct normal anatomy and at the same time to adjust safely for handling of the tibial cut.

In 1980, the Howmedica Universal Total Knee Instrumentation system was introduced, which established femoral component rotation "anatomically" by keying from or referencing to the posterior condylar axis and directing the rotation of the posterior aspects of the femoral component to lie parallel to the original position of the patient's posterior condyles.

Toward the mid 1980s, surgeons preferring to make proximal tibial cuts perpendicular to the overall tibial shaft axis were led by the analyses of John Moreland [2] to consider "externally rotating" the femoral component, that is, externally rotating relative to the posterior condylar axis line. These analyses recognized that for the knee in ex-

tension, the non-anatomical state of the classical cut made on the proximal tibia is offset by a corresponding and opposite non-anatomical resection for the distal femur. In other words, a perpendicular proximal tibial cut can be expected to remove more lateral tibia than medial tibia, and this is balanced in extension by the fact that the distal femoral cut removes greater bone medially than laterally. (An assumption is implicit that the case example is free of bony deformity.) The overall orientation of the femoral shaft and tibial shaft axis is as desired, and the variation of the prosthetic joint line orientation from anatomically normal has been deemed acceptable and desirable by a substantial proportion of arthroplasty surgeons.

In general, it can be said that the femoral component externally rotated away from the posterior condylar axis may be seen to more closely parallel the epicondylar axis. The rotational positioning of the femoral component to parallel the "epicondylar axis" has become a stated goal of many. Conceptually attempting to parallel or in any way reference the posterior condylar axis has always invited uncertainty in the presence of differential cartilage and/or bony wear. An instrument purporting to parallel the posterior condylar axis when there is common posteromedial wear rotates to some degree externally. In a valgus knee with very obvious wear on the posterior lateral condyle and also possibly an a priori hypoplastic condyle as part of the deformity, such a jig is directed to a position of internal rotation.

These considerations invited some additional appeal to referencing the epicondylar axis. Furthermore, cuts which parallel the epicondylar axis may naturally be well-behaved in providing proper soft-tissue balance and ligamentous stability, since the epicondyles are the origins of the collateral ligaments.

The introduction of the anteroposterior axis of Whiteside [13] added yet another axis to assist in the rotational alignment of femoral components. The AP axis is drawn as a line connecting the deepest point of the trochlear groove to a midpoint at the region of the posterior extent of the posterior intracondylar region. For those of us who have tried to draw this axis, it is usually obvious and seemingly reproducible. There is, however, a question of what to do with the patient whose trochlear groove is quite displaced due to patellofemoral joint pathology. In this situation and others, it really does appear that using the specifically termed Whiteside axis is a good bit like "eyeballing" the overall neutral rotation of the distal femoral bone. One has the concern of how specifically to align the instrument with this rotation, as most of the instrumentation we are putting onto the end of the femur obscures the view of the femoral bone, and hence the impression of where the axis is.

Tibial rotational landmarks, references for establishing tibial component rotation, are less distinct than what is present at the femur. At the tibia, however, similarly

25

simple definition of an anteroposterior or mediolateral axis seems available. Several possibilities are present. The following consistencies and limitations should be appreciated:

1. The overall appearance of the proximal joint surface of the tibia can be considered. In particular, a mid-transverse axis and/or a posterior cortical axis can be established. Bone loss, osteophyte formation, and general anatomical variability must be taken into account. Furthermore, the normal configuration of the posterior cortex extending further posteriorly on the medial than on the lateral side should be noted. Specifically, tibial fixation instruments which are designed to "key off" the posterior tibial cortex must be regarded with very strong suspicion. This normal configuration dictates that, in the absence of deformation from asymmetric bone loss or residual osteophytes, alignment parallel to the posterior tibial cortical "axis" will lead to abnormal tibial component positioning. The component tends to be rotated internally while the tibial bone itself is externally rotated. In this situation the tibial tubercle is lateralized and patellar tracking is destabilized. External rotation of the foot and ankle may be clinically apparent.

2. The next readily available anatomical structure is the patellotibial tuberosity, which typically lies lateral to an anterior midline. Generally, it would be inappropriate to aim a tibial plateau so that its neutral rotation axis pointed straight to the middle of the tibial tubercle.

3. Another anatomical landmark is the intermalleolar axis.

4. Still another landmark is the overall "long axis" of the foot as it is held up into neutral position of plantar flexion/dorsiflexion. These last two points, i.e., the intermalleolar axis and the "long axis" of the foot, are moderately variable – as much as 15°-20° or even more – in a significant number of people. Because of these aspects of anatomical and rotational variability, it is wise to clinically assess these landmarks preoperatively. One needs to know the starting point.

5. Another consideration for referencing tibial rotation might be the position established by the soft tissues. This technique involves acceptance of the tibial rotation defined by the soft-tissue attachments. By this method, preparation of some or most of the joint surfaces and also essentially all of the soft-tissue release have been performed, after which rotation of the tibia with regard to the femur is guided by soft tissues. The neutral position of the tibia is marked to parallel that of the femur in extension when longitudinal tension is applied across the joint. The neutral anteroposterior rotation position of the tibia is taken to be the natural resting position, which is achieved during this tension-stress testing.

It has been estimated that there are approximately 4 782 969 possible positions available for the combination of femoral and tibial components [14]. However, the systematic approach to analyzing and correcting the deformity has allowed surgeons to arrive at a generally acceptable method of knee arthroplasty. Unfortunately, given the vast array of possibilities, true reliability is difficult to obtain.

Current Methods of Optimizing Alignment

Traditionally, surgeons performing total knee arthroplasty have been concerned with optimizing the axial alignment of the lower extremity, i.e., varus and valgus. However, as the influence of alignment on implant survival [1-7] became known, a greater consideration to rotational and medial-lateral positioning of components developed. In an effort to improve overall alignment and to minimize situations of gross malalignment, the senior authors developed a system for computer-assisted total knee arthroplasty [15]. The current method of optimizing alignment involves utilization of the Knee Track Module (Stryker Navigation Systems, Stryker Howmedica Osteonics, Allendale, NJ) developed principally by the senior authors (K.A.K and W.M.M.)

An infrared sensor array located at the side of the operating room table is used by this system to localize emitters placed at specific locations on the lower extremity of the patient. A tracking pin is placed into the patient's ipsilateral iliac crest for the purpose of identifying the center of the femoral head. After the surgeon's choice of incision, the distal femur and proximal lateral tibial bony prominences are identified and similar tracking pins are placed. With the infrared emitters placed onto the tracking pins, the lower extremity can be manipulated in a circular fashion about the hip. Using an iterative Gaussian algorithm to solve the true non-linear system, the center of the femoral head can be identified by the computer. The center of the femoral head is calculated via a subroutine that assumes the head of the femur is spherical. Two hundred and fifty data points are collected in 20 s as the surgeon moves the lower extremity about the hip joint in a gentle spherical arc. The method of least squares is used to find the best-fit sphere given the data points collected. The center estimate is then determined using an iterative Gauss-Newton algorithm to solve the true non-linear system. This algorithm runs through 200 iterations to assure convergence. Finally, the center point is transformed into the femoral reference frame. Using the pointing device, the geometry of the distal femur is digitized. One must identify the medial and lateral epicondyles, the center of the knee, and the anteroposterior axis of Whiteside, as well as the condylar surfaces.

Likewise, the geometry of the proximal tibia is digitized as the surgeon identifies the sulcus between the tibial spines, the anteroposterior midpoint, and the medial and lateral malleoli, along with the center of the ankle.

Given all the defined points, the tibiofemoral and mechanical axes can be determined before any bone cuts have been made. This determination then allows accurate depiction of any correction needed to properly align the components. Additionally, this navigation system is able to identify intraoperatively the real-time relative position of the tibia in respect to the femur. That is, one is able to precisely determine tibiofemoral angle, the flexion-extension position, and the amount of relative internal or external rotation of the tibia with respect to the femur. Also, changes in the relative tibiofemoral compression-distraction and mediolateral or anteroposterior displacements can be determined by calculating the change in the directional vector from the tibial to the femoral reference frames.

The potential for error still exists with this system; however, it ranges from 0.1 to 1 mm for each of the three coordinates [14], which is considerably less than that obtained from any other system available. Armed with this knowledge, the operating surgeon is able to utilize jigs from any specific instrument system to make a more accurate cut. Upon final verification of cuts, a more accurate alignment of the lower extremity can be obtained than previously without the use of this device. Additionally, knowledge of flexion-extension gaps at all ranges of knee flexion allow for more accurate ligament balancing techniques.

The ability to optimize the axial, rotational, and medial-lateral translational alignment with the assistance of computerized navigational assistance should provide a better aligned and balanced extremity. We anticipate that yet more accurate alignment will result in even longer life spans of given prostheses.

Computer-assisted knee navigation is available for routine use. It allows for accurate positioning of jigs, the ability to correctly establish femoral component rotation, instantaneous feedback on overall alignment, and the ability to prevent implantation of malpositioned components. Overall, computer assistance results in decreased variability and the elimination of outliers (❑ Fig. 25-2) [12, 16].

Given the successes of the first series of cases [17], potential clinical benefits would include faster rehabilitation and better range of motion. Additionally, the advent of modern computers and the development of procedure-specific software have assisted in the process of optimizing alignment and hopefully will result in improved long-term outcomes.

Acknowledgements. We appreciate the kind assistance we received in producing this chapter and extend our thanks to Dr. S. Munjal and Dr. M.J. Phillips, State University of New York at Buffalo, Kaleida Health, Buffalo General Hospital, Buffalo, NY.

References

1. Maestro A et al (1998) Influence of intramedullary versus extramedullary alignment guides on final total knee arthroplasty component position. J Arthroplasty 13:552-558
2. Moreland JR (1988) Mechanisms of failure in total knee arthroplasty. Clin Orthop 226:49-64
3. Lotke P et al (1977) Influence of positioning of prosthesis in total knee replacement. J Bone Joint Surg [Am] 59:77-79
4. Windsor RE et al (1989) Mechanisms of failure of the femoral and tibial components in total knee arthroplasty. Clin Orthop Rel Res 248:15-20
5. Mont MA et al (1997) Intramedullary goniometer can improve alignment in knee arthroplasty surgery. J Arthroplasty 12:332-336
6. Delp SL et al (1998) Computer-assisted knee replacement. Clin Orthop 354:49-56
7. Ritter M et al (1994) Postoperative alignment of total knee replacement. Its effect on survival. Clin Orthop 299:153-156
8. Krackow KA (1990) The technique of total knee arthroplasty. Mosby, St. Louis
9. Chao E et al (1994) Biomechanics of malalignment. Orthop Clin North Am 25:379-386
10. Moreland JR et al (1987) Radiographic analysis of the axial alignment of the lower extremity. J Bone Joint Surg [Am] 69:745-749
11. Kettelkamp D et al (1972) A method for quantitative analysis of medial and lateral compression forces at the knee during standing. Clin Orthop 83:202-213
12. Mihalko WM et al (2004) Intramedullary and computer navigational femoral alignment in TKA. Trans. American Academy of Orthopedic Surgeons, San Francisco
13. Whiteside LA et al (1995) The anteroposterior axis for femoral rotational alignment in valgus total knee arthroplasty. Clin Orthop 321:168-172
14. Krackow KA et al (2003) Computer-assisted total knee arthroplasty: Navigation in TKA. Orthopedics 26:1017-1023
15. Krackow KA et al (1999) A new technique for determining proper mechanical axis alignment during total knee arthroplasty: progress toward computer-assisted TKA. Orthopedics 22:698-702
16. Mihalko WM et al (2004) Extramedullary, intramedullary and CAS tibial alignment techniques for TKA. Trans. American Academy of Orthopedic Surgeons, San Francisco
17. Phillips MJ et al (2003) Computer-assisted total knee replacement - results of the first 90 cases using the Stryker navigation system. In: Proceedings of conference on Computer-assisted orthopaedic surgery. Marbella, Spain

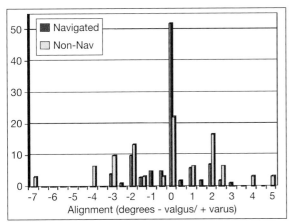

❑ **Fig. 25-2.** Postoperative radiographic alignment in patients undergoing TKA

26 Assess and Release the Tight Ligament

L. A. Whiteside

Summary

The structure of the knee is complex, and its behavior can be unpredictable even in the most experienced hands. However, the task of replacing the bone surfaces and balancing the ligaments can be made manageable by following a logical plan based on correct alignment throughout the arc of flexion and ligament release based on the function of each ligament. Optimal knee function requires correct varus-valgus alignment in all positions of flexion. This requires reliable anatomical landmarks for alignment both in flexion and extension. The long axes of the femur and tibia and the anterior-posterior axis of the femur are highly reliable and provide the guidelines for establishing stable alignment of the joint surfaces by placing the tibia and patellar groove correctly in the median anterior-posterior plane through the entire arc of flexion. Ligaments perform specific functions, and these functions differ in different positions of knee flexion. Knowing their function and testing their tension provides the information necessary to release only the ligaments that are excessively tight, leaving those that are performing normally. Fractional release does not destabilize the knee, because other ligaments are retained, and because the peripheral attachments of the ligament to other soft-tissue structures such as the periosteum or synovial-capsular tissue allow the released ligament to continue to function. Ligament release does not cause instability. Failure to align the knee and release the tight ligaments, however, does cause instability, unreliable function, and excessive wear. With this knowledge, good instruments, and sound implants, the surgeon can align, balance, and stabilize the knee even when severe bone destruction and ligament contracture are present.

Introduction

Although the knee has been studied intensively for decades, it continues to confound investigators and to frustrate knee surgeons. Its intricate ligaments and complex joint surfaces interact in ways that defy description. Nevertheless, the surgeon must repair and reconstruct the damaged and arthritic knee so that its performance is near normal, and this requires decisions and adjustments made with reasonable accuracy under the pressure and time constraints of the operating room. This chapter simplifies the geometry and kinematics of the knee enough that the knee can be understood and managed effectively. It establishes rules for resection and alignment that position the joint surfaces so that the ligaments can be balanced through the normal flexion arc; it illustrates stability tests that can be performed with ease, and it teaches safe guidelines for ligament release so that the ligament balancing can be performed quickly and effectively without destabilizing the knee.

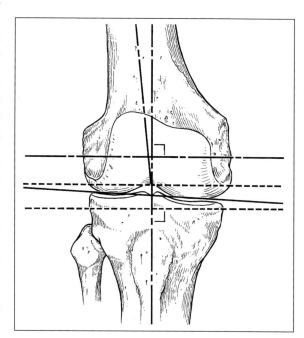

Fig. 26-1. In the extended position the joint surface slopes medially approximately 3°. Tibial resection is perpendicular to the long axis of the tibia and mechanical axis of the lower extremity. The resection surface is 3° valgus to the articular surface. Femoral resection is perpendicular to the mechanical axis, and 5° valgus to the long axis of the femur. The resection surface is approximately 3° varus to the articular surface. These 3° 'errors' in the femoral and tibial surface resections compensate for one another, and result in surface resections that are parallel to one another and perpendicular to the mechanical axis of the lower extremity. (Reprinted from [8] with permission from Springer-Verlag)

The long axis of the femur serves as the anatomical reference for alignment of the distal femoral cuts perpendicular to the mechanical axis and AP plane. Cutting the distal femoral surfaces at a 5° valgus angle to the long axis of the femur places the joint surface perpendicular to the AP plane in the extended position [1]. Likewise, cutting the upper tibial surface perpendicular to the long axis of the tibia also places the tibial joint surface perpendicular to the AP plane in extension (■ Fig. 26-1).

The AP axis serves as the anatomical landmark for femoral resection in flexion [1, 3, 5, 6]. The AP axis can be constructed by marking the lateral edge of the PCL and the deepest part of the patellar groove. A line drawn between these two points lies in the AP plane and passes through the center of the femoral head and down the long axis of the tibia (■ Fig. 26-2).

The ligaments stabilizing the lateral side of the knee all have differing functions in the flexed and extended positions [4, 6, 8, 9]. The lateral gastrocnemius tendon and capsule of the posterolateral corner, lateral collateral ligament (LCL), and popliteus tendon complex attach near the lateral femoral epicondyle and are stabilizers of the lateral side throughout the flexion arc. The lateral posterior capsule (PC) and iliotibial band attach far away from the epicondylar axis and are effective lateral stabilizers only in the extended position (■ Fig. 26-3a, b).

On the medial side, the medial collateral ligament (MCL, anterior and posterior portions) is attached to the epicondyle and is effective throughout the flexion

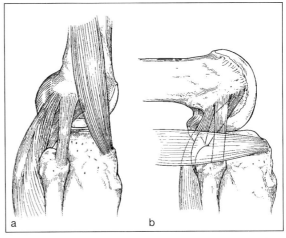

■ Fig. 26-3a, b. *a* Lateral view of the knee showing the major lateral static stabilizing structures with the knee extended. The lateral gastrocnemius tendon, lateral collateral ligament, lateral posterior capsule, popliteus tendon, and iliotibial band all cross the joint perpendicular (or nearly so) to its surface, and are capable of stabilizing the knee in the extended position. (Reprinted from [4] with permission from Lippincott Williams and Wilkins.) *b* Lateral view of the knee showing the major lateral static stabilizing structures with the knee flexed 90°. The lateral gastrocnemius tendon, posterolateral capsule, lateral collateral ligament, and popliteus tendon are the only effective lateral stabilizing structures with the knee flexed to this position. The iliotibial band is parallel to the joint surface, and the posterior capsule is slack. (Reprinted from [4] with permission from Lippincott Williams and Wilkins)

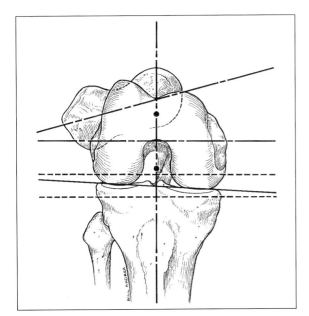

■ Fig. 26-2. With the knee flexed 90°, the joint surface resections are parallel to the epicondylar axis and perpendicular to the AP axis of the femur. The femoral neck is anteverted approximately 15° to the epicondylar axis. When the knee is in functional position in flexion (walking up stairs or standing from a seated position), the positions of the femoral neck and epicondylar axis remain unchanged, and in the normal knee the tibia is vertical. (Reprinted from [8] with permission from Springer–Verlag)

arc [5, 7, 8, 10, 14]. The epicondylar attachment is broad enough that there is a difference in function of the anterior and posterior portions of this ligament in flexion and extension. The medial posterior capsule attaches far from the epicondylar axis, and is tight only in extension. The posterior cruciate ligament is attached slightly distal and posterior to the epicondylar axis, so it slackens in full extension and tightens in flexion (■ Fig. 26-4a, b).

By using the three accessible anatomical axes, the femoral and tibial components can be positioned so that the knee is in correct varus-valgus alignment throughout the flexion arc. The ligaments then can be balanced by determining which ligaments are contracted based on their function in flexion and extension. Simply stated, ligaments that attach to the femur on or near the epicondyles are effective both in flexion and extension, and those that attach distant from the epicondylar axis are effective either in flexion or extension, but not in both positions. To extend this concept further, it can be stated that the portions of the ligament complexes that attach anteriorly in the epicondylar areas stabilize primarily in flexion, and those that attach posteriorly in the epicondylar areas stabilize primarily in extension. Ligaments that attach far posteriorly on the tibia are most effective in extension, and those attaching anteriorly are primarily tensioned in flexion.

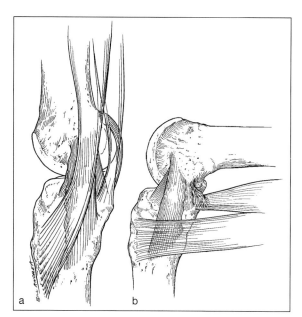

Fig. 26-4a, b. *a* On the medial view, the medial collateral ligament (deep and superficial) is the primary medial stabilizer that is tight in extension. The anterior fibers are slackened in full extension and the posterior fibers (posteromedial oblique ligament) are differentially tightened in extension because of their position in the medial femoral condyle. The lateral posterior capsule also is tight. Active medial stability is added by the medial hamstrings through the pes anserinus and semimembranosus. (Reprinted with permission from Elsevier.) *b* Viewed from the medial side with the knee flexed, the medial stabilizing structures are the deep and superficial medial collateral ligament. The anterior fibers of the medial collateral ligament are taut and the posterior fibers are relatively lax because of their attachment more posteriorly on the femur. The posterior capsule is slack and is not effective in flexion. The semimembranosus and pes anserina are parallel with the joint and are incapable of supplying active stability in flexion. (Reprinted with permission from Elsevier)

Varus Knee

In the presence of articular surface deformity the joint surfaces themselves cannot be used as reference landmarks for measuring resection of the bone, so the anatomical references are especially important for correct varus-valgus alignment. The usual reliable landmarks for varus-valgus alignment of the femoral component in flexion include the posterior femoral condyles, the long axis of the tibia, and the tensed supporting ligaments. If the posterior femoral condyle wears and the tibial plateau collapses on the medial side of the knee, these normally reliable landmarks cannot be used. Instead, the AP axis of the femur is used as a reference line for the anterior and posterior femoral cuts and the long axis of the tibia is used for a reference line for the tibial cut, so that the joint surfaces are cut perpendicular to these two reference lines [3, 11] (Fig. 26-5).

Once the joint surfaces have been resected correctly to establish normal varus and valgus alignment in flexion and extension, the trial components are inserted and lig-

ament function is assessed in flexion and extension. The anatomical basis for the different functions of the anterior and posterior portions of the medial collateral ligament, the posterior capsule, and the posterior cruciate ligament has been at least partially established [5, 7, 8, 10, 14]. Because the medial collateral ligament attaches to the medial femoral condyle through a band about 1.5 cm wide, and spreads across a much broader surface on the medial tibial flare as the anterior portion and posterior oblique portion of the medial collateral ligament, each cannot function identically in flexion and extension. Instead the anterior portion tightens and the posterior oblique portion of the medial collateral ligament loosens as the knee flexes. When the knee fully extends the posterior oblique portion tightens and the anterior portion slackens. The posterior capsule slackens early in knee flexion, and tightens only in full extension. The posterior capsule normally has no effect on varus and valgus stability in the flexed knee. The posterior cruciate ligament also is not a varus and valgus stabilizer in the normal

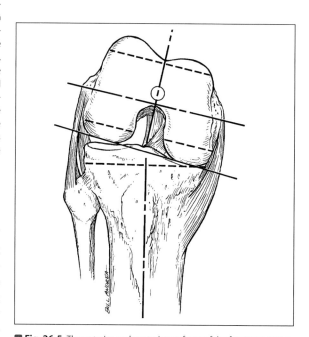

Fig. 26-5. The anterior and posterior surfaces of the femur are resected perpendicular to the anteroposterior axis and parallel to the epicondylar axis. Similar to the long axis of the femur, the anteroposterior axis is used as a reliable reference axis to align these cuts. This axis is identified by marking the lateral edge of the posterior cruciate ligament and the deepest part of the patellar groove. The articular surfaces are resected perpendicular to the anteroposterior axis and parallel to the epicondylar axis. In most cases of varus knee the posterior femoral condyles maintain their normal 3° medial down-slope, and can be used for alignment of the femoral component in flexion. In this case, a 3° external rotational guide would be used to engage the posterior femoral condyles to place the anterior and posterior femoral surfaces in neutral alignment. The long axis of the tibia is used as a reference for the upper tibial resection. This surface is resected perpendicular to the tibial long axis when viewed from the front, and with a 4°-7° posterior slope when viewed from the side. (Reprinted from [14] with permission from Lippincott Williams and Wilkins)

knee because of its distance from the medial and lateral condylar surfaces.

With this information the medial ligament structures of the knee can be released individually according to the position in which excessive tightness is found: release of the anterior portion of the medial collateral ligament to correct inappropriate medial ligament tension in flexion (◘ Fig. 26-6), release of the posterior oblique portion of the medial collateral ligament (◘ Fig. 26-7) and posterior medial capsule to correct inappropriate medial ligament tension in extension, and release of the posterior cruciate ligament to correct excessive femoral roll-back in flexion. The posterior cruciate ligament is an important secondary varus and valgus stabilizer in flexion and, in the absence of the medial collateral ligament, also is likely to function as an important medial stabilizing structure in extension.

Tight PCL

Because the PCL is a medial structure, it often is contracted in the varus knee and stretched in the valgus knee. The tight PCL causes excessive roll-back of the femur [2]. When palpated with the knee in flexion, it feels extremely tight. A simple and effective means of releasing the PCL is to remove the polyethylene trial component and elevate the bone attachment of the PCL directly from the tibia [8] (◘ Fig. 26-8a, b).

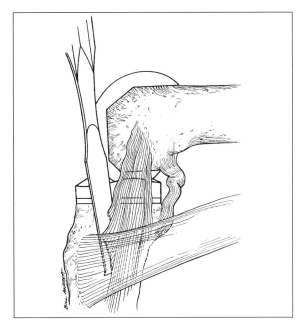

◘ **Fig. 26-6.** The taut anterior fibers are released subperiosteally. These fibers attach fairly far distally (8-10 cm), and the osteotome is passed far enough to completely release the anterior fibers. The attachment of the pes anserinus and posterior oblique fibers of the medial collateral ligament are left intact. (Reprinted from [14] with permission from Lippincott Williams and Wilkins)

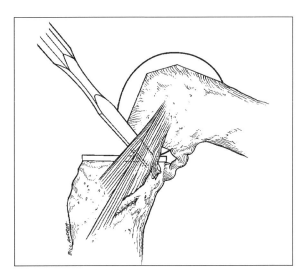

◘ **Fig. 26-7.** In this case, only the posterior portion of the medial collateral ligament should be released first. A curved half-inch osteotome is used to elevate all but the anterior portion of the medial collateral ligament. The osteotome is directed approximately 45° downward and tapped gently to release the posteromedial oblique fibers from the tibia and from the tendon of the semimembranosus. (Reprinted from [14] with permission from Lippincott Williams and Wilkins)

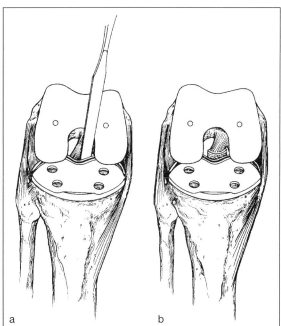

a   b

◘ **Fig. 26-8a, b.** *a* The posterior cruciate ligament is released with a small segment of bone from its posterior tibial attachment. A quarter-inch osteotome is used to make several small cuts around the posterior cortical margin, and then the bone piece is levered loose. (Reprinted with permission from Elsevier) *b* The bone piece slides proximally 0.5-1 cm, slackening the posterior cruciate ligament. The synovial membrane remains intact, and the ligament remains unfrayed by the release. (Reprinted with permission from Elsevier)

Valgus Knee

Correction of alignment and elimination of articular surface deformity now can be achieved with modern instruments and alignment devices even in the most difficult valgus knees. Using the anteroposterior axis of the distal femoral surface or the epicondylar axis of the femur virtually has eliminated the rotational alignment problem of the femoral component and has paved the way to a rational approach to ligament balancing in the valgus knee [11]. Using the central axis of the femur and tibia as reference lines for valgus angle ensures highly reproducible alignment in the frontal plane [3, 11]. Using the distal surface of the medial femoral condyle as the point of reference for distal femoral resection ensures that the distal surface of the femur will be in correct position relative to the medial ligaments and the patella (**□** Fig. 26-9). This ensures that the patellar groove, intercondylar notch, and condylar surfaces all are positioned correctly in extension.

For alignment in flexion either the anteroposterior axis or the epicondylar axis of the femur is used as anatomical reference for resection of the anterior sur-

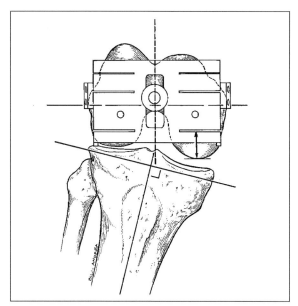

□ Fig. 26-10. The cutting guide for femoral resection is aligned so the surfaces are resected perpendicular to the AP axis of the femur (a) and parallel with the epicondylar axis (b), resecting the thickness of the implant from the intact medial femoral condyle, and much less from the deficient lateral side. This places the joint surfaces in anatomical position to correct the valgus position in flexion, and places the patellar groove correctly with the mechanical axis of the lower extremity. The tibial surface is resected perpendicular to the long axis of the tibia. The lateral ligaments are still tight, and the tibia is held in a valgus malalignment by the ligament contractures. (Reprinted from [9] with permission from Lippincott Williams and Wilkins)

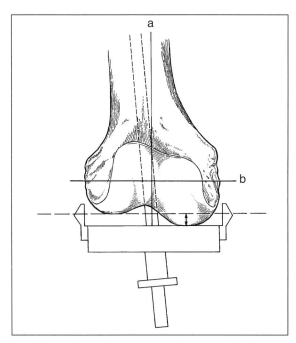

□ Fig. 26-9. The intramedullary alignment rod lies slightly medial to the center of the patellar groove, and the cutting guide is set at a 5° valgus angle. This will align the joint surface perpendicular to the mechanical axis of the femur (a), and parallel to the epicondylar axis (b). The cutting guide seats against the high (medial) side, which is the reference for resection of the joint surfaces. The thickness of the implant is resected distally from the medial side. In some cases resection of the thickness of the implant from the medial side results in minimal or no resection from the lateral side of the distal femur. Regardless of the lateral bone deficit, the medial surface should be used as the reference surface, and augmentation of the lateral surface should be done to make up for the deficit. (Reprinted with permission from Elsevier)

faces of the femur (**□** Fig. 26-10). The posterior femoral condyles are unreliable as references for femoral component alignment because of lateral femoral condylar deficiency. Correct resection of the femoral surfaces prior to ligament balancing produces a laterally conveying joint space in flexion [17].

With the surfaces in correct alignment, ligament balancing requires a rational approach for correct balance in flexion and extension. Consideration of the effects of the functions of the lateral stabilizing structures throughout the arc of flexion offers a basis from which to formulate this approach [4, 6, 8, 9]. The lateral collateral ligament is regarded as a stabilizing structure both in flexion and extension, and has rotational as well as valgus stabilizing effects. The popliteus tendon complex also has passive varus stabilizing effects in flexion and extension, and also has a prominent role in external rotational stabilization of the tibia on the femur. These two structures would be appropriate to release for a knee that is excessively tight laterally both in flexion and extension [12].

The iliotibial band is aligned perpendicular to the joint surface when the knee is extended, and therefore can provide lateral knee stability when the knee is extended. But when the knee is flexed to 90°, the IT band is parallel to the joint surface and cannot stabilize the knee to varus stress. The lateral posterior capsular structures are tight only in full extension and are slack when the knee is flexed. Release of either the posterior capsule or the IT band would have a rational basis only for a knee that is tight laterally in extension. Release of either would have little effect on lateral knee stability in the flexed position.

Thus, after total knee arthroplasty, the knee that is tight laterally in flexion and extension will be almost completely corrected by release of the lateral collateral ligament and popliteus tendon. No other structures afford lateral stability in flexion, so release of these two structures is all that is needed to correct the effects of the lateral ligament contracture in flexion (◘ Fig. 26-11a). However, in extension the IT band and the lateral posterior capsule are effective lateral stabilizers, and may still need release (◘ Fig. 26-11b). Knees that start out with tight lateral structures in flexion and extension often will require further work to correct lateral tightness in extension after release of the popliteus tendon and lateral collateral ligament. Because the IT band is easily accessible, it is the next lateral stabilizing structure to be released if

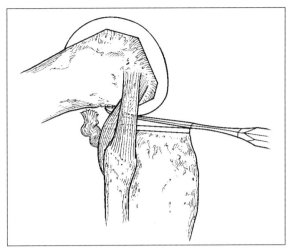

◘ **Fig. 26-12.** In a few cases the knee remains tight laterally only in full extension after release of the iliotibial band. In these cases the lateral posterior capsule is the next structure to be released. The lateral posterior capsule is released by removing the polyethylene spacer and inserting the curved osteotome behind the knee against the femoral attachment of the posterior capsule, then gently tapping the end of the osteotome. This release does not affect stability of the lateral side of the knee in flexion. (Reprinted with permission from Elsevier)

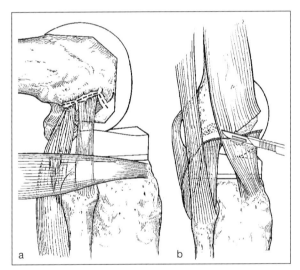

◘ **Fig. 26-11a, b.** *a* Now that the lateral collateral ligament, popliteus tendon, and posterolateral corner have been released, they retract partially, but remain attached to the surrounding capsule and dense overlying synovial membrane, and so continue to function as lateral stabilizers. Release of the popliteus tendon, lateral collateral ligament, and rarely the posterolateral corner capsule always corrects lateral ligament tension in flexion because these are the only structures that stabilize the lateral side of the knee in flexion. The iliotibial band and posterior capsule remain as stabilizers in extension and may still apply deforming forces, but only in the extended knee. (Reprinted with permission from Elsevier.) *b* If the knee remains tight laterally in extension, the iliotibial band should be released. In this case the release is done just above the joint line, extrasynovially, so that the iliotibial band elongates but remains attached to the synovial membrane and can continue to support the lateral side of the knee in extension. The posterior cruciate ligament, posterior capsule, and biceps femoris remain as lateral stabilizers in extension. (Reprinted with permission from Elsevier)

the knee remains tight laterally in extension. If the knee remains tight laterally even after the IT band release, then the posterior capsule can be released to finish correcting lateral ligament tightness [12] (◘ Fig. 26-12).

Because knee stability in extension is absolutely necessary for good function, these two extension stabilizers (IT band and lateral posterior capsule) should be released only as a last resort. If they are released first, before lateral laxity is tested in flexion, and the lateral collateral ligament and popliteus tendon are released to achieve ligament balance in flexion, then nothing will remain to provide crucial extension stability.

For reasons probably related to differences in deformity of the lateral side of the knee, the knee sometimes is tight laterally only in extension after the trial implants have been inserted or tensioners applied. In these cases the lateral collateral ligament and the popliteus tendon should not be released, but only the IT band and the lateral posterior capsule should be released to achieve ligament balance. Uncommonly, valgus knees require all static lateral stability structures to be released to adequately correct the deformity and ligament imbalance. In these cases the biceps femoris muscle, the gastrocnemius muscle, and the deep fascia provide support for the lateral side of the knee until capsular healing occurs.

Acknowledgements. The author thanks William C. Andrea, CMI, for his assistance with preparation of the illustrations, and Diane J. Morton, MS, for her assistance with preparation of the manuscript.

References

1. Anouchi YS, Whiteside LA, Kaiser AD, Milliano MT (1993) The effect of axial rotational alignment of the femoral component on knee stability and patellar tracking in total knee arthroplasty. Clin Orthop 287:170-177
2. Arima J, Whiteside LA, Martin JW, Miura H, White SE, McCarthy DS (1998) Effect of partial release of the posterior cruciate ligament in total knee arthroplasty. Clin Orthop 353:194-202
3. Arima J, Whiteside LA (1995) Femoral rotational alignment, based on the anteroposterior axis, in total knee arthroplasty in a valgus knee. J Bone Joint Surg [Am] 77:1331-1334
4. Kanamiya T, Whiteside LA, Nakamura T, Mihalko WM, Steiger J, Naito M (2002) Effect of selective lateral ligament release on stability in knee arthroplasty. Clin Orthop 404:24-31
5. Saeki K, Mihalko WM, Patel V, Conway J, Naito M, Thrum H, Vandenneuker H, Whiteside LA (2001) Stability after medial collateral ligament release in total knee arthroplasty. Clin Orthop 392:184-189
6. Whiteside LA (1993) Correction of ligament and bone defects in total replacement arthroplasty of the severely valgus knee. Clin Orthop 288:234-245
7. Whiteside LA (1995) Ligament release and bone grafting in total knee arthroplasty of the varus knee. Orthopedics 18:117-122
8. Whiteside LA (2000) Positioning the femoral component. The effect of proper ligament balance. Am J Knee Surg 13:173-180
9. Whiteside LA (1999) Selective ligament release in total knee arthroplasty of the knee in valgus. Clin Orthop 367:130-140
10. Whiteside LA (2002) Soft tissue balancing. J Arthroplasty 17 [Suppl 1]:23-27
11. Whiteside LA, Arima J (1995) The anteroposterior axis for femoral rotational alignment in valgus total knee arthroplasty. Clin Orthop 321:168-172
12. Whiteside LA, Kasselt MR, Haynes DW (1987) Varus-valgus and rotational stability in rotationally unconstrained total knee arthroplasty. Clin Orthop 219:147-157
13. Whiteside LA, McCarthy DS (1992) Laboratory evaluation of alignment and kinematics in a unicompartmental knee arthroplasty inserted with intramedullary instrumentation. Clin Orthop 274:238-247
14. Whiteside LA, Saeki K, Mihalko WM (2000) Functional medial ligament balancing in total knee arthroplasty. Clin Orthop 380:45-57
15. Whiteside LA, Summers RG (1983) Anatomical landmarks for an intramedullary alignment system for total knee replacement. Orthop Trans 7:546-547
16. Whiteside LA, Summers RG (1984) The effect of the level of distal femoral resection on ligament balance in total knee replacement. In: Dorr LD (ed) The knee: papers of the First Scientific Meeting of the Knee Society. University Park Press, Baltimore, pp 59-73
17. Yoshii I, Whiteside LA, White SE, Milliano MT (1991) Influence of prosthetic joint line position on knee kinematics and patellar position. J Arthroplasty 6:169-177

27 The Technique of PCL Retention in Total Knee Arthroplasty

T. J. Williams, T. S. Thornhill

Summary

The posterior cruciate ligament is the strongest ligament about the knee and a significant contributor to the flexion space and flexion balance in total knee arthroplasty (TKA). The authors feel that the posterior cruciate ligament should be retained and balanced during primary knee arthroplasty and, when applicable, in revision total knee arthroplasty. It is essential, however, to balance the posterior cruciate ligament and use a tibial femoral geometry that is compatible with PCL retention. The technique for PCL balancing is straightforward, but the tests to determine proper PCL balance are different in fixed-bearing vs mobile total knee arthroplasties. This chapter reviews the anatomy of the PCL, its importance in balancing the flexion space, and the techniques for assuring proper PCL balance in fixed- and mobile-bearing total knee arthroplasties.

Introduction

In the normal knee, the posterior cruciate ligament (PCL) prevents posterior translation of the tibia on the femur. Along with the anterior cruciate ligament, it forms part of the four-bar linkage system allowing normal knee function.

However, its function in patients with total knee arthroplasty remains debated, with most authors divided into one of two camps: cruciate retainers and cruciate substituters. While no current research shows a significant difference in outcome or function between cruciate-substituting and cruciate-retaining knees, it is the authors' preference to preserve the posterior cruciate ligament when possible in primary total knee arthroplasty (TKA). This chapter will highlight the rationale for preserving the PCL and demonstrate the technique for correct balancing of a fixed-bearing and rotating-platform total knee arthroplasty performed with retention of the PCL.

Functional Anatomy

The origin of the posterior cruciate ligament (PCL) is on the lateral aspect of the medial femoral condyle. It inserts on the posterior aspect of the tibia in line with the intercondylar space and spreads out to a broad attachment approximately 1 cm below the joint line [1]. It increases in cross-sectional area from its tibial attachment to its femoral origin [2].

Functionally, in the normal knee, the PCL serves to prevent posterior translation of the tibia and in the intact knee contributes to normal anatomical femoral roll-back as well as to the "screw-home" mechanism seen in extension. Beyond 90° of flexion, the PCL tightens, encouraging femoral roll-back, which has the effect of increasing the quadriceps moment arm and enhancing the ability to engage in activities such as stair climbing.

Rationale for Retaining the PCL

In posterior-stabilized total knees, the PCL is usually replaced by a post-and-cam mechanism that attempts to substitute for the sacrificed PCL. In cruciate-retaining designs, the intact PCL was thought to encourage more normal kinematics, maintain femoral roll-back, and increase range of motion [3-5]. Regrettably, this has not borne out in *in vitro* kinematic studies, and Komistek et al. have shown that neither posterior-stabilized nor cruciate-retaining knees preserve femoral roll-back [6,7]. In fact, posterior cruciate-retaining knees demonstrated paradoxical anterior femoral translation in some cases. Adequate balancing of the PCL and use of a conforming tibial insert may rectify this paradoxical movement, and early concerns of excessive polyethylene wear may be eradicated with more contact area [5] and/or mobile-bearing knees.

Similarly, range of motion has not been shown to be significantly improved with cruciate-retaining knees in all studies [8]. In our own series, however, as well as in that of Ritter et al., increased flexion in PCL-retaining knees was seen when the tight PCL was recessed [5,9].

Originally, conforming polyethylene in PCL-retaining knees was considered to limit femoral roll-back and potentially create high stresses at the component-host interfaces. It is now well recognized that flat tibial inserts in a cruciate-retaining knee create high contact stresses, yielding significant early wear and polyethylene failure. In fact, PCL designs with moderately conforming polyethylene trays have shown little problem with issues of wear or early loosening [3, 4]. We advocate the use of conforming polyethylene tibial trays in PCL-retaining knees, particularly rotating-platform knees.

One of the main reasons for preferring cruciate-retaining knees is the preservation of bone stock, particularly in younger patients likely to undergo revision in their lifetime. In the PCL-substituting knee, a large bone block is removed from the intercondylar notch in order to house the post-and-cam mechanism. This bone is obviously left in place in the cruciate-retaining designs. In addition, PCL-substituting designs typically require more distal femoral condylar resection than PCL-retaining knees, as removing the PCL opens the flexion space and necessitates increased distal femoral resection in order to balance the flexion and extension space. Those in favor of cruciate-substituting knees would argue that this is of little concern since most revisions are ultimately cruciate sacrificing and the central condylar portion would be removed at time of revision regardless of the original knee replacement. However, it has been our experience that in some cases, revision of knees with intact PCLs may be performed with a cruciate-retaining design. Frequently, these knees have condylar bone loss and the central intercondylar bone may be the only good bone stock available. Even if these knees are converted to cruciate-substituting knees, the intercondylar notch makes excellent bone graft.

The rationale for PCL retention is best appreciated by considering the flexion space of the knee. The goal is to have a rectangular space that equals the extension space. The flexion space is determined on the medial side by the medial collateral ligament (MCL), which courses from the femur to the tibia. The MCL is broad and strong. In contradistinction, the lateral collateral ligament (LCL) supports the lateral side of the flexion space along with the popliteus tendon, the lateral capsule, and the iliotibial band. The LCL is short and round and courses from the femur to the fibula. An intact PCL, acting as a tether in the middle of the flexion space, mitigates the discrepancy between the MCL and LCL. In addition, the PCL and the MCL create a balanced medial flexion space, which is the center of rotation of the tibiofemoral joint as the knee flexes

Moreover, posterior-stabilized knees have a risk of posterior dislocation, especially if proper balancing techniques are not performed. This is most common in the valgus knee, where lengthening of the tight lateral structures in the absence of a PCL destabilizes the lateral flexion space, allowing the cam-and-post mechanism to dissociate as the knee flexes.

While patellar clunk syndrome is uncommon, it can still be a problem in certain cruciate-substituting de-

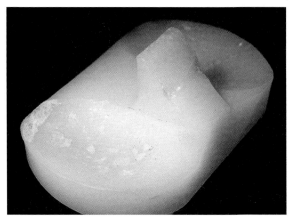

Fig. 27-1. Peg wear in a salvaged posterior-stabilized knee

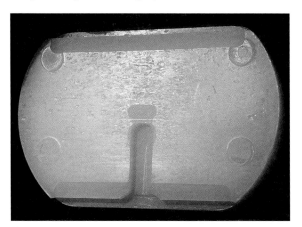

Fig. 27-2. Backside wear in a posterior-stabilized knee

signs. One of the emerging problems in cruciate-substituting knees is peg wear and backside tibial wear that can lead to osteolysis and loosening (Figs. 27-1, 27-2) [10, 11]. Peg wear can be posterior, anterior, or on the side of the polyethylene peg. Posterior peg wear is common when the knee is left loose in flexion. It is a common misconception that a PCL-substituting TKA can be left loose in flexion in order to improve motion. In fact, Ranawat (personal communication) routinely leaves the flexion space 2 mm smaller than the extension space in PCL-substituting TKA. Laxity in flexion can increase posterior peg wear as well as polyethylene damage and wear caused by abnormal sliding. Anterior peg wear is usually due to component hyperextension caused by extension laxity and/or increased posterior tibial slope that requires component hyperextension in order for the patient's knee to fully extend. Wear on the side of the peg is usually due to rotational malalignment in a fixed-bearing design.

Backside wear has been reported with many modular designs. There are many factors that can lead to backside wear, including a poor or damaged locking mechanism, oxidized polyethylene, a poor tibial surface finish, and excessive constraint. In the authors' experience, this is more common in cruciate-substituting designs due to the increased constraint conferred by the cam-and-post mechanism.

Technique

Exposure can be performed by any of several techniques with or without patellar eversion or disruption of the quadriceps mechanism. It is important to have adequate exposure to protect the skin, to identify the important landmarks, and to achieve proper soft-tissue balance and component alignment.

After exposure is obtained, preliminary soft-tissue balance is performed, based on the patient's soft-tissue status and preoperative deformity. For instance, a preliminary medial soft-tissue release is performed on varus knees. This process continues throughout the performance of the procedure, with continuous fine-tuning carried out until the final components are cemented in place. Our initial steps even start with the exposure. We initially carefully dissect a medial sleeve of tibial periosteum to start balancing the medial side of the knee. In a valgus knee, this may be a very small sleeve; just enough to obtain exposure. In the varus knee, this sleeve may be extended posteriorly to perform an initial release of the medial soft-tissue sleeve.

Our earliest balancing maneuvers also include removal of peripheral osteophytes, particularly those that may tent the collateral ligaments or the PCL. We also trim the osteophytes out of the anterior femoral notch to assess the integrity of the PCL and the true anatomy of the femur, which may help with rotation and component placement. We consider adequate exposure of the PCL from its femoral origin to its tibial insertion essential to its proper balancing (◘ Fig. 27-3).

The menisci are then initially resected and, in varus knees, a curved osteotome is passed around the medial side of the joint at the level of the tibia until the posterior-medial aspect of the tibia is reached. At this point the tibia may be delivered in front of the femur by hyperflexing the knee and externally rotating the tibia. Next, the patello-femoral ligament and any remaining meniscal attachments (especially the posterior horns) are released and removed, which greatly aids in exposure.

The bony cuts are then performed using the jigs from the surgeon's implant system of choice. These are based on the bony anatomy. Either tibial or femoral cuts may be completed first, according to surgeon preference. Regardless of which is done first, it is critical for balancing that the cuts be accurate. The tibial cut is perpendicular to the mechanical axis of the tibia. The axis is not between the malleoli, but lies in the center of the talus, which is medial to the intermalleolar point. The cutting guide must be positioned accordingly.

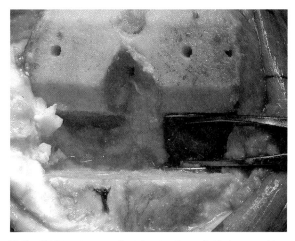

◘ **Fig. 27-4.** Laminar spreader tightening the medial flexion space. Note how the MCL and PCL frame the medial flexion space and how the lateral space passively balance

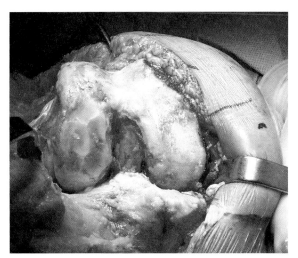

◘ **Fig. 27-3.** The posterior cruciate ligament exposed prior to the bony cuts

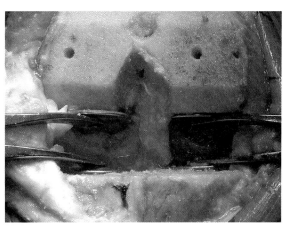

◘ **Fig. 27-5.** Second laminar spreader placed laterally and tightened to demonstrate that the lateral side of the flexion space is more lax than the medial side. This facilitates lateral roll-back

When the femoral cuts are made, rotation is critical. In most varus knees the posterior femoral reference point is used and the component is externally rotated 3° to that axis. This is confirmed by the transepicondylar and transtrochlear lines. In the valgus knee, hypoplasia of the lateral femoral condyle renders the posterior axis inaccurate, and one must rely on the transepicondylar and transtrochlear lines. Proper femoral component rotation is essential to achieve proper PCL balance.

Once the bony cuts have been completed, laminar spreaders are spaced medially and laterally and tensioned to confirm and balance the medial and lateral flexion space. This provides an opportunity to look for the presence of posterior osteophytes and to make an initial assessment of the flexion gap (◘ Figs. 27-4, 27-5). Any remaining menisci and osteophytes that may impinge upon the PCL are removed. The trial components are placed and PCL balancing is assessed.

Assessment of proper PCL tension is different in fixed-bearing and rotating-platform TKAs. In a fixed-bearing knee, proper tension in extension is established using varying tibial insert thicknesses. The knee is then flexed. If the knee is too loose in flexion a thicker or more conforming insert is used to establish balance in flexion. This will necessitate additional distal femoral resection and/or extension releases. If the knee is balanced in extension and tight in flexion, PCL recession is indicated. In a fixed-bearing knee, tightness in flexion is manifested by excessive roll-back on the medial side as the knee is flexed. Moreover, the tibial trial component will lift off anteriorally as the knee is flexed. This test is performed with the trial components in place and the knee flexed. If the tibial trial component can be "pulled out", then the PCL is too loose and a thicker polyethylene should be used (◘ Fig. 27-6). If the anterior edge of the trial insert "lifts off", then the PCL is too tight and needs to be balanced or, if appropriate, a thinner polyethylene is used (◘ Fig. 27-7).

In flexion the posterior femoral condyle should be in the middle portion of the tibial plateau (see ◘ Fig. 27-8).

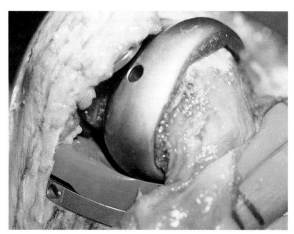

◘ **Fig. 27-8.** Proper tension following PCL recession. Note the central medial dwell point and no "liftoff" of the tibial trial

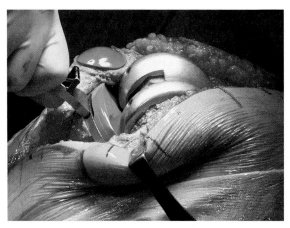

◘ **Fig. 27-6.** The "pull-out" test, indicative of excessive laxity in flexion

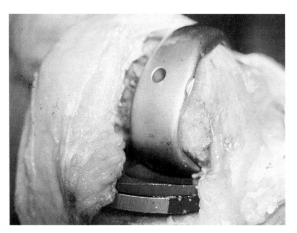

◘ **Fig. 27-7.** A positive "liftoff" test. Note the medial femoral condyle positioned posteriorly in flexion, and the anterior lip of the tibial trial lifting in flexion. These indicate a tight PCL

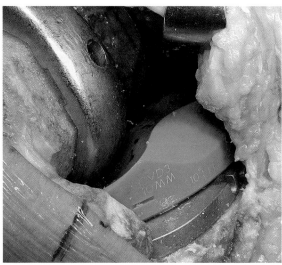

◘ **Fig. 27-9.** The "too much metal sign", indicating a tight PCL in a rotating platform TKA

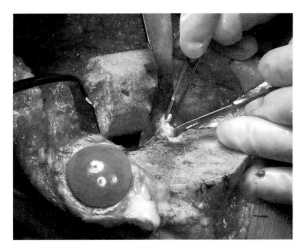

Fig. 27-10. Recession of the PCL from the tibia

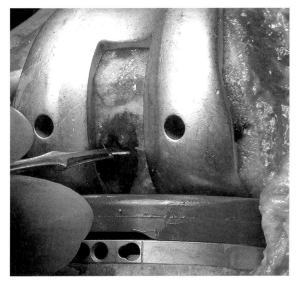

Fig. 27-11. Selective release of tight anterolateral fibers of the PCL during trial reduction

In a rotating-platform knee, tightness of the PCL will force the medial side of the platform to rotate posteriorly in flexion and the trial polyethylene may "spin out" laterally. As this test is performed with the extensor mechanism in position, the lateral "spin-out" may not be apparent but the excessive roll-back medially exposes the medial portion of the metal plate ("too much metal sign"; ◻ Fig. 27-9). If this happens, the PCL is too tight and needs to be balanced.

Recession of the PCL may be performed from either the femur or the tibia, or both. In general a tight PCL is palpated to determine if the entire ligament is tight or if there is selective tightness of certain fiber bundles (usually the anterolateral bundles). If the entire ligament is tight, recession is preferred from the tibia, as the entire ligament is recessed and the broad expanse of the insertion on the tibia prevents inadvertent complete release

(◻ Fig. 27-10). If there is selective tightness, recession from the femur with the trial components in place is preferred, as titration of the release is easier (◻ Fig. 27-11). These techniques require the use of a conforming insert, as the recessed PCL heals over several weeks and the conforming geometry confers the proper pattern of motion while the PCL heals. In a flat-on-flat design excessive sliding may result in paradoxical motion that has been observed on fluoroscopic studies.

After adequate balancing of the PCL, re-insertion of the trial components and reassessment of balancing in both flexion and extension is performed. There should be a balanced tension in flexion and extension, with a central dwell point medially and no liftoff or lateral "spin out".

Interestingly, many surgeons who routinely remove the PCL have avoided the cam-and-post designs and use "deep-dish" or more conforming inserts in order to achieve balance. In the authors' opinion, preservation of the present, albeit not normal, PCL provides an important tether and balance to the flexion space that preserves bone stock and facilitates soft-tissue balance.

References

1. Van Dommelen BA, Fowler PJ (1989) Anatomy of the posterior cruciate ligament. Am J Sports Med 17:24-29
2. Harner CD, et al (1995) The human posterior cruciate ligament complex: an interdisciplinary study: ligament morphology and biomechanical evaluation. Am J Sports Med 23:736-745
3. Rand JA (1996) Posterior cruciate retaining total knee arthroplasty. In: Morrey BF (ed) Reconstructive surgery of the joints, vol 2, 2nd edn. Churchill Livingstone, New York, pp 1401-1408
4. Barnes CL, Sledge CB (1993) Total knee arthroplasty with posterior cruciate ligament retention designs. In: Insall JN, Windsor RE, Scott WN, Kelly MA, Aglietti P (eds) Surgery of the knee, vol 2, 2nd edn. Churchill Livingstone, New York, pp 815-827
5. Scott RD, Thornhill TS (1994) Posterior cruciate supplementing total knee replacement using conforming inserts an cruciate recession: Effect on range of motion and radiolucent lines. Clin Orthop 309:64-68
6. Dennis DA, Komistek RD, Hoff WA, Gabriel SM (1996) In vivo knee kinematics derived using an inverse perspective technique. Clin Orthop 331:107-117
7. Stiehl JB, Komistek RD, Dennis DA, et al (1995) Fluoroscopic analysis of kinematics after posterior cruciate-retaining knee arthroplasty. J Bone Joint Surg [Br] 77:884-889
8. Hirsch HS, Lotke PA, Morrison LD (1994) The posterior cruciate ligament in total knee surgery: save, sacrifice, or substitute? Clin Orthop 309:64-68
9. Ritter MA, Faris PM, Keating EM (1988) Posterior cruciate ligament balancing during total knee arthroplasty. J Arthroplasty 3:323-326
10. Callaghan JJ, O'Rourke MR, et al (2002) Tibial post impingement in posterior-stabilized total knee arthroplasty. Clin Orthop 04:83-88
11. Puloski S, McCalden RW et al (2001) Tibial post wear in posterior stabilized total knee arthroplasty: an unrecognized source of polyethylene debris. J Bone Joint Surg [Am] 83:390-397

28 Posterior Cruciate Ligament Balancing in Total Knee Arthroplasty with a Dynamic PCL Spacer

A. B. Wymenga, B. Christen, U. Wehrli

Summary

PCL balancing in total knee arthroplasty (TKA) is diffi-cult to achieve with a bone-referenced technique. With a newly developed dynamic PCL spacer the flexion gap size of the knee, anterior tibia translation and distraction force were measured. We found that the flexion gap of the knee is a dynamic space which increased in size from an average of 17.3 mm with 100 N tension to 20.5 mm with 200 N tension. The anterior translation increased from 0.6 mm to 4.3 mm. The ratio between increase of the flex-ion gap and anterior tibia translation was 1:2. Total knee arthroplasty with the dynamic PCL spacer provided nor-mal stability in the anteroposterior direction, a good range of flexion, and a correct contact position of the femur onto the posterior 55%-60% of the tibia in patients operated on with this technique.

Introduction

Total knee arthroplasty (TKA) with retention of the pos-terior cruciate ligament (PCL) is an operation with excel-lent long-term results [1]. However, complications may occur if the PCL is not adequately balanced. A loose PCL may cause instability and pain [2-4] and a tight PCL may cause limited flexion, high polyethylene stresses, and wear [4, 5].

In recent studies of the normal knee with MRI the me-dial femoral condyle was shown to act as a circle that does not move anteroposteriorly in a broad band of motion. There is no roll-back from 10° to 120° of flexion. The contact point on the tibia is maintained at approximately 2-5 mm posterior from the middle of the medial tibia plateau, which is at 54%-60% of the anteroposterior di-ameter of the medial tibia [6,7]. The medial compartment is thus comparatively constrained. This contact point of the medial condyle should be restored during the knee implantation in order to restore normal kinematics.

In the knee the PCL is the main restraint to posterior translation of the tibia at greater flexion angles. The PCL is tensioned only in flexion and its main function is to prevent posterior tibial subluxation [8]. As such, the PCL controls the contact point of the medial femoral condyle on the tibia from approximately 60° to 120° of flexion.

The goal of our newly developed PCL-balancing tech-nique is to achieve the correct PCL tension and with this correct pretension to define the optimal bone cuts to create an adequate flexion space. Fulfilling these two pre-requisites will automatically provide a normal contact point of the medial femoral condyle on the tibia plateau with subsequent good flexion and normal anteroposteri-or stability of the knee in flexion. A dynamic PCL spacer, the "BalanSys PCL Tensioner", was developed by two of us (BC and UW).

This chapter describes the ligament-guided PCL balancing technique with a dynamic PCL spacer and the dynamics of the flexion gap size in relation to PCL tension and anterior tibial translation. The first clinical results with this operation technique are presented, together with kinematic data from laboratory experiments sup-porting the new approach of PCL balancing.

PCL-Balancing Technique with the Dynamic PCL Tensioner

The principle of the technique is based on creation of the correct amount of flexion space for the prosthesis with a pretensioned PCL. The PCL is not released; rather, addi-tional bone cuts of a few millimeters are performed or the thickness of the polyethylene is adjusted. The PCL is balanced only after the medial and lateral ligaments are balanced in extension and in 90° of flexion and after a rectangular flexion gap is created.

The BalanSys TKA is a ligament-guided knee system which uses a double-spring tensioner. The operative tech-nique is performed with the "tibia-cut-first" technique with which the tibia cut and the ventral and dorsal femur cuts are made first and the extension cut of the femur is based on the polyethylene size chosen for the flexion space.

Following the tibia osteotomy of 6-8 mm with 7° pos-terior slope and preservation of the PCL insertion, the necessary medial or lateral releases are made in extension

183   **28**

Chapter 28 · Posterior Cruciate Ligament Balancing in Total Knee Arthroplasty – A. B. Wymenga et al.

with a tensor in the knee joint exerting 150-200 N tension. An intramedullary femur guide is used to indicate the direction of the femur cut. Following the releases in extension, the tibia cut should be parallel to the plane of the distal femur cut. This indicates a correct mechanical axis, and no further releases are performed.

Thereafter the knee is flexed and a double tensor is inserted with 100-150 N. The femur finds its rotational position through the ligament tension of the central PCL and the collateral ligaments. The femur cutting guide is inserted over an intramedullary rod and rotated parallel to the tibia cut, creating a rectangular flexion space. The anterior and posterior femur osteotomies are performed. The size of the femoral component is matched with the original medial femoral condyle dimensions, and approximately 9 mm (prosthesis thickness) is cut from the posterior femoral condyle. This leaves the joint line on the medial side of the knee at the same level.

Now the PCL is balanced with the BalanSys PCL Tensioner with an adjustable spacer block. On the adjustable spacer the corresponding polyethylene sizes are marked 8, 10.5, 13, and 15.5 mm. Thickness of the tibial tray (2 mm) and femoral component (9 mm) of the knee system are included. When the PCL tensioner is opened the PCL spacer increases in size. The surgeon can read on the handle of the device how much tension is being applied (scale from 0 to 250 N). On the femur side a sliding plateau is

mounted which enables anterior tibia translation when the spacer is gradually opened. Since the fiber course of the PCL is oblique from tibia inferior-posterior to the medial femoral condyle superior-anterior, the opening of the joint space with a tensor causes the tibia to move forward when the PCL is tensioned (Figs. 28-1, 28-2).

At the beginning of the tensioning by the BalanSys PCL Tensioner the joint opens in a proximal-distal direction without translation as the PCL is not tensioned. As soon as the PCL is tensioned, the oblique fibers will pull the tibia forward. We currently use a 2- to 3-mm anterior translation for the correct pretension of the PCL. The relative positions of femur and tibia with the spacer in situ are accepted as the correct position.

Now the surgeon has to check whether the prosthesis can be fitted into the created flexion space.

- If the indicated PE thickness on the BalanSys PCL Tensioner is 8 mm, this is accepted.
- If the flexion space is too small (e.g., 5 mm PE) the flexion space should be enlarged. The surgeon can choose to make an additional tibia cut of 3 mm or to use a smaller femur size (increments of 3 mm). After this additional cut is made, the flexion space can harbor the tibia tray, the 8 mm PE, and the femur component and, given the volume of the prosthesis material, the PCL is automatically pretensioned after implantation of the material.

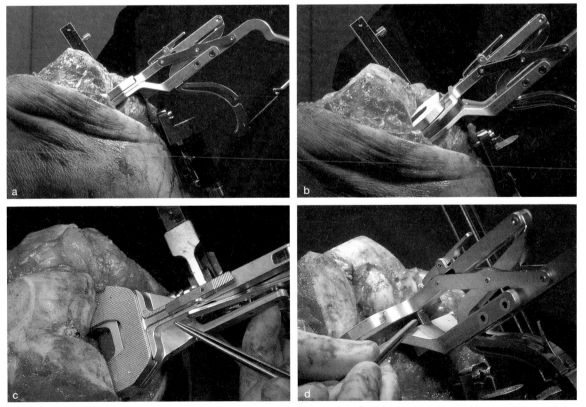

 Fig. 28-1a-d. Tensioning the PCL during surgery with the BalanSys PCL Tensioner. *a* Without tension; *b* with tension. In *c* the anterior translation can be read, and in *d* the gap size can be read

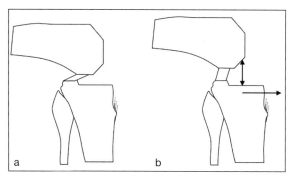

Fig. 28-2a, b. Orientation of the PCL and relative movements of the femur onto the tibia. As the flexion gap increases by applied tension, the tibia is pulled anteriorly by the PCL

can only downsize the femur in order to gain more flexion space since a tibia re-cut would cause instability in extension. In case of a loose flexion space a larger polyethylene size can be used with a re-cut of the distal femur.

Results

Flexion Gap Dynamics Measured with the BalanSys PCL Tensioner

In a prospective study at the Department of Orthopedic Surgery, Spital Bern Ziegler, 82 patients received a total knee arthroplasty with a PCL-sparing technique. The BalanSys PCL Tensioner was used to balance the PCL and create the correct flexion space.

— If the flexion space is larger than 8 mm the surgeon can choose a larger PE size. If the flexion space size is between two PE sizes (e.g., 9 mm) a larger size (10.5 mm) can be chosen but an additional 1.5-mm bone cut has to be made.

After the PCL balancing is finished the extension cut on the distal femur is made, guided by a tensor with 150 N and anticipating the same polyethylene thickness as chosen in flexion. If a bone-referenced technique is used and all bone cuts are made before flexion-space testing, the adjustment possibilities are more limited. With a tight flexion space and a correct extension space the surgeon

The size of the flexion gap was measured with 100 N, 150 N, and 200 N. Also the anterior translation of the tibia was measured with the spacer. The results are summarized in ◻ Table 28-1.

There is a large variation in the amount of opening of the flexion space and the applied tension. In some patients the flexion space opens up to 14 mm with 200 N, whereas in others the joint space is only 6.5 mm. This may depend on the amount of tibia resection, the pre-existing laxity and morphotype of the patient, and the angulation of the PCL fibers, which may run a more vertical or horizontal course in some patients. Also, the weight of the extremity has an influence (◻ Figure 28-3).

◻ **Table 28-1.** Relation of flexion gap, tension, and anterior tibial translation

Tension BalanSys PCL tensioner	100 N	150 N	200 N
Flexion gap size in mm[1] (SD, range)	6.3 (0.6, 5.5-10.0)	7.6 (1.1, 5.0-11.0)	9.5 (1.8, 6.5-14.0)
Anterior translation in mm (SD, range)	0.6 (0.6, 0.0-2.5)	2.2 (1.7, 0.0-8.5)	4.3 (2.0, 0.0-10.0)

[1] Flexion gap size expressed in mm polyethylene; for real flexion gap size 2 mm tibia tray and 9 mm femoral component thickness should be added.

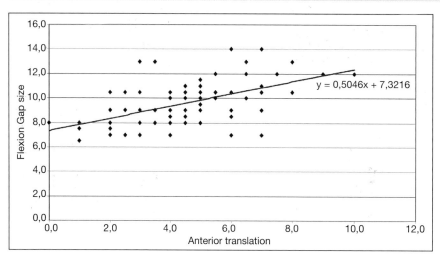

◻ **Fig. 28-3.** Relation between the increase of the flexion gap (mm) and anterior translation (mm) of the tibia with use of the BalanSys PCL Tensioner measured from 0 to 200 N tension

Chapter 28 · Posterior Cruciate Ligament Balancing in Total Knee Arthroplasty – A. B. Wymenga et al.

185   **28**

More important, however, is the anterior translation. We found on average a 1:2 ratio between the increase of the joint space and the anterior translation when the tension was increased from to 0 to 200 N. There was some variation from knees having a 1:1.5 ratio to a more than 1:2 ratio, as can be seen in Fig. 28-2. From these data it is clear that the flexion space of a knee with an intact PCL is not defined as a fixed space but rather as a space depending on the tension and the direction of the PCL fibers and the anteroposterior position of the tibia. The greater the PCL tension, the larger the space becomes and the more anterior translation of the tibia occurs.

It is also clear that small adjustments of the flexion space have a significant influence on the anteroposterior position of the femur. If, for instance, an additional 3-mm bone cut of the tibia is made, the contact position of the femur will change (based on the 1:2 ratio) 2 × 3 = 6 mm, which can be the difference between a too posterior and a correct contact position of the femur. For example, if a 2.5-mm-larger PE insert is used, the femur will move 5 mm posteriorly, which could make the knee too tight.

Anteroposterior Laxity Measured in 90° of Flexion in Clinical Patients with a TKA Implanted with the PCL Tensioner

In a prospective study (results prepared for publication) at the Department of Orthopedic Surgery, Spital Bern Ziegler, 141 patients (37 male and 104 female) were treated with a BalanSys TKA between May 2001 and May 2003. Mean age of the patients was 71 years (49-89). All patients were treated for osteoarthrosis. In 54 patients with valgus knees a lateral approach and in 87 patients with a varus knee a medial approach was used. These patients were evaluated with the Rolimeter (Aircast Europe Ltd.) [9-12]

Table 28-2. Anteroposterior laxity measured with rolimeter in 90° of flexion

Measure	Preoperative	Postoperative
Median	6.7	5.0
Mean	7.0	5.2
SD	2.9	2.0
Range	0-17	2-10

in order to measure anteroposterior laxity of the knee in 90° of flexion preoperatively and postoperatively in the operating room after implantation of the prosthesis. The results are shown in Table 28-2.

In a subset of these patients (*n*=65) the average flexion after surgery was 117.5°, indicating that with an adequate PCL, balancing can give a very stable knee in flexion with an anteroposterior drawer of only 5 mm and, despite this, a good range of motion.

Kinematics of TKA with the BalanSys PCL Tensioner in Laboratory Experiments

In a laboratory experiment five TKAs were implanted in fresh-frozen knee specimens using the BalanSys PCL Tensioner (results prepared for publication). The procedures were supported by a navigation system (PRAXIM, Grenoble, France). A relatively conforming, fixed-bearing insert was tested and then, in the same specimen, an AP-gliding meniscal-bearing insert was tested. After recording of the knee kinematics with passive motion, the PCL was cut and kinematics were recorded with a non-functional PCL. To quantify AP translation of the femur relative to the tibia (results in Fig. 28-4), the reference point on the femur was chosen as the intersection

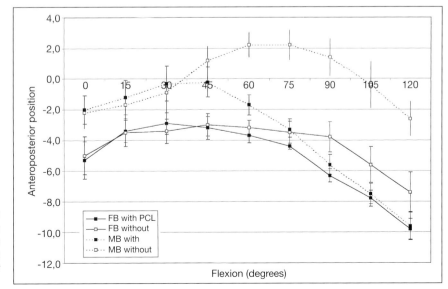

Fig. 28-4. Average (*n*=5, mean +/-1 SEM) femoral AP translation of five knee specimens with a mobile- (*MB*) and a fixed-bearing (*FB*) TKP both before and after resection of the PCL

of the femur rotation axis (femoral component: single radius design) and a central sagittal plane through the femoral component.

The fixed- and meniscal-bearing configurations show a correct contact point posterior to the middle of the tibial plateau in AP direction, even in extension (◻ Fig. 28-4). In extension the meniscal variant is 2 mm anterior compared with the fixed-bearing variant. In flexion both bearing types resulted in roll-back between 60° and 120° of flexion with a correct contact point similar to the normal knee in 90° of flexion [6].

After the PCL has been cut the kinematics are disturbed and the femur contact point moves forward. The effects for the fixed-bearing insert are limited, whereas the effects for the AP-gliding meniscal-bearing insert are quite considerable. These data illustrate the effectiveness of PCL balancing with the BalanSys PCL Tensioner and confirm the importance of a well-functioning PCL, especially in AP-gliding meniscal-bearing knees.

Discussion

A new concept of flexion-gap balancing with the BalanSys PCL Tensioner was developed. With the use of this dynamic spacer, the PCL can be adequately tensioned; the required amount of flexion gap for the prosthesis can be precisely determined and, if necessary, adjusted with small bone cuts or an increase of PE size. Patients from a case series operated on with this technique had an average of 117.5° of flexion with normal anteroposterior laxity, indicating a functional PCL.

The flexion gap is dependent on PCL tension and the anterior translation of the tibia. A small increase of the flexion space causes a comparatively large anterior translation of the tibia with a ratio of 1:2. This is caused by the obliquely oriented PCL fibers that pull the tibia anterior with the opening of the flexion gap. A few millimeters difference of bone resection can change the contact point of the femur on the tibia considerably. If the flexion gap is accepted without sufficient tension of the PCL the femur automatically slides forward. If the PCL is too tight the contact position is too posterior.

These findings may explain why it was difficult in some laboratory experiments to achieve normal PCL function with a PCL-retaining TKA [13]. Mahoney et al. [14] found a normal PCL strain in only 37% after TKA. They also concluded that the PCL strain was increased by 50% by inserting a 2.5-mm-thicker polyethylene insert. Most [15] and Sorger [16], however, were able to balance PCL and the flexion gap in laboratory tests and to restore normal 'roll-back'. Li [17] found a partial restoration of the roll-back beyond 60° of flexion. If the PCL was cut he found reciprocal anterior translation, showing the importance of the PCL.

Also in clinical series with fixed-bearing knees variable results are found. The PCL function can be analyzed by measuring the contact point of the femur on the tibia in flexion and AP-laxity in flexion. Misra [18] compared PCL resection and retention with a fixed-bearing condylar prosthesis and found roll-back in only 20% of both groups, indicating that PCL balancing was not achieved. Matsuda [19] achieved only good anteroposterior stability in half of the patients with a PCL-retaining prosthesis. Dejour [20] found anteroposterior instability in 41% of the patients with posterior cruciate-retaining (PCR) TKA, indicating a non-functioning PCL. Straw [21] found anteroposterior laxity in 54% of patients with PCR TKA. Kim [22], however, was able to achieve a contact point of 55% with PCR TKA, which is similar to that in the normal knee [6]. In mobile-bearing knees PCL balancing seems to be even more critical. Morberg [3] found a high rate of failures after AP-gliding mobile-bearing total knee arthroplasty due to flexion instability caused by inadequate PCL balancing. Archibeck [23] found a low rate of clinical posterior instability and measured an average contact point of 45% (22%-98%) in meniscal-bearing knees. This contact point shows that the PCL balancing was not perfect in all patients. Hartford [24] found anterior sliding of the meniscal bearing in 70% of patients, indicating a non-functional PCL; the patients with roll-back had better knee scores and better flexion. Anteroposterior-gliding mobile bearings and flat fixed bearings depend more on soft-tissue restraints, whereas more fixed conforming designs are more self-stabilizing [25]. Also with fluoroscopic analysis in vivo in PCR TKAs frequently show a paradoxical anterior sliding in flexion [26, 27], but results seem to vary between individual surgeons [26, 28]. Bertin found a consistent posterior contact point in PCR TKA [29]. Better flexion was found in patients with a posterior contact position.

From these studies it is clear that PCL balancing and the creation of a normal contact point of the femur on the tibia are difficult to achieve in PCL-retaining TKA with a bone-referenced technique. The flexion gap is not a static space but a dynamic space that is controlled mainly by the oblique PCL fibers that link flexion gap size and tibia translation in a 1:2 ratio. With the newly developed dynamic PCL spacer it is possible to adequately balance the PCL in a reproducible way.

Conclusions

A ligament-guided PCL-balancing technique was developed with a new device, the BalanSys PCL Tensioner. This dynamic PCL spacer controls the PCL tension and also determines exactly the required flexion space size. Changes in flexion space have a large effect on anterior translation of the tibia, which may explain the difficulty

Chapter 28 · Posterior Cruciate Ligament Balancing in Total Knee Arthroplasty – A. B. Wymenga et al.

187   **28**

with PCL balancing in the past. The flexion space is adjusted with small 1- to 2-mm bone cuts and the PCL is not released. We were able to achieve a high rate of anteroposterior stability with an average ROM of 117.5° in patients operated on with this technique, indicating a functional PCL. Laboratory tests confirmed normal kinematics and normal contact points with the new PCL-balancing technique.

Acknowledgements. We acknowledge the co-authorship of A. J. Schuster and S. R. Thomann (Department of Orthopedic Surgery, Spital Bern Ziegler, Switzerland), T. Wyss (Balgrist Spital, Zurich, Switzerland) and W. Jacobs (St. Maartenskliniek, Nijmegen, The Netherlands).

References

1. Gill GS, Joshi AB, Mills DM (1999) Total condylar knee arthroplasty: 16- to 21-year results. Clin Orthop 367:210-215
2. Waslewski GL, Marson BM, Benjamin JB (1998) Early, incapacitating instability of posterior cruciate ligament-retaining total knee arthroplasty. J Arthroplasty 13:763-767
3. Morberg P, Chapman-Sheath P, Morris P, Cain S, Walsh WR (2002) The function of the posterior cruciate ligament in an anteroposterior-gliding rotating platform total knee arthroplasty. J Arthroplasty 17:484-489
4. Pagnano MW, Hanssen AD, Lewallen DG, Stuart MJ (1998) Flexion instability after primary posterior cruciate retaining total knee arthroplasty. Clin Orthop 356:39-46
5. Migaud H, Tirveilliot F (2003) Preservation, resection or substitution of the posterior cruciate ligament in total knee replacement. In: Lemaire R, Horan F, Scott J, Villar R (eds) Proceedings of the EFORT congress. European Instructional Course Lectures 6:176-184
6. Freeman MA, Pinskerova V (2003) The movement of the knee studied by magnetic resonance imaging. Clin Orthop 410:35-43
7. Komistek RD, Dennis DA, Mahfouz M (2003) In vivo fluoroscopic analysis of the normal human knee. Clin Orthop 410:69-81
8. Gollehon DL, Torzilli PA, Warren RF (1987) The role of the posterolateral and cruciate ligaments in the stability of the human knee. A biomechanical study. J Bone Joint Surg [Am] 69:233-242
9. Balasch H, Schiller M, Friebel H, et al (1999) Evaluation of anterior knee-joint instability with the rolimeter. Knee Surg Sports Traumatol Arthrosc 7:204-208
10. Ganko A, Engebretsen L, Ozer H (2000) The rolimeter: A new arthrometer compared with Kt 1000. Knee Surg Sports Traumatol Arthrosc 8:36-39
11. Pässler H, Ververidis A, Monauni F (1998) Beweglichkeitswertung an Knieen mit Vkb-Schaden mit Hilfe des Kt 1000 und Aircast Rolimeter. Unfallchirurg 272:731-732
12. Schuster AJ, McNicholas MJ, Wachtl SW, McGurty DW, Jakob RP (2004) A new mechanical testing device for measuring anteroposterior knee laxity. Am J Sports Med (in press)
13. Corces A (1989) Strain characteristics of the posterior cruciate ligament in total knee arthroplasty. Orthop Trans 13:527-528
14. Mahoney OM, Noble PC, Rhoads DD, Alexander JW, Tullos HS (1994) Posterior cruciate function following total knee arthroplasty. A biomechanical study. J Arthroplasty 9:569-578
15. Most E, Zayontz S, Li G, Otterberg E, Sabbag K, Rubash HE (2003) Femoral rollback after cruciate-retaining and stabilizing total knee arthroplasty. Clin Orthop 410:101-113
16. Sorger JI, Federle D, Kirk PG, Grood E, Cochran J, Levy M (1997) The posterior cruciate ligament in total knee arthroplasty. J Arthroplasty 12:869-879
17. Li G, Zayontz S, Most E, Otterberg E, Sabbag K, Rubash HE (2001) Cruciate-retaining and cruciate-substituting total knee arthroplasty: An in vitro comparison of the kinematics under muscle loads. J Arthroplasty 16 [Suppl 1]: 150-156
18. Misra AN, Hussain MR, Fiddian NJ, Newton G (2003) The role of the posterior cruciate ligament in total knee replacement. J Bone Joint Surg [Br] 85:389-392
19. Matsuda S, Miura H, Nagamine R, Urabe K, Matsunobu T, Iwamoto Y (1999) Knee stability in posterior cruciate ligament retaining total knee arthroplasty. Clin Orthop 366:169-173
20. Dejour D, Deschamps G, Garotta L, Dejour H (1999) Laxity in posterior cruciate sparing and posterior stabilized total knee prostheses. Clin Orthop 364:182-193
21. Straw R, Kulkarni S, Attfield S, Wilton TJ (2003) Posterior cruciate ligament at total knee replacement: essential, beneficial or a hindrance? J Bone Joint Surg [Br] 85:671-674
22. Kim H, Pelker RR, Gibson DH, Irving JF, Lynch JK (1997) Rollback in posterior cruciate ligament-retaining knee arthroplasty. A radiographic analysis. J Arthroplasty 12:553-561
23. Archibeck MJ, Berger RA, Barden RM, Jacobs JJ, Sheinkop MB, Rosenberg AG, Galante JO (2001) Posterior cruciate ligament-retaining total knee arthroplasty in patients with rheumatoid arthritis. J Bone Joint Surg [Am] 83:1231-1236
24. Hartford JM, Banit D, Hall K, Kaufer H (2001) Radiographic analysis of low contact stress meniscal bearing total knee replacements. J Bone Joint Surg [Am] 83:229-234
25. Walker PS, Ambarek MS, Morris JR, Olanlokun K, Cobb A (1995) Anterior-posterior stability in partially conforming condylar knee replacement. Clin Orthop 310:87-97
26. Dennis DA, Komistek RD, Mahfouz MR, Haas BD, Stiehl JB (2003) Multicenter determination of in vivo kinematics after total knee arthroplasty. Clin Orthop 416:37-57
27. Banks S, Bellemans J, Nozaki H, Whiteside LA, Harman M, Hodge WA (2003) Knee motions during maximum flexion in fixed- and mobile-bearing arthroplasties. Clin Orthop 410:131-138
28. Nozaki H, Banks SA, Suguro T, Hodge WA (2002) Observations of femoral rollback in cruciate-retaining knee arthroplasty. Clin Orthop 404:308-314
29. Bertin KC, Komistek RD, Dennis DA, Hoff WA, Anderson DT, Langer T (2002) In vivo determination of posterior femoral rollback for subjects having a Nexgen posterior cruciate-retaining total knee arthroplasty. J Arthroplasty 17:1040-1048

29 Achieving Maximal Flexion

J. Bellemans

Summary

Despite all recent advances in total knee arthroplasty surgery, limited flexion remains a subject of frustration for many knee surgeons and patients. Frequently, it is the physiotherapist, the patient, or the designing engineers who get the blame. In our experience however, the most frequent reasons for limited knee flexion after TKA are surgical technical factors. Extension-flexion gap balancing, adequate posterior clearance, and the avoidance of anterior overstuffing are indeed factors that can be controlled perfectly intraoperatively when recognized by the surgeon. Failure to do so will inevitably result in loss of flexion, despite the best physiotherapy, the most motivated patient, and the most optimal implant with regard to regaining flexion.

Table 29-1. Most frequent reasons for limitation of flexion following TKA

Extension gap–flexion gap mismatch, due to
Extension space >flexion space PCL too tight
Excessive femoral component (internal or external) rotation
Insufficient tibial slope
Inadequate posterior clearance, due to
Osteophytes
Soft-tissue remnants
Posterior tibial overhang
Decreased posterior off-set
Anterior overstuffing
Patellar thickening
Femoral or tibial anteriorization
Retinacular tightness
Quadriceps shortening
Inadequate physiotherapy
Inadequate implant

Introduction

Many variables determine the final outcome after total knee arthroplasty. Not all of these factors can be influenced by the surgeon; most are actually beyond the surgeon's control. The patient's preoperative status, severity of the disease, associated co-morbidity, multiple joint involvement, motivational status, etc., are all important issues with great impact on the clinical and subjective results after TKA. All this is equally true with regard to maximal flexion that is obtained by the patient after TKA [1-5].

Nevertheless, there is growing evidence that concerning maximal postoperative flexion obtained by the patient, as well as design-related aspects of the implanted TKA system, surgical technical factors do play an important role [6-11]. In this chapter I will review the surgical and design-related factors which I consider to be most important in regaining flexion after TKA.

With regard to surgical technical factors, these can be subdivided into three important categories: (Table 29-1). The first category is related to inadequate flexion and extension gap balancing, with relative tightness of the flexion gap leading to potential overstuffing of the flexion space and mechanical blocking of further flexion.

The second group of technical factors concerns issues related to the posterior area of the knee joint. The third group deals with issues related to the anterior aspect of the knee.

Together with increased awareness of these surgical factors, implant designers have recently shown increased attention towards implant design-related factors that may influence maximal range of motion postoperatively. The renewed interest in the importance of femoral roll-back, as well as increased knowledge about the in vivo kinematic behavior of contemporary TKA systems, has played an important role in this process [8-10,12-17].

This, together with an increased awareness of the physiological and anatomical characteristics that allow the normal knee to obtain maximal flexion, has led to the design and development of more optimal knee arthroplasty components with regard to maximizing postoperative flexion [6, 7, 10].

Inadequate Flexion and Extension Space Balancing

One of the most important issues in contemporary surgical TKA techniques is an adequate creation of the flexion

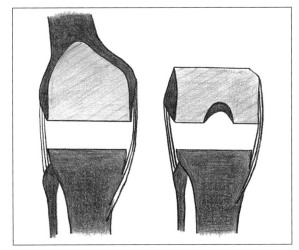

Fig. 29-1. Equally sized flexion and extension spaces

and extension spaces. These spaces are defined as the opening of the knee joint space after completion of the bone cuts, while the knee is held in extension (extension space) or flexion (flexion space). These spaces are subsequently filled up by the prosthetic components, and their size is therefore critical, since a space that is too small may make it difficult to squeeze the components into the created space without causing excessive tension on the soft-tissue structures. Likewise, when the space is too large, underfilling of the space by the prosthetic components will occur, with insufficient soft.tissue tension and instability as a result.

Since most contemporary knee arthroplasty designs have an identical metal thickness on their extension and flexion regions, the flexion and extension spaces created should therefore be equal in size (❏ Fig. 29-1) Moreover, they should be rectangular to allow for comparable tension in the medial and lateral soft tissues. Some lateral laxity or wideness of the flexion and extension spaces may be accepted, however, since the normal knee is also a bit more lax on the lateral than on the medial side.

Despite the fact that the amount of bone resection is controlled by the surgeon, reality shows that unequal flexion and extension spaces are not seldom obtained during TKA surgery. More specifically, if the flexion space is smaller than the extension space it may lead to problems with obtaining satisfactory postoperative flexion, if the situation is not addressed and corrected during surgery. In theory, a thinner tibial insert could be used to avoid overstuffing the flexion space, but this would lead to underfilling of the extension space with inadequate soft-tissue tension to provide sufficient joint stability in extension.

However, several more appropriate options are available to the surgeon when attempting to correct this situation of a tight flexion space. For example, downsizing the femoral component while maintaining the same anterior reference point will increase the flexion space without altering the extension space, and may correct the problem. Increasing the tibial slope will also open up the flexion space for the prosthetic components, since the femorotibial contact points can move posteriorly during flexion. During extension femorotibial contact occurs anterior and is therefore little influenced by increasing the tibial slope.

Finally, release of the posterior cruciate ligament (PCL) will predominantly increase the flexion space and is another way to compensate for flexion space tightness. Such release can be performed by resecting the PCL, or by gradually releasing it from its bony attachments on the tibia or the femoral condyle. When this option is chosen by the surgeon, a PCL-substituting implant should be used.

Apart from these general principles that can be applied in case of flexion space tightness, the surgeon should realize that a number of very specific factors may be the cause of the tightness.

PCL Shortening

Shortening of the PCL is such a factor; it can be encountered in severe osteoarthritis or after previous high tibial osteotomy due to fibrotic scarring (❏ Fig. 29-2). PCL shortness can usually be diagnosed by two intraoperative signs: (a) the presence of excessive femoral roll-back during flexion testing with the trial components in situ, and (b) anterior liftoff of the tibial insert from the trial base plate during flexion testing. It is obvious that in these situations, releasing the PCL is the method of choice for correcting the problem.

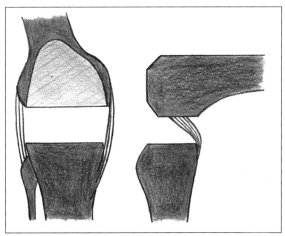

Fig. 29-2. Shortening of the PCL leads to tightness of the flexion space

Femoral Component Malrotation

Malrotation of the femoral component is another single variable that may be responsible for flexion space tightness. It is well known that excessive internal rotation of the femoral component may cause lateral patellar tilting and subluxation, but it may also lead to asymmetric flexion space tightness at the medial side, leading to excessive tension and pain in the medial soft tissues when the knee is flexed (◘ Fig. 29-3). Likewise, excessive external femoral component rotation will lead to lateral flexion space tightness with excessive tension built up in the lateral soft tissues during flexion (◘ Fig. 29-4).

Errors in femoral component rotation occur relatively frequently and are very difficult to correct or compensate for once the bone cuts have been made. Furthermore, the presence of femoral component malrotation may be overlooked during surgery, since full passive flexion may still be possible in the anesthetized patient. Once the patient is awake, however, pain in the excessively tensioned collateral soft tissues will prevent him or her from moving the knee into deep flexion. The best way to avoid this problem is therefore to carefully assess the soft-tissue tensions during full range of motion, by digital palpation of the collateral structures and by varus or valgus stress testing with the knee in flexion.

In the case of excessive femoral component internal rotation, release of the anterior fibers of the medial collateral ligament from the tibial insertion can be performed in an attempt to improve the situation, since releasing these fibers will open the medial flexion space without influencing the extension space [18]. Likewise, excessive femoral component external rotation can be addressed by releasing the popliteus tendon and lateral collateral ligament, leading to opening of the lateral flexion space. If the iliotibial band is left intact, such release will not influence the extension space [18].

In cases of very severe femoral malrotation, however, it is obvious that revising the bone cuts to the correct rotation will be required. The use of wedges or cement is frequently necessary in these cases in order to maintain implant contact with the revised bone cuts.

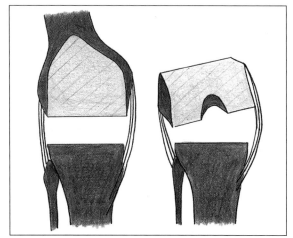

◘ Fig. 29-3. Excessive femoral component internal rotation, leading to medial tightness of the flexion space

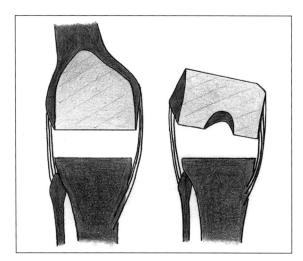

◘ Fig. 29-4. Excessive femoral component external rotation, leading to lateral tightness of the flexion space

Insufficient Tibial Slope

Most people consider the degree of tibial slope an important factor in maximizing postoperative flexion after TKA, despite the fact that few hard data are available to substantiate this. The introduction of more conforming knee designs in particular has led to the general belief that some down-sloping of the tibial component is advisable, since it avoids the so-called kinematic conflict that is present during knee flexion, where femoral roll-back is prohibited by the up-sloping posterior lip of the tibial insert. Down-sloping the tibial component may therefore reduce such conflict, and may allow the knee to go into deeper flexion.

Recent work by our group has indeed demonstrated a beneficial effect of increasing tibial slope with regard to maximal flexion [11]. In a cadaver simulation of previously obtained in vivo kinematics of contemporary PCL-retaining TKA patients, an average gain of 1.7° flexion for every degree of extra tibial slope was seen. In other words, increasing the slope by 6° leads to an average increase of flexion by 10°.

With regard to tibial slope, however, it is important to note that altering the slope also influences anterior stability of the knee [19]. Excessive down-sloping may therefore lead to anterior instability and so-called mid-flexion laxity. We therefore believe that the increase of the tibial slope should not exceed 7°.

Posterior Clearance

The posterior aspect of the knee joint is crucial for the ability to regain maximal flexion following TKA. Recent work by us has demonstrated that maximal obtainable flexion in patients with modern PCL-retaining TKA is ultimately determined by impingement of the tibial insert against the back of the femur [9, 10] (◘ Fig. 29-5).

Such impingement obviously occurs faster when femoral osteophytes are not adequately removed, or when protruding bone beyond the femoral condyles is left behind (◘ Fig. 29-6). Likewise, soft-tissue remnants in the backside of the knee, such as meniscal remnants or hypertrophic synovial tissue, should be removed adequately for the same reasons. According to the same principle, posterior tibial component overhang should be avoided.

Posterior Condylar Offset

Restoring the posterior condylar offset is another important factor with respect to maximizing postoperative flexion. In an analysis of 150 consecutive PCL-retaining TKA patients, we demonstrated a significant correlation between operative restoration of posterior condylar offset and maximal postoperative flexion. For every 2-mm decrease in posterior condylar offset, the maximal obtainable flexion was reduced by a mean of 12.2° (◘ Fig. 29-7).

Especially in TKA using anterior referencing for femoral component positioning, the surgeon may have the tendency to reduce femoral condylar offset, since most surgical technical guides suggest the use of a smaller femoral component when in between two sizes. By downsizing, overfilling of the flexion space with prosthetic material is avoided, and flexion is believed to be facilitated by greater laxity.

Our observations do not confirm this reasoning, however. As well as risking an excessive flexion gap, downsizing with anterior referencing leads to a decreased posterior condylar offset and therefore to reduced flexion because of earlier impingement (◘ Fig. 29-8).

Femoral Roll-back

Posterior insert impingement is theoretically avoided by femoral roll-back. Today, however, there is abundant evidence that the majority of contemporary PCL-retaining TKAs do not show roll-back, but instead demonstrate so-called paradoxical roll-forward of the femoral component during flexion [9, 10].

In a recent study using three-dimensional computer-aided design video-fluoroscopy, we measured the amount of femoral roll-back in 121 knees, treated with 16 different types of arthroplasties with clinically excellent results,

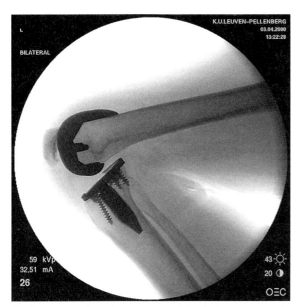

◘ **Fig. 29-5.** Mechanical impingement of the tibial insert against the back of the femur, blocking further flexion

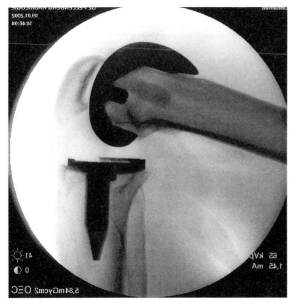

◘ **Fig. 29-6.** Protruding bone beyond the femoral component's posterior condyles, blocking further flexion

◘ **Table 29-2.** Quantitative influence of surgical factors on maximal flexion

Factor	Effect
Tibial slope	1.7° extra flexion for every degree tibial slope
Posterior condylar offset	6° extra flexion for every millimeter posterior condylar offset
Femoral roll-back	1.4° extra flexion for every millimeter femoral roll-back

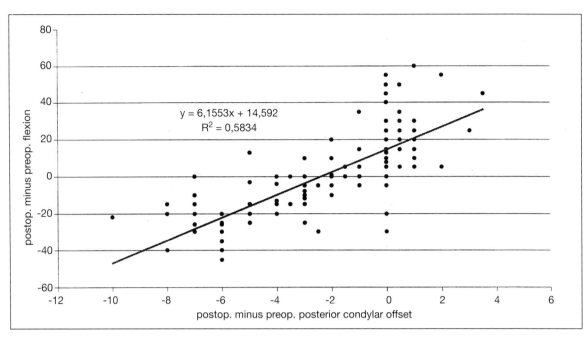

Fig. 29-7. Correlation of restoration of posterior condylar offset (postoperative minus preoperative) with postoperative flexion gain (+)/loss (-). Overlapping points are not shown. (Reprinted, with permission, from [10])

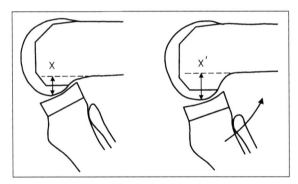

Fig. 29-8. Decreased posterior condylar offset (left) leads to earlier impingement and limited flexion (x@x'). (Reprinted, with permission, from [10])

during maximal knee flexion in a lunge activity. A highly significant correlation was noted between the amount of femoral roll-back and maximum weight-bearing knee flexion, with an average of 1.4° greater flexion for each millimeter of additional femoral roll-back (Table 29-2).

Anterior Clearance

While the posterior area of the knee is important with respect to avoiding early impingement and thereby maximizing postoperative flexion, the importance of the anterior aspect of the knee should not be underestimated. Overstuffing the anterior compartment may lead to excessive tension on the anterior structures during flexion, with the risk of limited postoperative range of motion.

Increasing the patellar thickness for example, will lead to increased tension in the extensor mechanism, with anterior knee pain during flexion due to painful stretching of the quadriceps and patellar tendon, and limitation of flexion as a result. The same negative effect is obtained when the femoral component is positioned too anterior, or when the anterior aspect of the component is thicker than the amount of bone that was resected.

Tibial component anteriorization should equally be avoided, since it will lead to patellar tendon and fat pad impingement against the frontal part of the insert during flexion, causing anterior knee pain and restricted range of motion.

Finally, an adequate release of the potentially shortened lateral retinacular expansion should be performed in order to facilitate maximal flexion. Especially in the valgus knee with lateral tracking of the patella, such shortening needs to be addressed.

Conclusion

Achieving maximal flexion after TKA is a continuous challenge for both the patient and the surgeon. Despite the fact that the parameters influencing the achievement of maximal flexion have not been very well understood for a long period of time, recent work by our group and others has substantiated the importance of several surgical and design-related factors. Many of these factors can indeed be controlled by the arthroplasty surgeon and are appropriately addressed during the surgical procedure.

When faced with a patient showing poor flexion following TKA, the surgeon ought to defer blaming the patient or his physiotherapist or the implant designer until he is convinced that the above-mentioned surgical technical factors have been addressed appropriately.

References

1. Anouchi Y et al (1996) Range of motion in total knee replacement. Clin Orthop Rel Res 331:87-92
2. Kim J et al (1994) Squatting following total knee arthroplasty. Clin Orthop Rel Res 313:177-186
3. Lizaur A et al(1997) Preoperative factors influencing the range of movement after total knee arthroplasty for severe osteoarthritis. J Bone Joint Surg [Br] 97:626-629
4. Jordan L et al (1995) Early flexion routine. An alternative method of continuous passive motion. Clin Orthop Rel Res 315:231-233
5. Schurman D et al (1985) Total condylar knee replacement. A study of factors influencing range of motion as late as two years after arthroplasty. J Bone Joint Surg [Am] 67:1006-1014
6. Akagi M et al (1997) Improved range of flexion after total knee arthroplasty. Bull Hospital Joint Dis 56:225-232
7. Akagi M et al (2000) The bisurface total knee replacement: a unique design for flexion. J Bone Joint Surg [Am] 82:1626-1633
8. Banks S et al (2003) Knee motions during maximum flexion in fixed and mobile bearing arthroplasties. Clin Orthop Rel Res 410:131-138
9. Banks et al (2003) Making sense of knee arthroplasty kinematics: news you can use. J Bone Joint Surg [Am] 85:64-72
10. Bellemans J et al (2002) Fluoroscopic analysis of the kinematics of deep flexion in total knee arthroplasty. The influence of posterior condylar offset. J Bone Joint Surg [Br] 84:50-53
11. Robyns et al (2003) Effect of tibial slope on flexion in total knee arthroplasty. Proc Am Acad Orthop Surg 4:258
12. Bertin K et al (2002) In vivo determination of posterior femoral rollback for subjects having a NexGen posterior cruciate-retaining total knee arthroplasty. J Arthroplasty 17:1040-1048
13. Dennis D et al (1998) In vivo anteroposterior femorotibial translation of total knee arthroplasty: a multicenter analysis. Clin Orthop Rel Res 356: 47-57
14. Stiehl J et al (2000) In vivo kinematic comparison of posterior cruciate ligament retention or sacrifice with a mobile bearing total knee arthroplasty. Am J Knee Surg 13:13-18
15. Stiehl J et al (1990) Detrimental kinematics of a flat on flat total condylar knee arthroplasty. Clin Orthop Rel Res 365:139-148
16. Uvehammer J et al (2000) In vivo kinematics of total knee arthroplasty: flat compared with concave tibial joint surface. J Orthop Res 18:856-864
17. Walker P, Garg A (1989) Range of motion in total knee arthroplasty. A computer analysis. Clin Orthop Rel Res 262:227-235
18. Whiteside L (2004) Ligament balancing in total knee arthroplasty. Springer-Verlag Berlin Heidelberg New York Tokyo
19. Bonnin M (1990) La subluxation tibial antérieure en appui monopodal dans les ruptures du ligaments croisés antérieure. Etude clinique et biomécanique. Thèse Med., Lyon, n° 180

30 Assess and Achieve Maximal Extension

R. S. Laskin, B. Beksac

Summary

Inability to obtain full extension following knee arthroplasty is due to a combination of many factors. Some factors are not under the control of the surgeon, and are related to patient morphology and disease. Others are related to prosthesis design. Many, however, are directly related to the surgical technique and are therefore controllable by the surgeon. By attention to detail, the surgeon can have a direct effect on these factors and can maximize extension.

Introduction

The major goal of total knee arthroplasty is relief of pain. Almost as important, however, is the restoration of function, and that function depends primarily on an adequate arc of motion in the knee. Extension and flexion following a knee arthroplasty are dependent upon a multitude of factors related to surgical technique, the implant used, the physical therapy program, and the patient him- or herself. This chapter will discuss these factors and describe methods that the authors have used to maximize motion in extension. A subsequent chapter will deal with the subject of obtaining full flexion.

Why Do We Need Full Extension?

During normal gait, the knee is at full extension at the time of heel strike and then gradually flexes during stance phase and swing phase [1]. A patient whose knee cannot come into full extension must contract his quadriceps to prevent the knee from buckling during early stance, and this increases the work of walking. Whereas most patients after knee replacement have sufficient quadriceps strength to compensate in this manner when they first begin walking, with continued walking quadriceps fatigue can result in a limp and anterior thigh pain [2]. When the knee does not come to full extension, the limb is functionally short. This can cause a limp as well as pain in the back and in the ipsilateral hip and ankle. For all these reasons, there-

fore, the goal for the total knee surgeon is to obtain full extension in the reconstructed knee.

How Do We Determine if the Knee Is Fully Extended?

At the onset, the authors would like to distinguish between two terms. Extensor lag refers to an inability to actively extend the knee to the point where it can be passively extended (it is the difference between passive and active extension). A flexion contracture, on the other hand, is an inability to bring the leg to full extension passively. Although regaining muscle power is important after knee replacement, very few patients have an extensor lag following primary surgery. It is a flexion contracture that we are most concerned with during knee replacement.

To examine for full extension, the patient should be recumbent with both legs exposed and the heel on the table. If the knee is fully extended, the examiner should not be able to pass any of his hand behind the knee in the popliteal space. The greater the flexion contracture, the more fingers the examiner should be able to pass under the knee.

Full passive extension of the knee can appear limited if there is hamstring spasm or tightness (for instance, in the patient with discogenic disease), especially if the knee is tested with the hip flexed. It is for this reason that assessing extension while the patient is sitting with his leg hanging off the side of the examining couch often results in a false increase in the appearance of a flexion contracture. If an exact measurement of extension is required, a lateral cross-table radiograph can be taken with the ankle supported on a small box.

The standard method of recording knee range of motion assigns zero degrees to the fully extended knee. A knee that has a 5° flexion contracture and can, for example, flex to 125° of flexion should be listed as having a range of motion of 5°-125°. The use of minus numbers should be reserved for degrees of recurvatum at the knee.

During surgery, these tests are difficult to perform because the leg is encased in sterile drapes. A test has been used by the senior author that eliminates this problem: The leg is lifted from the ankle and the ankle joint itself is passively dorsiflexed. Axial pressure is then applied to the sole of the foot. If there is a flexion contracture, the knee will suddenly flex. If the knee is at full extension, however, there will be motion.

Although the presence of pain can lead to a false evaluation of joint motion, this relates predominantly to flexion. In a study performed at the senior author's institution, patients who were to undergo knee arthroplasty had an evaluation made of knee motion prior to and after the administration of their epidural anesthetic. Although an average of 15° more motion was obtained in flexion once the patient's pain sensation had been eliminated, there was no significant change in extension.

What Factors in the Arthritic Patient's Knee Can Cause a Block to Full Extension?

Lack of full extension is commonly seen in patients with advanced arthritis who are candidates for knee arthroplasty. In the author's database of over 1500 patients undergoing TKA, the average block to full extension in patients with osteoarthritis was 5°. In patients with rheumatoid arthritis the mean flexion contracture was 10.5°, while in patients with post-traumatic arthritis it was 14°. It is fairly intuitive that this pre-operative contracture must be corrected at surgery if a postoperative contracture is to be avoided.

For patients with a flexion contracture less than 10°-15°, the culprit is usually anterior or posterior osteophytes (❏ Fig. 30-1). Anterior tibial osteophytes are normally removed when the proximal tibia is resected; however, posterior femoral osteophytes, which can tent the

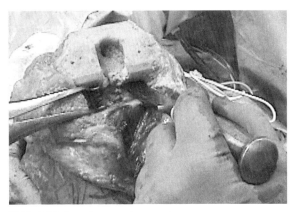

❏ **Fig. 30-2.** Removing posterior osteophytes

posterior capsule, are not easily visible during the surgical exposure [3].

Posterior femoral osteophytes can be most easily removed once the proximal tibia and posterior femur are resected. A laminar spreader is placed medially, and the knee, in 90° of flexion, is distracted. A curved osteotome and angled curettes will remove the posterior osteophytes from the medial femoral condyle (❏ Fig. 30-2). The position of the laminar spread is then changed to the medial side and a similar procedure is performed to remove any lateral femoral condylar osteophytes. Finally, a check should be made for any remaining osteophytes behind the posterior cruciate ligament.

For patients with a flexion contracture >15°, further releases are normally necessary. The next step should be elevation of the posterior capsule from the femur. The knee should be flexed maximally and laminar spreaders again placed between the femur and tibia. The posterior capsule of the knee can then be elevated for 1-2 cm from the proximal femur using a periosteal elevator [3]. For flexion contractures greater than 45° this same approach can be used to elevate the tendinous origins of the gastrocnemius muscle medial and laterally.

In 1991, the senior author reported his results using a technique of transverse sectioning of the posterior capsule [4], a technique that had initially been described by Insall [5]. The safety of this procedure was based on the assumption that, in flexion, the posterior neurovascular structures displaced posteriorly away from the posterior capsule. In actuality, the reverse is true, as described by Zaidi [6] in 1995. With knee flexion, the neurovascular bundle is displaced anteriorly and can lie tethered against the posterior capsule. For this reason, posterior capsule sectioning should not be routinely used, lest inadvertent popliteal artery and vein damage occur.

An apparently simple surgical solution to correct a block to full extension would be to remove extra bone from the distal femur, i.e., a segment of bone greater than the distal thickness of the femoral component that will be inserted. Whereas an extra resection of 3-4 mm can at

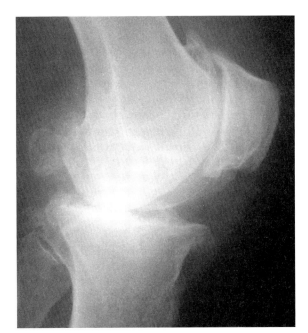

❏ **Fig. 30-1.** Multiple osteophytes

times be beneficial to help correct a block to full extension, further resection than this should usually not be performed. Doing so raises the joint line and adversely affects knee kinematics. It can also result in an extensor lag and, in the extreme, damage to the collateral ligament insertions on the femur.

What Factors in the Implant Itself May Lead to a Block to Full Extension?

All currently available total knee components, if they are properly aligned and positioned in the knee, allow complete knee extension. However, the surgeon has to be knowledgeable of the configuration of the tibial component in choosing the degree of posterior tibial slope that is to be created. For example, if the anterior portion of the tibial component is "built up", as is the case with some ultracongruent inserts, a posterior slope of the resection will lead to anterior impingement and a block to full extension. In these cases full extension is normally obtained by resecting the tibia at 90° to its anatomical axis in the sagittal plane, rather than the usual 3°-5° backslope.

What Factors of Surgical Technique May Lead to a Block of Full Extension?

Problems with the surgical technique itself can result in a block of full extension even in a patient who had full extension prior to the knee replacement. This occurs because of stuffing of the extension space.

The borders of the extension space are the resected surface of the distal femur and proximal tibia. The thickness of the space is related to the amount of bone and cartilage that has been removed and the elasticity of the surrounding capsular structures. It is this space which must be filled with implants of proper thickness if the knee is to be stable in extension. Likewise, overfilling of this space can lead to a potential block of full extension.

In most situations, the surgeon will remove bone equal in thickness to the distal thickness of the femoral component to be inserted. Doing this positions the prosthetic joint line at its proper proximal-distal level and enhances knee kinematics and patellar tracking [7]. Since the distal thickness of different implants vary (normally between 8 and 12 mm), the amount of resection will vary dependent upon the implant itself.

The thickness of proximal tibia that is removed varies. Most implant systems include some type of stylus device that senses the highest point on the "normal" tibial plateau and then positions the tibial cutting block a certain distance (normally 8-10 mm) below this. This method is applicable to many situations in which there is a "normal" (or at least

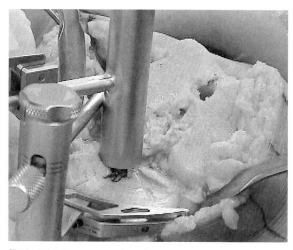

Fig. 30-3. Sensor, posterolaterally

a less abnormal) side remaining on the tibial surface, i.e., the lateral side in a patient with a varus deformity.

If one uses this method, the stylus must be placed at the lowest point of the normal side of the joint to judge the proper resection plane. For a varus knee, the stylus is placed laterally. Anatomically, the lateral tibial plateau is convex from front to back , and the lowest point is posterior, not in the center of the plateau (Fig. 30-3). Placing the stylus in the center of the plateau will result in insufficient bone being removed and will lead to a stuffed extension space. For a valgus knee, reference is made from the medial tibial plateau. Anatomically, that plateau is concave anterior to posterior so that the stylus there can be placed in the center of the surface.

The method of using the stylus on the lowest point of the good side becomes ineffectual in the patient with inflammatory arthritis, where both the medial and lateral sides are often affected to the same degree.

In order to avoid this problem, the senior author has adapted a method [8] which is a combination of the measured resection and extension space filling methods. The distal femur is resected as described above. The knee is then extended and tensed medially and laterally with laminar spreaders. A spacer block, equal to the sum of the distal dimension of the femoral component and the thinnest tibial component, is then set at the level of the cut surface of the femur. The inferior surface of the block marks the level for the tibial resection.

A block to full extension can also occur if the components are malpositioned. Although small degrees of malposition usually cause no statistical difference in the arc of motion [9], larger amounts can result in a flexion contracture. For example, the senior author has seen cases where flexion of the femoral component greater than 15°-20° from the anatomical axis of the femur in the sagittal plane rendered the knee unable to extend fully.

A situation often occurs where the knee fully extends with the trial implants in place and a thigh tourniquet inflated. However, after the tourniquet is released and the incision is closed, there appears to be a flexion contracture. This pseudo flexion contracture is secondary to a hemarthrosis. As such, in most cases it abates as the postoperative hemarthrosis abates.

Will a flexion contracture that remains at the end of the operation prior to tourniquet release gradually stretch out with time? Although there have been reports of this occurring [10, 11] this has not been the authors' experience. The degree of extension that is present with the implants in place and with the tourniquet inflated is most often the maximum extension that the patient will finally obtain.

On occasion, one encounters a patient who has undergone a revision operation during which his surgeon has "changed the polyethylene", inserting a thinner component in order to preclude a flexion contracture. One must seriously question whether full extension was ever obtained at the original surgery. The soft tissues of the knee are viscoelastic. If one presses hard enough with the patient under anesthesia it may appear that the knee is extending; however, as soon as the pressure is removed the knee will "spring back" into a mild flexion contracture. During testing of the knee, it should be allowed to come to full extension without pressure being placed on the patella lest a false evaluation be obtained.

Although full extension is the goal, there are situations in which full extension is not possible without marked shortening of the femur. Such might be the expected situation if knee arthroplasty were performed in patients with flexion contractures >60° [12]. Such situations were occasionally encountered in the early years of TKA, when patients would present to the surgeon after having been chair bound and nonambulatory for many years. With the knowledge of joint replacement that now exists among the medical and lay communities, seeing a patient at that late stage has become uncommon. For such a patient, pre-operative traction can often decrease the contracture to below 45°. The senior author has elected in those uncommon situations either to perform a femoral shortening and to accept an extensor lag or to allow a residual 10°-15° flexion contracture to remain rather than risking stretch injuries of the neurovascular structures.

The use of Botox injections into the hamstring muscles has recently been suggested for patients with severe flexion contractures secondary to cerebral palsy. This treatment may offer some promise for the patient with a severe pre-operative contracture in whom full extension is not possible at surgery without excessive femoral shortening.

Postoperative Factors

Despite proper surgery, a block to full extension may occur following surgery. If, for example, the patient uses pillows or other bolsters under the knee on a repeated basis during the first few postoperative weeks, a flexion contracture can develop. A flexion contracture can also develop if the patient is allowed to sleep in a continuous passive motion (CPM) machine. Observations of patients sleeping in a CPM unit will often reveal that the knee joint moves from the axis of flexion of the machine and never comes to full extension. This problem has become less prevalent now that CPM machines are not routinely used 23 h a day, a method that was recommended during the 1980s.

Problems in Adjacent Joints

There are patients with bilateral knee osteoarthritis and severe angular or flexion deformities who, because of concomitant medical problems, undergo the knee arthroplasty during two separate hospital stays, rather than simultaneously. The knee that has been operated upon first becomes longer than the contralateral side. To compensate for the leg length discrepancy, the patient will walk with the operated knee slightly flexed, and over a period of several months this can lead to a flexion contracture. The treatment is to place a lift on the shoe of the nonoperated leg until the time of its surgery. A similar problem can occur if the patient has a severe hip flexion contracture secondary to coxarthrosis. It most cases it is beneficial to treat the hip first to allow full extension and then, at a later time, perform the knee arthroplasty.

References

1. Perry J (1990) Pathologic gait. Instr Course Lect 39:325-331
2. Tew M, Forster IW (1987) Effect of knee replacement on flexion deformity. J Bone Joint Surg [Br] 69:395-399
3. Lombardi AV (2001) An algorithm for PCL in TKA. Clin Orthop Rel Res 392:75-87
4. Laskin RS The PS total knee prosthesis in the knee with severe fixed varus deformity.
5. Insall JN, Scott WN, Ranawat CS (1979) The total condylar knee prosthesis. A report of two hundred and twenty cases. J Bone Joint Surg [Am] 61:173-182
6. Zaidi SH, Cobb AJ, Bentley G (1995) Danger to the popliteal artery in high tibial osteotomy. J Bone Joint Surg [Br] 77:384-386
7. Yoshii I, Whiteside LA, White SE, Milliano MT (1991) Influence of prosthetic joint line position on knee kinematics and patellar position. J Arthroplasty 6:169-177
8. Laskin RS (1991) Soft tissue techniques in total knee replacement. In: Laskin RS (ed) Total knee replacement. Springer-Verlag, London, pp 41-53
9. Ritter MA, Stringer EA (1979) Predictive range of motion after total knee replacement. Clin Orthop 143:115-119
10. Tanzer M, Miller J (1989) The natural history of flexion contracture in total knee arthroplasty. A prospective study. Clin Orthop 248:129-134
11. Mc Pherson EJ, Cushner FD, Schiff CF, et al (1994) Natural history of uncorrected flexion contractures following total knee arthroplasty. J Arthroplasty 9:499-502
12. Lu H, Mow CS, Lin J (1999) Total knee arthroplasty in the presence of severe flexion contracture: a report of 37 cases. J Arthroplasty 14:775-780

31   Understanding the Rheumatoid Knee

K. K. Anbari, J. P. Garino

Summary

Total knee arthroplasty in the rheumatoid patient presents unique challenges, including the systemic nature of the patient's disease, the presence of significant soft-tissue deformities and osteopenic bone, and an increased risk of complications such as wound healing and persistent contractures. In order to maximize the probability of a successful outcome, the surgeon must optimize the patient's pre-operative medical status, pay meticulous attention to soft-tissue balancing and contracture release in the operating room, and closely monitor the patient's postoperative course. Adherence to these principles optimizes the results of total knee arthroplasty in the rheumatoid patient, making this a very rewarding procedure for both patient and surgeon.

Introduction

The knee joint is affected in approximately 90% of patients with chronic rheumatoid arthritis [1]. Total knee arthroplasty (TKA) provides the rheumatoid patient with substantial alleviation of pain and deformity. However, the rheumatoid knee presents several challenges to the surgeon in the operating room as well as in the pre- and postoperative stages. Rheumatoid arthritis is a systemic disease that affects multiple organ systems, and rheumatoid patients frequently take several immunosuppressive medications that must be addressed in the perioperative period. The surgeon encounters several important issues when planning knee arthroplasty, including the timing of knee surgery relative to other arthritic joints and the choice of anesthesia. At the time of surgery, the rheumatoid knee is characterized by osteopenic bone, valgus deformity with a frequently incompetent medial collateral ligament, and soft-tissue contractures. The level of constraint of the prosthesis is an important decision. Extreme care must be given to soft-tissue balancing. Postoperatively, the rheumatoid patient may be affected by wound-healing problems, infection, and loss of full extension. This chapter discusses the issues of importance to the surgeon performing knee arthroplasty in the rheumatoid patient.

Preoperative Considerations and Planning

The systemic involvement in rheumatoid patients is an important issue in the preoperative period. Several organ systems are affected by the disease as well as by the immunosuppressive medications commonly used to treat it. Approximately 10% of rheumatoid patients undergoing total knee arthroplasty are taking maintenance corticosteroids [1].

Systemic Manifestations of Rheumatoid Arthritis

Rheumatoid patients should routinely undergo a complete medical evaluation prior to knee arthroplasty. This evaluation should also include a complete blood count, urinalysis, urine culture, electrolytes, and an electrocardiogram [2]. The evaluation should include examining the patient for remote sites of potential infection such as the oral cavity. The skin over the knee in rheumatoid patients may be thin and atrophic secondary to chronic steroid therapy or as a manifestation of the disease process. Rheumatoid arthritis is considered to be a catabolic, wasting disease. Therefore, many rheumatoid patients may be malnourished even if they are not clinically underweight [3].

Management of Corticosteroids

It has been common practice to administer stress-dose steroids at the time of surgery to patients who take chronic maintenance steroids. The purpose of this is to prevent adrenal insufficiency, particularly in patients who take relatively high doses of steroids (more than 20-30 mg hydrocortisone daily) [2]. It is our practice to administer 100 mg hydrocortisone iv before surgery and then Q8H for three doses after surgery. However, the need for routine exogenous steroid administration has been questioned in one study. Friedman et al. [4] reported on 28 patients taking chronic steroids who underwent 35 major orthopedic surgeries. Patients were given only their usual doses of oral steroids without supplementation. No patients had evidence of adrenal insufficiency on physical exam or laboratory criteria.

Management of Other Immunosuppressive Medications

There exists conflicting evidence regarding the decision to discontinue non-steroid rheumatoid medications at the time of surgery. Grennan et al. [5] described a prospective randomized study of 388 rheumatoid patients undergoing orthopedic surgery. The study found that certain remittive agents such as penicillamine, hydroxychloroquine, and cyclosporine were associated with statistically significant increased risk of wound problems. However, patients who continued to take methotrexate had no increase in wound complications and experienced fewer rheumatoid flares than those who did not receive methotrexate. In contrast, Bridges et al. [6] reported on 38 rheumatoid patients undergoing elective orthopedic surgery. There were four infections in 19 procedures performed on patients who took methotrexate around the time of surgery, compared with no complications in 34 procedures for patients who discontinued methotrexate 4 weeks before surgery. Other sources recommend discontinuing methotrexate and other similar agents 1-2 weeks before surgery and restarting them 1-2 weeks after surgery [2]. It remains our practice to discontinue these medications for 2 weeks before surgery and to restart them 1 week thereafter.

There is scant information in the literature about the treatment of the newer anticytokine agents such as etanercept in the perioperative period. One case report [7] describes disseminated joint infections and fatal septic shock in a rheumatoid patient on etanercept who had a history of bilateral hip and knee prostheses. The authors caution that etanercept may mask the signs of acute infection and inflammation, and that a patient on this agent should be monitored closely for early symptoms of infection and be treated aggressively.

Timing of Knee Arthroplasty Relative to Other Orthopedic Surgery

The rheumatoid patient presenting with end-stage knee arthritis may also suffer from joint pain and deformity in the spine, upper extremities, hips, and feet.

Cervical Spine. It is important for the arthroplasty surgeon to evaluate the rheumatoid patient for evidence of cervical spine disease. It is estimated that 88% of rheumatoid patients have some degree of cervical spine involvement

[8]. The most common manifestations of this are atlantoaxial subluxation, basilar invagination, and subaxial subluxation. The surgeon should obtain a thorough history, looking for worrisome signs such as neck pain extending to the head, upper or lower extremity weakness, urinary or bowel incontinence, dysphagia, and loss of fine motor coordination. The physical examination should include neurological motor and sensory testing of the upper and lower extremities. Any positive finding should be further investigated with cervical spine radiographs including AP, flexion and extension lateral, and odontoid views. Because of the devastating complications that may arise from spinal instability, stabilization of the cervical spine takes first priority in the rheumatoid patient. It is important to note that despite the progressive nature of cervical rheumatoid disease, only 15% of rheumatoid patients require cervical spine surgery [9]. Our practice has been to obtain cervical spine radiographic series if there are any concerns in the history or physical, and subsequently to refer the patient for orthopedic spine evaluation if the radiographs demonstrate instability. Finally, cervical spine involvement complicates the options for anesthesia as discussed below.

Upper Extremity. It is usually advisable for the rheumatoid patient to undergo lower extremity joint reconstruction before shoulder or elbow reconstruction to avoid stressing upper extremity prosthetic joints with the use of crutches or a walker. Furthermore, addressing lower extremity joints promptly may spare the debilitated patient from becoming wheelchair bound and preserve mobility. Occasionally, a rheumatoid patient may have such severe limitation of upper extremity or hand function that use of assistive devices after knee arthroplasty may be impossible. In these cases, we turn our attention to the upper extremity first.

Hip Versus Knee Reconstruction. When both the hip and the knee need surgical reconstruction, it is usually preferable to begin with the hip [3, 8]. Rehabilitation of a hip arthroplasty may proceed with a diseased ipsilateral knee more effectively than rehabilitation of a knee with a diseased ipsilateral hip. However, there are important exceptions. First, a rheumatoid knee with severe valgus deformity would jeopardize the stability of an ipsilateral hip because of the resulting hip internal rotation and adduction. In this circumstance, it may be safer to proceed with knee arthroplasty first. Second, a patient with severe bilateral knee flexion contractures would have difficulty standing erect until both knees are reconstructed. Such a patient would be a good candidate for bilateral knee arthroplasty if medically appropriate. We have found that in selected cases, simultaneous ipsilateral hip and knee arthroplasty could be given consideration as well.

Anesthesia for Knee Arthroplasty in the Rheumatoid Patient. Administering safe anesthesia can be challenging in the rheumatoid patient because of the systemic nature of the disease and the multiple medications used to treat it. An anesthesiologist with experience in this situation is crucial to a good outcome. If intubation is necessary, fiberoptic management of the airway may be advisable to avoid excessive manipulation of the cervical spine [10]. The thoracic, lumbar, and sacral portions of the spine are usually spared in rheumatoid patients, making regional spinal anesthesia ideal in these patients. Regional anesthesia also provides the advantages of blunting the neurohormonal response to surgery and offering effective postoperative analgesia.

Intraoperative Options

The surgeon faces several important choices when deciding on the optimal prosthesis and surgical technique for a rheumatoid knee. This section reviews the literature and gives the authors' perspective.

Cemented Versus Cementless. The evidence in the literature has been inconsistent regarding whether cementless fixation has a role in the treatment of the rheumatoid knee. There are several studies with a relatively small number of patients that show adequate results for cementless knees in the intermediate term, but with some concerns, nonetheless. Schroder et al. reported on 41 cementless knees in rheumatoid patients with an average follow-up of 54 months [11] and described one tibial revision and five tibias with radiolucencies. While these authors quoted a favorable success rate of 97% (40/41) after 4-5 years, these results were not long term. Another study of 103 cementless knees implanted in patients with rheumatoid arthritis or osteoarthritis described two tibial revisions for aseptic loosening, two tibias with asymptomatic loosening, and four tibias with lucent lines at a follow-up period of 3 years [12]. Rosenqvist et al. [13] showed that more than half of 34 porous-coated anatomical (PCA) knee arthroplasties demonstrated radiographic evidence of displacement, and all knees had a radiolucent zone at an average of 17 months. Analysis of 3054 rheumatoid knees from the Swedish Knee Arthroplasty Register for which data on cementation were available showed statistically significant reduction in loosening as well as revision rate in the cemented knees [14]. Bogoch and Moran commented on the issue of cementless knees for rheumatoid patients [15]. They stated that in the absence of convincing evidence favoring cementless knees and because of the good long-term results with cemented knees, cemented knee arthroplasty was preferred in this patient population. Our practice is to perform cemented knee arthroplasty in this population because of

consistently good results as well as the ability to mobilize the debilitated rheumatoid patient with immediate weight-bearing.

Patellar Resurfacing. We favor routine resurfacing of the patella in all rheumatoid patients, based on extensive evidence in the literature. Remaining articular cartilage on the undersurface of the patella may provide an antigenic stimulus in the rheumatoid knee that allows the synovial inflammation to persist, leading to anterior knee pain [16]. In a large study involving more than 27000 total knee replacements from the Swedish Knee Arthroplasty Register [17], there was a higher proportion of satisfied patients in the patellar resurfacing group, both for rheumatoid patients and overall. An interesting study examined in a prospective fashion 35 rheumatoid patients who underwent simultaneous bilateral TKA with resurfacing of one randomly chosen patella while leaving the contralateral one unresurfaced [18, 19]. At 2-year minimum follow-up, Hospital for Special Surgery knee scores and range of motion were similar in the two sets of knees [18]; this result was corroborated at 6-year minimum follow-up [19]. However, the authors evaluated parameters specific to the patellofemoral joint at 6-year follow-up that they did not at 2-year follow-up, namely, tenderness over the patellofemoral joint and pain with using stairs. They reported that patellofemoral tenderness and pain with stairs were found in eight and nine unresurfaced knees, respectively, out of 26 knees remaining in the study. None of the resurfaced knees had these symptoms. They therefore recommended routine patellar resurfacing based on these results. Finally, even when another group of authors [20] resurfaced the patella selectively (i.e., only when the surgeon found loss of cartilage under the patella, exposed bone, gross surface irregularity, or abnormal tracking), they found a higher proportion of anterior knee pain in the unresurfaced group versus the resurfaced group at a mean of 6.5 years. These authors similarly recommended routine resurfacing of the patella.

Posterior Cruciate-Retaining Versus -Substituting Designs. While both cruciate-retaining and cruciate-substituting designs have excellent results in the osteoarthritic knee, outcomes in rheumatoid knees have been less consistent. The concern with cruciate-retaining prostheses is that the inflammatory process in rheumatoid arthritis compromises the PCL, exposing the patient to the risk of late rupture of the PCL and posterior instability. To be sure, cruciate-retaining prostheses have strong proponents in the literature. Schai et al. [21] reported on 81 rheumatoid knee arthroplasties using cruciate-retaining components followed for 10-13 years. The authors reported 13-year survivorship of 97%. Furthermore, they did not observe any late instability from PCL attenuation or rupture. Two knees were revised for reasons unrelated to the cruciate-retaining design (failed metal-backed patella and severe synovitis necessitating synovectomy). Archibeck et al. [22] described 72 cruciate-retaining TKAs in 51 rheumatoid patients for a mean of 10.5 years. Nine of 72 knees required revision operations, but six of these revisions were performed for failure of a metal-backed patellar component. The rate of 10-year survival was 93% with the end point being femoral or tibial revision. Two of the 72 knees had posterior instability. Therefore, the authors of both of these reports preferred cruciate-retaining TKA, even in the rheumatoid patient. The findings of these reports were contradicted by Laskin and O'Flynn [23], who reviewed the outcomes of 98 rheumatoid knees treated with cruciate-retaining prostheses at minimum 6-year follow-up. Fifty percent of 98 knees demonstrated posterior instability of 10 mm or more, compared with 1% of 80 rheumatoid knees treated with a posterior-stabilized prosthesis. Eleven patients in the cruciate-retaining group required revision for instability, and the PCL was not identifiable in any of them during the revision surgery. These authors advocated posterior-stabilized TKA in rheumatoid knees. Basic science research demonstrates that the PCL in rheumatoid knees shows evidence of degeneration and collagen breakdown using light and electron microscopy, respectively, and that the PCL is biomechanically less elastic and less resistant to rupture than in normal knees [24-26]. We favor substitution of the PCL in all rheumatoid patients because of the consistently excellent results obtainable with this design and because of insufficient evidence that cruciate-retaining TKA provides significant advantages to the patient.

Surgical Technique

While some rheumatoid patients have ligamentous laxity with no fixed deformity, rheumatoid knees often present with severe soft-tissue contractures [1]. Additionally, rheumatoid bone is usually weakened secondary to disuse osteopenia and steroid intake. This section describes the surgical technique for rheumatoid TKA with special attention to the difficult areas of exposure, angular deformity, weak bone, and flexion contracture (Fig. 31-1).

The Typical Rheumatoid Knee. The surgeon must be mindful of the compromised bone quality in the rheumatoid knee. The bone may be directly involved in the inflammatory process by infiltration of the rheumatoid granulation tissue into subchondral bone, and prostaglandin release by nearby synovial tissue can lead to bone resorption and osteopenia in the rheumatoid knee [1]. The stiffness of proximal tibial cancellous bone in rheumatoid patients is approximately 675 N/mm, compared with 1287 N/mm for normal bone and 1116 N/mm for osteoarthritic bone [15]. Therefore, excessive retraction or manipulation of the extremity during surgery can lead to inadvertent fractures. Furthermore, rheumatoid knees more often than not have an angular deformity. In a study of 99 rheumatoid knees [27], 38% were in valgus, 31% in varus, and 30% had no angular deformity. Forty-four percent of all knees studied had a flexion contracture over 10°.

Exposure. We use the standard anterior midline skin incision followed by a medial parapatellar arthrotomy. A complete synovectomy is recommended to minimize the likelihood of a recurrent inflammatory synovitis after TKA. The fatty tissue between the anterior femur and synovium should be preserved to avoid adhesions. The patella is everted, and the rest of the knee exposure is performed in the usual manner.

If exposure of the knee proves to be difficult, and proximal and distal extension of the arthrotomy does not pro-

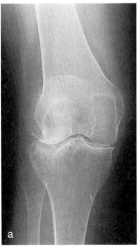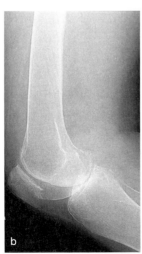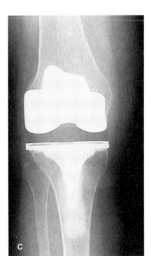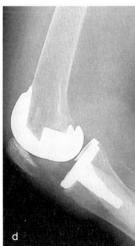

Fig. 31-1a-d. Total knee arthroplasty in a 46-year-old rheumatoid patient. *a, b* AP and lateral radiographs of the knee preoperatively. *c, d* AP and lateral radiographs of the knee 3.5 years postoperatively

vide adequate exposure, a quadriceps snip (proximal and lateral extension of the quadriceps arthrotomy) is sometimes necessary. This allows easier eversion of the patella. The quadriceps snip is repaired securely at the end of surgery and it does not typically result in postoperative quadriceps weakness [27]. A complete patellofemoral turndown is very rarely required; this involves extending the capsular incision laterally and distally, starting at the proximal end of the medial parapatellar arthrotomy. This technique provides unparalleled exposure but it commonly results in quadriceps weakness and an extensor lag.

Medial Release. Some degree of medial dissection is necessary to allow enough exposure to perform the surgery in any knee. The extent of medial release is dependent on the pre-existing varus deformity, and as mentioned above, varus alignment is not uncommon in rheumatoid knees. The medial release begins with raising a periosteal flap on the proximal medial tibia and extending distally and posteriorly as necessary. This involves raising the deep portion of the medial collateral ligament, elevation of the semimembranosus insertion, and removal of medial osteophytes. It is sometimes necessary to elevate a medial soft-tissue flap more distally on the tibia to achieve adequate medial release. Despite these releases, the knee may, rarely, remain asymmetric with lateral laxity and medial tightness. In this case, we use a constrained condylar knee prosthesis.

Lateral Release. Valgus deformity is comparatively more common in the rheumatoid population and can present a challenge to achieving soft-tissue balance. The lateral structures, including the iliotibial band, lateral collateral ligament (LCL), popliteus tendon, and lateral joint capsule are contracted in a valgus knee with relative laxity of the medial structures. After femoral and tibial lateral osteophytes have been resected, the tightest structure is usually the iliotibial band, and it should be released from its tibial insertion. The posterolateral capsule is subsequently detached from the femur with a periosteal elevator. If more release is necessary (such as when the valgus deformity is greater than 15°), the popliteus tendon, followed by the LCL, may be released from their femoral origin. Rarely, the femoral origin of the lateral head of the gastrocnemius may require release by sharp dissection with the knee in flexion [27]. In the course of this dissection, the inferolateral geniculate branch should be cauterized to prevent excessive bleeding. The purpose of these releases is to match the relative laxity of the medial side of the knee and achieve a rectangular gap in flexion and extension. This may not always be possible in severely deformed knees and may necessitate the use of a constrained prosthesis. As described below, this becomes particularly important in combined valgus and flexion contracture deformities.

Bone Cuts. After soft-tissue releases have been performed as required by the deformity, the bone is prepared to accept the prosthesis. We use the measured resection technique, removing an amount of bone equal to the dimensions of the prosthesis. The distal femur is cut in 6° of valgus, based on an intramedullary guide rod. The anterior and posterior cuts are made in a few degrees of external rotation, as determined by Whiteside's line and the transepicondylar axis. The tibia is cut with an extramedullary guide, removing 8-10 mm of the proximal tibia.

Flexion Contracture. The flexion and extension gaps can now be assessed. The bone cuts provide access to the posterior aspect of the knee, and posterior osteophytes are removed with a curved osteotome. This occasionally is all that is required to correct a mild flexion contracture. If more correction is necessary, a periosteal elevator is used to release the capsule from the posterior femur [28] (◘ Fig. 31-2).

The attachments of the cruciate ligaments are released completely from the intercondylar notch. To achieve even more correction, the origin of the gastrocnemius muscle is dissected from the posterior distal femur. If necessary, the release can be brought medially and laterally around the femur to the posterior aspects of the insertions of the collateral ligaments without sacrificing the integrity of the ligaments. At this point, the next step in achieving flexion-extension balance is resecting more distal femoral bone. This should be used as a last resort after the posterior structures are fully released, since resecting more distal femur elevates the joint line and can

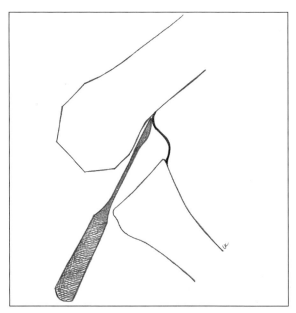

◘ **Fig. 31-2.** Posterior capsular release for flexion contracture after osteophyte removal. (Drawn by Lisa Khoury, MD; University of Pennsylvania Health System)

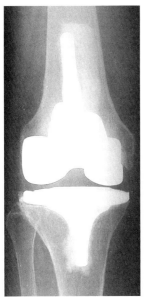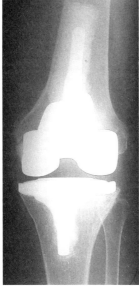

Fig. 31-3. Bilateral total knee arthroplasty using constrained prostheses and stems in a 68-year-old rheumatoid patient. Instability with standard components was found to be excessive, and constrained femoral components with stems were used

result in lax collateral ligaments, particularly in mid flexion. If these releases achieve good, stable extension but result in looseness in flexion, the surgeon may consider upsizing the femoral component and using augments posteriorly. This would add stability to the knee in flexion. Doing so would be appropriate as long as the femoral component remains well sized in the mediolateral dimension.

If the knee can achieve adequate extension only by sacrificing stability in flexion, then we have a low threshold to using a constrained device in this case. Of course, constraint has the disadvantage of transferring shear and rotational stresses to the bone-cement interface, which can adversely affect implant longevity. Therefore, we would resort to it only when the flexion laxity is severe and would lead to a functional disability, and after a full posterior release has been performed. We also favor the use of stems with a constrained device.

With loss or incompetence of the medial collateral ligament, the stresses normally attenuated by this structure can lead to premature loosening. Stem use has been shown to be advantageous when higher levels of constraint are necessary [29] (Fig. 31-3).

It is important to guard against losing extension postoperatively in these knees. This may be accomplished by casting the knee in extension and by diligent physical therapy to maintain extension [1].

Implantation and Closure. When the surgeon is satisfied with the soft-tissue balancing and trial components, the knee is irrigated and the components are cemented. The arthrotomy is repaired. We do not typically use a drain. A meticulous closure is done while minimizing trauma to the subcutaneous tissues.

Postoperative Rehabilitation

The reconstructed knee is examined at the end of the procedure to determine if there is any residual flexion contracture. If the knee easily comes to full extension, a soft dressing is applied and a continuous passive motion device is used in the recovery unit. But if the last few degrees of extension can be achieved only with passive pressure applied anteriorly by the surgeon, the knee should be placed in a cylinder cast. We also utilize a cylinder cast when the soft tissue overlying the prosthesis is thin and tenuous; this enhances the potential for uneventful wound healing. The cast can be removed at 3-7 days postoperatively, and then physical therapy for gentle range of motion is started. The physical therapist should pay particular attention to maintaining full extension, particularly in knees that were contracted chronically prior to surgery. The surgeon must be vigilant regarding signs or symptoms of infection. There is a significantly increased risk of deep prosthetic infection in rheumatoid patients compared with osteoarthritic patients [30]. Prolonged drainage from a seroma or hematoma should be treated aggressively with débridement to prevent bacterial seeding of the prosthetic joint.

Results

Overall, the results of knee arthroplasty in the rheumatoid population have been excellent. Robertsson et al. [14] desribed the results of 4143 primary tricompartmental knee replacements from the Swedish Knee Arthroplasty Register. They reported a cumulative revision rate of 5% at 10 years. A survey of patient satisfaction from the same group of patients [17] demonstrated higher satisfaction rates among rheumatoid patients than among patients with osteoarthritis. These findings may be secondary to the lower demand placed on the prosthesis by sedentary rheumatoid patients. Therefore, despite the multiple challenges inherent in knee arthroplasty in the rheumatoid patient, excellent pain relief and durable restoration of function can be expected from the procedure.

References

1. Chmell MJ, Scott RD (1999) Total knee arthroplasty in patients with rheumatoid arthritis. Clin Orthop 366:54-60
2. MacKenzie CR, Sharrock NE (1998) Perioperative medical considerations in patients with rheumatoid arthritis. Rheum Dis Clin North Am 24:1-17

3. Stuchin SA, Johanson NA, Lachiewicz PF, Mont MA (1999) Surgical management of inflammatory arthritis of the adult hip and knee. Instructional Course Lectures 48:93-109
4. Friedman RJ, Schiff CF, Bromberg JS (1995) Use of supplemental steroids in patients having orthopaedic operations. J Bone Joint Surg [Am] 77:1801-6
5. Grennan DM, Gray J, Loudon J, Fear S (2001) Methotrexate and early postoperative complications in patients with rheumatoid arthritis undergoing elective orthopaedic surgery. Ann Rheum Dis 60:214-217
6. Bridges SL, Lopez-Mendez A, Han KH, Alarcon GS (1991) Should methotrexate be discontinued before elective orthopedic surgery in patients with rheumatoid arthritis? J Rheum 18:984-988
7. Baghai M, Osmond DR, Wolk D, Wold LE, Haidukewych GJ, Matteson E (2001) Fatal sepsis in a patient with rheumatoid arthritis treated with etanercept. Mayo Clin Proc 76:653-656
8. Dunbar RP, Alexiades MM (1998): Decision making in rheumatoid arthritis. Rheum Dis Clin North Am 24:35-54
9. Pellicci PM, Ranawat CS, Tsairis P, et al (1981) The natural history of rheumatoid arthritis of the cervical spine. J Bone Joint Surg [Am] 63:342-350
10. Matti MV, Sharrock NE (1998) Anesthesia on the rheumatoid patient. Rheum Dis Clin North Am 24:19-33
11. Schroder HM, Aaen K, Hansen EB, Nielsen PT, Rechnagel K (1996) Cementless total knee arthroplasty in rheumatoid arthritis. A report on 51 AGC knees followed for 54 months. J Arthroplasty 11:18-23
12. Nielsen PT, Hansen EB, Rechnagel K (1992) Cementless total knee arthroplasty in unselected cases of osteoarthritis and rheumatoid arthritis. A 3-year follow-up study of 103 cases. J Arthroplasty 7:137-143
13. Rosenqvist R, Bylander B, Knutson K, Rydholm U, Rooser B, Egund N, Lidgren L (1986) Loosening of the porous coating of bicompartmental prostheses in patients with rheumatoid arthritis. J Bone Joint Surg [Am] 68:538-542
14. Robertsson O, Knutson K, Lewold S, Goodman S, Lidgren L (1997) Knee arthroplasty in rheumatoid arthritis; a report from the Swedish Knee Arthroplasty Register on 4381 primary operations 1985-1995. Acta Orthop Scand 68:545-553
15. Bogoch ER and Moran EL (1999) Bone abnormalities in the surgical treatment of patients with rheumatoid arthritis. Clin Orthop 366:8-21
16. Burnett RS and Bourne RB (2003) Indications for patellar resurfacing in total knee arthroplasty. J Bone Joint Surg [Am] 85:728-745
17. Robertsson O, Dunbar M, Pehrsson T, Knutson K, Lidgren L (2000) Patient satisfaction after knee arthroplasty: a report on 27,372 knees operated on between 1981 and 1995 in Sweden. Acta Orthop Scand 71:262-267
18. Shoji H, Yoshino S, Kajino A (1989) Patellar replacement in bilateral total knee arthroplasty. A study of patients who had rheumatoid arthritis and no gross deformity of the patella. J Bone Joint Surg [Am] 71:853-856
19. Kajino A, Yoshino S, Kameyama S, Kohda M, Nagashima S (1997) Comparison of the results of bilateral total knee arthroplasty with and without patellar replacement for rheumatoid arthritis. A follow-up note. J Bone Joint Surg [Am] 79:570-574
20. Boyd AD Jr, Ewald FC, Thomas WH, Poss R, Sledge CB (1993) Long-term complications after total knee arthroplasty with or without resurfacing of the patella. J Bone Joint Surg [Am] 75:674-681
21. Schai PA, Scott RA, Thornhill TS (1999) Total knee arthroplasty with posterior cruciate retention in patients with rheumatoid arthritis. Clin Orthop 367:96-106
22. Archibeck MJ, Berger RA, Barden RM, Jacobs JJ, Sheinkop MB, Rosenberg AG, Galante JO (2001) Posterior cruciate ligament-retaining total knee arthroplasty in patients with rheumatoid arthritis. J Bone Joint Surg [Am] 83:1231-1236
23. Laskin RS and O'Flynn HM (1997) Total knee replacement with posterior cruciate ligament retention in rheumatoid arthritis: problems and complications. Clin Orthop 345:24-28
24. Alexiades M, Scuderi G, Vigorita V, et al (1983) A histological study of the posterior cruciate ligament in the arthritic knee. Am J Knee Surg 64A:1328-1333
25. Neurath MF (1993) Detection of Luse bodies, spiraled collagen, dysplastic collagen, and intracellular collagen in rheumatoid connective tissues: an electron microscopic study. Ann Rheum Dis 52:278-284
26. Hagena FW, Hoffman GO, Mittlemeier T, et al (1999) The cruciate ligaments in knee replacement. Int Orthop 249:9-12
27. Aglietti P, Buzzi R (2002) Correction of combined deformity. In: Scuderi GR, Tria A (eds) Surgical techniques in total knee arthroplasty, 1st edn. Springer-Verlag, Berlin Heidelberg New York
28. Lotke PA, Simon RG (2002) Flexion contracture in total knee arthroplasty. In: Scuderi GR, Tria A (eds) Surgical techniques in total knee arthroplasty, 1st edn. Springer-Verlag, Berlin Heidelberg New York
29. Garino JP, Lotke PA (1999) Fixation techniques in revision total knee surgery: stem designs, rationale, and fixation. In: Lotke PA, Garino JP (eds) Revision total knee arthroplasty, 1st edn. Lippincott-Raven, Philadelphia
30. Sculco TP (1998) The knee joint in rheumatoid arthritis. Rheum Dis Clin North Am 24:143-156

31

32 Management of Extra-Articular Deformities in Total Knee Arthroplasty

K. G. Vince, V. Bozic

Summary

Limb alignment, whether "intra-", or "extra-" articular is the key to success of an arthroplasty. Malalignment of a knee replacement may result in component loosening, prosthetic wear, instability and patellar complications. It is the alignment of the entire limb, from the hip to the knee to the ankle and referred to as the mechanical axis, that is important, not just the alignment of the knee joint. Component position in the plane of motion of the joint is less important, but correct rotational positioning is essential.

A "neutral mechanical axis" or straight line through the centers of the hip, knee, and ankle results from the angular position of the tibial and femoral components. The joint must then be stabilized with either ligamentous releases or mechanically constrained implants. Extra-articular deformities pose technical challenges.

Bone deformities may be corrected outside or inside the arthroplasty. In the first case, a corrective osteotomy may be performed at the site of the deformity (a fracture malunion or the apex of a rickets deformity) or closer to the joint where it may be performed concurrent with the arthroplasty. If an extra-articular deformity is corrected inside the joint, aggressive and even innovative soft-tissue procedures or a constrained implant will be required to stabilize the knee.

Introduction

Extra-articular deformity is no less important than deformity of the joint itself for surgeons considering knee arthroplasty, but it does pose unique technical challenges [1-6]. Limb alignment is the key to controlling forces across the knee- forces that are usually responsible for failure of the arthroplasty. These deformities may have genetic (tibiae vara), metabolic (rickets), or traumatic origins (fracture malunion or osteotomy) They may be considered "extra-articular" when present in the femur proximal to the epicondyles or distal to the tip of the fibula [1] (beyond the attachments of the collateral ligaments). They must not compromise the arthroplasty; it must be remembered that it is the alignment not of the knee, but of the entire limb that matters.

Lotke and Ecker established the importance of alignment in 1977 [7] and John Insall, instrumental in developing ligament balancing techniques, confirmed this observation with 10-12 years follow-up [8]. The problems of malalignment are manifold. Varus is associated with tibial loosening, breakage, wear, and osteolysis. Valgus exacerbates instability and patellar maltracking. More recent studies reveal how patellar complications (originating in maltracking), knee stiffness, and instability result from rotational malalignment.

Alignment may be restored in the presence of extra-articular deformity through corrective osteotomy at the site of deformity, compensatory osteotomy distant from the deformity, and intra-articular correction through positioning of components. The preferred technique depends on the specifics of the deformity.

Intramedullary instrumentation and rotational landmarks, so useful in routine knee replacement surgery, fail in the presence of extra-articular deformity. Extramedullary instruments and recent navigation systems enable surgeons to accurately "look beyond" extra-articular deformities and visualize the articulations above and below the knee.

Understanding Alignment: the Anteroposterior Radiograph

The point has been made that if one considers the "six degrees of freedom" in terms of potential component positioning, the potential for error is immense [9]. Extra-articular deformity can confound the positioning of tibial and femoral components in all directions. The word "alignment" is most commonly associated in the minds of surgeons with the varus and valgus angles on an anteroposterior radiograph. This can be expressed as either the "anatomical" or the "mechanical" axis of the knee joint. The former refers to the angle formed by the intersection of the axes of the intramedullary canals of the tibia and the femur. This is a useful and pragmatic frame of reference, as this is precisely what we see on a conventional radiograph, what we expose surgically, and where we place instruments during an arthroplasty. It is only useful, however, because it approximates the more important "mechanical axis".

The mechanical axis is the angle formed by two lines: one that connects the centers of the hip and the knee and another that connects the centers of the knee and the ankle. This "mechanical axis" is more important, because it is not influenced by deformity between these joints. There is general agreement that the goal of arthroplasty surgery is to re-establish a "neutral mechanical axis", an angle of 180° or a "straight line" that passes through the center of each joint (◘ Fig. 32-1).

Mechanical alignment can also be expressed, not as the angle of intersection of the mechanical axis of the femur and tibia but as the point where a line from the center of the hip to the center of the ankle intersects the knee joint line or its theoretical extension into space [10]. Deformity would then be expressed as a linear measurement, or deviation from the center of the knee and not as an angle. This is less useful in planning surgery. We must acknowledge, however, that these are all "static" and structural evaluations that neglect potentially formidable dynamic effects [11].

Normal knee alignment (assuming ligamentous integrity), as viewed on an anteroposterior radiograph, is comprised of the respective angles of the articular surfaces of the distal femur and proximal tibia. Similarly, the alignment of an arthroplasty results from the positioning of the respective components. With ligament compromise, the sum of the distal femoral articular surface and tibial articular surface, plus the ligamentous instability, will equal the alignment. Extra-articular deformity, whether from fracture, osteotomy, or unusual anatomy, adds to this equation.

Surgical Alignment

Moreland and colleagues quantified normal lower extremity alignment in a study of UCLA resident physician volunteers [12] (Fig. 32-1). This raises the question as to whether knee arthroplasties should be aligned in "normal alignment" or some mechanically more advantageous alternative, such as a neutral mechanical axis. The idea that patients are somehow restored to normal alignment by knee arthroplasty is suspect. Indeed, many individuals become arthritic because a "normal" tendency to varus (or valgus) has overloaded one compartment, leading to cartilage failure. Accordingly, the releases that confer stability to a re-aligned joint are also non-anatomical, though highly effective at reducing load on the knee joint and enhancing durability. This means that, irrespective of deformity, we must ultimately place the tibial component at right angles to the axis of the tibia and the femoral component at right angles to the "mechanical" axis of the femur, i.e., the line drawn from the center of the femoral head to the center of the knee joint.

Radiographic Assessment of Alignment

How can alignment be assessed most accurately? Small X-ray cassettes and non-weight-bearing films are both inaccurate. Radiographs must show enough of the medullary canal to approximate the anatomical (let alone the mechanical) axis. Similarly, unless the patient is bearing weight we will not appreciate the effects of instability, pseudo laxity, and cartilage loss on alignment. While the full-length radiograph shows the hip, knee, and ankle (i.e., the mechanical axis), vagaries of rotational positioning may compromise these studies as well [13].

Extra-articular deformity requires the full-length radiograph. The tibia is resected at right angles to its long axis and the femoral cut is planned at right angles to the mechanical axis, to the line drawn from the center of the femoral head to the center of the knee. The divergence between the femoral mechanical axis and the intramedullary canal will be the desired amount (of valgus) that is selected on an intramedullary femoral guide. The discrepancy between the angle of the distal femur and the proximal tibia will usually be eliminated by ligament

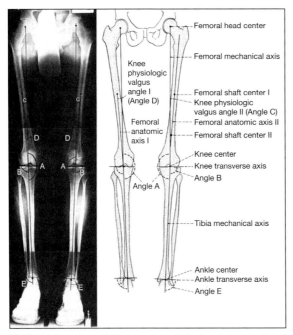

◘ **Fig. 32-1.** Mechanical alignment is established as the intersection of a line from the center of the hip to the center of the knee, and another from the center of the knee to the center of the ankle. Anatomical axis is the intersection of the intra-medullary axes of the tibia and femur. (From [12], Fig. 3)

releases, occasionally by constrained implants, and rarely by ligament reconstruction.

Lateral Alignment

Sagittal alignment of the limb and components (as viewed on a lateral radiograph) is perplexing, although less problematic, because the forces act in the plane of motion of the joint. Flexion contracture and recurvatum, though important, usually require soft-tissue rather than osseous correction. The positions of the femoral component are typically described as flexion or extension, and those of the tibia as anterior or posterior slope.

The tibial component is, in most systems, implanted with some degree of posterior slope, meaning that the posterior portion of the articulation is lower than the anterior. This effect can be achieved by either the orientation of the bone cut or the design of the component as a means of decreasing tension in the collateral ligaments during flexion. Anterior slope is universally regarded as deleterious. Posterior-stabilized prostheses will be relatively intolerant to flexion of the femoral component, because the anterior flange of the femoral component will soon impinge on the front of the tibial post [14].

Rotation

In 1993, Berger and Rubash used computerized tomography (CT) to illustrate malrotation and the role of the epicondylar axis [15], and in 1998 they quantified the relationship between internal rotation of the femoral component (relative to the epicondylar axis) and internal rotation of the tibial component (relative to the tibial tubercle) [16] as an explanation of patellar complications. Whiteside validated the axis of the trochlear groove in 1995 (now widely referred to as "Whiteside's line") as a simple guide for rotational positioning of the femoral component in primary arthroplasty [17]. Poilvache and Insall popularized the epicondylar axis for rotational positioning in 1996 [18].

Extra-articular rotational malunions can be difficult to understand, predict, or correct at primary arthroplasty except by corrective osteotomy at the site of the malunion. Developmental torsion should probably not be corrected at primary surgery, except as indicated by the epicondylar axis. In general, rotation malunions that are located beyond the attachments of the collateral ligaments should not be corrected by changing the rotational position of either the tibial or femoral component in the knee. This is a difficult determination, however, and disastrous patellar complications may result from the combination of excessive valgus and internal rotation of both tibial and femoral components (❑ Fig. 32-2).

Surgical Planning for Correction of Extra-articular Deformity

Deforming and stabilizing forces influence every arthroplasty. Malalignment is the most potent deforming force, while stability results from soft-tissue integrity or, occasionally, mechanically constrained devices. A surgical plan that does not consider both of these forces will fail. Extra-articular deformities differ in degree of angulation and distance from the knee joint. Wolff and colleagues demonstrated trigonometrically that the closer the deformity is to the knee, the greater is its importance [1]. This conclusion should not distract our attention from the mechanical axis. Deformities cannot be ignored simply because they are distant from the knee joint. They must be evaluated on the extent to which the limb deviates from a neutral mechanical axis.

Bone deformity must in some way be corrected by cutting bone: This will be either an osteotomy at the deformity or compensatory positioning of the arthroplasty components. The former approach requires a separate surgical procedure but enables a standard arthroplasty. The latter eliminates the osteotomy but complicates the arthroplasty significantly.

Extra-articular Correction

Extra-articular correction of extra-articular deformities has generally been reserved for "severe" deformities. Lonner and colleagues at the University of Pennsylvania described the technique in femoral deformities measuring 14°-40°, and carefully considered multi-planar deformity [5]. Radke and Radke reported their experience with osteotomies for tibial deformities exceeding 15° [4].

The appeal of correcting an extra-articular deformity with an osteotomy either prior to or concurrent with the arthroplasty is obvious. The alignment of either the femur or tibia itself will be restored to normal, potentially in three planes, and the arthroplasty can be implanted anatomically, with a conventional approach to ligament balancing. In some cases, the knee will be restored to a neutral mechanical axis by the osteotomy, and no ligament releases will be required. The disadvantages include the separate surgical procedure with risks of infection, hardware failure, etc. Fixation devices may complicate intramedullary instrumentation or fixation with stem extensions during the arthroplasty.

When the deformity is remote from the joint, an osteotomy will require intramedullary or plate fixation independent from the prosthesis. If close to the joint, it may be exposed through (an extension of) the arthroplasty incision and fixed with a stem extension from the prosthesis. It is preferable to correct the deformity at its apex; although a compensatory osteotomy closer to the joint may

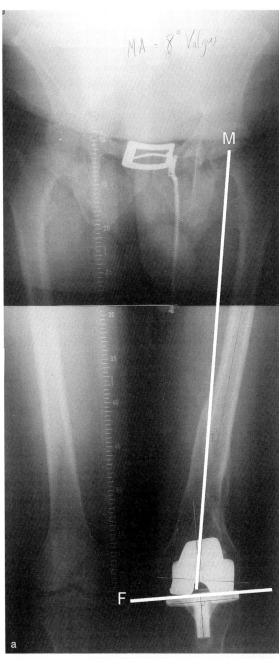

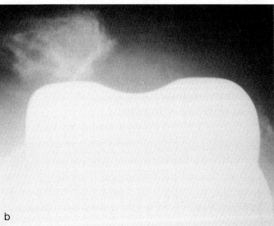

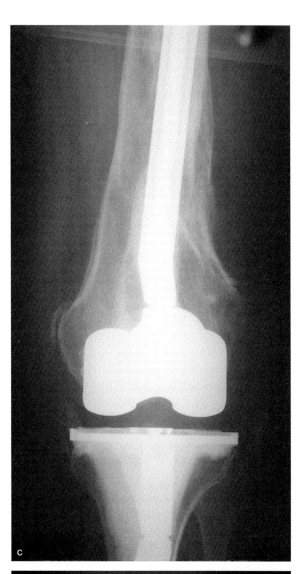

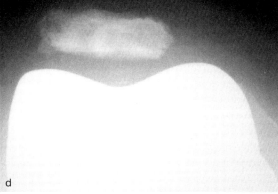

◘ **Fig. 32-2a-d.** *a* Full-length AP radiograph of failed primary TKA. Mechanical axis (*M*) and femoral cut (*F*) indicate that the original surgeon failed to recognize the effect of the old distal femur fracture. *b* Patellar subluxation resulted from an oblique patellar osteotomy, internal rotation positioning of the tibial and femoral components, and excessive valgus. *c* By inserting the uncemented stem extension into the femur, proximal to the old fracture, mechanical re-alignment was restored. Femoral and tibial rotation was corrected. Conventional releases restored stability. *d* Correction of the previous patellar osteotomy further contributed to central patellar tracking

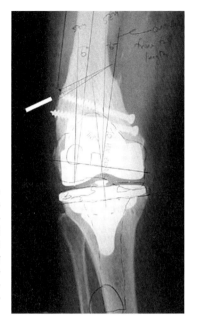

◘ **Fig. 32-3.** Malunion of a distal femoral fracture. At the time of revision, this was treated with a wedge resection corrective osteotomy and fixation with an intramedullary stem extension (osteotomy indicated at *white line*)

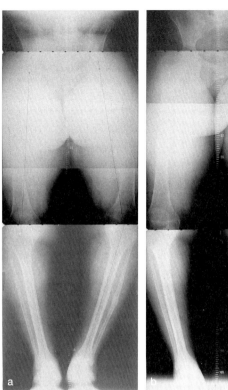

◘ **Fig. 32-4a, b.** *a* Preoperative full-length radiograph demonstrating severe varus angulation of the mechanical axis (*lines*) related to old femoral malunion from a motor-vehicle accident. Patient was obese, had knees that required bilateral arthroplasty, and was unable to accept blood transfusion for religious reasons. *b* Postoperative radiograph of same patient with intra-articular correction of extra-articular deformity by cutting the distal femur at right angles to the mechanical axis of the femur (center of femoral head to center of knee joint). This required an exaggerated valgus angulation of the distal femur that could not be corrected with standard releases. Corrective osteotomy or ligament advancements, while excellent strategies, were avoided due to the risk of blood loss. Fixation requirements with constraint were achieved with short, fully cemented, and so-called stubby stem extensions that allowed the necessary valgus femoral position

be performed through the arthroplasty incision, the resultant intramedullary angulation will render fixation with an intra-medullary stem extension impossible.

Osteotomies are planned conventionally. The axes of the medullary canals proximal and distal to the deformity are drawn, the angular correction is calculated, and then this is accomplished usually with a closing-, and sometimes with an opening-wedge technique. Correction with external fixation devices or osteoclasis techniques require a staged approach because of the risk of infection. Many surgeons avoid external fixation techniques whenever arthroplasty is anticipated (◘ Fig. 32-3).

Intra-articular Correction

Two clinical situations where it is best to leave the site of deformity untouched are previous osteomyelitis (as in an old open femur fracture with skin compromise) or delayed healing (as in an old mid-shaft tibial fracture that healed with great difficulty). Restoration of a neutral mechanical axis is nonetheless crucial and can be accomplished with compensatory positioning of the arthroplasty components, a technique favored by Insall [6]. Wang and colleagues applied this technique to deformities of up to 20° in the femur and up to 30° in the tibia, with combined rotational deformities as great as 20° [6]. As a practical guide, Wang et al. concluded that intraarticular correction was feasible (a) if the necessary corrective distal femoral resection did not violate the attachment of either collateral ligament, and (b) if the mechanical axis of the tibia, when extended proximally, passed through the articular surface of the tibia. Soft-tissue balance in the knee may become aberrant, requiring aggres-

sive releases, possibly ligament advancements [19], and maybe mechanical constraint (◘ Fig.32-4).

Planning and Technique for Intra-articular Correction

Planning and execution of the intra-articular correction of extra-articular deformity begins and ends with the full-length "hip, knee, ankle" radiograph. The mechanical axes of the tibia and femur, drawn on the radiograph, define the mechanical axis of the limb. Another line, drawn perpendicular to the mechanical axis of the femur at the knee, will determine the desired angular position of the femoral component and the angle, if not the level, of the distal femoral bone cut. The anatomical axis of the femoral canal represents the position of an intramedullary cutting guide, and the angle formed between these mechanical and anatomical axes of the femur will be the "angle of resection", or the angle at which an intramedullary cutting guide is set. Accuracy can be evaluated intra-operatively by placing a block with a hole in it on the distal osteotomy, introducing a guide rod, and determining whether this rod (representing the mechanical axis of the femur) is directed at the center of the femoral head.

The resultant ligament alterations are complex. If, for example, a varus femoral deformity of 15° has been corrected in this way, with a distal valgus cut that is 15° in excess of the usual orientation of the arthroplasty technique, there will be inordinate laxity on the lateral side of the knee joint in extension that may not be present in flexion. An aggressive medial release will be required, with a concomitant ligament advancement on the lateral side (proximally on the femur for extension). If this is not feasible, constraint will be required.

The problem is a little less complex when tibial deformity is corrected. Because tibial resection affects both flexion and extension gaps symmetrically, the aggressive release and possible ligament advancement will have comparable effects on both the flexion and extension gaps.

Ligament advancement techniques as originally described by Krackow, or with slight modification, may be effective [20]. Advancement techniques depend on the integrity of the ligament itself (plastic deformation is a contraindication). In concept, medial laxity can be improved by detaching the medial collateral ligament from the femur by sawing it off with a disc of epicondyle. The ligament is reinforced with a heavy nonabsorbable suture (no. 5) employing a Krackow stitch [21]. A standard bone screw is placed 1 cm beyond the intended attachment point of the ligament and the free end of the heavy suture is tied over this screw. The screw and the ligament are positioned more proximally to tense the ligament in extension and more anteriorly to increase tension in flexion. If both the flexion and extension gaps require tightening, the ligament is re-attached proximally and anteriorly. The epicondyle is further secured with two small fragment bone screws and ligament washers. This reconstruction usually obviates the need for constrained implants, but in selected patients a constrained prosthesis will splint the reconstruction, while the reconstruction will ensure that the non-linked constrained implants remain articulated.

Fixation is straightforward when primary components suffice, but difficult when both an unusual orientation of the component to the bone and stem extensions are required. Stem extensions will be necessary because of poor bone quality, or when the possible need for a constrained articulation will become difficult. Certainly, uncemented press-fit stems are unlikely to fit into the medullary canal, in view of the fixed angular relationship between the standard prosthesis and the intramedullary canal. In these cases a shorter stem that is fully cemented in the bone will be necessary. The size and shape of the stem may require modification.

When old malunions of supracondylar fractures are close to the knee, the intra-articular correction method may be used in conjunction with very long press-fit stem extensions (200-240 mm). If it is possible for these stems to span the deformity and reach proximally into the unaffected bone, we can be assured that the anatomical alignment of the femoral component will be the same as that cast into the prosthesis (usually 6° of valgus).

Other conditions, perhaps less well recognized, can create significant extra-articular deformities that lead to loosening or instability. Anything that decreases the offset of the hip joint will be a problem. Hip dysplasia with a valgus neck-shaft angle or a proximally and laterally subluxed femoral head, especially if exacerbated by abductor weakness, will decrease the valgus alignment required at the knee. Similarly, a total hip arthroplasty with a lateralized acetabular component or diminished femoral component offset will reduce the amount of valgus desired at the knee joint. Metabolic and developmental disorders lead to extreme bowing of the femur, such that the intramedullary guides in the distal femur underestimate the overall alignment of the limb. Paget's disease, for example, may present severe problems, which if not recognized will result in poor component position [22]. Deformities of the rheumatoid hindfoot have implications for alignment but should probably be corrected prior to knee arthroplasty. Valgus deformity at the knee is often associated with rupture of the tibialis posterior tendon and difficult valgus instability of the subtalar joint. This too requires attention prior to arthroplasty.

Conclusions

Limb alignment, rather than simply knee-joint alignment, is of paramount importance to the function and durability of an arthroplasty, especially in the presence of an extra-articular deformity. By definition, these deformities are located beyond the attachments of the collateral ligaments and may be dealt with in one of three ways: (a) corrective osteotomy at the apex of the deformity, (b) compensatory osteotomy distant from the deformity but accessible from the arthroplasty exposure, or (c) intra-articular correction by component positioning, usually requiring aggressive soft-tissue balancing techniques or a constrained implant. Although the deformities distant from the joint are regarded as less important than those close to the joint, it is the mechanical alignment of the limb rather than the location of the deformity that must be considered.

32

References

1. Wolff AM, Hungerford DS, Pepe CL (1991) The effect of extra-articular varus and valgus deformity on total knee arthroplasty. Clin Orthop 271:35-51

2. Wang JW, Wang CJ (2002) Total knee arthroplasty for arthritis of the knee with extra-articular deformity. J Bone Joint Surg [Am] 84:1769-1774

3. Ritter MA, Faris GW (2003) Total knee replacement following extra-articular deformities. Orthopedics 26:969-970

4. Radke S, Radke J (2002) Total knee arthroplasty in combination with a one-stage tibial osteotomy: a technique for correction of a gonarthrosis with a severe (:15 degrees) tibial extra-articular deformity. J Arthroplasty 17:533-537

5. Lonner JH, Siliski JM, Lotke PA (2000) Simultaneous femoral osteotomy and total knee arthroplasty for treatment of osteoarthritis associated with severe extra-articular deformity. J Bone Joint Surg [Am] 82:342-348

6. Mann JW 3rd, Insall, JN. Scuderi, GR (1997) Total knee arthroplasty in patients with associated extra-articular deformity. Orthop Trans 21:59

7. Lotke PA, Ecker ML (1977) Influence of positioning of prosthesis in total knee replacement. J Bone Joint Surg [Am] 59:77-79

8. Vince KG, Insall JN, Kelly MA (1989) The total condylar prosthesis. 10- to 12-year results of a cemented knee replacement. J Bone Joint Surg [Br] 71:793-797

9. Hungerford DS (2000) The consequences of malalignment: forewarned is forearmed. Orthopedics 23:981-982

10. Kennedy WR, White RP (1987) Unicompartmental arthroplasty of the knee. Postoperative alignment and its influence on overall results. Clin Orthop 221:278-285

11. Andriacchi TP (1994) Dynamics of knee malalignment. Orthop Clin North Am 25:395-403

12. Moreland JR, Bassett LW, Hanker GJ (1987) Radiographic analysis of the axial alignment of the lower extremity. J Bone Joint Surg [Am] 69:745-749

13. NehratJiang CC, Insall JN (1989) Effect of rotation on the axial alignment of the femur. Pitfalls in the use of femoral intramedullary guides in total knee arthroplasty. Clin Orthop 248:50-56

14. Callaghan JJ, O'Rourke MR, Goetz DD, Schmalzried TP, Campbell PA, Johnston RC (2002) Tibial post impingement in posterior-stabilized total knee arthroplasty. Clin Orthop 404:83-88

15. Berger RA, Rubash HE, Seel MJ, Thompson WH, Crossett LS (1993) Determining the rotational alignment of the femoral component in total knee arthroplasty using the epicondylar axis. Clin Orthop 286:40-47

16. Berger RA, Crossett LS, Jacobs JJ, Rubash HE (1998) Malrotation causing patellofemoral complications after total knee arthroplasty. Clin Orthop 356:144-153

17. Whiteside LA, Arima J (1995) The anteroposterior axis for femoral rotational alignment in valgus total knee arthroplasty. Clin Orthop 321:168-172

18. Poilvache PL, Insall JN, Scuderi GR, Font-Rodriguez DE (1996) Rotational landmarks and sizing of the distal femur in total knee arthroplasty. Clin Orthop 331:35-46

19. Vince K, Spitzer A, Berkowitz R (1997) Ligament advancement in total knee arthroplasty. Presentation at Knee Society Interim Meeting (and Combined Specialty Day Meeting) of the Annual Meeting of the American Academy of Orthopedic Surgeons, San Francisco, CA, February 16

20. Vince KBD, Newton DOD (1991) Plastie ligamentaire interne dans l'arthroplastie prosthetique du genou. Maitrise Orthopedique 89:6

21. Krackow KA, Thomas SC, Jones LC (1986) A new stitch for ligament-tendon fixation. Brief note. J Bone Joint Surg [Am] 68:764-766

22. Gabel GT, Rand JA, Sim FH (1991) Total knee arthroplasty for osteoarthrosis in patients who have Paget disease of bone at the knee. J Bone Joint Surg [Am] 73:739-744

33   Use of a Tensiometer at Total Knee Arthroplasty

T. J. Wilton

Summary

Soft-tissue alignment of the knee is important in total knee replacement. Achieving perfectly aligned and well-balanced soft tissues is more difficult than achieving good bony alignment. A mechanical balancer/tensiometer is an invaluable tool for this purpose and should be available to any surgeon performing knee arthroplasty.

Introduction

Soft-tissue alignment of the knee is widely regarded as critical to the success of total knee replacement. Achieving perfectly aligned and well-balanced soft tissues is, if anything, more taxing than achieving good bony alignment and many solutions have been proposed. It is also to some extent uncertain whether the soft tissues should be "balanced" in both flexion and extension, since the normal non-arthritic knee has a tendency to more laxity in the lateral collateral structures than in the medial structures [1].

However, most authors have agreed that the preferred option is to achieve a rectangular flexion and extension gap with the bony cuts appropriate to the overall valgus alignment that has been chosen.

If this alignment is to be achieved a number of prerequisites exist:

1. The bony alignment that is required/appropriate must be known, and this may need to be tailored to the individual patient.
2. It must be possible to reproduce the bony alignment accurately.
3. The soft-tissue alignment must be quantifiable in some way.
4. The soft-tissue alignment needs to be adjustable, preferably in a gradual rather than step-wise fashion.
5. Such soft-tissue adjustments themselves need to be adjustable independently in flexion and extension.

The bony alignment is not within the purview of this chapter, but suffice it to say that varus/valgus alignment and rotational alignment of the components are intimately intertwined with the soft-tissue tension and bal-

ance. Furthermore, for a given soft-tissue sleeve, since most surgeons achieve bony alignment within a ±2° error band for each component, the inherent soft-tissue imbalance created solely by the surgeon may be in the order of ±4°. Fortunately, the surgeon is unlikely to create a maximal error on both tibial and femoral components in the same case, and if this does occur it is unlikely to be in the same direction for both components at once. With these many reasons for uncertainty over the soft-tissue alignment, it must be clear that one absolute essential during total knee replacement will be a reliable and accurate means of measuring soft-tissue balance. Various methods have been used over the years, but they can be broadly grouped as:

1. Using blocks/spacers (or the implants) and performing stress tests
2. Using distractors such as laminar spreaders in the medial and lateral compartments
3. Using a tensiometer of one sort or another

Using blocks and spacers, or even the implants themselves, coupled with stress testing, is simple, quick, and always available. This method is, unfortunately, rather imprecise, very subjective, and particularly difficult to use accurately in flexion due to the rotational freedom of the hip joint.

The use of distractors such as laminar spreaders in the medial and lateral compartments is not prone to these difficulties of rotation at the hip joint but does lead to the possibility of separate and different forces being applied to distract the medial and lateral compartments. This may represent a problem because the soft tissues are themselves extensible visco-elastic structures. It is therefore possible to create a false impression of a well-balanced rectangular flexion gap by applying a greater distraction force to one compartment than to the other (◘ Fig. 33-1). This difficulty applies with whatever instrument system is used if a separate distraction force is applied to the medial and lateral compartments, unless such forces are measured and can be seen to be applied evenly to the two compartments.

Such an instrument would be a form of tensiometer, although the term tensiometer could also be used to de-

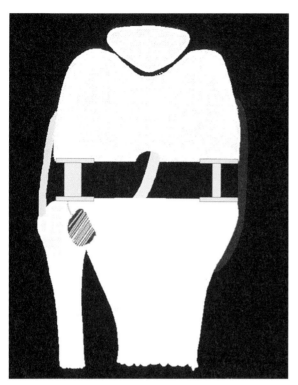

☐ **Fig. 33-1.** Rectangular flexion gap created by applying greater distraction force laterally than medially

scribe a balancer, whereby a single force is applied to the knee joint, distracting the whole joint and allowing the soft tissues themselves to indicate the presence or absence of soft-tissue balance.

An example of such a soft-tissue balancer/tensiometer is the Monogram balancer. The principle of this balancer is shown in ☐ Fig. 33-2, where it can be seen that release of the soft tissues on the tight side of the knee in

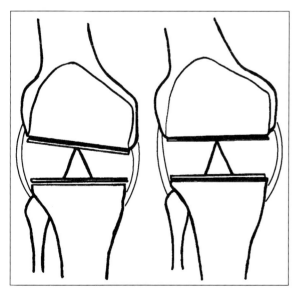

☐ **Fig. 33-2.** *Left*: Balancer distracted in flexion gap showing tight medial structures. *Right*: Balancer distracted in flexion gap showing balanced medial and lateral structures

Fig. 33-2, left, will ultimately allow the two distractible plates of the device to become parallel once the soft-tissue tension on the two sides of the knee is equal (Fig. 33-2, right).

A further possibility has recently gained currency – namely electronic or computerized tensiometers using load cells of various kinds to indicate the forces applied across the knee at the time of arthroplasty.

Use of the Tensiometer During TKR

Mechanical balancers of this kind give invaluable feedback peroperatively and offer two main benefits compared with the alternative methods. First, the soft-tissue balance is quantified. This means that the surgeon can know precisely the amount of imbalance at the start of the procedure, the degree to which release of the individual structures remedies any imbalance present, and the amount of imbalance remaining at the end of the procedure.

Second, the feedback thus gained allows a much more sophisticated approach to adjusting the alignment and balance so that the surgeon can choose to adjust the femoral rotation and/or readjust the varus/valgus alignment at a late stage of the operation if this is required to produce a perfectly balanced knee.

Using such a balancer we have demonstrated that the overwhelming majority of knees can be fully and perfectly balanced in extension, assuming a tibiofemoral mechanical alignment of 5°-7° is chosen [2]. In addition, the great majority of varus osteoarthritic knees can be perfectly balanced in *both* flexion and extension [3].

In contrast, significant numbers of valgus knees are left with a degree of imbalance in either flexion or extension, or both, despite careful attempts to balance the tissues. The proportion of such imbalanced knees will vary with the severity of cases treated, but also with surgical technique. Undoubtedly, it is easier to balance a valgus knee perfectly in flexion and extension if the knee is operated on through a lateral approach. This probably reflects the fact that a medial approach to such knees compounds the pre-existing soft-tissue imbalance between medial and lateral.

It is not clear how much soft-tissue imbalance is acceptable. Insall and colleagues noted [4] that even two extremely expert TKR surgeons who felt that they had balanced knees perfectly at operation were found by careful measurements to be nevertheless leaving some 50% of knees with minimal imbalance (up to 1 mm difference) and some 5%-10% of knees with 2 mm or more mediolateral difference.

In our own study [5] of knees perfectly balanced in extension, we found that 2° or more of residual coronal imbalance *in the flexion gap* was associated with a significantly less good outcome with respect to joint position sense.

A retrospective review of all TKRs performed at our institution from 1978 to 1987 found evidence of mild residual soft-tissue imbalance after operation in up to 40% of cases [6]. In a subsequent review of these cases a greater number of those with such soft-tissue imbalance were found to have undergone mechanical failure [2]. It seems, therefore, that relatively little imbalance, perhaps in flexion or extension or both, may be enough to threaten a good outcome after TKR. This proposal is supported by Ishii et al. [7], who found that knee replacements flexed significantly less well if they were left with any degree of coronal soft-tissue imbalance and that this finding was independent of the posterior tibial slope, posterior femoral offset, and even the degree of laxity in the knee both at the time of surgery and thereafter.

Two fundamentally different methods exist for balancing the varus/valgus plane at TKR:

1. Determining the bony alignment in extension and the femoral component rotation by bony landmarks, and then balancing the soft tissues by careful graduated ligament release
2. Determining the coronal alignment and soft-tissue balance and then choosing the rotational alignment of the femoral component which gives a balanced rectangular gap with that particular soft-tissue sleeve

The difficulty with the former method is that soft-tissue balancing cannot always give infinitely variable adjustments, and in some cases the balancing will be overdone or underdone. The problem with the balanced gaps method is that in some cases good soft-tissue balance is obtained at the expense of accepting some degree of malrotation of the femoral component. This has been demonstrated recently [1], and there is clearly a potential risk of producing poor patellofemoral tracking as a result of such compromise.

Apart from poor patellofemoral tracking, what may be the disadvantage of a less well balanced knee? A recent study [7] has looked specifically at the relationship between coronal balance, overall soft-tissue laxity, and range of motion after TKR. The authors found that coronal imbalance, rather than the degree of total soft-tissue laxity, was by far the more important determinant of postoperative improvement in range of motion. This study clearly suggests that an accurate method of ensuring perfect coronal balance at the time of operation will be important in improving range of motion and therefore function after TKR. Such a method is uniquely provided by a Tensiometer.

Failure to balance adequately also leaves the arthroplasty free to rock excessively in varus and valgus with walking, so that impact loading in the polyethylene is accentuated. The possibility of gross imbalance leading to subluxation and dislocation is obvious, but more subtle imbalance probably leads to excessive wear and loosening far more frequently.

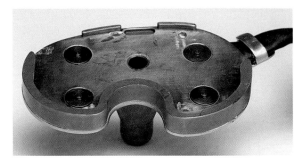

Fig. 33-3. Electronic balancer: tibial trial with load cells implanted in it

An electronic balancer with load cells can give accurate feedback during surgery and may allow not only coronal, but also sagittal soft-tissue balancing to be measured. One such device is in development at our institution (Fig. 33-3). A similar device, "The E knee" (C. Colwell Jr., 2003, personal communication), has been described in the literature and has now been implanted as a device to give real-time feedback of loads across the knee replacement during use after implantation [8].

A mechanical balancer such as the Monogram balancer (Fig. 33-4) can allow very accurate measurement of the rectangularity of the flexion and extension gap and allows the surgeon to decide whether one or two degrees of imbalance is acceptable. In practice, however, release of some soft-tissue structures may achieve more dramatic soft-tissue correction than others. The lateral collateral ligament in particular is found to give substantial correction when divided or released. Furthermore, the release of some structures such as the popliteus tendon or PCL produces changes in three dimensions rather than two. Such a device may also confirm that the PCL, when tight, does give rise to varus/valgus imbalance and can prevent the release of other structures from realizing their full potential to correct soft-tissue imbalance.

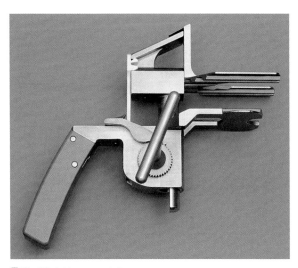

Fig. 33-4. Monogram balancer

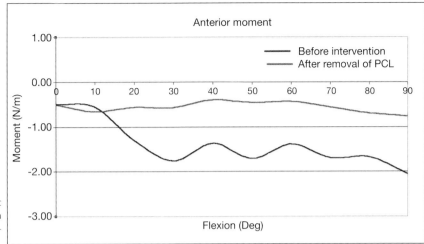

Fig. 33-5. Read-out from electronic balancer demonstrating the effect of a tight PCL and the improvement following resection of PCL

In contrast, use of an electronic force plate/transducer array can allow adjustment of the whole sagittal space, so that subtle alterations in tightness in full or mid-flexion may be identified and corrected. The surgeon can learn of tightness of the PCL that is creating an excessively tight flexion gap and indeed may examine the relative merits of releasing the PCL or of altering the posterior slope of the tibial cut. ◻ Figure 33-5 shows a chart of the AP moment on the tibial component, demonstrating how it may be improved by release of the tight PCL.

The use of Fuji film to demonstrate contact pressures and to map contact areas has increased progressively over the past 20 years but is confined largely to static systems and to in vitro experiments.

The use of digital pressure monitoring systems was perhaps first explored in a major way using the Tekscan system, and the accuracy of such systems to investigate dynamic as well as static diarthrodial joint systems has been investigated and validated [9].

With a re-usable system to use intraoperatively as an instrument to give feedback on soft-tissue balancing, the utopian goal of a knee arthroplasty balanced perfectly in three dimensions and also perfectly aligned should be realizable. Regarding the Monogram balancer, Winemaker [10] suggested that a perfectly balanced and perfectly aligned knee can be achieved in every case, simply using a mechanical device. This is a very attractive technique involving cutting the extension gap, then producing perfect balance by soft-tissue release in extension, followed by adjusting the femoral rotation to produce a perfectly rectangular gap.

This technique may fail in two respects: (a) If there are large posterior osteophytes on the femur which are removed only at the last step (excision of posterior condyles), this may alter the soft-tissue balance which has already been established. (b) Occasionally, (frequency depends upon case severity) release of a very tight varus knee may mean that the flexion gap cannot be perfectly balanced. Reliance on the soft tissues to determine femoral component rotation can then give rise to serious femoral malrotation. For this reason we abandoned attempts to incorporate this technique in the balancer-based instrument system after trials with a prototype Monogram balancer in our institution up to 1996, for fear of occasional balancer-based malalignments.

Such problems should not apply with electronic or digital pressure monitoring tensiometer systems. These systems therefore offer considerable potential to allow perfect balance of the soft tissues and a properly aligned implant. Perhaps the most valuable aspect of using such a device is the invaluable feedback to the surgeon, allowing him to refine his own operative technique and to be constantly aware of the subtle variations in soft-tissue balance which are attributable to different structures around the knee.

A mechanical balancer/tensiometer is an invaluable tool and should be available to any surgeon performing knee arthroplasty. Perhaps, however, to achieve perfection we may all need to avail ourselves of more sophisticated electronic tensiometers!

References

1. Hanada H, Whiteside LA, Steiger J, Dyer P, Naito M (2004) Stability, alignment and contact stress in two techniques of TKA. Poster Presentation, 71st AAOS conference, March 2004
2. Wilton TJ, Sambatakakis A, Attfield F (1994) Soft-tissue balancing at the time of knee replacement: Rationale and method. Knee 1:111-116
3. Attfield SF, Warren-Forward M, Wilton T, Sambatakakis AJ (1994) Measurement of soft tissue imbalance in total knee arthroplasty using electronic instrumentation. Med Eng Phys 16:501-505
4. Griffin FM, Insall JN, Scudieri GR (2000) Accuracy of soft tissue balancing in total knee arthroplasty. J Arthroplasty 15:970
5. Attfield SF, Wilton TJ, Pratt DJ, Sambatakakis A (1996) Soft-tissue balance and recovery of proprioception after TKR. J Bone Joint Surg [Br] 78:540-545
6. Sambatakakis A, Wilton TJ, Newton G (1991) Radiographic sign of persistent soft tissue imbalance after knee replacement. J Bone Joint Surg [Br] 73 751-756

7. Ishii Y, Matsuda Y, Ishii R, et al (2003) Coronal laxity in extension in vivo after total knee arthroplasty. J Orthop Sci 8:683-692
8. D'Lima D, Patil S, Steklov N, Slamin J, Collwell C Jr (2005) In vivo knee forces after total knee arthroplasty. Chitranjan Ranawat Award at Knee Society Open Meeting AAOS, February 26. Clin Orthop Rel Res (in press)
9. DeMarco AL, Rust DA, Bachus KN (2000) Measuring contact pressure and contact area in orthopaedic applications: Fuji Film vs Tekscan. Poster presentation, 46th ORS Annual Meeting, March 2000
10. Winemaker MJ (2002) Perfect balance in total knee arthroplasty – the elusive compromise. J Arthroplasty 17:2-10

33

34 Specific Issues in Surgical Techniques for Mobile-Bearing Designs

P. T. Myers

Summary

Mobile-bearing knee arthroplasty promises better kinematics, improved range of motion, and implant longevity. Various designs have evolved since the procedure was first introduced in the late 1970s. Successful mobile-bearing arthroplasty relies on obtaining movement as closely as possible around the original mechanical axes and within the normal soft-tissue envelope of the knee. Retaining tension of the collateral and posterior cruciate ligaments is essential, along with preserving the joint line. If these are not achieved then it is unlikely that the mobile component will move, thus compromising the result.

Introduction

Mobile-bearing knee arthroplasty (MBKA) involves having a mobile polyethylene (PE) insert between the femoral component and the tibial tray (□ Fig. 34-1). The concept was developed with the intention of more closely mimicking the kinematics of the intact knee, improving range of motion, and reducing point loading of the PE component in the hope of reducing wear and im-

proving longevity [1]. To date, none of these goals have been definitively achieved by any of the MBKA models available. There is also a recognized potential risk of increased backside wear [2,3]. However, it remains the desire of surgeons to achieve the best results for their patients, and in searching for the optimal knee replacement, there will be continued use and development of the MBKA. While there is no strong evidence indicating that MBKA is significantly better than fixed-bearing knees, there is similarly no evidence to the contrary. Indeed, studies have shown that a mobile-bearing (MB) implant is more tolerant of technical errors of malalignment and does show less point loading in flexion in some models [4-6]. Certainly, there is sufficient evidence to support continued use and development of the MBKA [6]. While the surgical principles are similar for the implantation of fixed and MB components, some aspects relating to rotation, alignment, and tension are important and worth considering separately in the context of a MBKA.

Types of Mobile-bearing Knee Replacements

The various types of MBKA available can be categorized according to the PE movement allowed and the functioning of the posterior cruciate ligament (PCL):
1. Polyethylene movement allowed by the implant
   - Rotation only
   - Translation only
   - Rotation and translation
   - No constraints
2. Posterior cruciate ligament
   - Released
   - Released and stabilized (by the implant)
   - Retained

The mechanisms restraining the movement of the PE component, by posts, rotating stems, grooves, rails, or others, all imply some opportunity for increased PE wear. This potential complication may prove to be a problem in the future.

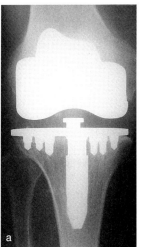
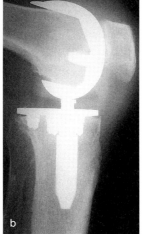

□ **Fig. 34-1a, b. AP** (*a*) and lateral (*b*) radiographs of a mobile-bearing knee arthroplasty

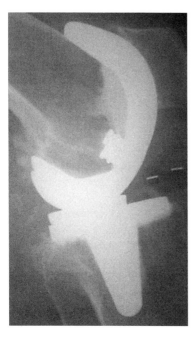

Fig. 34-2. Lateral view showing anterior dislocation of mobile-bearing component

Those implants which allow more freedom of movement of the PE component will require the knee itself to be more stable. If the mobile component has few or even no limitations on its motion and the PCL has been released, then the component may move more than is required or even dislocate (see ◘ Fig. 34-2). Excessive movement of a PE component can result in symptomatic clicking with movement. These aspects must be considered at the time of surgery.

Surgical Issues to Be Considered with MBKA Designs

Space for Movement of the Implant

At the time of implantation of the trial components and, more importantly, of the definitive implant, there must be a clear space for the movement of the mobile bearing. If the PE is required to rotate or translate beyond the margins of the tibial component, then this should be possible. Clearance of soft tissues and bone at the margins of the implant should be achieved with the surgical exposure but must be checked at the time of implantation. Components that allow anterior and posterior translation should be shaped so as not to impinge anteriorly on the fat pad and the overlying patella tendon, or posteriorly on the PCL. It may be necessary to excise some of the patella fat pad to allow full anterior movement of the PE in extension. Patients may feel anterior discomfort in full extension with some implants that are more bulky and impinge on the anterior soft tissues as they translate in terminal extension.

Constraint

The constraint on the MB component should be within the parameters that will allow it to move and yet remain stable. Excessive constraint will diminish range of motion. Conversely, laxity across the MB component may result in symptoms ranging from a clunking sensation with movement to frank instability and even dislocation of the implant. An implant that allows translation requires some block to posterior movement of the tibia to prevent the implant from dislocation. The PCL provides the natural resistance to this motion, and so it should ideally be left intact [7]. Otherwise, the MB component must have some form of block on the tibia (a post or an anterior stop) and a limiting mechanism on the femoral side (deep dish articulation or femoral post). Aspects of ligament balancing in a MBKA will be dealt with later in this chapter.

The Importance of Joint Line Position

Optimal functioning of any knee arthroplasty relies on the interaction between the geometry of the implant and the soft-tissue restraints. In order that the soft tissues can simultaneously allow movement and control stability, the prosthesis must have a similar contour and move around axes similar to those of the native joint. Hence, the position of the joint line in the replaced knee must be as close as possible to the original position in both flexion and extension in order to allow normal soft-tissue tension and stability [7, 8].

Much of the controversy, difficulty, and clinical problems surrounding knee arthroplasty could be avoided if more attention were paid to the joint line position. This applies equally to fixed and MBKA [8]. The majority of patients undergoing knee arthroplasty do not have severe ligament contractures or deficiency, and few have gross deformity. Consequently, the need for "ligament balancing" should be uncommon, or at least restricted only to more difficult cases. The perceived need to balance ligament tension and equalize flexion and extension gaps is largely the result of ignoring the principles of restoring original joint geometry and joint line position. If these fundamental principles are followed, then the complicating issues tend not to arise. For example, if in a knee with minimal or no medial bone loss the tibial cut is made just below the medial tibial surface, removing, say, 2 mm of bone, and the minimal tibial component thickness is 10 mm then the joint line has effectively been raised by 8 mm. There are two possible methods to accommodate this error; either the distal femoral cut must take more bone, thus also forcing the posterior condyles to be cut short to allow "equal flexion and extension gaps", or, if correct femoral bone cuts are made, then the joint will be too tight and "ligament balancing by releases" will have to

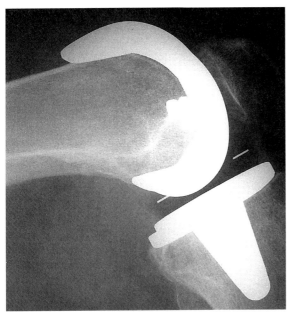

Fig. 34-3. Lateral radiograph showing a raised joint line as evidenced by the height above the fibular head and the level of the patella

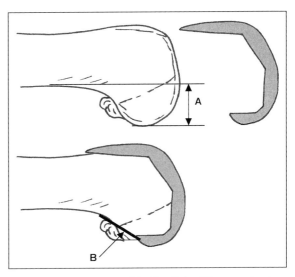

Fig. 34-4. The posterior condyle offset (*A*) should be restored as closely as possible by the implant. The line for removal of posterior bone (*B*) should include the remaining proximal portion of the posterior condyle as well as the posterior osteophytes

be undertaken (see ◻ Fig. 34-3). Neither of these would have been necessary if the joint line had been correctly placed initially.

Achieving Range of Motion

Extension. For an MBKA to achieve full extension the following operative factors need to be addressed.
- Adequate bone cuts should be made to allow full extension, and the PCL must not be tight, particularly if there has been a flexion deformity preoperatively.
- There must be no obstruction to anterior movement of the mobile component (see above).
- The extensor mechanism must function correctly, requiring:
  - Sufficient length and strength of the muscle/tendon unit to achieve full extension
  - Adequate strength of the quadriceps repair
  - Stability of the patella
  - Adequate lever arm effect of the patella tendon, i.e., the joint line must not be so high as to reduce the mechanical advantage of the patella.
- Posterior osteophytes, if present, should be removed.
- Occasionally, the posterior capsule will need to be released to allow full extension.

Flexion. The factors that can assist in gaining optimal flexion include:
- Allowing the MB component to glide and/or rotate as required to allow for the altered kinematics resulting from deficiency of the anterior cruciate ligament

- Restoring the posterior tilt of the tibia and possibly increasing it by 1°-2°
- Restoring the length of the posterior femoral condyles. This is also known as the posterior condyle offset [9] (see ◻ Fig. 34-4).
- Resecting the posterior osteophytes of the femoral condyles and shortening the posterior condyles to the same size as the prosthesis. (This is required because the sagittal radius of the posterior condyles of the prosthesis is usually smaller than that of the normal knee; see Fig. 34-4.)
- Ensuring the PCL is not excessively tight
- Maintaining the joint line at the correct height

Rotation. Correct rotational alignment of the implants in the longitudinal axis is paramount to the success of any knee arthroplasty. While the MB component may "self-correct" any small errors of rotation of the tibial component, it may be compromised if there are rotational errors in positioning of the *femoral* component.
Aspects affected by incorrect rotation of the femoral component include:
- Patella position: Excessive internal rotation may require an extensive lateral release; the patella may dislocate; excessive tension may lead to pain or restricted flexion. External rotation may cause the patella to be too loose, predisposing to subluxation or dislocation.
- The collateral ligaments will be either too tight or too loose (depending on the direction of the rotational error), leading to a number of potential problems such as:
  - Varus or valgus malalignment or instability in flexion

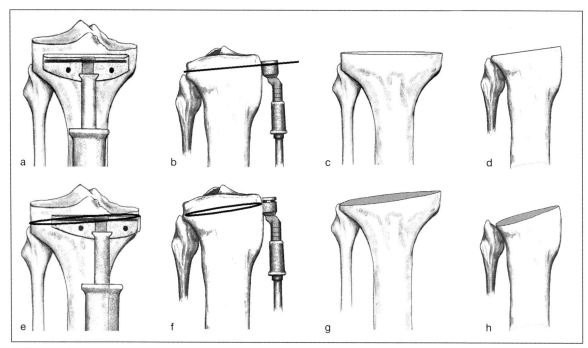

◘ Fig. 34-5a-h. Correct rotational alignment of the tibial cutting block produces a neutral varus/valgus alignment with a posterior tibial slope (*a-d*). However, incorrect rotational alignment of the tibial jig with posterior tilt will cause a varus or valgus malalignment (*e-h*)

– Dislocation of the MB component
– Excessive contact pressures predisposing to PE wear
– A perceived need to "balance" the ligaments by releasing the "tight" side, thus creating an unstable joint

Incorrect rotation to a minor degree of the *tibial* component can be accommodated by a rotating MB component, and this is probably one of the perceived advantages of the MBKA [5]. However, there are two situations where tibial implant rotation errors can be a problem: (a) Excessive rotation of the tibial base plate may result in the mobile PE component overhanging the margins of the base plate, leading to a risk of dislocation and/or point loading and possible fracture of the component. (b) Malrotation of the tibial base plate can change the effective varus-valgus alignment of the tibia if there is anteroposterior tilt incorporated into the cut. This can be difficult to appreciate at the time of surgery (see ◘ Fig. 34-5).

Author's Preference

Exposure

A tourniquet is used (without exsanguination) and a midline skin incision is deepened to the retinaculum. The quadriceps tendon is split longitudinally, with a small medial margin left for repair and a very definite angle made at the superomedial corner of the patella to ensure accurate reattachment. The parapatellar retinacular and capsular incision extends medial to the tibial tuberosity and the medial periosteum is reflected. The menisco-tibial attachments are released to the posterior aspect of the tibia. The fat pad is released from the tibia and the lateral meniscus and the lateral capsule are dissected from the tibia and reflected laterally. The patella is dislocated and everted. The knee is flexed and the soft tissues are released as required to obtain full flexion. The fat pad is not resected.

Bony Preparation

Rotational alignment is important to minimize liftoff in flexion and possible spinout of the MB. Referencing from the posterior condyles is most common but is inaccurate if the articular cartilage has been eroded or in the valgus knee. Aligning with the epicondyles is ideal but intraoperative identification is often not accurate. This is even more difficult with mini-incision techniques. Whiteside's line is perpendicular to the epicondylar axis in 97% of cases [10]. Osteophytes are removed and the appropriate jigs are used to prepare the distal femur. Computer navigation systems are becoming more advanced and accurate but are not in general use. The primary benefit of these systems is that they force the surgeon to look very closely at the bony architecture and to constantly check and recheck alignment and position of bony cuts.

In most implant designs the length of the prosthesis posterior condyles is less than the length of the native condyles. This is due to the reduced posterior sagittal ra-

34

dius. The bony condyle plus any posterior osteophytes must be removed to allow the PE to move around the femoral component, thus maximizing flexion. It is important that the condyle length be maintained, as this determines the flexion gap and the capacity for flexion (see Fig. 34-4).

In cases with a long-standing fixed-flexion deformity posterior capsular release may be required, and this is usually done by releasing proximal to the posterior condyles after resection of the osteophytes.

Tibial alignment and rotational positioning is the most difficult step of knee arthroplasty surgery. For implants which require a posterior tibial tilt (usually 3°) it is imperative that the alignment and rotation be precise. Any error of rotational alignment of the tibial cut by virtue of the tibial tilt causes an alteration of the varus/valgus alignment. A mobile bearing may self-correct for rotational malposition; however, the altered varus or valgus alignment results in a widened flexion gap in one compartment which could lead to dislocation of the PE component (see Fig. 34-5). An external alignment tibial jig is preferred for varus-valgus determination because the medullary canal of the tibia is often curved [11]. The amount of bone to be resected must be measured from the more normal side and should equal the thickness of the tibial component. This ensures that the original joint line is maintained. Ligament tension in flexion and extension should be checked before the jig is completely removed. Close attention must be paid to the alignment of the tibial cut and it must be checked before implantation of the trial tibial component.

Posterior Cruciate Ligament

Most MBKA designs retain the PCL [12] as a means of controlling the constraint on the PE and thus (theoretically) allowing it to move. If the PCL is sacrificed then the anteroposterior stability of the joint is controlled only by the PE constraint on the tibia. If the PE is to translate, then the PCL must remain intact. To reflect the PCL, the tibia is levered anteriorly and an osteotome is used to carefully reflect an osteoperiosteal flap, preserving the original lower portion of the PCL origin. If the PCL is subsequently tight in flexion then partial release from the femur is all that is required.

Patella

It is the author's preference not to routinely resurface the patella. In cases where there is articular cartilage degeneration to bone in the patellofemoral joint, a patellar button is cemented in place. Otherwise, the patella is just débrided of osteophytes.

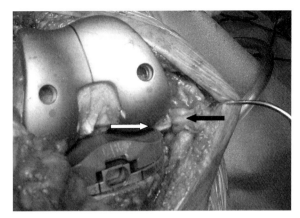

Fig. 34-6. Operative photograph showing that the joint line is maintained in flexion. The meniscal rim (*black arrow*) is adjacent to the prosthesis contact surface (*white arrow*)

Trial Implantation

The trial components are then inserted, and stability and range of motion are checked. Aspects which are specifically checked include:
1. In extension:
   - That full extension is obtained
   - Position of the joint line
   - Varus-valgus alignment of the knee
   - Stability
2. In flexion:
   - That adequate flexion is obtained
   - That the patella is tracking normally and is stable
   - Stability
   - Position of the joint line. Determining the position of the meniscal rim in relation to the prosthesis contact surface best assesses this (see Fig. 34-6).
   - There should be no liftoff of the PE insert which could be a result of inadequate posterior condyle resection. (Other potential causes of PE liftoff such as an inadequate flexion gap or a tight PCL were assessed earlier at the time of the tibial resection.)
   - The PE insert is mobile with no soft-tissue impingement. At this stage some of the fat pad may need to be removed.

Implantation and Closure

The joint is then thoroughly irrigated and the definitive implants are inserted, usually uncemented. The wound is closed in layers over a reinfusion drain system. A simple extension knee splint is applied in recovery, and the patient begins rehabilitation within 24 h, with passive flexion to 90°. The splint is removed when straight leg raising is accomplished.

Conclusions

Future studies will determine whether MBKA is ultimately more beneficial to the patient than a fixed-bearing implant. Subjective issues of patient satisfaction and function are paramount, although factors such as actual movement, component stresses, and wear characteristics need to be further assessed. Ultimately, surgeons will consider these various issues and will also be influenced by the ease and accuracy of implantation of the device.

In general terms, the principles of performing MBKA are the same as those for a fixed-bearing arthroplasty. However, attention to precise positioning is required for the MB component to be able to move as designed. Whether this translates to a better functional result for the patient as a result of the technique or the bearing mobility is yet to be determined. It is evident that MBKA has a place in the management of degenerate knee conditions, as no major problems have been reported in the past 30 years. Research and development should continue to produce better kinematic knee designs, and hopefully the potential benefits of MBKA will be realized.

Knee arthroplasty has progressed exponentially in the past 50 years. The future promises improvements in design, materials, fixation, and lubrication. Genetic and biological technologies may have a role in future knee replacement surgery. The challenge will be whether to remove otherwise normal structures and have their function replaced by the prosthesis, or to retain as much of the normal knee as possible and have the prosthesis function within that framework.

Acknowledgements. I would like to thank Mr. Adrian Wilson, M.B.B.S., B.Sc., F.R.C.S., F.R.C.S. Orth, and Mr. Mark Watts, B.Sc., App.H.M.S.(Ex-Sc) Hons, for their assistance with this chapter.

References

1. Menchetti PPM, Walker PS (1997) Mechanical evaluation of mobile bearing knees. Am J Knee Surg 10:73-82
2. Wasielewski RC (2002) The causes of insert backside wear in total knee arthroplasty. Clin Orthop 404:232-246
3. Chapman-Sheath PJ, Bruce WJ, et al (2003) In vitro assessment of proximal polyethylene contact surface areas and stresses in mobile bearing knees. Med Eng Phys 25:437-443
4. Cheng CK, Huang CH et al (2003) The influence of surgical malalignment on the contact pressures of fixed and mobile bearing knee prostheses - a biomechanical study. Clin Biomech (Bristol, Avon). 18:231-236
5. Stukenborg-Colsman C, Ostermeier S, et al (2002) Tibiofemoral contact stress after total knee arthroplasty: comparison of fixed and mobile-bearing inlay designs. Acta Orthop Scand 73:638-646
6. Price AJ, Rees JL, et al (2003) A mobile-bearing total knee prosthesis compared with a fixed-bearing prosthesis. A multicentre single-blind randomised controlled trial. J Bone Joint Surg [Br] 85:62-67
7. Morberg P, Chapman-Sheath P, et al (2002) The function of the posterior cruciate ligament in an anteroposterior-gliding rotating platform total knee arthroplasty: J Arthroplasty 17:484-489
8. Beverland D (2002) Advanced mobile-bearing surgical technique: Orthopedics 25 [Suppl 2]:s265-271
9. Bellermans J, Banks S, et al (2002) Fluorscopic analysis of the kinematics of deep flexion in total knee arthroplasty. Influence of posterior condylar offset: J Bone Joint Surg [Br] 84:50-53
10. Whitesides LA, Arima J (1995) The anteroposterior axis for femoral rotational alignment in valgus total knee arthroplasty. Clin Orthop 321:168-172
11. Tosun N, Aydinlioglu A, et al (2003) Anatomical characteristics of the tibial medullary canal and their implications for intreamedullary fixation. J Int Med Res 31:557-660
12. Vertullo CJ, Easley, et al (2001) Mobile bearings in primary knee arthroplasty. JAAOS 9:355-364

34

35 Optimizing Cementing Technique

G. R. Scuderi, H. Clarke

Summary

Supported by the long-term clinical success and survivorship analysis, cemented total knee arthroplasty continues to be the gold standard against which alternative means of fixation need to be compared. Fundamental to implant longevity is meticulous technique, bone preparation, and handling of the cement. Fixation of polymethylmethacrylate to the cancellous bony surface is achieved by the irregular configuration of the bony surface and the penetration of the cement into the bone. Well-fixed cemented components have shown very little micromotion at the fixation interface, with little displacement over the years. A well-designed and properly positioned cemented total knee arthroplasty has a greater than 90% chance of surviving more than 15 years.

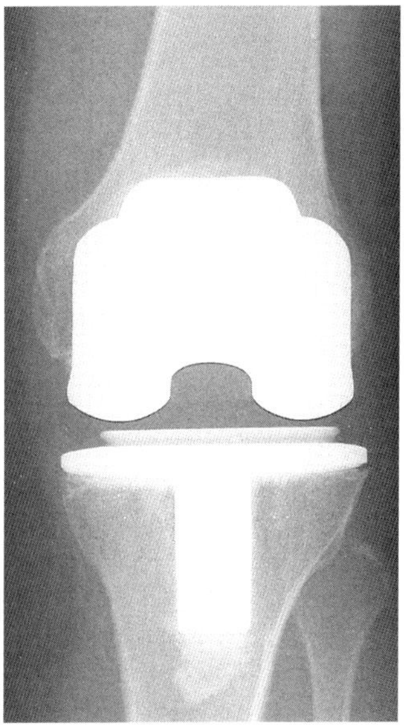

Fig. 35-1. The AP radiograph demonstrates a pristine cement mantle at 15 years

Introduction

Supported by the long-term clinical success and survivorship analysis, cemented total knee arthroplasty continues to be the gold standard against which alternative means of fixation need to be compared. A well-designed and properly positioned cemented total knee replacement has a greater than 90% chance of surviving more than 15 years [11] (Fig. 35-1). This success consistently surpasses the results of cementless total knee replacement [9].

Polymethylmethacrylate (PMMA) is a derivative of acrylic acid that is formed by the combination of a monomer liquid mixed with a polymer powder that leads to an exothermic reaction as it changes into a solid state. All cements are not identical. The polymerization process takes several minutes with the change from the liquid state, through a doughy period, and into a solid material [30]. The liquid or wetting stage is usually short, while the doughy stage is more variable and susceptible to outside factors such as ambient temperature or humidity in the operating room. The final stage to a solid state is not significantly influenced by outside factors, but may vary from one brand to another.

Bone preparation is critical for adequate penetration of the cement into the cancellous surface. PMMA acts as an intermediary between the prosthesis and the bone. The cement is not an adhesive agent and performs best under compressive loads [30].

Cement Technique

Fundamental to implant longevity is meticulous technique, bone preparation and handling of the cement [26]. Fixation of PMMA to the cancellous bony surface is achieved by the porosity of the bone and the penetration of the cement into the bone. Since bone penetration is critical to the intrusion of PMMA into the cancellous bone, the resected bone surfaces are cleansed with pulsatile irrigation to remove blood, fat, and bone debris. Proper preparation allows for uninhibited penetration of the cement into the bone. Our preference is to use Simplex cement (Howmedica, Rutherford, NJ) in a doughy tactless state. This permits easy handling and manual pressurization of the cement into the porous bone. The ideal cement penetration into the bone is 1-2 mm. With soft rheumatoid bone, deeper cement penetration may occur. On the other hand, with hard sclerotic bone, the bone surface

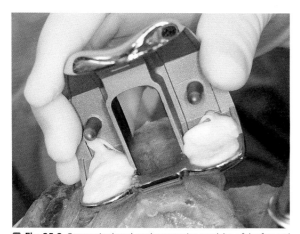

Fig. 35-2. Cement is placed on the posterior condyles of the femoral component prior to impaction

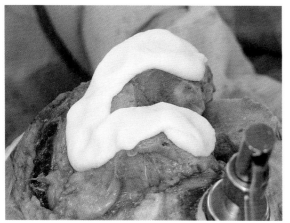

Fig. 35-3. The doughy cement is placed in a "horseshoe" fashion around the distal femur

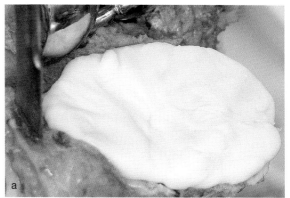

a

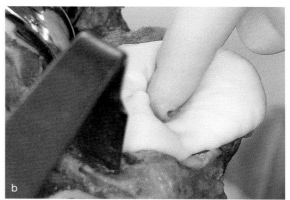

b

Fig. 35-4a, b. Since the entire tibial component is cemented, cement is placed on the proximal tibial surface (*a*) as well as pushed into the central fixation hole (*b*)

should be drilled or abraded to allow the cement to grasp the bone surface.

This cement technique has not changed for over two decades [25]. The components are cemented in a sequential fashion, and we choose to mix two separate batches of cement. With the first batch of cement, an all polyethylene patellar component along with the femoral component is cemented in place. While the patellar component is held in place with the patellar clamp, a small amount of cement is placed on the posterior condyles of the femoral component (**Fig. 35-2**). The remainder of the cement is placed in a horseshoe-shaped fashion over the anterior and distal surface of the prepared femur (**Fig. 35-3**). The femoral component is then impacted in place and the excessive cement is removed. The precise femoral cuts allow a tight fit between the bone and prosthesis such that the resultant cement mantle is approximately 1 mm thick. The tibial component is then cemented in place with the second batch of cement. The entire tibial component, including the central stem, is cemented in place (**Fig. 35-4 a, b**). All excess cement must be removed from around the components to prevent cement particles from breaking loose (**Fig. 35-5**). The presence of entrapped cement between the articular surfaces leads to third-body wear and damage to the polyethylene. The postoperative radiograph should demonstrate a perfect cement mantle around the components (**Fig. 35-6**).

The importance of initial prosthetic fixation has been emphasized in the past, since it has been shown that prostheses that continuously migrate will eventually loosen. The most decisive time is during the operative procedure and influenced by the surgical technique and prosthetic design. While cementing the femoral component has been standardized, there appears to be some variation to cementing the tibial component. Some tibial tray designs have a cruciate-shaped central stem, which allows "hybrid" fixation [23]. This means that the undersurface of the tray is cemented while the stem is press-fit into the metaphyseal bone. This is design specific, since other central stem designs have an I-beam configuration, which should be completely cemented. Prosthetic designs such as the Total Condylar and Posterior Stabilized Prostheses (Zimmer, Warsaw, IN) were designed for routinely cementing the entire tibial component including the central stem [23]. In order to do so, cement is pushed into the central stem hole in the tibia and the cement is manually pressurized on the tibial plateau. It has always been our

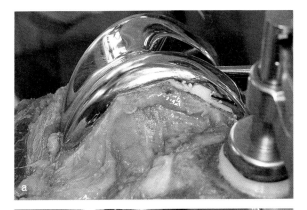

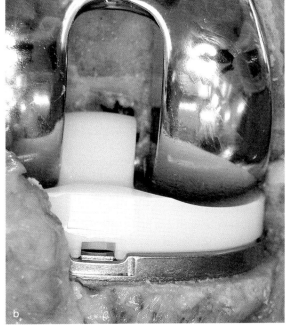

☐ **Fig. 35-5a, b.** With the components fully seated, all excess cement is removed from around the femoral (a) and tibial (b) components in an effort to prevent particles from breaking free and getting trapped in the articulation

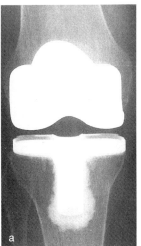 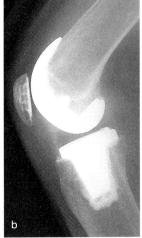

☐ **Fig. 35-6a, b.** The anteroposterior (a) and lateral (b) radiographs demonstrate an ideal cement mantle

recommendation that the tibial component be completely cemented. "Hybrid" or surface tibial cement fixation has little merit and is prone to unacceptable rates of loosening. Gunderson et al. have shown a 9% tibial loosening rate with surface cementation compared with no tibial component loosening with a fully cemented tibial component [13]. This result led those investigators to abandon the surface cementation technique. Bert further supports cemented stems with an in vitro study showing that a 1-mm cement mantle surrounding the central stem improves stability of the tibial component [4]. Additionally, Ryd [21] and Albrektsson [2] have shown that, when compared with cementless fixation, the addition of cement to the implant has reduced micromotion. This reduction in micromotion greatly influences the final outcome because if there is little inducible displacement of a prosthesis at 6 weeks, there will be little inducible displacement after 1 year and little migration after 2 years [26].

Modes of Cement Failure

Though component loosening was the most frequent reported cause of failure with early designs, it is not accurate to blame it entirely on cement fixation. Early prosthetic designs with limited sizes and instrumentation did not allow the kinematics, alignment, and soft-tissue balancing to be optimized. The original linked prostheses were highly constrained, placing stresses on the bone-cement interfaces. This resulted in high rates of loosening [12]. The introduction of less-constrained surface-replacing cemented prostheses, designed with greater attention to knee kinematics, seems to have resolved some of the earlier problems. Despite the better than expected results with cemented TKR, cases of aseptic loosening do occur. There are those who believe that micromotion at the bone-cement interface progresses to macromotion with eventual bone loss and component loosening, while others speculate that the underlying bone, when subjected to uneven stresses, subsides, leading to component loosening. This is particularly the case with varus malalignment of components. Subsidence is a problem of surgical technique and the underlying cancellous bone, not of cement fixation.

Concerns about constraint and increased stress at the bone-cement interface have been a recurring issue in the debate about PCL retention versus substitution in TKA. Advocates of PCL retention are concerned that the increased constraint with PCL-substituting designs results in increased stresses on the bone-cement interface. In fact, the interaction of the femoral cam and tibial spine with the Insall Burstein Posterior Stabilized Knee (Zimmer, Warsaw, IN.), imparts a compressive force on the tibia that negates tibial component liftoff [14]. Furthermore, metal backing of the tibial component has been shown to transmit the load better to the underlying bone [3].

Clinical Results

The clinical success of cemented TKR supports its continued use. Posterior cruciate-retaining designs such as the kinematic total knee prosthesis (Howmedica, Rutherford, NJ) have had long-term success [10]. In a 5- to 9-year follow-up study of this prosthetic design, the investigators have reported 90% good or excellent results. Though there were eight patellar complications in this study, there were no loose femoral or tibial components. Similarly, in a review of his last 1000 consecutive primary TKRs with a PCL-retaining design, Scott had no femoral or tibial components loosen [23].

The total condylar prosthesis, which sacrificed the PCL, was one of the first modern cemented knee prosthesis. Along with Ranawat [18], Vince et al. [31] have reported excellent results with this prosthetic design, supporting the belief that cemented TKR is a durable and predictable procedure. Despite the success of the total condylar prosthesis, the posterior-stabilized prosthesis was introduced [14]. The intent was to design a prosthesis that improved stair-climbing, increased range of motion, and prevented tibial subluxation. The early and midterm results were very favorable. Aglietti and Buzzi [1] reported 90% good and excellent results at 3- to 8 year follow-up. Scott and co-workers [24] demonstrated 98% excellent and good results at 2- to 8-years. In 1992, Stern and Insall [27] reported on the long-term results of the posterior-stabilized prosthesis. The 9- to 12-year results with an all-polyethylene tibial component produced 87% good and excellent results, which were comparable to the long-term results with the total condylar prosthesis. Analysis of the failures in the posterior stabilized series shows that there were five infections, three loose femoral components (1.5%), and six loose tibial components (3%). Metal backing of the tibial component improved fixation. In a 10- to 12-year follow-up study of the posterior-stabilized prosthesis with a metal-backed tibial component Colizza et al. [6] reported 96% excellent and good results. Despite the occurrence of two loose femoral components, there were no loose tibial components. The remaining two failures included one knee revised for recurrent hemarthosis of unknown etiology and another for postoperative recurvatum. In both of these cases, the cemented components were well fixed. These results confirm the advantage of prosthetic conformity in minimizing polyethylene wear without compromising fixation.

Several other cemented posterior-stabilized designs have also yielded comparable results. Ranawat reviewed the 4- to 6-year results with the modular Press Fit Condylar PCL-substituting design (Johnson & Johnson, NJ) [18]. He reported 93% excellent and good results with no cases of component loosening.

Speculating that the level of activity would influence the longevity of cemented TKR, Diduch et.al. evaluated the long-term results and the functional outcome in patients who were 55 years of age or younger at the time of the index procedure [7]. All patients were rated good or excellent at an average follow-up of 8 years. The 18-year cumulative survivorship was 94%. This was a group of patients who regularly participated in physical activities, which placed high stresses on the cement interfaces. Though there was one case of polyethylene wear, there were no cases of component loosening.

Following the introduction of modular tibial components in 1987, there have been recent concerns that polyethylene wear on the backside of the tibial component would lead to osteolysis. Brassard et al. attempted to evaluate this theoretical concern with a long-term evaluation of the modular Insall Burstein Prosthesis [5]. In this radiographic review, there were no cases of massive osteolysis, but the authors did mention that three knees had local minimally progressive lesions which were not clinically significant. This series of metal-backed tibial components had an overall incidence of tibial component radiolucent lines of 11% compared with 49% seen with the all-polyethylene tibial component [5, 27]. Therefore, the introduction of modularity to this particular implant design did not appear to raise concerns about osteolysis.

Survivorship analysis has been a useful tool in determining the durability of an implant design. This method of analysis depends on the definition of implant failure. Success is usually defined as a prosthesis that is still in place, while failure is defined as a knee that has been revised or a revision has been recommended. The 12-year cumulative success of the Insall Burstein Posterior Stabilized Prosthesis with an all-polyethylene tibial component is 94% [27]. In more recent long-term studies of the Insall Burstein Posterior Prosthesis with a metal-backed tibial component, both best- and worst-case scenarios have been tested. The best-case scenario revealed a cumulative success of 96.4% at 11 years. In contrast, the worst-case scenario considers knees that are lost to follow-up as failures. This scenario yielded a cumulative success of 92.6% at 11 years [5, 6]. A further testimony to implant durability is a 94% survivorship at 18 years in an active patient population under the age of 55 years with a posterior-stabilized prosthesis [7].

Despite the long-term success of the original Insall Burstein design, incremental technical improvements and modifications have been made. These include the introduction of metal-backed and modular tibial components, modifications of the trochlear geometry to optimize patellofemoral kinematics and optimization of the spine-cam mechanism to reduce the risk of dislocation. Therefore, while the central principles of the Insall Burstein prosthetic design have been preserved, an evolution of this design has occurred. In the latest major redesign, the Insall Burstein Posterior Stabilized Prosthesis evolved into the NexGen Legacy Posterior Stabilized Prosthesis (Zimmer, Warsaw, IN) in 1997 (see Fig. 35-2). Recently we reviewed our initial cohort of patients with this prosthesis: 233

patients underwent 279 primary total knee arthroplasties between August 1997 and December 1999. Ten patients (ten knees) subsequently died, 16 patients (16 knees) were excluded because of severe medical disability, and 12 patients (13 knees) were lost to follow-up. Thus, 195 patients (240 knees) were available for analysis. The mean age at the time of operation was 66 years. The mean duration of follow-up was 48 months (range 24-72 months). Pre-operatively, the mean arc of motion was 107°, compared with 117° at the latest follow-up examination. The mean pre-operative Knee Society Knee Score was 48 points, compared with 96 points at the latest follow-up examination. The mean Knee Society Functional Score was 83 points at the latest follow-up examination. Radiographic evaluation revealed an incidence of minor radiolucent lines of 4%, and their presence was of no clinical significance. There was no evidence of loosening, osteolysis or polyethylene wear.

A comparison of current designs reveals that cemented TKA has a longer predicted survival than cementless implants. In a clinical and radiographic comparison of cemented and cementless fixation with the Miller-Galante Prosthesis (Zimmer, Warsaw, IN.), Rosenberg found no cemented implant that failed due to loss of fixation, while three cementless implants failed due to lack of tibial bone ingrowth [20]. While an early comparison study of cemented and cementless Porous Coated Anatomic prostheses (Howmedica, Rutherford, NJ) demonstrated comparable results, cementless fixation has shown a precipitous decline in successful results with longer follow-up [8, 15-17].

While some surgeons may seek other means of fixation, cemented TKR should be the gold standard against which alternative fixation techniques are compared. A well-designed cemented prosthesis, implanted with meticulous surgical technique, has proven to be predictable and durable with excellent long-term results.

References

1. Aglietti P, Buzzi R, Gaudenzi A (1988) Patellofemoral functional results and complications with the posterior stabilized total condylar knee prosthesis. J Arthroplasty 3:17-25
2. Albrektsson BEJ, Carlsson LV, Freeman MAR, et al (1992) Proximally cemented versus uncemented Freeman-Samuelson Knee arthroplasty. A prospective randomized study. J Bone Joint Surg [Br] 74:233-238
3. Bartel DL, Bicknell VL, Wright TM (1986) The effect of conformity, thickness and material on stresses in ultra-high molecular weight components for total knee replacement J Bone Joint Surg [Am] 68:1041-1051
4. Bert JM, McShane M (1998) Is it necessary to cement the tibial stem to improve tibial implant stability in cemented total knee arthroplasty. Presented at the Knee Society Specialty Day, New Orleans, LA, March 22
5. Brassard MF, Insall JN, Scuderi GR, Colizza W (2001) Does modularity affect clinical success? A comparison with a minimum 10-year follow-up. Clin Orthop 388:26-32
6. Colizza WA, Insall JN, Scuderi GR (1995) The posterior stabilized total knee prosthesis. Assessment of polyethylene damage and osteolysis after a ten-year minimum follow-up. J Bone Joint Surg [Am] 77:1713-1720
7. Diduch DR, Insall JN, Scott WN, Scuderi GR, Font-Rodriguez D (1997) Total knee replacement in young active patients. J Bone Joint Surg [Am] 79:575-582
8. Dodd CAF, Hungerford DS, Krackow KA (1990) Total knee arthroplasty fixation: comparison of the early results of paired cemented versus uncemented porous-coated anatomic knee prostheses. Clin Orthop 260:66-70
9. Duffy GP, Berry DJ, Rand JA (1998) Cement versus cementless fixation in total knee arthroplasty. Clin Orthop 356:66-72
10. Emmerson KP, Moram CG, Pinder IM (1996) Survivorship analysis of the kinematic stabilizer total knee replacement. A 10- to 14-year follow-up study. J Bone Joint Surg [Br] 78:441-445
11. Font-Rodriguez DE, Scuderi GR, Insall JN (1997) Survivorship of cemented total knee arthroplasty. Clin Orthop 345:79-86
12. Grimer RJ, Karpinski MR, Edwards AN (1984) The long-term results of the Stanmore total knee replacements. J Bone Joint Surg [Br] 66:55-62
13. Gunderson R, Mallory TH, Herrington SM (1998) Surface cementation of the tibial component in total knee arthroplasty. Presented at AAOS Annual Meeting, New Orleans, LA, March 19-23
14. Insall JN, Lachiewicz PF, Burstein AH (1982) The posterior stabilized condylar prosthesis: a modification of the total condylar design. J Bone Joint Surg [Am] 64:1317-1323
15. Moran CG, Pinder IM, Lees TA, Midwinter MB (1991) 121 Cases in survivorship analysis of the uncemented porous coated anatomic knee replacement. J Bone Joint Surg [Am] 73:848-857
16. Moran CG, Pinder IM, Midwinter MJ (1990) Failure of the porous coated anatomic (PCA) knee. J Bone Joint Surg [Br] 72:1092
17. Nafei A, Nielsen S, Kristensen O, Hvid J (1992) The press fit kinemax knee arthroplasty. High failure rate of noncemented implants. J Bone Joint Surg [Br] 74:243-246
18. Ranawat CS, Boachie-Adjei O (1988) Survivorship analysis and results of total condylar knee arthroplasty. Eight to eleven year follow-up period. Clin Orthop 226:6-13
19. Ranawat CS, Luessenhop CP, Rodriguez JA (1997) The press fit condylar modular total knee system: four to six year results with a posterior substituting design. J Bone Joint Surg [Am] 79:342-348
20. Rosenberg AG, Barden RM, Galante JO (1989) A comparison of cemented and cementless fixation with the Miller-Galante total knee arthroplasty. Orthop Clin North Am 20:97-111
21. Ryd L, Lindstrand A, Strenstrom A, Selvik G (1993) Porous coated anatomic tricompartmental tibial components. The relationship between prosthetic position and micromotion. Clin Orthop 251:189-197
22. Schai PA, Thornhill TS, Scott RD (1998) Total knee arthoplasty with the PFC system. Results at a minimum of ten years and survivorship analysis. J Bone Joint Surg [Br] 80:850-858
23. Scott RD (1996) Posterior cruciate ligament retaining designs and results. In: Insall JN, Scott WN, Scuderi GR (eds) Current concepts in primary and revision total knee arthroplasty. Lippincott-Raven, Philadelphia, pp 37-40
24. Scott WN, Rubinstein M, Scuderi G (1988) Results of total knee replacement with a posterior cruciate substituiting prosthesis. J Bone Joint Surg [Am] 70:1163-1173
25. Scuderi GR, Insall JN (1991) Cement technique in primary total knee arthroplasty. Tech Orthop 6:39-43
26. Scuderi GR, Insall JN (2001) Acrylic cement is the method of choice for fixation of total knee implants. In: Laskin RS (ed) Controversies in orthopedic surgery. Oxford University Press, Oxford, pp 163-172
27. Stern SH, Insall JN (1992) Posterior stabilized results after follow-up of nine to twelve years. J Bone Joint Surg [Am] 74:980-986
28. Stiehl JB, Komistek RD, Dennis DA, et al (1995) Fluroscopic analysis of kinematics after posterior cruciate retaining knee arthroplasty. J Bone Joint Surg [Br] 77:884-889
29. Toksvig-Larsen S, Ryd L, Lindstrand A (1998) Early Inducible displacement of tibial components in total knee prostheses inserted with and without cement. J Bone Joint Surg [Am] 80:83-89
30. Tria AJ (2002) Cement in primary total knee arthroplasty. In: Scuderi GR, Tria AJ (eds) Surgical techniques in total knee arthroplasty. Springer-Verlag, Berlin Heidelberg New York, pp 257-261
31. Vince KG, Insall JN, Kelly MA (1989) The total condylar prosthesis: 10- to 12-year results of a cemented knee replacement. J Bone Joint Surg [Br] 71:793-797

36 Assessment and Balancing of Patellar Tracking

J. H. Lonner, R. E. Booth, Jr.

Summary

Accurate patellar tracking should now be the norm with most contemporary total knee implants, but this is predicated not only on the use of a femoral implant with sound trochlear geometry that is favorable for patellar kinematics, but also on a meticulous soft-tissue technique. Additionally, malrotating or malpositioning the components can have devastating consequences for the patellofemoral compartment, as can overstuffing the anterior compartment, which may reduce the space available for the patella and predispose to subluxation. Considering the unfavorable results of revisional surgery for patellar maltracking, ensuring accurate patellar tracking at the time of the initial arthroplasty should be a priority.

Introduction

While patellofemoral complications after contemporary total knee replacement are diminishing [1], historically they have been considered the most common causes of dysfunction after total knee arthroplasty, accounting for as many as 50% of secondary surgeries [2]. The typical extensor mechanism problems encountered include patellar maltracking or instability, patellar fracture, osteonecrosis, extensor mechanism disruption, patellar clunk, or implant loosening or wear. The incidence of patellar maltracking (tilt, subluxation, or dislocation) has been reduced from the high of three decades ago, which was reportedly as much as 29% or 35% in some series [2-5], to less than 1% in contemporary series [6]. Patellar maltracking can occur as a result of several maladies, including flawed prosthetic design, soft-tissue imbalance, asymmetric patellar resection, overstuffing of the anterior compartment, malrotation or malposition of the femoral or tibial components, or patellar component malposition [7, 8]. Advancements in surgical technique and prosthetic design have reduced the incidence of patellar maltracking to an acceptable level [9]. This chapter will address the strategies for ensuring sound patellar tracking after total knee arthroplasty.

Prosthetic Design

Paramount is selection of an implant with design features that can positively affect patellar tracking [10-13]. An asymmetric femoral component with a trochlear groove oriented laterally with approximately 5°-7° valgus alignment can enhance engagement of the patella both in extension and in midflexion (◘ Fig. 36-1). An elevated lateral trochlear flange can also help contain the patella within the groove (◘ Fig. 36-2). The trochlear groove of the femoral prosthesis should have just enough constraint so that it engages the patella but does not predispose to increased patellofemoral contact forces and subsequent component wear, loosening, dissociation, or patellar fracture [14]. To accommodate either a resurfaced or an unresurfaced patella, the femoral component should ideally have a broad trochlear groove that extends proximally to accommodate the patella in full extension. Additionally, the trochlea should be directed towards the lateral side to engage the patella early in flexion. Distally, patellar tracking is enhanced when the trochlear groove is nar-

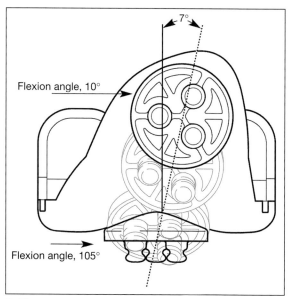

◘ **Fig. 36-1.** An asymmetrical femoral component oriented in 7° of valgus to optimize engagement of the patella (Printed with permission from Zimmer, Inc., USA)

Chapter 36 · Assessment and Balancing of Patellar Tracking – J.H. Lonner, R.E. Booth, Jr.

229   **36**

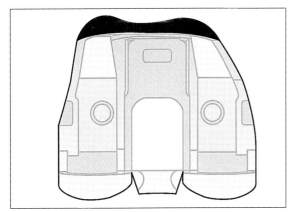

☐ **Fig. 36-2.** The asymmetrical trochlear groove with an elevated lateral trochlear flange can help contain the patella within the femoral prosthesis in extension and mid flexion. (Printed with permission from Zimmer, Inc., USA)

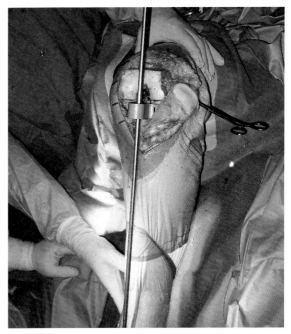

☐ **Fig. 36-3.** Following proximal tibial resection, an alignment rod is used to ensure that the resection is perpendicular to the long axis of the tibial shaft

rowed and deepened to contain the patella, limiting lateral subluxation in flexion [16]. Comparing the results of TKA in two disparate designs, Theiss et al. found that results were comparable except for the incidence of postoperative patellofemoral complications, which occurred in 10% with one design and in 0.7% with the other. The authors surmised that the discrepancy in the incidence of patellofemoral complications with the implants studied was related to design features, considering that surgical technique and patient demographics were comparable [13]. Patellar component geometry can also have an impact on patellofemoral performance. The authors favor a central dome patellar geometry, which, if appropriately implanted, can produce reliable patellar tracking, provided all other elements of the total knee replacement are performed appropriately. Alternative patellar designs include a medial offset dome, anatomical, and metal-backed mobile-bearing implants. An additional benefit of an all-polyethylene central dome patellar component geometry is that it can generally be retained during revision tibiofemoral arthroplasty if it is unworn and well positioned, even if there is manufacturer mismatch with the revision system [15].

Surgical Technique

Once a sound implant has been selected, the surgical technique must be meticulous. Proper tracking relies on restoration of a normal Q-angle. Axial and rotational position of the femoral and tibial components, as well as soft-tissue balance, can affect the force vectors around the knee and influence the relative Q-angle. Efforts to normalize the Q-angle are made at several steps during the surgical procedure.

Axial alignment of the tibial and femoral components is one variable that impacts on patellar tracking. The tibial component should be implanted perpendicular to the long axis of the tibial shaft in the coronal plane (☐ Fig. 36-3). The proximal tibial resection can be done with an extramedullary or intramedullary technique. In the authors' hands, extramedullary instrumentation is accurate and reproducible, and minimizes the problems associated with the use of intramedullary instrumentation, such as fat embolization, particularly in bilateral cases. Regardless of what method is used, the common error of varus tibial resection must be avoided. Valgus malalignment of the tibial or femoral components is also potentially problematic, particularly for patellofemoral kinematics. The distal femoral resection is made in 4°-7° of valgus relative to the anatomical axis of the femur. Tibiofemoral malalignment in excess of 10° valgus can increase the Q-angle and ultimately the risk of patellar subluxation or dislocation because of the increased lateral quadriceps vectors [16].

Component position can also help to neutralize the Q-angle. For instance, it is preferential to lateralize the tibial and femoral components slightly until they are flush with the respective lateral cortices of the metaphyseal surfaces (☐ Fig. 36-4), and to medialize the patellar prosthesis (☐ Fig. 36-5). Conversely, medializing the tibial or femoral components and lateralizing the patella can all cause relative increase in the Q-angle and subsequent tightening of the lateral soft tissues, predisposing to lateral patellar subluxation or dislocation. The patellar component should be medialized as much as possible to maximize engagement of the patella within the lateral-

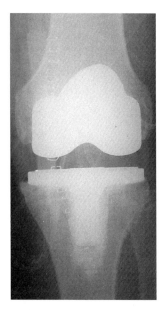

Fig. 36-4. AP radiograph demonstrating lateralization of the tibial and femoral components

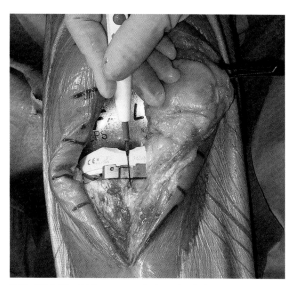

Fig. 36-6. The tibial component is aligned with the medial third of the tibial tubercle

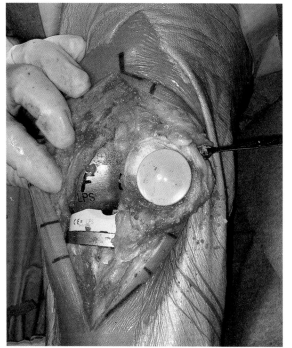

Fig. 36-5. Intraoperative photograph of the trial components in place. The patellar component has been medialized. The exposed lateral patellar facet is beveled to avoid osseous impingement

ponent subsidence with an implant that does not necessarily rest circumferentially on the tibial cortices, using a slightly downsized tibial component would reduce the prospect of soft-tissue impingement that can occur with excessive posterolateral tibial overhang, particularly on the popliteus tendon. Downsizing the tibial component can also avoid the common error of internal malrotation of the tibial component.

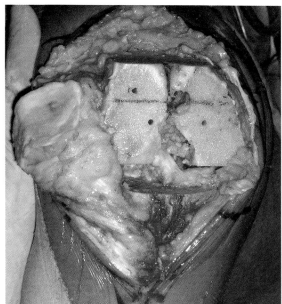

Fig. 36-7. A rectangular flexion gap has been created by several techniques. The tension gap technique was utilized. After tensioning of the collateral ligaments in flexion, anterior and posterior femoral resections were made. These resections are parallel to the epicondylar axis (horizontal purple line) and perpendicular to the Whiteside anteroposterior axis (vertical line)

ized trochlea of the femoral component and reduce the Q-angle.

Rotational alignment of the femoral and tibial component also impact on patellar tracking. Internal rotation of the tibial component can cause the tibia to rotate externally during knee flexion, forcing the tibial tubercle laterally. The tibial component should be rotated in line with the medial third of the tibial tubercle [16] (Fig. 36-6). This may cause posterolateral overhang when symmetrical tibial components are used. Despite fears of tibial com-

Chapter 36 · Assessment and Balancing of Patellar Tracking – J. H. Lonner, R. E. Booth, Jr.

231   **36**

Rotational alignment of the femoral component should be such that a rectangular flexion gap is achieved. Internal rotation of the femoral component in flexion can tighten the lateral retinacular sleeve and predispose to lateral patellar subluxation. This is particularly risky in a valgus-deformed knee. Several methods are available for gauging and confirming femoral component rotation (◘ Fig. 36-7). One technique is the tensioned gap technique, which is performed after removal of all periarticular osteophytes and balancing of the soft tissues. Restoring a balanced and rectangular flexion gap will generally result in an externally rotated femoral component. Another technique is a measured resection, referencing off the posterior femoral condyles, but in deformed knees this may be problematic, and additional reference points should be sought as a safeguard (◘ Fig. 36-8). The posterior condylar axis averages 3°-5° internal rotation relative to the transepicondylar axis. Therefore, the posterior femoral condylar resections should be externally rotated approximately 3° relative to the posterior condylar axis. In valgus-deformed knees, with lateral posterior condylar erosions or hypoplasia of the lateral femoral condyle, there is a tendency to under-rotate the posterior condylar referencing instrumentation, resulting in neutral or internally rotated anterior and posterior resections

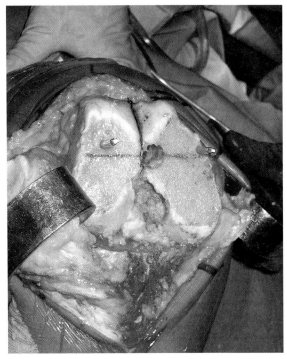

◘ **Fig. 36-9.** Intraoperative photograph showing two pins oriented in 3° of external rotation relative to the posterior condylar line in a severely valgus deformed knee. Deficiency of the posterior lateral condyle resulted in internal rotation of the pins relative to the epicondylar axis and Whiteside axis

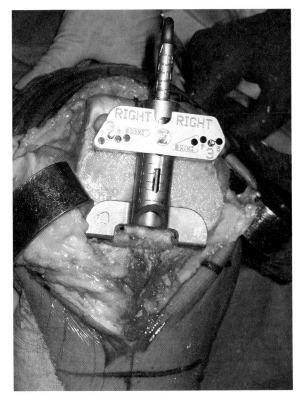

◘ **Fig. 36-8.** Alignment guide referencing from the posterior femoral condylar axis can be used effectively and accurately in most situations. Generally, the posterior condylar axis is oriented 3° from the epicondylar axis. This may not be true in deformed knees with either severe varus or severe valgus angulation

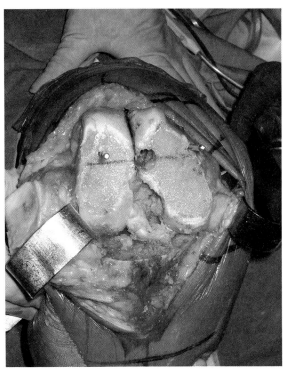

◘ **Fig. 36-10.** Replacement of the pins parallel to the epicondylar axis in a valgus-deformed knee, 7° externally rotated relative to the posterior condylar axis

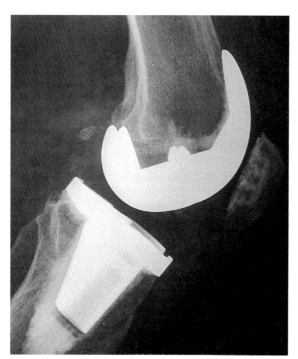

Fig. 36-11. Lateral radiograph displaying appropriate implantation of the femoral component with the anterior flange flush with the anterior femoral cortex

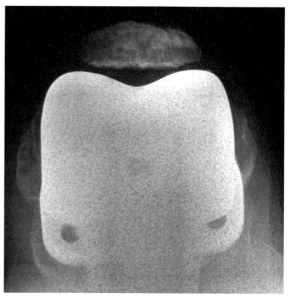

Fig. 36-12. Postoperative sunrise radiograph showing implantation of the patellar prosthesis parallel to the anterior patellar cortex. The original patellar thickness is restored

(**Figs. 36-9, 36-10**). Again, in these situations, alternative alignment references should be used. Two additional techniques are the so-called Whiteside anteroposterior axis and the transepicondylar axis. The AP axis of the femur is a line through the nadir of the center of the trochlear groove to the apex of the intercondylar notch (Fig. 36-10). A perpendicular line to that axis should be parallel to the epicondylar axis, which is a line drawn from the sulcus of the medial epicondyle to the prominence of the lateral epicondyle (Fig. 36-10) [17-20].

The femoral component should be implanted flush with the anterior femoral cortex without notching (**Fig. 36-11**). Generally, this can easily be done with an anterior referencing system. Overstuffing of the patellofemoral articulation can also predispose to patellar maltracking because the anterior soft-tissue envelope is incapable of housing both the anterior femoral flange and patellar components. This can happen with an under-resected patella, an asymmetrically resected patella (particularly when the lateral facet is under-resected, which leaves undue tension on the lateral retinaculum), or an anteriorized femoral component [21, 22].

The patellar cut should be parallel to the anterior patellar surface (**Fig. 36-12**). Additionally, resection of the patella in line with the anatomical landmark known as "the patellar nose" can help to ensure restoration of the normal composite patellar thickness or would make it 1-2 mm smaller than the original patellar thickness. The patella should be measured before and after cutting its

surface to ensure that it is appropriately resected. Generally, 12-15 mm of residual patellar bone after resection will result in adequate composite patellar thickness and avoid overstuffing of the patellofemoral joint.

Finally, soft-tissue imbalance can predispose to lateral patellar subluxation. This is particularly problematic in patients with severe preoperative valgus deformity, longstanding contracture of the lateral retinaculum, and other lateral soft-tissue restraints. In these circumstances, release of the lateral retinaculum may be necessary to ensure accurate patellar tracking. Additionally, in unusual circumstances, advancement of the vastus medialis may be necessary if the medial sleeve has been rendered lax because of severe deformity. In standard non-deformed knees, the need for lateral release has been reduced by improvements in implant design and refinement of surgical technique [9].

Assessment of patellar tracking is performed once the trial components are in place. While there is some potential binding effect of the tourniquet on the extensor mechanism, patellar tracking can usually be considered without deflating the tourniquet. In fact, slight longitudinal tension on the quadriceps mechanism may be a useful alternative to the "no thumbs" technique. The patella should track centrally without lateral tilt, subluxation, or dislocation. There is a tendency to overestimate the need for a lateral release because of loss of the check reign effect with standard quadriceps-violating incisions. A single suture in the medial retinaculum or towel clamp can help in judging whether a lateral release is necessary. The quadriceps-sparing techniques should reduce the need for lateral patellar retinacular releases.

If the patella is subluxing, then steps are taken to ensure that the components are appropriately aligned, the cuts accurate, and lateral soft tissues not contracted. If a lateral retinacular release is necessary, several different techniques are available. Regardless of which technique is used, attempts should be made to preserve the superolateral geniculate vessels if possible. Secondary surgery for patellar instability after total knee arthroplasty can produce significant improvements in pain, active knee extension, and function, but clinical outcomes are comparable to those of revision, rather than those of primary, total knee arthroplasty [23]. Therefore, efforts should be made at the time of the initial total knee arthroplasty to ensure that patellar tracking is accurate.

References

1. Sharkey PF, Hozack WJ, Rothman RH, Shastri S, Jacoby SM (2002) Why are total knee arthroplasties failing today? Clin Orthop 404:7-13
2. Brick GW, Scott RD (1988) The patellofemoral component of total knee arthroplasty. Clin Orthop 231:163-178
3. Cameron HU, Fedorkow DM (1982) The patella in total knee arthroplasty. Clin Orthop 165:197-199
4. Lynch AF, Rorabeck CH, Bourne RB (1987) Extensor mechanism complications following total knee arthroplasty. J Arthroplasty 2:135-140
5. Mochizuki RM, Schurman DJ (1979) Patellar complications following total knee arthroplasty. J Bone Joint Surg [Am] 61:879-883
6. Mont MA, Yoon TR, Krackow et al (1999) Eliminating patellofemoral complications in total knee arthroplasty. Clinical and radiographic results of 121 consecutive cases using the Duracon system. J Arthroplasty 14:446-455
7. Lonner JH, Lotke PA (1999) Aseptic complications after total knee arthroplasty. J Am Acad Orthop Surg 7:311-324
8. Malo M, Vince KG (2003) The unstable patella after total knee arthroplasty. Etiology, prevention, and management. J Am Acad Orthop Surg 11:364-371
9. Sodha S, Kim J, McGuire KJ, Lonner JH, Lotke PA (2004) Lateral retinacular release as a function of femoral component rotation in total knee arthroplasty. J Arthroplasty 19:459-463
10. Yoshii I, Whiteside LA, Anouchi YS (1992) The affect of patellar button placement and femoral component design on patellar tracking in total knee arthroplasty. Clin Orthop 275:211-219
11. Andriacchi TT, Yoder D, Conley A, Rosenberg A, et al (1997) Patellofemoral design influences function following total knee arthroplasty. J Arthroplasty 12:243-249
12. Chew JT, Stewart NJ, Hanssen AD, et al (1997) Differences in patellar tracking and knee kinematics among three different total knee designs. Clin Orthop 345:87-98
13. Theiss SM, Kitziger KJ, Lotke PS, Lotke PA (1996) Component design affecting patellofemoral complications after total knee arthroplasty. Clin Orthop 326:183-187
14. D'Lima DD, Chen PC, Kester MA, Colwell CW Jr (2003) Impact of patellofemoral design on patellofemoral forces and polyethylene stresses. J Bone Joint Surg [Am] 85 [Suppl]: 85-93
15. Lonner JH, Mont MA, Sharkey P, Siliski JM, Rajadhyaksha AD, Lotke PA (2003) Fate of the unrevised all-polyethylene patellar component in revision total knee arthroplasty. J Bone Joint Surg [Am] 85:56-59
16. Merkow RL, Soudry M, Insall JN (1985) Patellar dislocation following total knee replacement. J Bone Joint Surg [Am] 67:1321-1327
17. Berger RA, Rubash HE, Seel NJ, et al (1993) Determining the rotational alignment of the femoral component in total knee arthroplasty using the epicondylar axis. Clin Orthop 286:40-47
18. Whiteside LA, Arima J (1995) The anteroposterior axis for femoral rotational alignment in valgus total knee arthroplasty. Clin Orthop 321:168-172
19. Poilvache PL, Insall JN, Scuderi GR, Font-Rodriguez DE (1996) Rotational landmarks and sizing of the distal femur in total knee arthroplasty. Clin Orthop 331:35-46
20. Olcott CW, Scott RD (1999) The Ranawat Award. Femoral component rotation during total knee arthroplasty. Clin Orthop 367:39-42
21. Pagnano MW, Trousdale RT (2000) Asymmetric patella resurfacing in total knee arthroplasty. Am J Knee Surg 13:228-233
22. Krackow KA (1990) The technique of total knee arthroplasty. CV Mosby, St Louis MO
23. Chin KR, Bae DS, Lonner JH, Scott RD (2004) Revision surgery for patellar dislocation after primary total knee arthroplasty. J Arthroplasty 19:956-61

37 Specific Issues in Surgical Techniques for Unicompartmental Knees

L. Pinczewski, D. Kader, C. Connolly

Summary

The concept of unicompartmental knee arthroplasty (UKA) is not new. Although it was introduced in the 1960s, it did not gain popularity till the early 1990s. The new interest in UKA was attributed largely to the technological advances in biomaterial science, a refined surgical technique, and patient selection criteria with the introduction of a minimally invasive approach. UKA is performed using either resurfacing, resection, or mobile-bearing designs. The three designs share a common theme, which involves achieving ligament balance through bony resection. A novel technique was developed to pre-balance the knee joint and restore ligament tension prior to bony resection. This alternative approach minimizes bony resection and takes into consideration the fundamental differences between the basic principles of total knee arthroplasty and unicompartmental knee arthroplasty.

History and Development of Unicompartmental Knee Arthroplasty

The concept of unicompartmental knee replacement or resurfacing is not new. McKeever, in 1960 [28], and MacIntosh and Hunter, in 1972 [23], reported on the insertion of metallic spacers onto the worn-out tibial plateau. In the early 1970s, Gunston reported the use of polycentric femoral and tibial resurfacing for osteoarthritic knee joints which retained the cruciate ligaments and simulated normal joint kinematics [10-12]. Inspired by the work of Gunston and McKenzie, Engelbrecht designed the St. George sledge prosthesis in 1969 [8]. In 1972, Marmor introduced a modular unconstrained unicondylar device designed to provide different plateau thickness and to resurface single or both arthritic femorotibial compartments [24-27]. At the same time bicondylar designs such as the Geometric knee emerged [6], which consisted of two linked unicompartmental components. The bicompartmental design was later transformed into a tricompartmental design by adding an anterior femoral flange for the femoropatellar articulation. These procedures sacrificed the anterior cruciate ligament and retained or substituted for excision of the posterior cruciate ligament. Therefore, a certain degree of ligament balancing was required, which resulted in the development of instrumentation and surgical techniques for total knee arthroplasty.

Although selected authors initially reported positive results with unicompartmental knee arthroplasty (UKA) [17-19, 26, 35], high failure rates began to appear in the literature [15,16,20]. In highly specialized units, excellent results were achieved due to the combination of a high degree of surgical skill and experience. This translated into strict patient selection criteria and an intuitive understanding of ligament balance. However, Insall and co-workers reported their disappointment with medial UKA. Nevertheless, they advocated the procedure for the lateral compartment, which did not do well after tibial osteotomy [15,16]. In retrospect, it appeared that the lateral compartment was more suited to the available prosthetic designs and contemporary implantation techniques. As a result of Insall's studies, the use of UKA fell out of favor in the USA.

The demise in popularity of the UKA can be attributed to many factors [26]. The most significant factor was the use of a surgical approach similar to that for total knee arthroplasty (TKA). The surgical approach for UKA therefore demanded results equal to those with total knee arthroplasty. Furthermore, the retention of the major ligaments of the knee joint, combined with the lack of instrumentation to align components and guide resections, led to a high margin of error and a difficult and prolonged learning curve.

The Resurgence of Interest in Unicompartmental Knee Arthroplasty

The technological advances in material science during the 1980s have led to specific improvements in polyethylene quality and in the abrasive properties of metallic components. At the few centers that persevered with UKA, results were seen to improve with modification of prosthetic design to remove edge loading and thin polyethylene, with the use of a decreased constraint in the sur-

Chapter 37 · Specific Issues in Surgical Techniques for Unicompartmental Knees – L. Pinczewski et al.

235

37

gical design of components, but most importantly with better patient selection. It became clear that unicompartmental replacement was contraindicated for patients with inflammatory synovitis, multicompartment disease, and severe deformity with or without subluxation. It also became clear that UKA was an intra-articular procedure that could not be used to correct a significant nonarticular deformity such as tibia vara. Relative contraindications included anterior cruciate ligament degeneration, chondrocalcinosis, lateral meniscectomy, osteonecrosis, combined obesity and small bone size as may be seen in a subgroup of osteoarthritic women.

The renewed interest in UKA in the 1990s can be attributed to John Repicci, who pioneered the minimally invasive approach, without dislocating the patella or violating the suprapatellar pouch [33]. The aim was to offer the patient a lesser procedure than a TKA. Repicci's recognition of this in 1992 led to his concept of minimally invasive UKA being a restoration procedure supplementary to future TKA. This concept is valid, as the Repicci technique does not sacrifice significant tibial bone stock.

The minimally invasive approach to UKA has led to a reduction in postoperative morbidity, a decrease in rehabilitation time, excellent subjective results, and a good long-term outcome [3, 13]. In addition to better cost-benefit ratios for patients and health systems, these factors have driven orthopedic surgeons to reconsider UKA as a real option for their patients with unicompartmental knee osteoarthritis. Given that the most common cause of UKA failure is tibial loosening, resulting from polyethylene wear and component malposition, however, a re-evaluation of the surgical technique was required.

Current Surgical Options

There are currently three systems with different surgical techniques for the implantation of UKA.

Resurfacing Designs. Resurfacing designs such as the Repicci II Unicondylar Knee System (Biomet Inc. Warsaw, IN) use a free-hand resurfacing technique in which alignment is achieved without the use of instrumentation guides. The major advantage of this system is minimal bone resection, preserving the tibial buttress. This free-hand technique has been criticized, however, by many authors who believe that proper alignment often cannot be obtained without the use of instruments [2, 21, 34].

Resection Designs. Resection design systems integrate modular saw-cut components and jig-type guide instrumentation to help in making the correct bony resection. The use of intramedullary instrumentation systems allows for a more standard method of placing unicompartmental prosthetic components and ensures precise anatomical cuts and component fit [2]. It is a technique familiar to TKA surgeons. Although this type of guide instrumentation produces accurate resections, it does not deal with ligamentous balance, which is crucial to ensure a successful outcome regardless of design. The main disadvantage of resection designs is the considerable amount of bone loss, particularly from the medial tibial plateau. Combined with the use of pegs, screws, and fixation methods, this further compromises medial tibial bone stock, which may be a significant factor during later revision.

Berger reported excellent results with resection UKA utilizing a patellar dislocating approach [1].

However, the results of combining resection arthroplasty with a minimally invasive approach may increase the complexity of the procedure, requiring a higher degree of surgical skills and experience, with greater understanding of the basic principles of the technique, to achieve a successful outcome [9]. This may not be available to the multi-disciplinary orthopedic surgeon.

Mobile-bearing Designs. The Oxford Meniscal Prosthesis, a mobile-bearing design, has produced excellent long-term survivorship with low wear characteristics in experienced hands and with a patella dislocating approach [30-32, 37]. It is acknowledged that in order to obtain these excellent results, adherence to strict selection criteria and a high degree of surgical precision are required. Early experience with this technique illustrated the difficulty in achieving precise ligament balancing due to the small margin of error [22]. Another main drawback of the technique is the significant femoral and tibial resection required to accommodate even the thinnest mobile bearing.

The common theme of these apparently differing surgical techniques is that restoration of ligament balance is essential. Also, these three surgical techniques share a feature common to TKR, i.e., that bony resection precedes ligament balancing, which is achieved by comparing flexion and extension gaps as well as trial components. The algorithm for obtaining ligament balance in TKA by preliminary bony resection followed by sequential ligament release [29, 40, 41] is not suitable for UKA. As one of the pioneers of unicompartmental arthroplasty asserts, "A unicompartmental knee replacement is not half a total knee" [9].

An alternative approach is to restore the joint line and ligament tension as well as lower limb alignment prior to making any bony resection of the femur and tibia. This has the added advantage of minimizing bony resection and restoring the joint line with respect to the unaffected compartment and aligning components through the complete flexion and extension arc. This technique is compatible with a minimally invasive approach, as the patella should not be dislocated, since otherwise abnormal joint kinematics would occur.

Novel Technique

A novel technique was developed by the senior author (Accuris, Smith & Nephew Inc, Memphis, TN). This technique determines the appropriate joint line using an articular spacer (or 'shim'), prior to making any femorotibial resection. The articular spacer is designed to closely match the femorotibial anatomy (similar to a tibial joint spacer). Osteophytes are removed first to achieve normal ligament tension. When the spacer remains stable through a full range of knee motion, the proper joint line is defined. Thus it is possible to pre-balance the knee joint prior to bony resection. With the shim in situ, the tibial cut can be set to minimize the resection level from the restored joint line. An extramedullary tibial guide then allows a cutting block to be positioned accurately in all planes. The cutting jig will guide the resection of both the proximal tibia and posterior femur, providing a parallel flexion space. This technique results in minimal tibial resection and joint line restoration.

An important principle is resection of the proximal tibia at an appropriate varus/valgus angle. Cartier has shown that a tibial resection made at right angles to the mechanical axis of the tibia, similar to that of total knee arthroplasty, is rarely suitable for UKA due to the intra-articular obliquities of the medial compartment (◻ Fig. 37-1) [4]. UKA differs from TKA in that alignment can be corrected only to the normal tension of the knee ligaments. Thus the UKA surgical procedure can correct alignment only within the joint. Attempts to correct low-er limb alignment by exceeding normal ligamentous length have resulted in failure. Thus the proximal tibia must be resected along its epiphyseal plane. This has to be assessed individually for each joint but generally dictates a varus alignment of components in the sagittal plane and a 3°-5° posterior slope. This can be assessed intraoperatively using the jig as a guide. If the resected proximal tibial "biscuit" is uniform in both anterior/posterior and medial/lateral directions, then component stability should be maintained throughout a full range of motion.

The femoral instrumentation consists of a device that resects the femoral surface by reaming 3-4 mm of bone proximal to the restored joint line through full range of motion. The system utilizes a femoral reamer that locks into a tibial base plate. The reamer is firmly planted on the resected tibial plateau and the distal femur is reamed through its range of motion while normal ligamentous tension is maintained. Thus the joint's own ligaments and anatomy guide the bony resection (◻ Fig. 37-2). This minimizes femoral bony resection and, given that the replacement femoral component does not exceed 4 mm in thickness from the resected surface when applied, abnormal forces at the joint line are minimized (◻ Fig. 37-3). Also, over-correction, a known cause of UKA failure, is almost impossible. Conversely, slight under-correction of the angular deformity is known to protect the opposite compartment from excessive loading [5, 14, 38].

Prosthetic design has been modified to avoid the known causes of prosthetic failure. A tapered anterior aspect and rounded edges of the femoral component minimize the risk of patella impingement and abnormal polyethylene edge loading, respectively. Fixed-bearing UKA designs must be unconstrained to minimize shear stress at the cement-bone interface of the component. A potential significant improvement is the use of a ceramic femoral surface such as oxinium with a lower coefficient

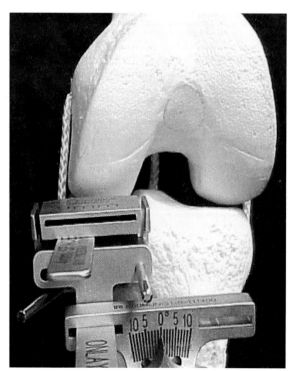

◻ **Fig. 37-1.** Resection guide for tibia and femur

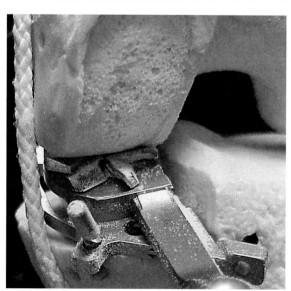

◻ **Fig. 37-2.** Femoral reamer

37

Chapter 37 · Specific Issues in Surgical Techniques for Unicompartmental Knees – L. Pinczewski et al.

237   **37**

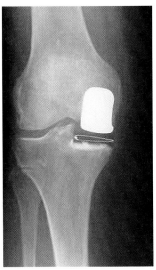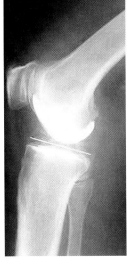

Fig. 37-3. Radiograph of unicompartmental knee replacement

of friction; this has variably been reported to decrease wear rates in biomechanical simulators by a factor of 2-10 [36, 39]. Debate exists regarding the use of a metal-backed tibial component versus an all-polyethylene component. It is accepted that a minimum polyethylene thickness of 6 mm must be implanted [7, 13, 26, 27]. The advantage of an all-poly tibial component is that a minimum 8 mm polyethylene thickness is implanted, and due to the lack of screws, pins, or pegs, any future revision is conservative regarding medial tibial bony loss [5, 13]. These technological advances should improve the wear characteristics of current designs and may significantly improve long-term survivorship.

However, these issues in surgical technique can be verified only by a prospective randomized study. Research should initially aim to verify the reproducibility of any technique utilizing the current minimally invasive approaches, and then be followed by a long-term study to confirm the place of unicompartmental arthroplasty in the management of osteoarthritis.

In summary, the principles of TKA are fundamentally different from those of UKA. TKA could be considered primarily a lower limb realignment procedure, UKA as a periarticular ligamentous balancing procedure.

References

1. Berger RA, Nedeff DD, Barden RM, Sheinkop MM, Jacobs JJ, Rosenberg AG, Galante JO (1999) Unicompartmental knee arthroplasty. Clinical experience at 6- to 10-year follow-up. Clin Orthop Rel Res 367:50-60
2. Bert JM (1991) Universal intramedullary instrumentation for unicompartmental total knee arthroplasty. Clin Orthop Rel Res 271:79 87
3. Cameron HU, Jung YB (1988) A comparison of unicompartmental knee replacement with total knee replacement. Orthop Rev 17:983-988
4. Cartier P (2000) Unicompartmental prosthetic replacement. In: Surgical techniques in orthopaedics and traumatology, pp 570-A-10. Editions Scientifiques et Medicales Elsevier SAS, Paris
5. Cartier P Sanouiller JL, Grelsamer RP (1996) Unicompartmental knee arthroplasty surgery: 10-year minimum follow-up period. J Arthroplasty 11:782-788
6. Coventry MB, Upshaw JE, Riley LH, Finerman GA, Turner RH (1973) Geometric total knee arthroplasty. I: Conception, design, indications, and surgical technic. Clin Orthop Rel Res 94:171-184
7. Deshmukh RV, Scott RD (2001) Unicompartmental knee arthroplasty: long-term results. [Review] [29 refs]. Clin Orthop Rel Res 392:272-278
8. Engelbrecht E (1971) Sliding prosthesis, a partial prosthesis in destructive processes of the knee joint [in German]. Chirurg 42:510-514
9. Grelsamer RP, Cartier P (1992) A unicompartmental knee replacement is not "half a total knee": five major differences. Orthop Rev 21:1350-1356
10. Gunston FH (1971) Polycentric knee arthroplasty. Prosthetic simulation of normal knee movement. J Bone Joint Surg [Br] 53:272-277
11. Gunston FH (1973) Polycentric knee arthroplasty. Prosthetic simulation of normal knee movement: interim report. Clin Orthop Rel Res 94:128-135
12. Gunston FH, MacKenzie RI (1976) Complications of polycentric knee arthroplasty. Clin Orthop Rel Res 120:11-17
13. Heck DA, Marmor L, Gibson A, Rougraff B (1993)T Unicompartmental knee arthroplasty. A multicenter investigation with long-term follow-up evaluation. Clin Orthop Rel Res 286:154-159
14. Hernigou P, Deschamps G (2004) Alignment influences wear in the knee after medial unicompartmental arthroplasty. Clin Orthop 432:161-165
15. Insall J, Aglietti P (1980) A five- to seven-year follow-up of unicondylar arthroplasty. J Bone Joint Surg [Am] 62:1329-1337
16. Insall J, Walker P (1976) Unicondylar knee replacement. Clin Orthop Rel Res 120:83-85
17. Johnell O, Sernbo I, Gentz CF (1985) Unicompartmental knee replacement in osteoarthritis: an 8-year follow-up. Arch Orthop Trauma Surg 103:371-374
18. Kozinn SC, Marx C, Scott RD (1989) Unicompartmental knee arthroplasty. A 4.5- to 6-year follow-up study with a metal-backed tibial component. J Arthroplasty 4 [Suppl]:S1-10
19. Kozinn SC, Scott R (1989) Unicondylar knee arthroplasty. [Review] [24 refs]. J Bone Joint Surg [Am] 71:145-150
20. Laskin RS (1978) Unicompartmental tibiofemoral resurfacing arthroplasty. J Bone & Joint Surg [Am] 60:182-185
21. Laskin RS (2001) Unicompartmental knee replacement: some unanswered questions. [Review] [21 refs]. Clin Orthop Rel Res 392:267-271
22. Lewold S, Goodman S, Knutson K, Robertsson O, Lidgren L (1995) Oxford meniscal bearing knee versus the Marmor knee in unicompartmental arthroplasty for arthrosis. A Swedish multicenter survival study. J Arthroplasty 10:722-731
23. MacIntosh DL, Hunter GA (1972) The use of the hemiarthroplasty prosthesis for advanced osteoarthritis and rheumatoid arthritis of the knee. J Bone Joint Surg [Br] 54:244-255
24. Marmor L (1973) The modular knee. Clin Orthop Rel Res 94.242-248
25. Marmor L (1977) Results of single compartment arthroplasty with acrylic cement fixation. A minimum follow-up of two years. Clin Orthop Rel Res 122:181-188
26. Marmor L (1988) Unicompartmental arthroplasty of the knee with a minimum ten-year follow-up period. Clin Orthop Rel Res 228:171-177
27. Marmor L (1988) Unicompartmental knee arthroplasty. Ten- to 13-year follow-up study. Clin Orthop Rel Res 226:14-20
28. McKeever DC (1960) Tibial plateau prosthesis. Clin Orthop 18:86-95
29. Mihalko WM, Whiteside LA, Krackow KA (2003) Comparison of ligament-balancing techniques during total knee arthroplasty. J Bone Joint Surg [Am] 85 [Suppl 4]:132-135
30. Murray DW (2000) Unicompartmental knee replacement: now or never? Orthopedics 23:979-980
31. Murray DW, Goodfellow JW, O'Connor JJ (1998) The Oxford medial unicompartmental arthroplasty: a ten-year survival study. J Bone Joint Surg [Br] 80:983-989
32. Psychoyios V, Crawford RW, O'Connor JJ, Murray DW (1998) Wear of congruent meniscal bearings in unicompartmental knee arthroplasty: a retrieval study of 16 specimens. J Bone Joint Surg [Br] 80:976-982
33. Repicci JA, Eberle RW (1999) Minimally invasive surgical technique for unicondylar knee arthroplasty. J South Orthop Assoc 8:20-27
34. Ridgeway SR, McAuley JP, Ammeen DJ, Engh GA (2002) The effect of alignment of the knee on the outcome of unicompartmental knee

replacement. [erratum in J Bone Joint Surg [Br] 2002 84:1091]. J Bone Joint Surg [Br] 84:351-355

35. Scott RD, Santore RF (1981) Unicondylar unicompartmental replacement for osteoarthritis of the knee. J Bone Joint Surg [Am] 63:536-544

36. Spector BM, Ries MD, Bourne RB, Sauer WS, Long M, Hunter G (2001) Wear performance of ultra-high molecular weight polyethylene on oxidized zirconium total knee femoral components. J Bone Joint Surg [Am] 83 [Suppl 2, Pt 2]:80-86

37. Svard UC, Price AJ (2001) Oxford medial unicompartmental knee arthroplasty. A survival analysis of an independent series. J Bone Joint Surg [Br] 83:191-194

38. Weale AE, Murray DW, Baines J, Newman JH (2000) Radiological changes five years after unicompartmental knee replacement. J Bone Joint Surg [Br] 82:996-1000

39. White SE, Whiteside LA, McCarthy DS, Anthony M, Poggie RA (1994) Simulated knee wear with cobalt chromium and oxidized zirconium knee femoral components. Clin Orthop Rel Res 309:176-184

40. Whiteside LA (1999) Selective ligament release in total knee arthroplasty of the knee in valgus. Clin Orthop Rel Res 367:130-140

41. Whiteside LA (2002) Soft tissue balancing: the knee. J Arthroplasty 17:23-27

V Technology

38 Computer-Assisted Surgery: Principles

J. B. Stiehl, W. H. Konermann, R. G. Haaker

Summary

Computer-assisted surgery has emerged as an important adjunct in total knee arthroplasty and will improve the precision of mechanical alignment and ligament balancing of most surgical techniques. Current methods utilize computed tomography, imageless methods, or fluoroscopic referencing for image acquisition. Evolving minimally invasive surgical approaches will benefit from the "virtual" imaging of computer-assisted navigation.

Introduction

Computer-assisted orthopedic surgery (CAOS) has recently been defined as the ability to utilize sophisticated computer algorithms to allow the surgeon to determine three-dimensional placement of total joint implants in situ [1]. A rapid ongoing evolution of technical advances has made it possible to move from cumbersome systems requiring preoperative computed tomography to more elegant systems that utilize image-free registration or the simple C-arm fluoroscopy at the time of surgery. Several reports on total knee replacement have cited the accuracy with which implants can be placed using computer-aided surgical navigation.

From a historical perspective, ROBODOC was the first modern attempt to use computers to place implants in bones. In this example, a cementless metal femoral stem was actively navigated into the proximal femoral canal. The goal was to improve the precision of implant placement and eliminate errors from a variety of sources including inaccurate plain radiographic templating, morphological anatomical variation, and problems related to the insertion of the implants. The ROBODOC system was conceived in 1986 by Bargar and Paul, and was developed over the next several years with grants from IBM. That team developed proprietary software for the CT imaging to obtain an accuracy of one pixel for the raw data. This advance allowed them to create three-dimensional CT reconstructions for choosing the implant sizes and planning the robotic surgical intervention. Originally, the fiducial markers for the robotic system were placed during a separate operative procedure. The marker was used to specifically orient the robotic tool into the inner canal of the proximal femur. This changed with the ability to register the unique anatomy of the patient intraoperatively. With improvements in software, the system could be referenced by using a digitizing probe for the key areas of the proximal femur. Small incisions were used about the midshaft of the femur for distal referencing [2, 3].

Components of Computer-assisted Navigation

In the early 1990s, other possibilities arose for computer navigation. While "active" or robotic navigation held promise, "passive" navigation developed with the possibility of remotely tracking the instruments and anatomy. The idea here was to reference the target object with "passive" markers. In this case, that would be the human hip or knee joint, which would then be tracked passively in space. For surgical navigation, computed tomography was first used to acquire a digital image representation of the anatomical structure to which the "passive" markers would be applied [4] (❑ Fig. 38-1).

C-arm fluoroscopy referencing followed, and ultimately "imageless" methods developed for total knee arthroplasty [5] (❑ Fig. 38-2). Optoelectronic tracking of the "passive" markers was developed, as that system was readily available from other industrial applications and was not affected by the surgical environment. Other referencing methods such as electromagnetic trackers and ultrasonography had certain disadvantages. The system required the use of multiple cameras that viewed markers in a three-dimensional fashion much as global positioning satellites are used for determining land navigation. As with the Global Postioning Satellite network, surgical navigation can be quite accurate, with most systems documented to an accuracy of 1-2 mm or degrees.

In order to determine the exact spatial orientation of the patient or any surgical instrument, at least three non-collinear points on a fixed body (dynamic reference

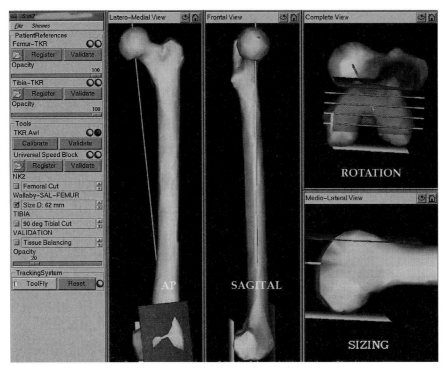

Fig. 38-1. The monitor view of a CT-based application demonstrates the portrayal of the femur where femoral component sizing, validation of the anterior distal femoral resection level, and the distal rotation of the femoral component can be realized. (From [16])

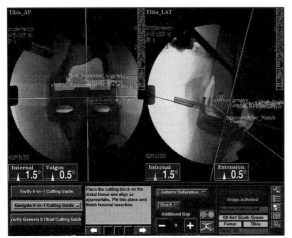

Fig. 38-2. Monitor view of the real fluoroscopic views that have been overlayed with the virtual CAD models of the implants. Note the detail of axes including the mechanical axis, coronal plane axis and the resection planes, including the resulting position of the planned prosthetic placement. (From [16])

base) must be recognized by a camera system which then inputs data into the computer for "virtual" referencing. The camera system generally will consist of two or three CCDs (charged couple devices) that pick up the light signal from the DRBs. The computer referencing protocol collects all components including the patient's anatomy and all registered surgical instruments. The DRBs may be active, consisting of light-emitting diodes (LEDs), or passive, where reflector balls are placed on the DRB and reflect infrared light originating from a light source on the camera. By differentiating the sphere arrangements

on the DRBs, the computer can then detect the specific DRB, such as the marker on the distal femur or a paddle probe.

Computer Referencing Methods

Registration is the process by which the computer recognizes the various three-dimensional objects that it must "virtually" characterize. For all DRBs the process is simply finding the appropriately defined DRB with the camera system and registering it with the computer (☐ Fig. 38-3).

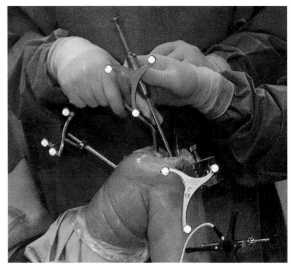

Fig. 38-3. Typical arrangement of DRBs with femoral, tibial, and "touch" pointer rigged with reflective balls that can be "viewed" by the camera system. (From [16])

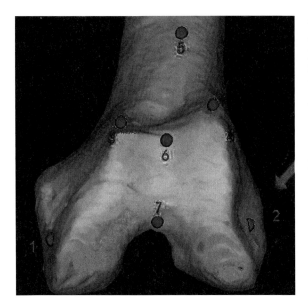

Fig. 38-4. Referencing of the CT 3D model requires point matching from the patient's distal femur which creates the virtual model on the computer for navigation. (From [16])

For instruments and implants, the exact dimensions and orientation of the referencing source are encrypted into the software. For the patient, the goal is to reference or "match" the anatomy of the patient into the computer model (Fig. 38-4).

There are two methods of performing this step. Paired-point matching takes prominent anatomical points that have been predetermined and then intraoperatively uses a space digitizer (pointer probe) that identifies or "matches" the same landmarks. The computer algorithm then matches these points to a "virtual" leg or pelvis built into the software system. Surface registration is a secondary referencing method whereby a small number of points may be digitized into the system to describe a surface contour such as the distal femoral condyle. An additional step is verification, which is cross-referencing additional points on the anatomy with the virtual object on the computer. From this information, the surgeon may judge the operational accuracy of the system.

The advantage of the CT scan for referencing is that it provides a three-dimensional data set for creating a patient-specific virtual model in the computer (see Fig. 38-4). However, acquisition of the CT scan adds additional logistical and financial factors to the process. The CT scan must be obtained preoperatively and must be digital in format for use on the computer [4]. Additional time will be required by the surgical team to manipulate the data, to pick the primary referencing points, for templating, etc. Also there are certain examples such as in navigated fracture reduction, where the bone topology of the CT scan will be intentionally altered during the surgical procedure. Other intraoperative referencing options include two-dimensional C-arm fluoroscopy or a direct imageless

anatomical approach. With fluoroscopy, the two-dimensional images may be used as portraying the virtual patient, while with the direct imageless system, the landmarks are established on a "universal" limb model [5] (see Fig. 38-2). Fluoroscopy requires specific calibration to maintain the desired accuracy of the imaging technique. It is known that the earth's magnetic forces will significantly distort the image acquired, and this must be accounted for. In practice, a calibrated grid with markers of known size and spatial relationship are combined with the image to create an accurate virtual portrayal on the computer. The images are then acquired with the patient's DRB in position to obtain the virtual model that allows navigation of the fluoroscopic image. The imageless applications require simply touch pointing the anatomical landmarks, which are then registered onto the computer. This has been quite effective and successful for navigating total knee arthroplasty and has now become the standard technique with most "open" systems. With any of these systems, the variability comes from the precision with which the surgeon inputs the desired points. The surgeon must be knowledgeable of the specific points required and know exactly where those points should arise. For example, with the Medtronic "Universal Knee" system, which is an imageless system, the proximal tibia center point has been defined as the midpoint of the proximal tibial surface on the medial-lateral and anterior-posterior dimension.

Total Knee Applications

Total knee arthroplasty requires attention to the entire complex of knee-joint mechanics, active muscle forces, and passive ligament structures. One has to appreciate that minimal malpositioning of intra- and extra-medullary tools may lead to considerable variations of implant positioning [6, 7]. Thus, reconstruction of the mechanical lower extremity axis, as well as soft-tissue balancing, is vital for good results. TKA survivorship of 80%-95% after 10 years is reported but this is significantly reduced in cases with more than 4° of varus or valgus alignment, as Rand and Coventry reported in their series with 71% and 73%, respectively, compared with 90% in cases where the component alignment was within the range of 4° [8]. In a similar study, Jeffrey et al. demonstrated that the loosening rate after 12 years was 3% in well-aligned TKA (less than 3° varus/valgus) and 24% in less optimal aligned cases (more than 4° varus/valgus) [9]. In addition, Fehring et al. have shown that chronic ligamentous instability causes a substantial number of revisions after primary total knee arthroplasty, on the order of 27% [10]. There is a compelling roll for better surgical technique to create the desired positioning and tensioning of prosthetics in total knee arthroplasty.

Historically, the first total knee navigation was done by Saragaglia and Picard in 1997 [11]. Following the navigation experience of others, they were interested in developing a method for total knee replacement. As landmarks of the knee joint are relatively accessible, point matching logically would be easy and this led to the totally imageless method of referencing. The direct imageless approach in total knee arthroplasty requires that the surgeon create the virtual computer model by digitizing the various points of the anatomy with a navigated probe. A novel approach has evolved for determining the hip center location whereby the center of rotation of the hip joint is determined kinematically by simply rotating the lower extremity in a large circular motion (◘ Fig. 38-5).

The computer automatically finds the smallest point of movement from the applied DRB, which in this case should be the center of the femoral head. The pelvis is held absolutely rigid for this maneuver. The mechanical axis of the lower extremity is defined by point matching the center of the distal femur, the center of the proximal tibia, and a factored point between the ankle malleoli for the most distal center. Other points such as the epicondyles, the joint surfaces, and the tibial tuberosity are referenced to provide the joint lines and appropriate rotational references [12,13]. Certain proprietary software applications have added surface matching to this direct method to supplement the anatomical features [14].

What are the typical objectives of navigation in total knee arthroplasty? The most obvious goal is to determine the mechanical axis of the lower extremity. This is particularly helpful in cases where ligament release may be extensive and an error may include inadequate release. Each of the joint surface cuts can be made based on the relationship to the mechanical axis. The anterior-posterior cuts of the distal femur may be done using an anterior or posterior cortical reference and the relationship to the transepicondylar axis. One of the recent applications allows for assessment of the gaps before the primary cuts have been made, assessing the precise distance as well as the eventual implant sizes (◘ Fig. 38-6).

Typical navigation will allow for assessing the mechanical alignment and femoral/tibial deviations throughout the range of motion. One may then measure the amount of laxity at each position of flexion through the range of motion. Optimal technique would place the final alignment at 0° for the mechanical axis. A posterior tibial slope should match the required implant. The distal femoral component position should be at 90° to the mechanical axis on the AP view and at 90° to the distal femoral axis on the sagittal plane view. The latter requires 4°-5° of flexion of the implant to the mechanical axis of the lower extremity. Transverse plane femoral rotation should be the prescribed 3°-4° for external rotation to the posterior condylar axis or on the transepicondylar axis.

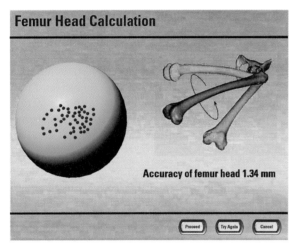

◘ Fig. 38-5. Kinematic verification of the femoral center is done by holding the pelvis rigid, rotating the lower extremity with femoral DRB attached, and computer viewing of the movement of the lower extremity. (From [16])

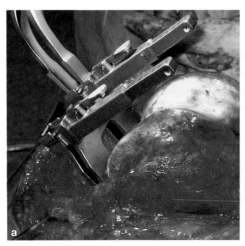
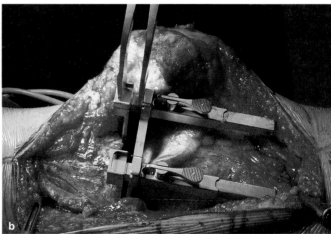

◘ Fig. 38-6a, b. Typical soft-tissue balancing systems available with currently available navigation systems allow assessment of gap dimension prior to resection and positional data that will guide implant sizing. (From [16])

The anterior cortical reference should match the final anterior cut to prevent notching of the distal femur. The mobile-bearing TKA technique typically uses the "tibial cut first" method for determining femoral rotation, which involves flexion spacing. Femoral rotation is based not on a measured distal femoral resection but on the results of a flexion space tensor. The femoral rotation in this scenario tends to reflect the initial flexion space rotation prior to ligament release, or may have an opposite variant rotation based on an extensive extensor release, such as may occur with a severe varus deformity.

CAS in Minimally Invasive Surgery

The applications to minimally invasive surgery will evolve from a unique combination of the above-noted techniques. The surgical problem with small incisions is that certain landmarks become inaccessible for direct point touch matching. While one may easily identify the lower extremity centers for the total knee quadriceps-sparing technique, accessory landmarks such as the epicondyles may not be readily obtained. Fluoroscopy provides images for which these additional landmarks may be point matched directly from the computer screen. The surgeon then has the option of either direct or indirect referencing of the various landmarks. Once referenced, the fluoroscopic images may be utilized for appropriate sizing and positioning of the implants, either with "stick models" of the surface cuts or with CAD model overlays (see Fig. 38-2). Future applications will include newer technologies such as electromagnetic sensors that can be made into miniature DRBs and the use of more sophisticated imaging systems such as three-dimensional C-arms and intraoperative CT scanners [15]. There are currently available technologies that will allow the surgeon unlimited capabilities where navigation may be combined with robotics and robotic-assisted ligament balancing (■ Fig. 38-7).

The interested surgeon must understand that both technologies of MIS and CAOS are recent innovations that are still evolving in terms of validation assessment and clinical efficacy. While both methods will potentially enhance total knee outcomes, only limited clinical studies are currently available. CAOS has clearly been shown to improve mechanical alignment of total knee arthroplasty in several clinical studies. However, the real advantage of CAOS may be in the ability to improve other aspects of surgical technique such as ligamentous balancing and refined component placement. The surgeon must also be cautioned to avoid attempting mastery of both technologies without adequate experience. A logical approach would be to choose one or the other and then gradually refine the technique over an extended period of time (■ Fig. 38-8).

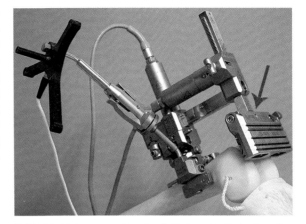

■ **Fig. 38-7.** Futuristic combination of robotic cutting devices (*arrow*) attached to navigation DRBs allows more precise bone resection along with an integrated ligament tensioner. (From [16])

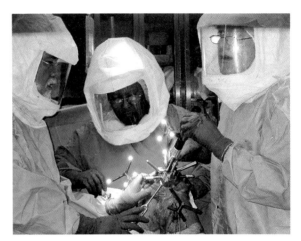

■ **Fig. 38-8.** Senior author demonstrates flexion spacing of a mobile-bearing total knee arthroplasty with the focus of attention to the computer monitor, which is out of the picture. (From [16])

References

1. Nolte LP, Langlotz F (2003) Basics of computer-assisted orthopaedic surgery (CAOS). In: Stiehl JB, Konermann WH, Haaker RG (eds) Navigation and robotics in total joint and spinal surgery. Springer-Verlag, Berlin Heidelberg New York Tokyo
2. Bargar WL, Bauer A, Boerner M (1998) Primary and revision total hip replacement using ROBODOC. Clin Orthop 354:82-101
3. Bargar WL (2003) Robotic surgery and current development with the ROBODOC system. In Stiehl JB, Konermann WH, Haaker RG (eds) Navigation and robotics in total joint and spinal surgery. Springer-Verlag, Berlin Heidelberg New York Tokyo
4. Weise M, Schmidt K, Willburger RE (2003) Clinical experience with CT-based Vectorvision system. In: Stiehl JB, Konermann WH, Haaker RG (eds) Navigation and robotics in total joint and spinal surgery. Springer-Verlag, Berlin Heidelberg New York Tokyo
5. Hagena FW, Kettrukat M, Christ RM, Hackbart M (2003) Fluoroscopy-based navigation in Genesis II total knee arthroplasty with the Medtronic "Viking" system. In: Stiehl JB, Konermann WH, Haaker RG (eds) Navigation and robotics in total joint and spinal surgery. Springer-Verlag, Berlin Heidelberg New York Tokyo

6. Konermann WH, Saur MA (2003) Postoperative alignment of conventional and navigated total knee arthroplasty. In: Stiehl JB, Konermann WH, Haaker RG (eds) Navigation and robotics in total joint and spinal surgery. Springer-Verlag, Berlin Heidelberg New York Tokyo

7. Krackow KA, Bayers-Thering M, Phillips MJ, Mihalko WM (1999) A new technique for determining proper mechanical axis alignment during total knee arthrplasty progress toward computer-assisted TKA. Orthopaedics 22:698-702

8. Rand JA, Coventry MB (1988) The accuracy of femoral intramedullary guides in total knee arthroplasty. Clin Orthop 232:168-173

9. Jeffrey RS, Morris RW, Denham RA (1991) Coronal alignment after total knee replacement. J Bone Joint Surg [Br] 73:709-714

10. Fehring TK, Odum S, Griffin WL, Mason JB, Nadaud M (2001) Early failures in total knee replacement. Clin Orthop 392:315-318

11. Saragaglia D, Picard F (2003) Computer-assisted implantation of total knee endoprosthesis with no preoperative imaging the kinematic model. In: Stiehl JB, Konermann WH, Haaker RG (eds) Navigation and robotics in total joint and spinal surgery. Springer-Verlag, Berlin Heidelberg New York Tokyo

12. Stulberg SD (2003) CT-free-based-navigation systems. In: Stiehl JB, Konermann WH, Haaker RG (eds) Navigation and robotics in total joint and spinal surgery. Springer-Verlag, Berlin Heidelberg New York Tokyo

13. Konermann WH, Kistner S (2003) CT-free navigation including soft-tissue balancing: LCS-TKA and vectorvision systems. In: Stiehl JB, Konermann WH, Haaker RG (eds) Navigation and robotics in total joint and spinal surgery. Springer-Verlag, Berlin Heidelberg New York Tokyo

14. Stindel E, Briard JL, Lavellee S, Dubrana F, Plawski S, Merloz P, Lefevre C, Troccaz J (2003) In: Stiehl JB, Konermann WH, Haaker RG (eds) Navigation and robotics in total joint and spinal surgery. Springer-Verlag, Berlin Heidelberg New York Tokyo

15. Langlotz F (2003) Navigation - where do we go from here? In: Stiehl JB, Konermann WH, Haaker RG (eds) Navigation and robotics in total joint and spinal surgery. Springer-Verlag, Berlin Heidelberg New York Tokyo

16. Stiehl JB, Konermann WH, Haaker RG (2003) Navigation and robotics in total joint and spinal surgery. Springer-Verlag, Berlin Heidelberg New York Tokyo

38

39 Computer-Assisted Surgery: Coronal and Sagittal Alignment

J. Victor

Summary

Computer-assisted total knee surgery has spread rapidly in the orthopedic community over the past 5 years. This technology has the potential to position the components of the total knee arthroplasty exactly in the desired position, hence avoiding outliers in postoperative alignment. This paper describes the currently available systems and their respective advantages and flaws. Accuracy and differential clinical outcomes are discussed, based upon the available literature.

Introduction

Today, total knee arthroplasty is considered a safe, reliable, and predictable procedure, allowing patients with knee arthritis to maintain their activities of daily life and moderate sports activities. Correct positioning of the components is a key factor in this success. Component malposition can cause pain [10], limited range of motion [5], instability [16], polyethylene wear, and loosening of the implant [7,23]. In the earlier days of total knee arthroplasty, much attention was given to the correction of limb alignment, as the detrimental effects of remaining malalignment were obvious and well documented, both clinically [1, 2, 7, 9, 12, 16, 17, 18, 21, 26, 29] and biomechanically [3, 8, 11].

Over the past decades, the characteristics of normal limb alignment were described [20] and with the advent of well-designed instrumentation systems, more reproducible results were obtainable. Also, the increased surgical training led to the perception among orthopedic surgeons that these problems of postoperative malalignment were behind us. However, recent literature proves the opposite [6,10,13,23]. A round table and multicenter evaluation of the French orthopedic community concluded that 31% of patients with major pre-operative coronal malalignment displayed a deviation of the mechanical axis of more than 5° postoperatively.

Jeffery et al. [13] noted good postoperative coronal alignment (mechanical axis deviation of less than 3°) in two thirds of their total knee arthroplasties. In one third

of the operated knees, mechanical axis deviation in the coronal plane was found. These knees had a mechanical loosening rate of 24% at 8 years, as opposed to 3% mechanical loosening for normally aligned knees.

Sharkey et al. [23] showed recently that malalignment and malposition of components still play a significant role in the failure mechanism of modern knee prostheses.

The increase of computer processor speed and technical evolution led to the development of computer assistance for orthopedic surgery (CAS). Many different systems were developed. Two mainstream technologies have prevailed in total knee surgery over the past 5 years: imageless CAS and image-based CAS, the latter being most often combined with fluoroscopy in total knee surgery. The typical characteristic of image-based CAS is that the system can create the spatial link between the image and the anatomical landmarks, the defined virtual points, planes, and axes. This additional information in the form of a fluoroscopic image allows the surgeon to double-check the information relating to the important reference planes and axes. However, these systems do have a significant disadvantage: The image intensifier is a tool that is normally not present in the operating theater during knee arthroplasty. It is bulky, needs to be draped, and poses a potential risk for contamination of the wound. It also increases surgical time and carries a potential radiation hazard. The imageless systems do not have these disadvantages; they are cheaper, easier to use, less bulky, and create no radiation hazard.

The aura of technological supremacy was, from the early beginning, inherently associated with CAS and many orthopedic surgeons expected, without critical analysis, a better positioning of the components, leading to fewer outliers in postoperative alignment. A hype was born, and through press releases the potential patients were informed of the supremacy of CAS.

In contrast, very few scientific papers were published in peer-reviewed journals. Even worse, the early studies on imageless systems did not show improved coronal alignment with the use of CAS [19, 22]. Some studies compared the computer-assisted TKAs with a matched control group [14] and were able to present better results with CAS, without completely avoiding outliers in the CAS group. Other studies showed good results with the use of CAS in TKA but had no control group [25].

Two recent prospective randomized trials that compared CAS with manual instrumentation in TKA reported excellent results for the CAS group with very few [24] or no [27] outliers. In the latter study we assessed the accuracy of the calculation of the kinematic center of rotation of the hip and compared the outcome between the patients that underwent TKA with and without image-based computer assistance.

Materials and Methods

A total of 100 patients were included in our study. No exclusion criteria regarding the amount of pre-operative malalignment, previous surgery, or primary diagnosis were applied.

Randomization was performed in permutation blocks of four. As such, the study was performed on a consecutive series of primary TKAs, where every operating day included two conventional and two CAS cases.

Pre-operative assessment included International Knee Society (IKS) knee and function score, measurement of range of motion (ROM), and radiological examination, including digital standing full-leg films (◘ Fig. 39-1), anteroposterior (AP), lateral, skyline, and condylar radiographs (Philips easyvision 4.2). The radiology technicians were instructed on how to align the limb with the patella pointing forward and the knee in maximum extension in order to obtain standardized full-leg radiographs.

In the conventional group, extramedullary alignment jigs were used on the tibia and intramedullary jigs on the femur. The full-leg standing films were used for

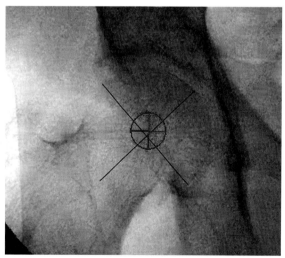

◘ **Fig. 39-1.** Kinematic center of the hip as calculated from mathematical algorithm (*center of small circle*). The crossing of the two *black lines* represents the anatomical center of the hip

pre-operative planning. The angle between the femoral mechanical axis (FMA) and femoral anatomical axis (FAA) was calculated and used on the distal femoral cutting jig.

In the CAS group, a fluoroscopy-based spatial navigation device, using active and passive reference frames (hardware: iON, Medtronic SNT, Louisville, CO; software: FluoroKnee, Smith & Nephew, Memphis, TN, and Medtronic SNT, Louisville, CO), was employed. This system includes the use of a fluoroscopic C-arm with a calibration frame to allow for positional calibration of the fluoroscopic image. The calibration frame carries light-emitting diodes to allow for tracking by the system's camera. In order to obtain ideal stability for the kinematic determination of the center of the hip, the patient was stabilized on the operating table using two padded posts, positioned against the iliac crests. No reference frame was attached to the iliac crest. Dual, bicortical pin fixation was chosen to eliminate the potential of insufficient rotational stability of the reference frame. Placement of the pins was percutaneous, after a small stab wound was made. At the beginning of the procedure a calibration shot was made with the C-arm and all instruments were validated. The fluoroscopic images were acquired (AP and three quarters of the hip, AP and lateral of the knee, AP and lateral of the ankle) and labeled. The limb was then moved in a circular fashion to obtain exact definition of the spherical motion that was described by the femoral reference frame. The computer calculated the kinematic center of rotation and positioned this calculated center on the already obtained fluoroscopic image of the hip.

Hemostasis, wound closure, and rehabilitation protocol were identical for both groups. At 6 weeks, the patients were seen in the clinic and standard digital radiographs (AP, lateral, skyline) and digital full-leg standing X-rays were obtained. All standard X-rays were made using fluoroscopic control to achieve correct orientation in the lateral and coronal plane. In those patients who had not yet achieved full extension at 6 weeks, the full-leg standing X-ray was taken at 3 months postoperatively. At this stage, IKS scores and ROM measurement were done for all patients.

On the fluoroscopic images of the hip with the superimposed calculated kinematic center of rotation that were obtained during surgery, the distance between the anatomical center of the hip and the calculated center of rotation was measured for every patient (see Fig. 39-1). Angles of femoral and tibial component position were noted on AP and lateral X-rays. The reference on the ateral radiograph was the posterior tibial cortex for the tibial component and the posterior femoral cortex for the femoral component. Overall mechanical coronal alignment was measured on the full-leg standing X-rays.

◘ Table 39-1. Demographic data and pre-operative distribution of variables

	CAS Mean	Range	Conventional Mean	Range
Age (years)	72	56-85	70	40-83
Weight (kg)	76	50-102	78	52-92
Length (m)	1.64	150-176	1.64	149-178
Male/female	13/37			
Varus/valgus	29/21		32/18	
Deformity (mech. axis)	8.4	0-16	7.5	0-19
Flexion	105	80-120	111	90-125
Ext. deficit	16	10-20	17	10-20
PS/CR	18/30		23/26	

Results

Three patients were excluded from the study: One patient in the CAS group died of unrelated causes, one patient in the CAS group was changed to conventional instrumentation because of a lead failure intraoperatively, and one patient in the conventional group suffered an ipsilateral hip fracture during the postoperative period. No patients were lost to follow-up. The pre-operative data are summarized in ◘ Table 39-1.

The intraoperative coronal alignment values, as computed during surgery by the CAS system before any bone cuts were made, and the measured pre-operative coronal alignments on the full-leg standing films were plotted against each other and are displayed in ◘ Fig. 39-2.

The mean distance between the computed kinematic center of rotation and the anatomical center of the femoral head was 1.6 mm (range 0-5 mm, standard deviation 1.46). The mean angular mistake on the femoral mechanical axis was 0.19° (range 0°-0.71°).

The tourniquet time was longer in the CAS group than in the conventional group (72 min versus 60 min, $p<0.0005$), as was the skin-to-skin time: 93 min versus 73 min ($p<0.0001$). The mechanical axis in the coronal plane was divided into three groups: 0°-2°, 3°-4°, and >4°. In the CAS group all knees ($n=49$) scored within 0°-2°. In the conventional group ($n=48$), 73.5% of the knees fell within 0°-2° and 26.5% within 3°-4°. No knees displayed a mechanical axis deviation of more than 4° (◘ Fig. 39-3). The difference in variance between the CAS group and the conventional group is significant: $p<0.0001$ (Fisher's exact test). This means that the postoperative alignment tends to be more variable in the conventional group than in the CAS group.

No significant differences were noted between the CAS patients and the conventional patients concerning blood loss, lateral femoral angle, lateral tibial angle, patellar shift, patellar tilt, knee score, function score, and ROM.

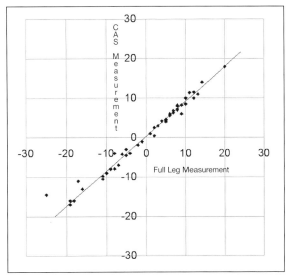

◘ Fig. 39-2. Plot of the pre-operative coronal alignment measurements on full-leg standing radiographs (*X-axis*) versus the intraoperative coronal alignment measurement by the image-based CAS system (*Y-axis*). Positive angular values represent mechanical axis varus alignment, negative angular values represent mechanical axis valgus alignment. Pearson correlation index $r=0.987$

IKS Knee score at 3 months postoperatively was 86 in the conventional group versus 87 in the CAS group. IKS function score was 68 at 3 months postoperatively in both groups.

Mean flexion at 3 months was 116° (100°-125°) in the conventional group versus 114° (90°-125°) in the CAS group. Fixed flexion contracture was present pre-operatively to an extent of :10° in four patients, 5°-9° in 49 patients, and <5° in 44 patients. Postoperatively, this was reduced in the conventional group to one patient, seven patients, and 41 patients, respectively, and in the CAS group to 0 patients, four patients, and 44 patients, respectively.

Complications in the conventional group included delayed wound healing (3), bleeding requiring evacuation of

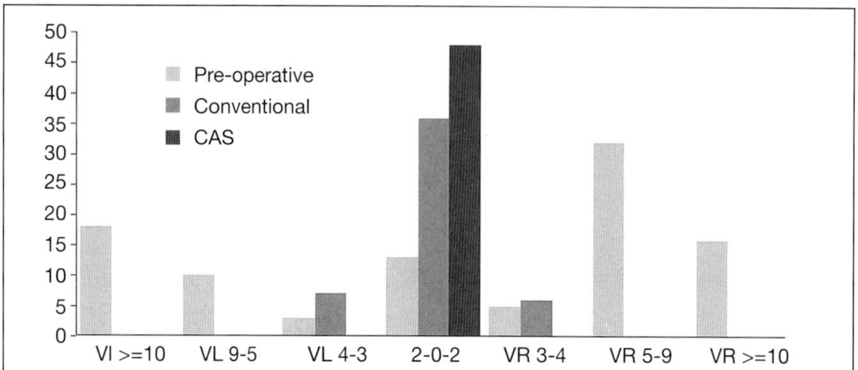

Fig. 39-3. Distribution of pre-operative, conventional postoperative, and CAS postoperative mechanical alignment, as measured on full-leg standing films

	VI >=10	VL 9-5	VL 4-3	2-0-2	VR 3-4	VR 5-9	VR >=10
Pre-operative	18	10	3	13	5	32	16
Conventional	0	0	7	36	6	0	0
CAS	0	0	0	48	0	0	0

hematoma (1), and symptomatic deep venous thrombosis (1). Complications in the CAS group were delayed wound healing (1), pin breakage (3), symptomatic deep venous thrombosis (1), urological (1), and reflex symptomatic dystrophy, successfully treated with epidural sympathetic block (1). Mean fluoroscopy time was 21 s (9-34 s), corresponding to a mean radiation of 0.19 Gy/cm².

Discussion

Malalignment in the coronal plane is still an important cause of early failure of TKA, despite improved surgical training and instrumentation [6,13,23]. The cause of postoperative malalignment is most often incorrect bone cuts. The error in performing the bone cut can be categorized as a 'reference error' or an 'execution error'. Conventional instrumentation uses bony references (anatomical landmarks) or ligament references. Reference errors with

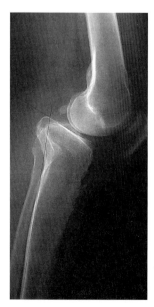

Fig. 39-4. Dysplastic nature of the proximal tibia with a largely abnormal slope of the proximal tibia. Using the 'natural' configuration of the tibial surface could lead to a major malalignment in the sagittal plane

anatomical landmarks occur because the references are not visible (as with the femoral head), are virtual in nature (as with the femoral mechanical axis), or are variable (dysplasia, bowing of long bones, morphotype variability) (Fig. 39-4).

The recent popularity of less invasive exposures for ZKA will certainly not reduce the incidence of reference errors. Ligament referencing is not an alternative for this problem and will not preclude these mistakes, as the tibial bone cut is used as a base reference and as the ligaments as such may be shortened or damaged during surgery.

One might assume that the use of computer assistance would rule out surgical errors, but this needs to be proven in controlled trials. The *total error* in CAS TKA will consist of the sum of the 'camera error', the 'algorithm error', and the 'execution error'. The latter will be similar to the situation with conventional instrumentation and is caused by displacement of the blocks during pinning or saw blade inaccuracy. The advantage of CAS is that block displacement can be detected prior to cutting and that the bone cut can be checked afterwards.

The 'camera error' and 'algorithm error' are specific for the hard- and software used and were the subject of this study. The first aim was to assess the accuracy of the kinematic determination of the center of rotation of the hip. Many navigation systems are employed in current orthopedic practice today, and most of them use a mathematical algorithm to define this center. Several in vitro tests have been carried out, mainly by the manufacturers but little has been published about the clinical performance [27]

The setup of this study allowed us to do this, as both kinematic and spatially linked radiographic data were available. The accuracy was excellent. The mean deviation between kinematic and radiographic center was 1.6 mm (range 0-5 mm). As stated before, this result is specific for the given hardware and software that was used. The software was very sensitive to pelvic motion, and the pelvis needed to be stabilized on the operating table with padded posts. It might be that algorithms less sensitive to pelvic motion are less accurate. With image-based systems, intraoperative control is possible. This is not the case with imageless systems, where the orthopedic surgeon has to rely on the information provided by the manufacturer, and accuracy can be deduced only indirectly in evaluating the postoperative alignment.

The second arm of the described study was a differential outcome analysis between the two groups. The limits of this study lie in the use of full-leg standing radiographs as an outcome tool for measuring alignment. Full-leg radiographs are far more reliable for measuring coronal alignment than the 14 × 17-inch films that are often used for this purpose [15, 25], the reason being that the angle between the femoral mechanical and femoral anatomical axis is variable [28]. One needs to see the femoral head before the femoral mechanical axis can be accurately determined. Full-leg radiographs have been used in previous studies [22] without correlation between the pre-operative measured values and the intraoperative computed values.

We were able to validate the use of full-leg standing radiographs for measuring coronal alignment in this study. The measured value on the film was compared with the computed intraoperative value, before the bone cuts were made. The figures matched exactly (1° or less) for 82% of the knees, as witnessed by the correlation index (see Fig. 39-2). Only two knees had a mismatch of more than 3° between the measured pre-operative value and the calculated intraoperative value. These patients had severe pre-operative fixed flexion contracture (>15°), explaining the inaccuracy of the pre-operative full-leg standing radiograph. As these fixed flexion contractures were corrected after surgery, one can conclude that the post-operative full-leg radiographs were reliable for measuring postoperative coronal alignment.

Our results are excellent in the CAS group: All knees displayed between 0° and 2° of mechanical alignment. This fact is paramount, as it is the main justification for the use of CAS in TKA. Previous studies did not report equally good results. Saragaglia et al. [22] took a wider error margin (0°-3°) and scored within this margin for 84% of the knees that were operated on with computer assistance (Orthopilot, Braun Aesculap, Tuttlingen). Two of 25 knees were 'big' outliers: 5° varus and 7° valgus in the mechanical axis. In the conventional group the results are comparable to ours: They reported 75% of the knees within the 0°-3° margin, versus 73.5% within 0°-2° for our series. Mielke et al. [19] compared 30 navigated cases (Orthopilot) with 30 matched patients who were treated conventionally. In the CAS group they reported 61.7% within 0°-2°; 6.7% in this group had a deviation of more than 4°. Two knees were 'big' outliers: 5° and 7° varus. In the conventional group, 10% of the knees displayed a deviation

of more than 4°. Jenny and Boeri [14] compared 40 navigated cases (Orthopilot) with 40 matched conventional cases. The error margin was defined between 0° and 3°; 95% of the CAS knees scored within this range, versus 85% of the conventional knees. Bäthis et al. [4] performed a randomized trial of 160 patients with the Brainlab Vector Vision system and achieved good mechanical alignment in the coronal plane (0°-3°) for 97% of the patients in the CAS group versus 74% in the conventional group.

Sparmann et al. [24] studied the outcome of using an imageless navigation system (Stryker Howmedica Osteonics, Allendale, NJ) prospectively on a large cohort of 120 navigated cases versus a control group of 120 conventional cases: 97.5% (117/120) in the CAS group displayed a mechanical alignment between 0° and 2°, versus 77.5% (93/120) in the conventional group. The CAS group had no outliers greater than 3°. The results from these authors are comparable to our own.

The position of the components on the lateral radiographs displays more variability. Several factors contribute to this. The measurements were taken on shorter films and are hence less accurate. During surgery, an

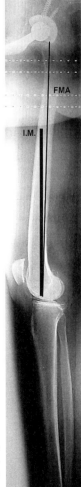

☐ **Fig. 39-5.** The virtual path of the intramedullary rod (*I.M., bold black line*) versus the femoral mechanical axis (*FMA, thin black line*) in the sagittal plane

attempt was made to mimic the natural slope of the tibia, taking the 4° of posterior slope in the polyethylene insert into account. The physiological variability is partially reflected in these figures. On the femur, we initially followed the mechanical axis in the sagittal plane that was calculated by the computer. These knees had a femoral component that was positioned more in extension than would have been the case with intramedullary alignment. Once we realized that the virtual path of our traditional reference, the intramedullary rod, was in a more flexed position than the mechanical axis in the sagittal plane, we changed our desired femoral component position with CAS to 6° of flexion (◘ Fig. 39-5)

In the CAS group no intramedullary rod was used. This is advantageous in cases where hardware remains

after fracture fixation, where there is deformity of the femur, or when there has been prior total hip surgery (◘ Fig. 39-6). As the intramedullary canal is not violated in the CAS group, one might expect less blood loss for these patients; this was not demonstrated. The explanation could be that the femoral hole that was made for the intramedullary rod in the conventional group was blocked with cement at the end of the procedure.

Conclusion

Correct alignment in the sagittal and coronal planes remains a challenge for the orthopedic surgeon performing TKA. The proven relation between malalignment and early failure is the main impetus for developing systems that avoid the outliers in alignment. From the start, it was hoped that computer-assisted surgery would fulfill this task. So far, the literature supports the use of some systems, as they are clearly superior to others. Our study showed excellent results with the use of an image-based system. The advantage of image-based technology is the potential for permanent control of every step in the procedure and the possibility to define landmarks kinematically as well as visually on the fluoroscopic image.

The downside of these systems is the radiation hazard and the practicality of using this machinery inside an operating theater. New imageless systems are promising, but their clinical accuracy remains to be determined in controlled trials. Also, the advent of minimally invasive surgery limits the possibility of acquiring the necessary reference points for imageless CAS. Every surgeon who starts to perfom computer-assisted surgery should make his own clinical accuracy checks on the hard- and software that he uses. The tools to assess outcome are full-leg standing X-rays or CAT scanning.

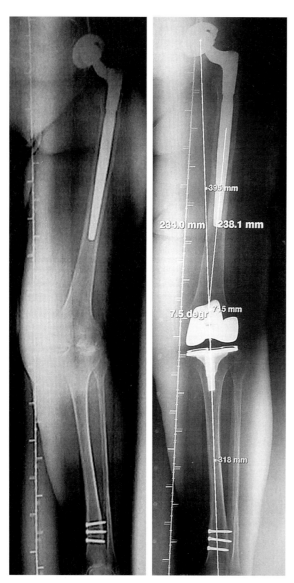

◘ **Fig. 39-6.** Pre- and postoperative alignment of a patient with a large femoral prosthesis proximally, treated with a surgically navigated TKA. Neutral alignment was obtained

References

1. Aglietti P, et al (1988) Posteriorly stabilised total condylar knee replacement: three to eight years follow-up on 85 knees. J Bone Joint Surg [Br] 70: 211-216
2. Bargren JH, et al (1983) Alignment in total knee arthroplasty. Clin Orthop 173:178-183
3. Bartel DL, et al (1982) Performance of the tibial component in total knee replacement. J Bone Joint Surg [Am] 64:1026
4. Bäthis H, et al (2003) Results of the Brainlab CT-free navigation system in total knee arthroplasty. In: Langlotz FL, Davies BL, Bauer A (eds) Computer-assisted orthopedic surgery: third annual meeting of CAOS international proceedings. Steinkopff Verlag, Darmstadt, pp 20-21
5. Bellemans J, et al (2002) Influence of posterior condylar offset. Fluoroscopic analysis of the kinematics of deep flexion in total knee arthroplasty. J Bone Joint Surg [Br] 84:50-53
6. Brilhaut J, et al (2003) Prothèse totale de genou et grandes déviations axiales. Ann Orthop l'Ouest 35:253-288
7. Gibbs AN, et al (1979) A comparison of the Freeman-Swanson (ICLH) and Walldius prostheses in total knee replacement. J Bone Joint Surg [Br] 61:358

8. Green GV, et al (2002) The effects of varus tibial alignment on proximal tibial surface strain in total knee arthroplasty. J Arthroplasty 17:1033-1039
9. Hamilton LR (1982) UCI total knee replacement: a follow-up study. J Bone Joint Surg [Am] 64:740-744
10. Hofmann S, et al (2003) Rotational malalignment of the components may cause chronic pain or early failure in total knee arthroplasty. Orthopade 32:469-476
11. Hsu HP et al (1989) Effect of knee component alignment on tibial load distribution with clinical correlation. Clin Orthop 248:135-144
12. Insall JI, et al (1979) The total condylar knee prosthesis: a report on two hundred and twenty cases. J Bone Joint Surg [Am] 61:173-180
13. Jeffery RS, et al (1991) Coronal alignment after total knee replacement. J Bone Joint Surg [Br] 73:709-14
14. Jenny JY, et al (2001) Computer-assisted implantation of a total knee arthroplasty: a case-controlled study in comparison with classical instrumentation. Rev Chir Orthop Reparatrice Appar Mot 87:645-652
15. Jessup DE, et al (1997) Restoration of limb alignment in total knee arthroplasty: evaluation and methods. J South Orthop Assoc 6:37-47
16. Kumar PJ, et al (1997) Severe malalignment and soft-tissue imbalance in total knee arthroplasty. Am J Knee Surg 10:36-41
17. Laskin RS (1990) Total condylar knee replacement in patients who have rheumatoid arthritis. A ten-year follow-up study. J Bone Joint Surg [Am] 72:529-535
18. Lotke PA, et al (1977) Influence of positioning of prosthesis in total knee replacement. J Bone Joint Surg [Am] 59:77-79
19. Mielke RK, et al (2001) Navigation in knee endoprosthesis implantation - preliminary experience and prospective comparative study in comparison with conventional technique. Z Orthop Ihre Grenzgeb 139:109-116
20. Moreland JR, et al (1987) Radiographic analysis of the axial alignment of the lower extremity. J Bone Joint Surg [Am] 69:745-749
21. Ritter MA, et al (1994) Postoperative alignment of total knee replacement. Clin Orthop 299:153-156
22. Saragaglia D, et al (2001) Computer assisted knee arthroplasty: comparison with a conventional procedure. Results of 50 cases in a prospective randomized study. Rev Chir Orthop Reparatrice Appar Mot 87:18-28
23. Sharkey PF, et al (2002) Why are total knee arthroplasties failing today? Clin Orthop 404:7-13
24. Sparmann M, et al (2003) Positioning of total knee arthroplasty with and without navigation support. A prospective, randomised study. J Bone Joint Surg [Br] 85:830-835
25. Stulberg SD, et al (2002) Computer-assisted navigation in total knee replacement: results of an initial experience in thirty-five patients. J Bone Joint Surg [Am] 84:90-98
26. Tew M, et al (1985) Tibiofemoral alignment and the results of knee replacement. J Bone Joint Surg [Br] 67:551-556
27. Victor J, et al (2004) Image-based computer-assisted total knee arthroplasty leads to lower variability in coronal alignment. Clin Orthop 428:131-139
28. Victor J, et al (1994) Femoral intramedullary instrumentation in total knee arthroplasty: the role of pre-operative X-ray analysis. Knee 1:123-125
29. Windsor RE, et al (1989) Mechanisms of failure of the femoral and tibial components in total knee arthroplasty. Clin Orthop 248:15-19

40 Computer-Assisted Surgery and Rotational Alignment of Total Knee Arthroplasty

G. M. Sikorski

Summary

Producing correct rotational alignment is important in total knee replacement. When bony landmarks are used, the transepicondylar axis (TEA) is the reference axis of choice for the femur. Referencing using soft-tissue balance or kinematics is today still speculative. The tibial component rotatory alignment should follow the achieved position of the femoral component. Good rotational alignment of both the tibial and femoral component is difficult to achieve with or without computer assistance.

Introduction

In a total knee replacement there is a complex relationship between prosthetic alignment, soft-tissue tensions, and the strains that are generated in the polyethylene as a result. The complexity of this relationship is increased by the effects of muscle contraction, by the aberrant kinematics of walking with a total knee replacement, and by static and dynamic forms of prosthetic loading. The objective in aligning a total knee replacement is to minimize and optimize the distribution of strains that are produced by activity, both in the polyethylene and at the various interfaces of the prosthesis.

At the moment we do not have the techniques to measure in vivo loads. Contact area mapping is an indirect approach and is bedeviled by multiple assumptions. So we are left to regard 'malalignment' and 'ligament balancing' as more or less unsubstantiated theoretical constructs. In the end, almost every statement in this chapter will need to be validated, at some future time, by direct measurement.

Correct rotational alignment of a total knee replacement (TKR) is required in order to obtain good and pain-free patellar tracking, functional knee kinematics, and implant longevity. This requires that the femoral component is located parallel to the plane of patellar tracking, that it provides a neutral axis around which the tibial component will rotate, and that the resultant pressure in the polyethylene is equally distributed.

Implications of Malalignment

Patellar Tracking. Excessive internal rotation of the femoral component alone [1] or combined with excessive internal rotation of the tibia [2] is known to be associated with anterior knee pain. When the internal rotation is severe, the patella can sublux or dislocate [2]. When during surgery the femoral component rotation is left in neutral or with a minor degree of external rotation, a lateral release of the patella is seldom required. The relationship with anterior knee pain is so strong that it seems likely that the debate as to whether or not the patella needs to be resurfaced will have to be revisited. Put simply, it is probable that if the femoral component rotation is correct then patellar resurfacing is not needed. If femoral component rotation is wrong then patellar resurfacing will not prevent anterior knee pain.

Soft-tissue Balance. Femoral and tibial component rotational alignments affect several aspects of soft-tissue balance. The effect on the lateral retinacular fibers of the patella has already been mentioned. In 90° of flexion the rotational alignment of the femoral component affects the symmetry of the flexion gap, with external rotation closing the lateral and opening the medial gap. Excessive external rotation of the femoral component (8° or more) produces tightness of the popliteus tendon, which can be alleviated by release of the popliteus [3]. A tight flexion gap may limit flexion and may cause excess wear on the polyethylene. A loose or excessive gap may precipitate laxity and even knee instability.

Femorotibial Kinematics. Paradoxically, internal rotation of the femoral component produces a valgus drift of the tibia in flexion [4] which might cause increased loading of the lateral compartment, although this has not been verified with any direct pressure measurements.

Obtaining Correct Femoral Component Rotation

In the majority of cases femoral rotational alignment is thought of as a relationship between the femoral component and femoral bony landmarks, which are more or less constant in their position. The consistency of the landmarks is not absolutely certain, however, and there is a suspicion that the relationship of these landmarks may change with increasing deformity.

Prosthetic alignment can also be considered in terms of soft-tissue tension balance or even as the result of kinematic analysis. The hypothesis is that if the 'soft-tissue balance' is correct then optimal wear characteristics result. This is a fairly speculative assumption because soft-tissue balance cannot be measured in an objective manner. Tensions and laxities that are produced at surgery are not necessarily the same as those produced during functional use of the knee. The kinematic hypothesis states that if we can produce normal knee kinematics then prosthetic alignment must be correct. Again, this remains to be proven. It is certainly theoretically possible to produce a construct that will have normal kinematics but with aberrant load distributions and shortened implant longevity.

Referencing to Bony Landmarks. Three sets of femoral landmarks have been used as references. Unfortunately, the relationship between them is not constant, nor is any one of them infallible. These landmarks are the posterior condylar axis (PCA), the anteroposterior axis (APA) of Whiteside, and the transepicondylar axis (TEA).

The PCA has been found to be about 4° externally rotated to the TEA, with a range of 0°-9° in one series. As the tibial joint line becomes more varus, the PCA rotates externally relative to the TEA [5]. The opposite happens in the valgus knee. Both are common findings in knee replacements for grossly valgus or varus patterns of disease (Fig. 40-1). The variability of the PCA makes it unsuit-

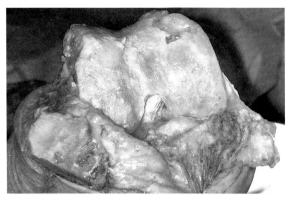

Fig. 40-2. Ostephytic obliteration of the intercondylar region causing difficulty with identification of the anteroposterior axis (Whiteside's line)

able for use as the primary reference axis for femoral rotation, at least in the knees with angular deformity.

The APA of Whiteside [6] is a line drawn along the sulcus between the medial and lateral femoral condyles. It can be difficult to define exactly, especially when there is gross degenerative disease and the region is deformed by a mixture of surface erosion and osteophyte formation (Fig. 40-2).

The TEA is a line drawn between the most prominent point of the lateral epicondyle and the sulcus of the medial epicondyle. If bending of the knee is modeled as an action around two axes, then flexion and extension occur around a fixed axis in the lower end of the femur, while rotation is around a longitudinal axis in the medial compartment of the tibia. The optimal flexion axis has been found to pass through the posterior condyles of the femur at the level of the TEA [7].

Identifying the reference points of the TEA is not always easy and in one study, variations of over 1 cm were found on the lateral side and of over 2 cm on the medial side [8]. The medial sulcus is not always present and the surface of the medial epicondyle can be planar or peaked (Fig. 40-3). However, it has been shown that, using the TEA, a more normal patellar tracking, lower patellofemoral sheer forces [9], and a more balanced flexion space are obtained, compared with surgical procedures where the PCA is used as reference [10].

In summary, we believe that the TEA is the best bony reference axis, but that it cannot be considered as perfect. It is interesting to note that with computer-assisted surgery and an awareness of all the imperfections, the average of the values provided by the TEA and APA can be used as the reference axis.

Referencing by Soft-tissue Balance. The soft-tissue alignment process starts with the distal femoral and tibial cuts in such a manner as to produce a parallel, balanced gap in extension. The knee is then bent to 90° with the tibia vertical, symmetrical distraction is produced, and the cuts that determine femoral rotation are made so as to

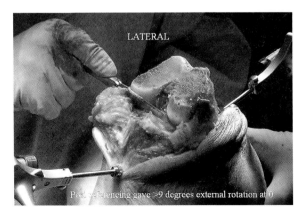

Fig. 40-1. Asymmetry of the femoral condyles, producing a sloping posterior condylar axis. This may lead to excessive external rotation in this varus knee with a deficient posterior medial condyle

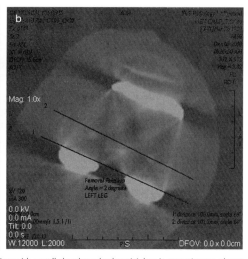

Fig. 40-3a, b. The medial epicondyle does not always have the 'typical' configuration with a well-developed sulcus (*a*), but is sometimes a planar medial epicondyle (*b*)

produce an equal, symmetrical flexion space. In effect, soft-tissue tension and the line of the tibial cut determine the rotatory position of the femoral component [11]. A single cadaver study has suggested that this method is more reliable than the traditional method using bony landmarks [12], although the general evidence supporting this technique is still a bit sparse.

Obtaining Correct Tibial Component Rotation

The major issue in tibial component alignment is whether the tibial component should be aligned in reference to tib-

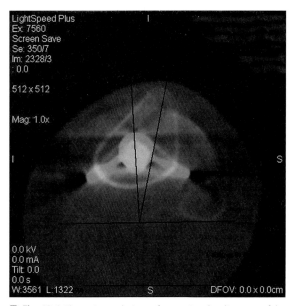

Fig. 40-4. The variant technique of measuring the alignment of the tibial tuberosity. The posterior line is tangential to the posterior cortex of the tibia and fibula

ial anatomical landmarks, or whether it should follow the alignment of the femoral component. The anteroposterior axis of the tibia (APT) is usually thought of as the axis represented by a line passing from the insertion of the posterior cruciate ligament to the medial third of the tibial tuberosity. The consistency of this in relation to other rotational parameters of the tibia is not known. If a line is taken perpendicular to the posterior surfaces of the tibia and fibula and another one through the medial part of the tibial tuberosity, a variant of the APT (APTv) is produced (**Fig. 40-4**). The relationship of this to ideal tibial alignment is inconsistent, however. In my unit postoperative CT scans of patients with TKRs are done routinely and their rotational parameters assessed. The APTv varied between 4° and 19° in ten patients who had perfect femoral rotational alignment (zero degrees to the TEA) and in whom femorotibial match was within 1° of neutral. The relationship between the TEA and the APT is similarly variable and may give rise to femorotibial rotational mismatch of over 10° [13]. For these reasons, there is a tendency to accept the femoral component position as the reference for the tibial plateau. The accuracy with which the two can then be matched in full extension is determined by the instrumentation provided by the manufacturers of the prostheses.

Postoperative Assessment of Adequacy of Rotational Alignment

CT scanning is an accurate way of measuring the component malrotation [14]. Assessment of the rotatory alignment of the femoral component and the axial rotational relationship of the femoral and tibial components is part of the Perth CT Protocol [15], which is used routinely in my unit following total knee replacements. In a group of 82 traditional and 69 computer-assisted total knee

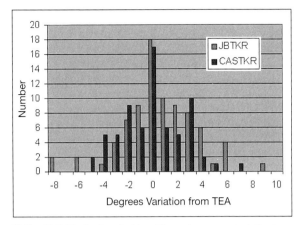

◻ **Fig. 40-5.** Distribution of achieved femoral component rotation in relation to the transepicondylar axis. *JATKR* conventional jig-assisted group, *CATKR* computer-assisted group

replacements, 63% ended up within 2° of the target TEA and the range of rotations produced varied between 9° internal and 8° external (◻ Fig. 40-5). The femorotibial mismatch in maximal extension showed an even greater variation, the range being 13° internal rotation of the tibia to 14° external. This is of great concern, as rotatory malalignment is a potential cause of premature polyethylene wear.

References

1. Barrack RL et al (2001) Component rotation and anterior knee pain after total knee arthroplasty. Clin Orthop 392:46-55
2. Berger RA et al (1998) Malrotation causing patellofemoral complications after total knee arthroplasty. Clin Orthop 356:144-153
3. Nagamine R et al (1995) Effect of rotation malposition of the femoral component on knee stability kinematics after total knee arthroplasty. J Arthroplasty 10:265-270
4. Anouchi YS et al (1993) The effects of axial rotation alignment of the femoral component on knee stability and patellar tracking in total knee arthroplasty demonstrated on autopsy specimens. Clin Orthop 287:170-177
5. Pagnano MW et al (2001) Varus tibial joint line obliquity: a potential cause of femoral component malrotation. Clin Orthop 393:68-74
6. Arima J et al (1995) Femoral rotational alignment, based on the antero-posterior axis, in total knee arthroplasty in a valgus knee. J Bone Joint Surg [Am] 77:1331-1334
7. Churchill DL et al (1998) The transepicondylar axis approximates the optimal flexion axis of the knee. Clin Orthop 356:111-118
8. Jerosch J et al (2002) Interindividual reproducibility in peri-operative rotational alignment of femoral components in knee prosthetic surgery using the transepicondylar axis. Knee Surg Sports Traumatol Arthrosc 10:194-197
9. Miller MC et al (2001) Optimizing femoral component rotation in total knee arthroplasty. Clin Orthop 392:38-45
10. Olcott CW et al (2000) A comparison of four intra-operative methods to determine femoral component rotation during total knee arthroplasty. J Arthroplasty 15:22-26
11. Romero J et al (2003) Significance of axial rotation alignment of components of knee prostheses. Orthopade 32:461-468
12. Katz MA et al (2001) Determining femoral rotation alignment in total knee arthroplasty: reliability of techniques. J Arthroplasty 16:301-305
13. Uehara K et al (2002) Bone anatomy and rotational alignment in total knee arthroplasty. Clin Orthop 402:196-201
14. Jazrawi LM et al (2000) The accuracy of computed tomography for determining femoral and tibial total knee arthroplasty component rotation. J Arthroplasty 15:761-766
15. Chauhan SK, Clark GW, Lloyd S, Scott W, Breidahl W, Sikorski JM (2004) A controlled cadaver study using a multi-parameter quantitative CT assessment of alignment (The Perth CT Protocol). J Bone Joint Surg [Br] 86:818-823

41 Imageless Computer-Assisted Total Knee Arthroplasty

J.-Y. Jenny

Summary

The OrthoPilot navigation system provides us with statistically improved accuracy in the alignment of a TKR compared with conventional manual techniques, without any additional preoperative imaging. According to a multicenter study, these results might be extended to all knee surgeons. The current version of the software allows control of the ligamentous balancing. The navigated prosthesis could have a longer survival through a more precise and more reliable quality of implantation and a more effective ligament balance, but longer follow-up is required. The cost-effectiveness of the imageless navigation technique should be compared with that of other systems, particularly ones with image-based navigation.

Introduction

Survival rates for modern total knee replacements (TKR) of 80%-95% after 10 years have been reported. The restoration of the physiological alignment of the lower limb is an accepted prognostic factor for long-term survival [1, 2].

Classical, surgeon-controlled instrumentations with intra- or extramedullary guides can lead to suboptimal implantation, with rates of unsatisfactory radiological implantation over 10% [3-12]. Computer-aided systems have been developed recently in order to improve the precision of implantation [13]. Image-guided systems allow virtual planning of the implantation and control of the orientation of bony resections during the operative procedure. However, these systems require a preoperative CT scan, which is not routinely provided in current practice. The imageless navigation system Orthopilot (Aesculap, Tuttlingen, Germany) is able to control the orientation of the bony resections without any additional preoperative imaging technique [14].

Correction of the coronal deformation is a major goal of the implantation of a TKR as well. It may be necessary to release retraction of the collateral ligament of the concave side in order to gain an optimal coronal correction. Some surgeons perform this release prior to the bone resections, which could not be optimally oriented without primary correction of the deformation. Others perform it only after implantation of the trial implants. The best timing and actual necessity for this procedure are not well-defined. Computer-assisted implantation can help to decide whether or not to perform a collateral ligament release and to measure the necessary amount of release (◻ Fig. 41-1).

Operative Technique

Three infrared localizers are implanted on screws in the distal femur and in the proximal tibia, and strapped on the dorsal part of the foot. The relative motion of two adjacent localizers is tracked by an infrared camera (Polaris, Northern Digital, Toronto, Canada). An intraoperative kinematic analysis is performed by mobilization of hip, knee, and ankle joints and implemented by the palpation of relevant anatomical landmarks with a pointer. The respective movement of two adjacent localizers is an-

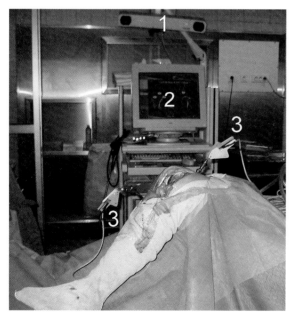

◻ **Fig. 41-1.** The system: *1* infrared camera, *2* monitor, *3* localizers

alyzed by dedicated mathematical algorithms to calculate the three-dimensional location of the respective centers of rotation of each joint. This allows the definition of the individual mechanical leg alignment.

A localizer is then fixed on the tibial resection block, and the software displays online the orientation of this block in comparison to the mechanical axes of the bone. The surgeon can fix the block with the desired orientation before performing the bony resection with a classical motorized saw blade. A navigated plate makes it possible to check the actual orientation of the resections in comparison to the expected one.

A laminar spreader is used to measure the flexion and extension gaps. Then a localizer is fixed on the femoral resection block, and the software displays online the orientation of this block in comparison to the mechanical axes of the bone. It is then possible to simulate influence of the orientation of the distal femoral resection on the ligamentous balance, and to find the best compromise after a potential ligamentous release. The surgeon can fix the block with the desired orientation (◻ Fig. 41-2) before performing the bony resection with a classical motorized saw blade. As for the tibia, a navigated plate makes it pos-

sible to check the actual orientation of the resections in comparison to the expected one.

Following implantation of the trial prosthesis and finally the implants, it is possible to navigate the actual axis correction, to control for full range of motion, and to test again the ligamentous balance.

Clinical Study – Orientation of Resections

Using log books from the operating room, all patients were selected in whom a navigated Search TKR (Aesculap, Tuttlingen, Germany) implantation had been performed at five participating centers (Bünde, Bleicherode, Hessisch-Lichtenau, Sendenhorst, Strasbourg) from 1999 to 2001. A historical control group was defined at the same centers; the inclusion criterion was a conventional manual implantation of the same prosthesis performed between 1995 and 1999 and prospectively followed up.

All patients had a preoperative clinical evaluation according to the Knee Society recommendations [15] and a radiological examination with standardized coronal long-leg stance X-ray and standard lateral X-rays, adapted from the technique described by Siu et al. [16]. Intraoperative complications, operating time, and postoperative complications were recorded. The radiological evaluation was repeated between the 6th and 12th postoperative weeks by an independent observer at each center. Coronal mechanical femorotibial angle and coronal and sagittal orientations of both femoral and tibial components were assessed. Results were expressed as mean ±1 SD. The TKR used was designed to be implanted with the following requirements: a coronal femorotibial mechanical angle of 0°, a coronal angle between the horizontal axis of the femoral or tibial implant and the mechanical femoral or tibial axis of 90°, and a sagittal angle between the horizontal axis of the femoral or tibial implant and the distal anterior femoral or proximal posterior tibial cortex of 90°.

Preoperative criteria were assessed in both groups with either the chi-square test (qualitative items) or the Mann-Whitney U-test (quantitative items) to assess comparability. Accuracy of implantation was compared in both study and control groups. The coronal mechanical femorotibial angle was considered the primary criterion. Numerical values for the five measured angles were compared using a Mann-Whitney U-test. These angles were also divided into two categories: optimal orientation (where deviation from the desired angle was ≤3°), and nonoptimal orientation (where deviation from the desired angle was 4° or more); the repartition into these two categories was compared in the two groups with a chi-square test. The number of fulfilled criteria for each patient was recorded, and the distribution was compared in

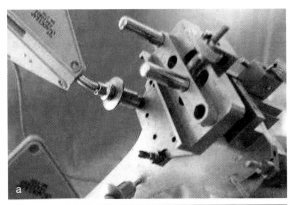

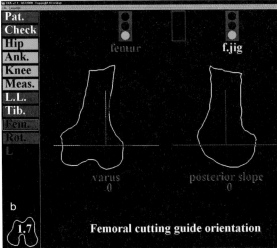

◻ **Fig. 41-2a, b.** Orientation of the femoral resection block: *a* The navigated block, *b* information displayed on the monitor

41

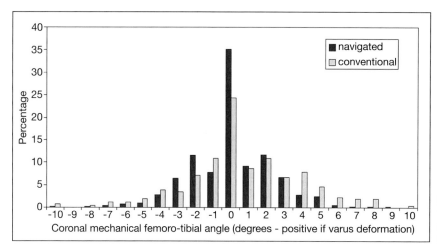

Fig. 41-3. Results: postoperative coronal mechanical femorotibial angle (positive angle if varus deformation)

the two groups with a chi-square test. All statistical tests were performed with a 0.05 level of significance.

There were 555 cases that met the eligibility criteria after navigated implantation, and 266 after conventional implantation: 205 men and 350 women, with a mean age of 70 years (range, 24-95 years). The preoperative radiological mechanical alignment varied from 30°of valgus to 42°of varus (mean: 6° of varus, SD 8°). The preoperative body mass index varied from 20.7 to 43.7 (mean: 30.0, SD 4.3). No significant difference between the groups was observed for all preoperative criteria studied.

All patients were operated on with the help of the navigation system, without any conversion to conventional technique. However, an older version of the software was used, with the need for an additional pelvic localizer fixed with a screw on the homolateral iliac crest.

The mean postoperative coronal mechanical femorotibial angle (■ Fig. 41-3) was 0.1°±2.3°in the navigated group and 0.6° ±3.3° in the conventional group (p=0.007); this angle was considered optimal in 491 (88%) navigated cases and in 192 (72%) conventional cases (p<0.001). The mean postoperative coronal orientation of the femoral component was 90.2° ±1.6° in the navigated group and 90.4° ±2.2° in the conventional group (p=0.51); this angle was considered optimal in 496 (89%) navigated cases and in 205 (77%) conventional cases (p<0.001). The mean postoperative sagittal orientation of the femoral component was 89.2° ±2.6° in the navigated group and 88.7° ±2.5° in the conventional group (p=0.02); this angle was considered optimal in 419 (75%) navigated cases and in 188 (71%) conventional cases (p<0.001).The mean postoperative coronal orientation of the tibial component was 89.8° ±1.4° in the navigated group and 89.6° ±1.9° in the conventional group (p=0.82); this angle was considered optimal in 510 (92%) navigated cases and in 222 (83%) conventional cases (p=0.001). The mean postoperative sagittal orientation of the tibial component was 90.0° ±2.2° in the navigated group and 89.6° ±2.6° in the conventional group (p=0.07); this angle was considered

optimal in 451 (81%) navigated cases and in 186 (70%) conventional cases (p<0.001). The prosthesis was considered optimally implanted (all fulfilled criteria) in 275 cases (50%) in the navigated group and in 82 cases (31%) in the conventional group (p<0.001).

The mean operating time was 108 min in the navigated group (range, 70-193 min; SD, 22 min) and 99 min in the conventional group (range,56-165 min; SD, 22 min; p<0.01).

Clinical Study - Ligamentous Balancing

We conducted a prospective study of 120 computer-assisted implantations of a gliding, posterior cruciate ligament-retaining TKA. The goal of implantation, in addition to correction of the axial deformation, was to obtain a medial laxity in flexion and in extension ≤3° and a lateral laxity in flexion and extension ≤5° [17]. All angular measurements were made intraoperatively by the OrthoPilot system following implantation of the trial prosthesis but prior to any ligamentous release

Twenty-five cases showed a coronal preoperative deformation ≤3°; 79 cases had a preoperative varus deformation (mean: 9°, range 4°-17°); 16 cases had a preoperative valgus deformation (mean: 6°, range 3°-12°). The preoperative deformation was reducible prior to any bone resection in 44 cases (37%), but a release of the concave ligament (always for varus knees) was necessary in only eight cases (7%) to implant the trial prosthesis; 112 cases remained available for analysis.

Optimal correction of the coronal deformation was obtained in 110 cases (98%): 92 knees were considered balanced in extension (82%); 78 knees were considered balanced in flexion (70%); 69 knees were considered balanced in extension and in flexion as well (62%).

Varus deformation over 10° required only medial collateral release in very selected cases. Valgus deformation over 10° required a routine lateral collateral release to correct the deformation.

Discussion

There is no general agreement in the literature about the optimal orientation of a TKR, and the critical point is that the instrumentation allows the surgeon to place the components in the orientation he or she decides. The accepted range for component orientation is also changing in the literature: between ±2° and ±4° from the optimal one. We chose the range of ±3° for all criteria, as this range is widely accepted in the literature and will allow easier comparison. Data were analyzed both quantitatively and qualitatively. However, the qualitative analysis seems to be clinically more relevant, as the outliers might have a worse clinical outcome [1, 2], and we decided to focus on this analysis.

The instrumentation systems most frequently used for TKR implantation are intra- or extramedullary rods which can be aligned along bone axes under visual guidance. The accuracy of such systems has been extensively studied. Rates of optimal implantation of about 70%-85% are generally reported [2, 4, 9] and are consistent with the results of our conventional group. As no significant difference was observed between the conventional and the navigated group for preoperative criteria, this conventional group can therefore be accepted as a control group for the quality of implantation in the navigated group.

We observed a significant improvement in the quality of limb axis correction in the navigated group, which was chosen as the primary criterion. However, it is a combined result of the orientation of the coronal femoral and tibial components, as well as of the ligamentous balance in extension. All individual criteria therefore have to be analyzed separately to assess the accuracy of implantation of the prosthesis as a whole.

Coronal orientation of the femoral component was statistically more accurate in the navigated group. Visual assessment of the longitudinal femur axis by extramedullary rods is made difficult by the larger soft-tissue cover and by the use of the blood-draining device [3]. Intraoperative X-ray location of the femoral head could be more accurate, but it is time and cost consuming and involves additional patient exposure. The intramedullary rod is the most accepted conventional technique [4, 6, 9], but the rate of inaccurate implantation has been reported to lie between 10% and 20%, which is consistent with our findings (23%). The orientation of the rod can be nonoptimal, depending on the diameter of the femoral canal, the location of the entry point in the coronal plane, and the length of the rod [9]. The navigation technique uses the calculated center of the femoral head to determine the direction of the femoral axis and can thus achieve a more accurate orientation.

Coronal orientation of the tibial component was statistically more accurate in the navigated group as well.

There is no general agreement in the literature about the superiority of intramedullary [5] or extramedullary [7] guiding systems, or both [10]. Extramedullary guides rely only on visual alignment, which can be difficult to achieve in a reliable way, especially in obese patients. Intramedullary guides can be deviated by post-traumatic or post-osteotomy conditions or by significant bowing of the tibia [8, 11, 12]. Both systems depend mainly on the visual definition of the center of the proximal tibia. Rates of inaccurate implantation of 10%-30% have been reported [5, 7, 8, 10, 18] and are consistent with our findings (17%). The navigation technique uses the calculated center of the knee and ankle joints to determine the direction of the tibial axis and thus achieves a more accurate orientation.

There is little in the literature about optimal sagittal orientation of the femoral and tibial components. However, results reported suggest a lack of accuracy in the conventional techniques as well, with ranges of 13°-30° for the femoral and of 11°-21° for the tibial component orientation [18, 19]. In the present study, the implantation was statistically more accurate in the navigated group, probably for identical anatomical reasons as for the coronal orientation, and especially the individual femoral curvature. Intramedullary rods tend to place the femoral component in a more flexed position, which could more easily avoid anterior notching of the femoral cortex, but could also lead to a remaining flexion contracture.

As accurate implantation for each criterion is desirable, probably the best way to study the accuracy of implantation of a TKR is to summarize the criteria fulfilled for each patient. The best results are achieved when the five parameters are in the "optimal" category. This was obtained for 54% of the patients in the navigated group and for only 31% of the patients in the conventional group. Navigated implantation allowed a significant improvement in the accuracy of implantation but did not preclude outliers. What could be the reasons for these errors?

Outliers for the coronal femorotibial mechanical angle can be explained by an excessive mediolateral ligament imbalance. This issue has not been studied, as the data were not available for the control group. The general impression was that this factor was not of major importance. However, it will be more precisely controlled by the new version of the software.

The accuracy of the system with infrared probes mounted on rigid plates and recording via a stereotactic camera is considered to be safe and reliable. With the current mathematical algorithm, the precision of the system for the angular alignment has been measured to less than 1° [13]. A potential source of error can be poor fixation of the localizer to bone, especially in the case of porotic bone. Since completion of the current study, the bone fixation system has been modified to allow more secure fixation.

41

Only cutting guides were navigated, but not the saws themselves. However, the existing guiding systems cannot completely avoid misguiding or bending the saw blade, especially when cutting in sclerotic areas. The new version of the system includes a navigated control of the area or resection for potential correction before implantation of the component. The use of high-precision tools for operations such as milling could address this issue.

The cementing technique could be another source of error. The cement thickness might be uneven in different parts of the bone-prosthesis contact area, leading to malalignment of the component on a perfectly resected bone surface. Navigation of the prosthetic components during implantation is desirable.

Computer-assisted TKR is an emerging technology. To our knowledge, there are few papers that report a significant clinical experience with other systems. Most systems currently available are based on a preoperative CT-scan analysis, which is not routine practice. The OrthoPilot system does not require additional preoperative imaging. As image-based systems did not demonstrate any superiority to non-image-based ones, the cost-effectiveness of the latter systems could be superior.

Surgeons' acceptance was high in this study. The software user's interface is friendly. Only small modifications of the well-known classical operative technique and instruments are necessary. In particular, the resection blocks are only slightly modified. There is no need for an additional technician to be present in the operating room, and the whole procedure can be performed by the conventional operating team. No navigated procedure had to be interrupted. The length of the skin incision was the same for both conventional and navigated procedures, including placement of navigation screws. The system works with a completely intraoperative analysis of the lower limb kinematics, without any additional imaging, and consequently with lower costs than other, image-guided systems. The surgeon decides himself or herself and without any limitation the optimal orientations of the bony resections according to the intraoperatively displayed information, and he or she can switch back at any time to the classical instruments if necessary. Mean operating time was 10 min longer with the navigated technique than with the manual one, but this increase was felt to be acceptable in view of the relevant displayed information. This additional time could be reduced with longer experience. Furthermore, some improvements in the system, such as avoidance of the pelvic localizer, could reduce the operating time. On the other hand, other expected developments such as rotational navigation or navigated soft-tissue balancing will increase this time. The cost-effectiveness of the system should be assessed more precisely.

Almost all cases seem to be suited for the navigated technique. Even very large coronal deformations have been treated successfully. The only contraindications to this navigated technique are hip and/or ankle arthrodesis, as the kinematic analysis cannot be performed, but such cases are very rare.

The follow-up of the navigated prostheses is currently too short for us to know if clinical outcome or survival rates will be improved. Longer follow-up is required to determine the respective advantages and disadvantages of both techniques.

This navigation system is a definite aid for optimal ligamentous balancing during TKR implantation. It allows precise and reliable gap measurement, and especially simulation of the ligamentous stability prior to any femoral resection. It also makes it possible to define precisely whether a ligamentous release is necessary or not. There is no need for a routine concavity release prior to bone resections to gain an optimal orientation of the bone resections for pre-implantation varus or valgus coronal deformations under 10°. Varus deformation over 10° needs only medial collateral release in very selected cases. Valgus deformation over 10° requires a routine lateral collateral release to correct the deformation.

Conclusion

The OrthoPilot navigation system resulted in statistically improved accuracy in the alignment of a TKR compared with conventional manual techniques. Because of the multicenter design of the study, these results might be extended to other knee surgeons. The help in ligamentous balancing might be a definite improvement. The navigated prostheses could have a longer survival. However, longer follow-up is required. This system could constitute an important step towards improving implantation technology. The given cost-effectiveness of the navigation technique used should be compared with that of other systems, particular ones that use image-based navigation.

References

1. Ryd L, Lindstrand A, Stentstrom A, Selvik G (1990) Porous coated anatomic tricompartmental tibial components. The relationship between position and micromotion. Clin Orthop 251:189-197
2. Jeffery RS, Morris RW, Denham RA (1991) Coronal alignment after total knee replacement. J Bone Joint Surg [Br] 73:709-714
3. Laskin RS (1984) Alignment of total knee components. Orthopedics 7:62
4. Engh GA, Petersen TL (1990) Comparative experience with intramedullary and extramedullary alignment in total knee arthroplasty. J Arthroplasty 5:1-8
5. Brys DA, Lombardi AV Jr, Mallory TH, Vaughn BK (1991) A comparison of intramedullary and extramedullary alignment systems for tibial component placement in total knee arthroplasty. Clin Orthop 263:175-179
6. Cates HE, Ritter MA, Keting EM, Faris PM (1993) Intramedullary versus extramedullary femoral alignment systems in total knee replacement. Clin Orthop 286:32-39

7. Dennis DA, Channer M, Susman MH, Stringer EA (1993) Intramedullary versus extramedullary tibial alignment systems in total knee arthroplasty. J Arthroplasty 8:43-47
8. Teter KE, Bregman D, Colwell CW Jr (1995) Accuracy of intramedullary versus extramedullary tibial alignment cutting systems in total knee arthroplasty. Clin Orthop 321:106-110
9. Teter KE, Bregman D, Colwell CW Jr (1995) The efficacy of intramedullary femoral alignment in total knee replacement. Clin Orthop 321:117-121
10. Ishii Y, Ohmori G, Bechtold JE, Gustilo RB (1995) Extramedullary versus intramedullary alignment guides in total knee arthroplasty. Clin Orthop 318:167-175
11. Maestro A, Harwin SF, Sandoval MG, Vaquero DH, Murcia A (1998) Influence of intramedullary alignment guides on final total knee arthroplasty component position: a radiographic analysis. J Arthroplasty 14:552-558
12. Ko PS, Tio MK, Ban CM, Mak YK, Ip FK (2001) Radiologic analysis of the tibial intramedullary canal in Chinese varus knees: implications in total knee arthroplasty. J Arthroplasty 16:212-215
13 Delp SL, Stulberg SD, Davies BL, Picard F, Leitner F (1998) Computer assisted knee replacement. Clin Orthop 354:49-56
14. Saragaglia D, Picard F, Chaussard C, Montbarbon E, Leitner F, Cinquin P (2001) Mise en place des prothèses totales du genou assistée par ordinateur: comparaison avec la technique conventionnelle. Rev Chir Orthop 87:18-28
15. Ewald FC (1988) The Knee Society total knee arthroplasty roentgenographic evaluation and scoring system. Clin Orthop 248:9-12
16. Siu D, Cooke TD, Broekhiven LD, Lam M, Fisher B, Saunders G, Challis TW (1991) A standardized technique for lower limb radiography. Practice, applications, and error analysis. Invest Radiol 26:71
17. Whiteside LA, Saeki K, Mihalko WM (2000) Functional medical ligament balancing in total knee arthroplasty. Clin Orthop 380:45-47
18. Mahaluxmivala J, Bankes MJ, Nicolai P, Aldam CH, Allen PW (2001) The effect of surgeon experience on component positioning in 673 Press Fit Condylar posterior cruciate-sacrificing total knee arthroplasties. J Arthroplasty 16:635-640
19. Mont MA, Fairbank AC, Yammamoto Y, Krackow KA, Hungerford DS (1995) Radiographic characterization of aseptically loosened cementless total knee replacements. Clin Orthop 321:73-78

42 Robotics

J. Bellemans

Summary

Today there is growing evidence that performing total knee arthroplasty using computer navigation can lead to a more accurate surgical positioning of the components and subsequent alignment of the knee prosthesis, compared with when a conventional operating technique without computer assistance and navigation is used. These computer navigation systems are readily available and are being used more and more in daily practice.

The use of robotic technology could theoretically take this accuracy one level further, since it uses navigation in combination with ultimate mechanical precision, which could eliminate or reduce the inevitable margin of error during mechanical preparation of the bony cuts by the surgeon. In this chapter we report the experiences gained so far with robotic technology in knee arthroplasty surgery.

Introduction

The introduction of robotic technology into orthopedic surgery dates from the late 1980s and led to the first robot-assisted hip replacement performed on a human patient in 1992, with subsequent commercialization of the system in 1994 under approval of the European Union [1]. Although most of the initial research and development was performed by schools and centers in Germany, the enthusiasm has since spread out not only over the whole European continent, but also over North America and the rest of the world. Today, for example, robots are used not only in hip arthroplasty but also in knee arthroplasty and cruciate ligament surgery, with different commercial systems available.

Generally speaking, robots can be categorized as passive, active, or semiactive. Passive robots hold the guide or jig in the correct place, but the actual cutting or drilling is performed by the surgeon or the operator. Active robots not only hold the cutting tool; they also autonomously make the appropriate cuts. Semiactive robots combine both principles, whereby the robot guides the cutting tool within a predefined trajectory (e.g., a plane on the proximal tibia), within which the surgeon can work under the constraints provided by the robot.

Although a number of groups are now exploring the potential role of semiactive robots in knee arthroplasty, the systems that are commercially available for knee surgery today are active robots [2]. Such active robots obviously require a high degree of safety and reliability and should give the surgeon adequate feedback about the ongoing process, such as the cutting path with respect to the preoperative planning, cutting forces, bone motion, etc., in order to allow the surgeon to detect if something is going wrong and subsequently allow him to intervene if necessary.

Two systems that fulfill these requirements have been made commercially available for knee arthroplasty, i.e., the ROBODOC system (Integrated Surgical Systems, Davis, Calif.) and the CASPAR system (U.R.S. Ortho Rastatt, Germany). Both systems have a comparable application protocol, with similar performance characteristics.

Application Protocol

The process of robot-assisted knee arthroplasty basically consists of four steps: placement of the fiducial marker pins, spiral CT-scanning of the patient's leg, preoperative planning and virtual implantation, and the actual surgical implantation.

Placement of the Fiducial Markers. Just as in classical computer-navigated TKA, fiducial markers need to be applied to the femur and tibia. These markers are used by the robot for spatial orientation and the necessary geometric calculations. These fiducial markers therefore need to be firmly fixed; this is usually achieved by double bicortical threaded pin fixation in a separate operation, which usually takes about 15 min.

Spiral CT-Scan. With the pins in place, a spiral CT-scan is obtained. The femoral head, the knee joint, the ankle joint, and the pins are scanned, usually while the patient is still under spinal or epidural anesthesia. The average time for acquiring such a CT-scan is usually 20 min. In case the operating theater is provided with on-site CT-scanning possibilities, both previous steps together with the actual robotic surgery can obviously be combined without having to displace and transfer the patient, which leads to a significant improvement in comfort for both the patient and the surgical team.

Preoperative Planning and Virtual Implantation. After the CT data have been transferred to the PC-based planning station, the necessary anatomical landmarks are identified at the level of the knee joint, as are the center of the femoral head and the center of the ankle joint, which are used for determination of the mechanical and anatomical axes (◘ Fig. 42-1). Subsequently, the calculation of the frontal, sagittal, and rotational alignment is performed by the system.

Next, the virtual implantation is performed on the screen by selecting a specific implant and size and positioning it onto the corresponding bone while changing or playing with the component translation and/or rotation until a satisfactory position is achieved (◘ Fig. 42-2).

Immediate graphical and numerical feedback on the alterations in alignment, as well as mediolateral and

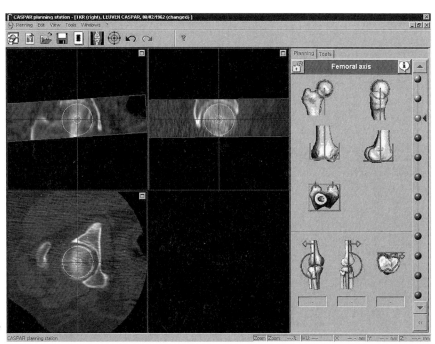

◘ **Fig. 42-1.** Determination of the anatomical landmarks

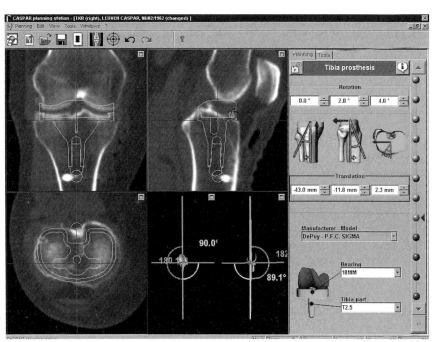

◘ **Fig. 42-2.** Virtual implantation of the tibial component

flexion/extension gap balancing, can be viewed on the screen. Other surgically relevant parameters such as the presence of femoral notching, over- or undersizing of the component relative to the bone size, or restoration of posterior condylar offset can be assessed and corrected instantly (◘ Fig. 42-3).

Once the optimal positions for the components have been obtained, the milling area can be specified and adapted in order to avoid milling into the soft-tissue regions, thereby reducing soft-tissue trauma (◘ Fig. 42-4). Finally, all data are saved and stored onto a memory disc,

which is subsequently transferred to the robot control unit (◘ Fig. 42-5).

The whole process of programming and virtual implantation takes 15-20 min on average, but it is unanimously appreciated as very enlightening to everyone being trained in robot-assisted knee arthroplasty, not only with regard to computer-assisted technology, but also with respect to conventional day-to-day TKA surgery.

Surgical Implantation. A standard incision with medial parapatellar arthrotomy and lateral dislocation of the

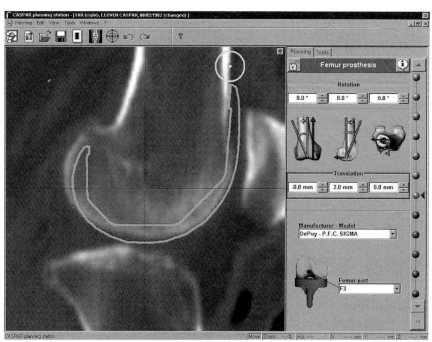

◘ **Fig. 42-3.** Virtual implantation of the femoral component

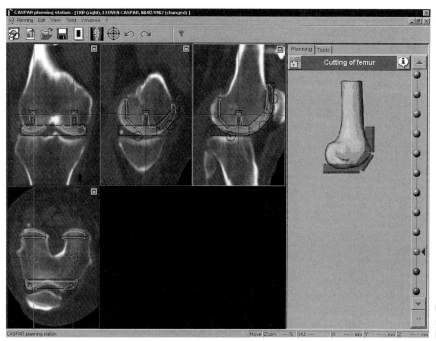

◘ **Fig. 42-4.** Determination and presetting of the milling areas indicated by the red linings

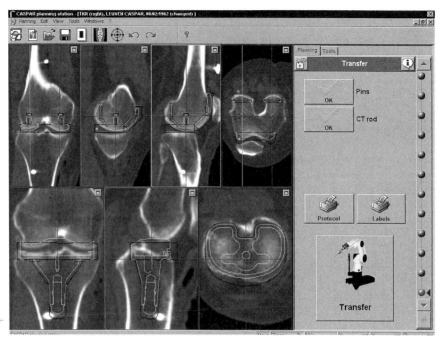

Fig. 42-5. Finalizing the virtual total knee implantation

patella is performed. Next, the leg is flexed and rigidly connected to the robot by two transverse Steinman pins inserted through the proximal tibia and the distal femur. These two pins are connected to a frame which is linked to the robot, while several retracting devices are mounted onto this frame for optimal exposure and soft-tissue retraction (Fig. 42-6). In order to detect and control undesired motion of the leg during the robotic surgery, reflective markers are attached to this frame as well. They are continuously monitored by an infrared camera system and will immediately stop the robot in case any type of undesired motion is detected.

Following verification of the fiducial markers, the robotic action is started by the surgeon. The robot uses a milling cutter to perform the bone resection, together with constant water irrigation for cooling purposes and for cleaning the milling debris. The surgeon maintains control over the milling process by a manually held button, which shuts off the robotic action as soon as the button is depressed. At any stage during the procedure, the surgeon can switch to conventional implantation techniques if desired. Once the bone cuts are finished, the robotic frame is disconnected, components are inserted, and the surgery is finished.

Experiences and Results

Twenty-one robot-assisted TKAs were performed with the CASPAR system at our institution between 2000 and 2002, with a typical and intense learning curve not only for the surgeon, but even more for the nursing staff and the radiologists involved. Unlike any other new operating technique, this type of robotic surgery has indeed posed many more challenges during the learning process. Not only the important increase in operating time, but also the sense of helplessness towards computer technology and software disfunctioning (caused by the operator or not) have been a constant area of concern and frustration during the learning phase, which required an adequate dose of perseverance for the team to succeed.

The 21 patients were randomly selected from our patient data base and underwent the robotic TKA surgery after prior consent, without any selection towards severity of the deformity, presence of osteoporosis, range of motion, or any other parameter. Despite the difficult learning curve, excellent results were obtained in all cas-

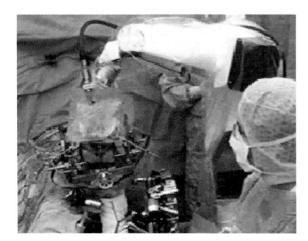

Fig. 42-6. Operative setup using the Caspar System

42

es that were finished successfully, with overall frontal alignment on full-leg standing X-rays within the 1° error of neutral alignment. In three cases the robotic process was aborted because of technical difficulties with recognizing the reflective marker positions, leading to a continuous error signaling on the screen. Each of these cases was successfully finished by converting to a conventional technique.

Experiences comparable to ours have been reported in the meantime by other groups. Siebert et al. recently published their results in 70 cases operated with the CASPAR system, with a mean difference between planned and obtained tibiofemoral alignment of 0.8°. Some outliers were noted, with a maximum of 4° compared with the planned alignment [3,4]. An average operating time of 135 (80-220) min was necessary to perform the surgery.

Borner et al. recently reported their results with the ROBODOC system and the Duracon total knee prosthesis in their first 100 cases. The procedure needed to be abandoned in only 5% of the cases and the surgeons switched to a conventional technique due to technical problems. Alignment was within the 3° margin for all cases, and operating time was between 90 and 100 min after the initial learning curve [5].

Discussion

It is clear today that excellent results can be obtained with robot-assisted total knee arthroplasty. The reported subjective outcome seems to be at least comparable to that with conventional TKA in the short-term follow-up, while evidence exists that coronal plane alignment and overall component positioning is much better using robotic technology compared with conventional TKA.

The advantages of robot assistance in surgery are the functional constraints that these systems can impose; i.e., increased precision is obtained by constraining the movement of the machining tool within well-specified margins. Total knee arthroplasty requires accurate machining of the bone surfaces of the tibia and femur, and the accuracy of the location and orientation of these surgical cuts is crucial to obtaining proper implant alignment, joint kinematics, and ligament balancing. Moreover, in cementless TKA, the surface flatness of the cuts has to be sufficient to maximize the chances for bone ingrowth and successful long-term fixation of the components [6,7].

Recent work by our group has shown that a milling robot can achieve this necessary high precision. The surface flatness of tibial bone cuts prepared by a robot-assisted procedure ranged between 0.15 and 0.29 mm, versus 0.16-0.42 mm during conventional surgery using an oscillating saw [8-10].

This advantage of robot-assisted surgery is clinically important, since the maximal distance between the bone

and the prosthetic component that allows for bone ingrowth to occur is 0.3-0.5 mm [6,7,10]. Moreover, in every case with conventional sawing a depression of the middle aspect of the prepared surface was noted; this was never seen in the robot-assisted cases [10].

Finally, temperature rise during the robot-assisted procedures can be controlled by altering or adapting the milling speed, which is another advantage over conventional bone preparation using a power saw, whereby a rise in temperature is frequently generated and may exceed the critical threshold of 44°-47°C, beyond which bone damage is known to occur, leading to compromised cementless or even cemented fixation [6,7,10,11].

These last-mentioned advantages of robotic TKA over conventional surgery also speak for robotic systems as compared with contemporary navigation systems. Although current navigation systems are significantly improved in comparison to the first-generation systems, which were beneficial to the surgeon mainly in improving frontal plane alignment, they still require the use of standard old-fashioned types of bone preparation methods with a well-known margin of imprecision.

The latest generation of navigation systems also have a number of important advantages over robotic systems, however. The versatility that is allowed during the actual procedure, for example, is an important benefit compared with the virtual implantation that is performed with the current robotic systems and that leaves the surgeon with no or very limited adaptations possible during the actual in vivo surgery, at least not without abandoning the robotic procedure and switching to conventional surgery. Also, latest-generation navigation systems allow for online and numerically quantified assessment of soft-tissue status and subsequent soft-tissue balancing, a feature which, again, is not readily available with the current robotic systems. Finally, today's navigation systems are much cheaper than the currently available robotic systems, not only in purchase costs but also with regard to operational costs related to the disposable ancillaries that are required for each procedure.

With the decreased complexity and greater user friendliness for radiology and operating room staff, navigation systems have therefore been much more popular than robots so far in the minds of surgeons and hospital administrators. The recent problems with regard to the distribution and sale of the CASPAR systems (financial problems and stipulations of the manufacturing company) have further added to the reluctance and reservation of many orthopedic surgeons to select robotic technology when performing orthopedic surgery.

Furthermore, some less encouraging data have recently been published on total hip replacement with active systems such as the ROBODOC, demonstrating higher complication rates compared with conventional total hip arthroplasty, more specifically with regard to dislocation rate, amount of muscle damage, duration of surgery, and revision rate [12].

It is for these reasons that most laboratories and companies involved in orthopedic robotics have started focusing more and more on semiactive robotic systems, which may combine to a better extent the surgical versatility and adaptability of navigation systems with the advantages of almost perfect machining and bone preparation offered by robotic systems. Such semiactive robots would theoretically be much cheaper and more user-friendly than the current active robot systems, and therefore would be more successful in daily application.

References

1. Bargar W (2004) Robotic hip surgery and current development with the Robodoc system. In: Stiehl JB, Konermann WH, Haaker RG (eds) Navigation and robotics in total joint and spine surgery. Springer-Verlag, Berlin Heidelberg New York Tokyo, pp 119-121
2. Van Ham G et al (1998) Machining and accuracy studies for a tibial knee implant using a force-controlled robot. Comput Aided Surg 3:123-133
3. Mai S et al (2004) Clinical results with the robot assisted Caspar System and the Search-Evolution Prosthesis. In: Stiehl JB, Konermann WH, Haaker RG (eds) Navigation and robotics in total joint and spine surgery. Springer-Verlag, Berlin Heidelberg New York Tokyo, pp 355-361
4. Siebert W et al (2002) Technique and first clinical results of robot-assisted total knee replacement. Knee 9:173-180
5. Borner M et al (2004) Clinical experiences with Robodoc and the Duracon Total Knee. In: Stiehl JB, Konermann WH, Haaker RG (eds) Navigation and robotics in total joint and spine surgery. Springer-Verlag, Berlin Heidelberg New York Tokyo, pp 362-366
6. Bellemans J (1999) Osseointegration in porous coated knee arthroplasty. Acta Orthop Scand 70:1-35
7. Bellemans J et al (1999) Osseointegration of porous coated knee arthroplasty. Arch Am Acad Orthop Surg 2:62-67
8. Toksvig-Larsen S et al (1991) Surface flatness after bone cutting: a cadaver study of tibial condyles. Acta Orthop Scand 62:15-18
9. Denis K et al (2002) How correctly does an intramedullary alignment rod represent the longitudinal tibial axes? Clin Orthop Rel Res 397:424-433
10. Denis K et al (2001) Influence of bone milling parameters on the temperature rise, milling forces and surface flatness in view of robot-assisted total knee arthroplasty. Int Congress Series 1230:300-306
11. Eriksson R et al (1984) the effect of heat on bone regeneration: an experimental study in the rabbit using the bone growth chamber. J Oral Maxillofac Surg 42:705-711
12. Honl M et al (2003) Comparison of robot assisted and manual implantation of a primary total hip replacement. A prospective study. J Bone Joint Surg [Am] 85:1470-1478

43 The Unicompartmental Knee: Minimally Invasive Approach

T. V. Swanson

Summary

The development of minimally invasive surgery may be changing the indications for unicompartmental knee arthroplasty. While UKA has never enjoyed consistent enthusiasm in the orthopedic community, minimally invasive techniques are bringing the procedure back into favor. Although exuberant enthusiasm for new techniques is common, the minimally invasive UKA has now proved successful in several surgeons' hands and is likely here to stay. However, further evaluation is needed to better identify the correct indications for the procedure.

Introduction

Unicompartmental knee arthroplasty (UKA) has enjoyed varying degrees of enthusiasm since its inception in the early 1970s. Many factors leading to unpredictable results were eventually identified. However, with appropriate indications and surgical technique, favorable outcomes can be achieved. Historically, unicompartmental knee replacements were performed through the same medial parapatellar incision used for total knee replacements. Extensile incisions, extensor mechanism trauma with eversion of the patella, and tibial retraction imparted the same degree of soft-tissue trauma to the unicompartmental knee as the total knee. Not until the advent of minimally invasive surgical techniques in the early 1990s did unicompartmental knee replacement experience a renewed enthusiasm among orthopedic surgeons.

Changing Indications for UKA

Kozinn and Scott described the classic indications for UKA in 1989 [1] (◘ Table 43-1). Using these stringent criteria, results improved significantly, although these criteria excluded 90-95% of patients with knee arthritis [2, 3].

◘ **Table 43-1.** Changing Indications for UKA

	Classic indications	Evolving indications
Age (years)	>60	>50 as temporizing measure; >60 as definitive procedure
Weight (kg)	<82	Yet undefined
Activity level	Low demand	Non-laborers
Arthritis location	Purely medial or lateral	Purely medial or lateral
Diagnosis	Non-inflammatory, non-crystalline	Non-inflammatory, non-crystalline; Ahlback stage 1, 2, or 3 (not 4) osteoarthritis
Range of motion		
Flexion	>90°	>90°
Flexion contracture	<5°	<15°
Deformity		
Varus	<10°	Passively correctible to within 5° of neutral mechanical axis
Valgus	<15°	
ACL	Intact without mediolateral subluxation	OK if attenuated or absent due to attrition; no gross clinical instability
Patellofemoral joint	No symptoms; minimal chondromalacia	Minimal symptoms; no sclerosis of patellar facet; mild/moderate degenerative changes OK if asymptomatic
Symptoms	Unicompartmental; abate with rest	Unicompartmental

Because the durability and longevity of UKA never quite equaled that of TKA, the advantages of UKA over TKA were minimal (retained proprioception, slightly improved motion, better kinematics, quicker recovery, easier revision) [1, 4, 16, 20]. With the advent of minimally invasive techniques for UKA, the magnitude of the surgery and recovery time were both significantly reduced. Hospitalization can often be reduced to 1-2 days, and recovery time to 2-4 weeks [11, 12, 15], with a resultant expansion of the indications for UKA to include it as a temporizing measure in younger patients with unicompartmental arthritis [5, 7, 12] (Table 43-1). Some centers claim that up to 30% of their knee arthritis patients now receive UKAs [6].

Requirements for Minimally Invasive UKA

The success of any minimally invasive joint replacement derives from reduced soft-tissue trauma, both superficial and deep. Achieving this objective requires: (a) incision placement in the most optimal location, (b) specialized instrumentation which can be used through smaller incisions, and (c) appropriate positioning of the extremity at each step of the procedure to expose the necessary anatomy through the limited incision.

Incision Placement

While a midline incision is used for total knee replacement and standard-incision UKA, the incision is medialized directly over the femoral condyle for minimally invasive UKA. This allows for easy access to the femoral condyle and tibial plateau. It is important to realize that the patella need be subluxated only slightly away from

the compartment being replaced, thereby imparting significantly less trauma to the extensor mechanism than dislocation and eversion of the patella (◘ Figs. 43-1a, b).

Specialized Instruments

While instruments resembling total knee instruments were used for years, the advent of minimally invasive UKA has necessitated a re-design of instruments. Some minimally invasive UKA instrumentation still accesses the intramedullary canal. However, invasion of the canal does make the procedure less "minimally invasive." Instruments, in general, have been downsized and fitted with extended handles to allow easier manipulation within the limited space available.

Extremity Positioning

Extremely important in minimizing the amount of soft-tissue retraction is positioning the limb to facilitate exposure of the anatomy being addressed during each step of the procedure (sometimes referred to as a "mobile window"). Hyper-flexion is often helpful for cutting the proximal tibia or the posterior femoral condyle. Extension to 60°-70° is often useful for exposing the distal and anterior femoral condyle. Full extension of the knee allows inspection of the patellofemoral joint. Placing a valgus stress on the flexed knee helps open up the medial joint space for removing meniscal remnants or bone debris, or for trimming posterior femoral osteophytes. Varus stress on the slightly flexed knee allows visualization of the lateral compartment. One must learn which position facilitates exposure for each step of the procedure.

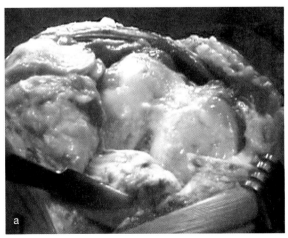
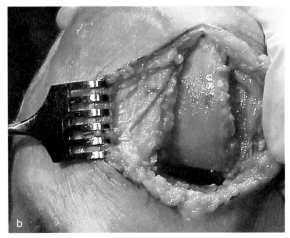

◘ **Fig. 43-1a, b.** *a* Standard medial parapatellar approach with eversion of the patella vs. *b* minimally invasive incision directly over the medial compartment

Surgical Technique for Minimally Invasive UKA

Surgical Approach

Although lateral minimally invasive UKA is occasionally performed, the following technique will focus on medial compartment arthroplasty. Minimally invasive UKA can generally be performed through an 8- to 10-cm incision when measured with the knee flexed (5-6 cm when measured in extension). With the knee flexed, make an incision from the superomedial corner of the patella to the superomedial corner of the tibial tubercle (see ◾ Fig. 43-2). The incision generally does not need to extend more than 2 cm below the joint line. Carry the incision sharply through retinalcular tissue immediately adjacent and parallel to the patella and patellar tendon. For easier retraction of the extensor mechanism, a small split of the vastus medialis obliquus fibers may be made at the superior corner of the patella, or the retinacular incision can be carried proximally into the quadriceps tendon 1-2 cm.

Visualization is critical. Excise any part of the fat pad that may obstruct visualization. In contrast to the more extensive soft-tissue releases performed with TKA, only the capsule and deep fibers of the medial collateral ligament should be released from the proximal tibia. At this point, the knee can be extended slightly and a varus stress placed on the joint to inspect the lateral compartment. Extend the knee fully to evaluate the patellofemoral joint.

With the knee extended, place a valgus stress on the knee to determine the amount of varus that is passively correctible. The knee alignment should correct to within 5° of a neutral mechanical axis to proceed [16-18].

Tibial Preparation

Although several minimally invasive UKA instrument systems are currently available, the author's preference is

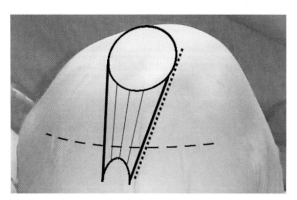

◾ **Fig. 43-2.** Incision placement from superomedial corner of patella to superomedial edge of tibial tubercle

the Accuris instrumentation system (Smith & Nephew Orthopaedics, Memphis, Tenn.). These instruments allow accurate placement of the components using "surface referencing" of the femur (without violating the intramedullary canal). Furthermore, they allow for placement of the femoral component in the kinematically correct position so as to track centrally on the tibial component throughout the range of flexion-extension.

Place a shim of appropriate thickness in the medial joint to correct the mechanical tibiofemoral axis to within 5° of neutral; thicker shims provide more correction and result in less tibial resection (◾ Fig. 43-3). Flex the knee to 110° and apply the cutting assembly to the shim. Normally, the shim can be used to establish the correct tibial posterior slope. However, if the patient has a slight flexion contracture or an attenuated ACL, it may be advantageous to cut the tibia with slightly less posterior slope [7, 8].

Align the tibial cutting guide in the coronal plane either perpendicular to the mechanical axis or parallel to the joint line. Minimize the number and depth of pin penetration into the proximal tibia to avoid tibial stress fracture [9]. Two types of tibial components are available – inlay and onlay. For the onlay technique, both the posterior femoral and proximal tibial cuts are made with this cutting jig, establishing a flexion gap of appropriate thickness. Because unicompartmental arthritis often involves the anteromedial joint [10], the shim may become too tight in flexion. In this case, remove 3 mm of additional bone from the posterior femur by cutting on top of the guide rather than through the slot. Make the sagittal tibial cut adjacent to the tibial attachment of the ACL (◾ Fig 43-4).

For the tibial inlay technique, a template is placed over the proximal tibia, and a 90° burr is used to remove the desired depth of bone, leaving a cortical rim around the tibial implant. Remove the cutting guide, and with the knee flexed, apply a gentle valgus stress to the knee by letting it rotate medially. This will open up the medial space to facilitate removal of bone fragments, meniscal remnants, and posterior femoral osteophytes. Alternatively, the compartment can be visualized with valgus stress on the extended knee. A tibial trial of appropriate size can be selected by measuring the anteroposterior dimension of the cut tibial surface, or by sizing the trial directly from the resected tibial plateau. The tibial trial is pinned in place.

Femoral Preparation

With a trial insert in the tibial component, extend the knee and mark the anterior-most contact point on the femur. Remove the trial insert and attach a powered concave milling device to the tibial trial. The knee is taken through a range of motion from flexion to full extension, allowing the milling device to remove 3-4 mm of bone

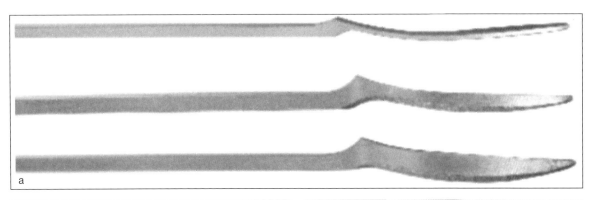

a

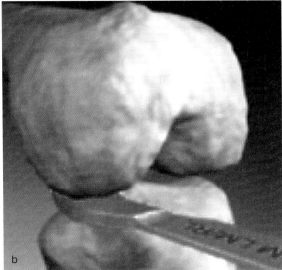

b

◘ **Fig. 43-3a, b.** *a* Shims used to correct coronal alignment in UKA. *b* Shim in medial compartment after passive correction of tibiofemoral varus deformity

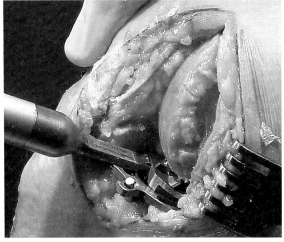

◘ **Fig. 43-5.** Femoral milling device. Attached to the tibial trial, it prepares the distal femur so that the femoral component contacts the center of the tibial component throughout the range of motion of the knee

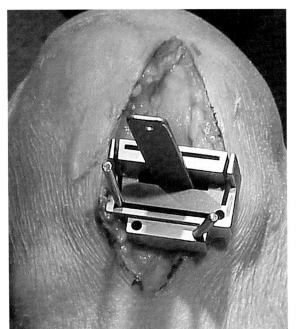

◘ **Fig. 43-4.** Proximal tibial and posterior femoral cutting guide in place. Using a single guide for both cuts establishes the correct flexion space

along the kinematic path of the tibial component (◘ Fig 43-5).

Once prepared, size the femur, and place a trial component in the track created by the milling device. This ensures that there will be no femoral component tilt (which can cause edge loading of the component) in either flexion or extension and that the femoral condyle will track in the center of the tibial component throughout the range of motion (to prevent eccentric loading of the tibial component). After placing the femoral trial and testing range of motion, prepare the lug hole and fin slot through the femoral trial.

Cementing

Fixation is critical to the longevity of the arthroplasty. Drill several 2-mm fixation holes into the cut surfaces of the femur and tibia. Cement the tibial component first. Remove excess cement from the back of the component with the knee flexed using right-angled instruments. Another method of cement removal is to place a thin sponge behind the tibial component. Once it is impacted into place, remove the sponge; excess cement will often stick to the sponge.

43

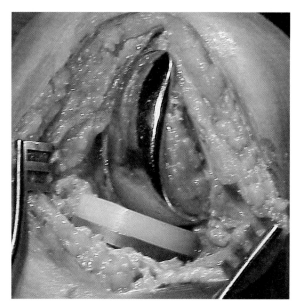

◘ **Fig. 43-6.** Final implants cemented in place

Cement the femoral component in place, and remove excess posterior cement with the knee flexed and anterior cement with the knee extended. Remove osteophytes, and release the tourniquet once the cement is set(◘ Fig 43-6).

Closure

One of the reasons that minimally invasive surgery is so efficient is that wound exposure and closure are very quick. The retinaculum can usually be closed with a running strong, braided suture, followed by closure of the subcutaneous layer and skin.

Pain control can be aided with use of a bupivacaine catheter in the knee joint for 24-48 h postoperatively. The author also routinely injects the knee capsule with $\frac{1}{2}$% bupivacaine with epinephrine, morphine sulfate, ketorolac, and methylprednisolone acetate. Full weight-bearing and range of motion exercises are begun immediately.

Results

John Repicci is generally credited with advancing the technique of minimally invasive UKA. Between 1992 and 1996, he performed more than 700 minimally invasive UKAs in well-selected patients utilizing a 3-inch incision. He routinely performs arthroscopy pre-operatively to evaluate the knee and performs thr arthroplasty with the knee dangling in flexion from the leg holder. Eighty percent of the operations were done on an outpatient basis, and 90% of the patients had regained independent function by 2 weeks postoperatively [11].

In the same publication, Repicci compared 50 patients who underwent standard-incision UKA in 1992 and 1993 with the next 50 patients who underwent minimally invasive UKA. Although not a randomized study, the two groups were equally matched demographically. The minimally invasive group had less postoperative drainage, was discharged earlier, and required significantly less physical therapy than the standard-incision group (0.2 visits per patient vs. 12.0 visits per patient). All three factors translated into a significant cost savings of approximately $9000 per patient ($7000 vs $16 000) [11].

Since then, Repicci has reported 8-year follow-up in 136 UKAs using his minimally invasive technique. He found good and excellent results in 86% of these patients and correlated disease progressions with degree of osteoarthritis at implantation. Although highly successful in his hands, his technique is basically a freehand technique, requiring considerable skill, which makes the procedure less reproducible for surgeons who do not perform a significant number of UKAs [12]. A recent study from Sweden shows that a steep learning curve leads to a significantly higher number of clinical failures [13].

Keys prospectively compared ten minimally invasive Oxford UKAs with ten standard-approach UKAs performed on an alternating basis. He found that ability to straight-leg raise, flex to 90°, climb stairs, and go home from the hospital were all achieved approximately 3 days earlier in the minimally invasive group. Component malpositioning was not seen. Both groups were clinically similar with respect to knee flexion and Knee Society scores by 3 months postoperatively [14].

Price and colleagues compared 40 minimally invasive Oxford UKAs with 20 standard incision UKAs and 40 TKAs. They found that the minimally invasive group recovered the ability to straight-leg raise, flex to 70°, and climb stairs twice as quickly as the standard-incision group and three times quicker than the TKA group. Additionally, they found no differences in implant position in the two UKA groups [15].

However, Fisher and colleagues compared implant position in 88 minimally invasive UKAs with 64 standard-incision UKAs and 54 TKAs. The minimally invasive UKA group had slightly more varus limb alignment and tibial component varus and also showed more variability in alignment and tibial component position than the other two groups. Although the differences were small, they were statistically significant [16].

As with many surgical procedures, successful UKA is highly dependent upon instrumentation [17]. Although proper tibial component positioning is relatively straightforward, proper femoral component positioning is challenging. The unicompartmental femoral component can be malpositioned by translation or rotation about any of the three major axes. Translational errors can result in inadequate femoral coverage, patellar impingement against the

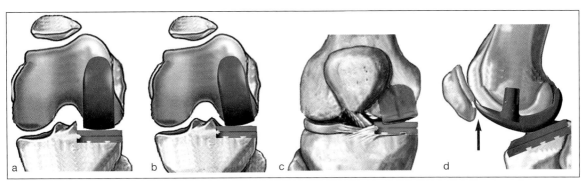

■ Fig. 43-7a-d. Results of malpositioned femoral component: *a* Well-positioned component in all planes. *b* Rotational malalignment causing edge loading and eccentric loading in flexion. *c* Rotational malalignment causing edge-loading and eccentric loading in extension. *d* Rotational and translational malalignment causing patellar impingement against the anterior femoral flange

anterior femoral flange, eccentric tracking on the tibial component, or over/under-correction of pre-operative deformity. Rotational malpositioning is more common and can result in inadequate femoral coverage, patellar impingement, eccentric loading, or edge loading of the tibial component in either flexion or extension (■ Fig. 43-7a-d).

Instrumentation is extremely important to correctly position implants, particularly when working through small incisions. Most modern UKA instrument systems utilize extramedullary alignment for the tibia. Femoral instrumentation utilizes either intramedullary or surface referencing. Although intramedullary instrumentation is extremely important for TKA, the goals of UKA are different than those of TKA. While TKA requires accurate correction of pre-operative deformity with proper bone cuts and ligament releases, the goal of UKA is to fill the space created by passive correction of the deformity [16,18]. Minimal ligament release is required with UKA, and if significant pre-operative deformity exists, the patient likely is not a candidate for UKA. Therefore, intramedullary instrumentation is not as critical for proper alignment of the UKA femoral component. Additionally, invasion of the femoral canal makes the procedure less "minimally invasive" and can lead to fat embolization and systemic ill effects.

Kinematic surface referencing of the femur consistently aligns the femoral component correctly in all three planes and around all three axes of rotation. The system removes the least amount of bone necessary to resurface the compartment without violating the intramedullary canal. Further assistance in component positioning may eventually be provided by computer navigation. Jenny and Boeri recently reported improved alignment in 30 computer-navigated UKAs compared with 30 matched pairs in nearly all aspects measured [19].

References

1. Kozinn SC et al (1989) Unicondylar knee arthroplasty (current concepts review). J Bone Joint Surg [Am] 71:145-150
2. Stern SH et al (1993) Unicondylar knee arthroplasty: an evaluation of selection criteria. Clin Orthop 286:143-148
3. Deshmukh RV et al (2002) Unicompartmental knee arthroplasty for younger patients. Clin Orthop 404:108-112
4. Meek RM et al (2004) Minimally invasive unicompartmental knee replacement: rationale and correct indications. Orthop Clin North Am 35:191-200
5. Engh GA (2002) Orthopaedic crossfire - can we justify unicondylar arthroplasty as a temporizing procedure? In the affirmative. J Arthroplasty 17 [Suppl 1]:54-55
6. Scott RD (2003) Unicondylar arthroplasty: redefining itself. Orthopedics 26:951-952
7. Mont MA et al (2004) Different surgical options for monocompartmental osteoarthritis of the knee: high tibial osteotomy versus unicompartmental knee arthroplasty versus total knee arthroplasty: indications, techniques, results, and controversies. Instr Course Lect 53:265-283
8. Hernigou P et al (2004) Posterior slope of the tibial implant and the outcome of unicompartmental knee arthroplasty. J Bone Joint Surg [Am] 86:506-511
9. Brumby SA et al (2003) Tibial plateau stress fracture: a complication of unicompartmental knee arthroplasty using 4 guide pinholes. J Arthroplasty 18:809-812
10. White SH et al (1991) Anteromedial osteoarthritis of the knee. J Bone Joint Surg [Br] 73:582-586
11. Repicci JA et al (1999) Minimally invasive surgical technique for unicondylar knee arthroplasty. J South Orthop Assoc 8:20-27
12. Romanowski MR et al (2002) Minimally invasive unicondylar arthroplasty (eight-year follow-up). J Knee Surg 15:17-22
13. Lindstrand A et al (2000) The introduction period of unicompartmental knee arthroplasty is critical. J Arthroplasty 15:608-616
14. Keys GW (2000) The reduced invasive approach for medial Oxford II meniscal bearing replacement. J Bone Joint Surg [Br] 82 (Suppl 1):24
15. Price AJ, Webb J, Topf H, Dodd CA, Goodfellow JW, Murray DW (2001) Rapid recovery after Oxford unicompartmental arthroplasty through a short incision. J Arthroplasty 16:970-976
16. Fisher DA et al (2003) Implant position in knee surgery: a comparison of minimally invasive, open unicompartmental, and total knee arthroplasty. J Arthroplasty 18 [Suppl 1]:2-8
17. Jenny JY et al (2002) Accuracy of implantation of a unicompartmental total knee arthroplasty with 2 different instrumentations: a case-controlled comparative study. J Arthroplasty 17:1016-1020
18. Argenson J-NA et al (2002) Modern unicompartmental knee arthroplasty with cement. J Bone Joint Surg [Am] 84:2235-2239
19. Jenny JY et al (2003) Unicompartmental knee prosthesis implantation with a non-image-based navigation system: rationale, technique, case-control comparative study with a conventional instrumented implantation. Knee Surg Sports Traumatol Arthrosc 11:40-45
20. Iorio R et al (2003) Unicompartmental arthritis of the knee (current concepts review). J Bone Joint Surg [Am] 85

44 Minimally Invasive: Total Knee Arthroplasty

S. B. Haas, A. P. Lehman, S. Cook

Summary

Numerous long-term clinical studies have demonstrated the success of total knee arthroplasty in regard to improving both pain and function. The typical exposure for a total knee arthroplasty employs an extensile approach through a medial parapatellar arthrotomy. The incision through the quadriceps tendon can lead to a long and painful recovery. The authors began performing minimally invasive total knee arthroplasties through a modified midvastus approach in 2001 as an alternative to the traditional approach. If the patella is not everted or the quadriceps tendon not transected, the extensor mechanism suffers less surgical trauma. Total knee arthroplasties done utilizing this technique achieve not only knee motion faster, but also a greater ultimate range of motion without an increase in complications.

Introduction/Background

Total knee arthroplasty (TKA) is a very successful treatment for end-stage arthritis of the knee. Long-term results for both pain relief and function are excellent [1-4]. The approach most commonly used to expose the knee is the medial parapatellar arthrotomy [5]. This approach was first described by Von Langenbeck in 1874 [6], and it has a successful track record with long-term follow-up. However, the incision through the quadriceps tendon and patellar eversion can lead to a long and painful recovery.

Another approach used for TKA, the midvastus approach, does not require incision of the quadriceps tendon [7]. Several studies have demonstrated a number of clinical improvements with this approach when directly compared with a standard medial parapatellar arthrotomy, including faster recovery of quadriceps strength, less postoperative pain, and a lower lateral retinacular release rate [8-12]. While the standard midvastus approach had numerous benefits, it still involved patellar eversion, which in some cases was difficult to perform. Eversion of the patella also leads to more splitting of the muscles and stretching of the quadriceps and patella tendons. Eversion of the patella via a medial parapatellar or midvastus ap-

proach also causes twisting of the patella tendon and nonphysiological stress at the tibial tubercle. In some cases this leads to pealing or avulsion of the tendon.

In 2001, in order to decrease the trauma to the extensor mechanism, the authors began performing minimally invasive total knee arthroplasty (MIS-TKA) utilizing a modified midvastus approach. We named it the "mini-midvastus" approach. The modification involved in this approach is that the patella is not everted, but rather dislocated laterally during the procedure. By not everting the patella, it is not necessary to split the VMO as far medially, and less stress is placed on the extensor mechanism.

Another potential advantage of this exposure is that it can be performed through a smaller skin incision. The incision with a traditional medial parapatellar arthrotomy must be carried proximally to the extent of the split in the quadriceps tendon. This is not necessary with the mini-midvastus technique. In fact, we have found that, with improvements in instrumentation, a total knee arthroplasty can be safely performed through an 8.5- to 12-cm skin incision without excessive retraction or the need for undermining the skin.

Instrumentation

Traditionally, instruments used for TKA have dictated the length of the incision. Smaller, modified instrumentation has been an integral part in the development of the MIS-TKA technique. Not only were the guides and cutting blocks made smaller; the corners of instruments were rounded and separate sets were made for both the right and the left knee.

The first change made was to the tibial cutting guide. Because of the proximity of the patellar tendon, the lateral wing of the tibial cutting guide is rarely used during the tibial cut with standard instrumentation. Hence, the tibial guide was made without a lateral wing. Instead, both a left and a right guide were made to wrap around the medial aspect of the tibia (□ Fig. 44-1). This modification allows the lateral tibial plateau to be cut from anterior to posterior as well as from medial to lateral.

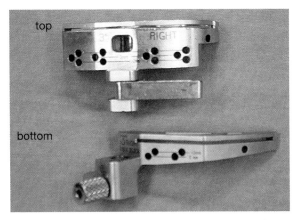

Fig. 44-1. (top) Standard Genesis II (Smith and Nephew, Memphis, TN) tibial cutting block. (bottom) MIS Genesis II (Smith and Nephew, Memphis, TN) tibial cutting block

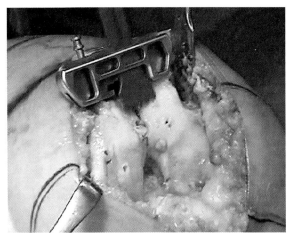

Fig. 44-3. Preparing femur with MIS distal cutting block

The femoral cutting blocks and valgus alignment guides were also modified. Again, a separate guide was made for each side. The anterior femoral cutting guide, distal femoral cutting block, and the 4-in-1 femoral finishing block were made narrower in the medial-to-lateral dimension and the corners were rounded (■ Fig. 44-2). This allows easy placement of the guides without impingement on the patella laterally.

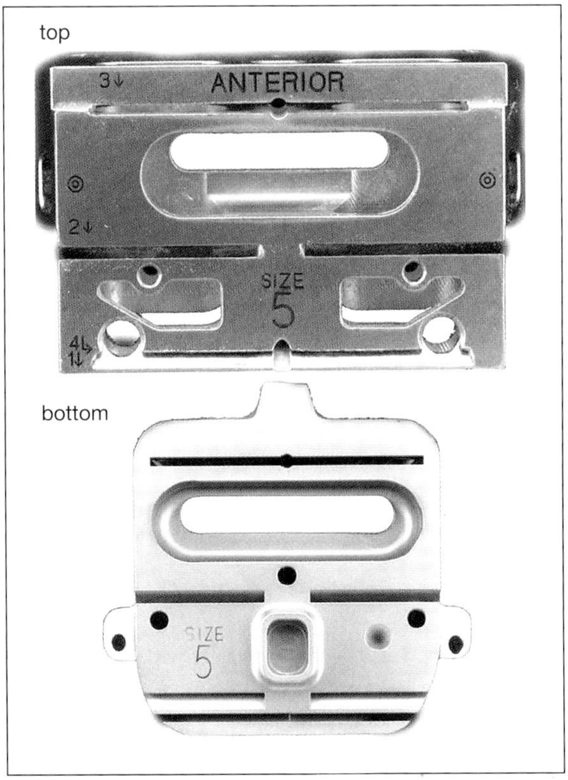

The remainder of the instruments, including the anterior resection stylus, the distal resection stylus, the housing resection block for posterior stabilized knees, and the femoral sizing guide, are also smaller in order to fit a smaller incision. Additionally, the anterior stylus is angled to allow placement under the skin proximally when referencing the anterior femoral cut, and the distal femoral cutting block is wedge-shaped and retracts the skin edges without the need for additional retractors (■ Fig. 44-3).

Surgical Technique

With the leg fully extended, a longitudinal incision is made over the anterior aspect of the knee along the medial border of the patella. The incision is generally between 8.5 and 12 cm and extends from the superior pole of the patella proximally to the proximal half of the tibial tubercle distally. If additional exposure is required, the incision can begin 1 cm proximal to the superior pole of the patella. A medial arthrotomy is then performed from the proximal border of the patella to about 5 mm medial to the tibial tubercle. The suprapatellar pouch is identified, separated from the underside of the quadriceps tendon, and preserved. The distal extent of the VMO is identified at the superomedial corner of the patella. The fascia of this muscle is incised obliquely along the line of the muscle fibers for approximately 1-2 cm (■ Fig. 44-4). The muscle fibers are then bluntly spread by hand.

While the leg is kept fully extended, the patella is retracted laterally. A portion of the fat pad is excised both medially and laterally. The anterior horn of the medial meniscus is divided and excised. Subperiosteal dissection is performed around the proximal medial tibia in standard fashion. The anterior cruciate ligament and the anterior horn of the lateral meniscus are excised. A small

Fig. 44-2. (top) Standard Genesis II (Smith and Nephew, Memphis, TN) femoral A-P cutting block. (bottom) MIS Genesis II (Smith and Nephew, Memphis, TN) femoral A-P cutting block

44

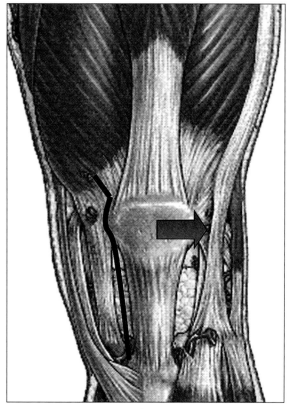

Fig. 44-4. Arthrotomy with mini-midvastus approach extends from tibial tubercle to superior patella and then to the muscle of the vastus medialus. The muscle fibers are not cut

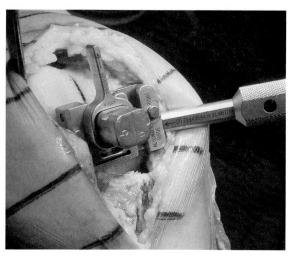

Fig. 44-5. Preparing femur with right-sided MIS valgus/rotation guide. The stylus is aligned with the AP axis line (Whiteside's line)

window is made along the anterior surface of the distal femur in order to reference the anterior cortex.

The TKA continues in routine fashion from this point. In patients with tight extensor mechanisms, an abundance of patellar osteophytes, or large patellae, the patella can be cut first to facilitate exposure. However, in patients with osteoporotic bone, care must be taken to avoid intraoperative damage to the cut patella surface with retractors. If it is not opted to cut the patella first, the femur should be prepared first with the patella retracted laterally but not everted.

Importantly, femoral preparation should be accomplished with the knee flexed to only 70°-90°. Limiting knee flexion allows the soft-tissue window to be mobile, and thus to move proximally without difficulty in order that the anterior femoral cortex can be referenced. Hyperflexion should be avoided, because this will not only tighten the extensor mechanism but also limit exposure. A thin, bent Hohman retractor is placed laterally to retract the patella. A 9.5-mm intramedullary drill is used to enter the femoral canal from a starting point in the notch just anterior to the posterior cruciate insertion on the femur. An intramedullary referencing guide is placed in the femoral canal after the marrow contents have been sucked out. The appropriate valgus angle collar, with or

without posterior condylar referencing paddles, should be placed in the rod. If the posterior paddles are utilized, the knee must be flexed to 100° during insertion. After rotation is set, the posterior paddles are removed and the leg is returned to between 70° and 90° of flexion.

Rotation for the anterior cut is determined utilizing the traditional landmarks of the anteroposterior axis (Whiteside's line), the epicondylar axis, or the posterior condylar axis (**Fig. 44-5**). The authors prefer to use Whiteside's line as the primary reference to femoral rotation and the posterior condylar axis as a secondary reference.

Following determination of femoral rotation, an anterior stylus is used to reference the preliminary anterior femoral resection. The stylus is placed in the small window that was created during exposure and flush on the highest point of the anterior femoral cortex. The saw blade will cut under the skin, but a right-angle retractor may be used to elevate the skin if desired.

At this time, the distal femoral resection is performed. Additional retractors are usually not necessary for placement of the guide. Because of the guide's wedge shape, it typically will provide adequate retraction by itself. Once the cutting block is placed on the anterior femur and secured in place, the distal femoral cut is made.

The size of the femoral component is determined using a sizing guide. The knee may require more flexion in order to place the guide in the correct position under the posterior condyles. The appropriately sized femoral cutting block is placed on the distal femur and secured. A thin, bent Hohman retractor is placed medially to protect the medial collateral ligament, as well as laterally to retract the patella. The femoral cuts are made in the following order: posterior condyles, posterior chamfer, anterior resection, and anterior chamfer.

The tibia is prepared next. Either intramedullary or extramedullary tibial alignment guides can be utilized. The authors prefer an extramedullary technique. We typically reference the guide over the tibial crest proximally and over the second metatarsal distally. A stylus is used to measure the amount of tibia to be removed from the least deficient tibial condyle. For a varus knee, the stylus is placed on the anterior aspect of the lateral tibial plateau. In general, we set the stylus to measure 11 mm of proximal tibial bone resection. Again, the two thin, bent Hohman retractors are in place medially and laterally, protecting the medial collateral ligament and the extensor mechanism, respectively. An Aufranc retractor is also placed posteriorly. The saw blade should initially be directed in a posterior direction. Then it should be directed laterally.

After the tibial cut is made, extension of the knee can provide a better perspective when the cut surface is inspected for cortical ridges. After the tibial bone is removed, the posterior horns of both the medial and lateral menisci are removed along with the posterior cruciate ligament (if a posterior-stabilized knee system is being utilized). We prefer to place a laminar spreader in the joint while the knee is in 90° of flexion in order to distract the surfaces and provide exposure of the posterior elements of the knee. Any posterior osteophytes should be removed with an osteotome at this time (◘ Fig. 44-6). The tibial preparation should be completed by measuring the surface and drilling and broaching the tibial canal to fit the prosthesis.

Spacer blocks are placed at this time in order to measure the extension and flexion gaps. If there is asymmetry, the appropriate releases should be performed to create a balanced knee. If a posterior-stabilized knee is being used, the posterior-stabilized resection block is placed on the distal femur and the femoral preparation is completed at this time.

Following tibial preparation, the patella is prepared. Unless it is required earlier for adequate exposure, it is

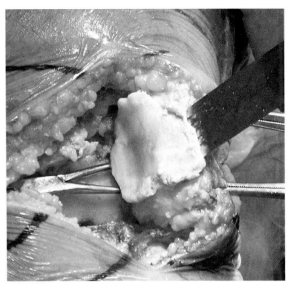

◘ **Fig. 44-7.** Patella rotated approximately 90° for patella preparation. Knee is extended, and femoral and tibial bone cuts have been made

easier to wait until after both the femoral and tibial cuts have been made to perform this step. With the knee in full extension, the leg is shortened and the extensor mechanism is relaxed. The patella is easily rotated 90°s and cut in routine fashion (◘ Fig. 44-7).

Once all the surfaces have been prepared, the trial components are placed. In order to clear the femoral condyles with the tibial trial, the knee must be maximally flexed, and in addition to thin, bent Hohman retractors medially and laterally, an Aufranc retractor can be placed posteriorly to subluxate the tibia anteriorly. The femoral trial is placed with the knee in 90° of flexion. Once the size of the polyethylene insert is confirmed and the placement of the trial is deemed satisfactory, the trials may be removed and the final implants placed using the same technique. The authors prefer to use cemented implants; however, cementless implants can also be used. The tibial component should be placed first in order to have access to the posterior aspect of the knee to allow complete removal of excess cement. The use of an asymmetric, anatomical tibial component is recommended, since the larger lateral side of the tibial component in symmetric designs often leads to impingement on the lateral femoral condyle during insertion, posterolateral overhang, and difficulty with cement removal. Once the tibial component has been placed, the femoral and patellar components are placed. Retraction of the proximal tissues for cement removal must be avoided with the knee flexed. Excess cement anteriorly in the suprapatellar pouch can be more easily removed with the leg in extension. The trial polyethylene insert is placed, and the leg is kept in full extension to pressurize the cement while it is polymerizing. The final polyethylene insert is placed after the cement has hardened. If a posterior-stabilized insert is used, in-

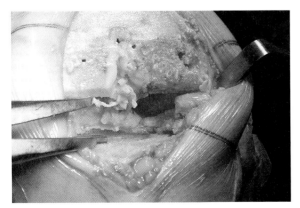

◘ **Fig. 44-6.** Laminar spreader is placed after bone resection. Good visualization for resection of meniscus and PCL and for posterior osteophyte removal

sertion of the final polyethylene should begin with the knee in 90° of flexion. The knee should then be brought into full extension to engage the locking mechanism. We prefer to use a high flexion insert in most cases.

The authors recommend that the tourniquet be deflated after the cement has polymerized in order to achieve hemostasis. Once all bleeding has been controlled, the wound is copiously irrigated and closure is begun. Two deep drains are placed. The arthrotomy is closed by initially placing 0-Vicryl sutures in the VMO fascia and tendon. Three to five sutures will usually suffice. The remainder of the arthrotomy, the subcutaneous tissues, and skin are closed in standard fashion.

Results

The initial 40 MIS-TKAs performed by the senior author (S.B.H.) were evaluated and compared with an age- and sex-matched cohort (control group) of patients who received a TKA through a standard medial parapatellar arthrotomy by the same surgeon [13]. All patients received the same posterior stabilized condylar knee (Genesis II, Smith and Nephew, Memphis, TN). Both groups also received the same postoperative physical therapy protocol, including a continuous passive motion machine in the recovery room.

There were no statistically significant demographic differences between the two groups. The Knee Society preoperative knee and function score averages were 28 and 23, respectively, in the MIS-TKA group and 33 and 24 in the control group. At 1 year postoperatively, the averages were 97 and 92 in the MIS-TKA group and 91 and 90 in the control group.

Preoperative range of motion was similar in both groups. However, at 6 weeks postoperatively, the mean flexion was significantly higher in the MIS-TKA group (114°) than in the control (96°). This difference persisted at 1 year, when the mean flexion in the MIS-TKA group improved to 125° and the control group improved to only 116°.

Although most patients selected for MIS-TKA during the first year weighed fewer than 100 kg, 10% were heavier. Over the past 3.5 years we have refined the selection criteria. Patients weighing less than 90-100 kg are the best candidates for MIS-TKA and women are generally easier to treat than men. Large muscular men are the most difficult and are generally more difficult than overweight women. A standard medial parapatellar approach is used for patients with preoperative flexion contracture greater than 20° and flexion less than 80°. Poor-quality skin or multiple previous incisions generally require a larger incision; however, the MIS arthrotomy may be utilized. During the past year, over 70% of all TKAs were performed using an MIS/mini-midvastus approach. While larger and

heavier patients are not ideal candidates for MIS-TKA with a mini-midvastus approach, MIS instruments allow many of these patients to have TKA performed through less extensive medial parapatelar arthrotomy without patellar eversion and with a smaller incision.

Between September of 2001 and September of 2003, the senior author performed 389 MIS-TKAs using the mini-midvastus approach. This represented 66% of all TKAs performed during that time period. The mean weight and height were 79.5 kg (46-126) and 165 cm (132-187 cm) and preoperative flexion was 109° (80°-150°). The mean postoperative flexion at 6 weeks and 3 months was 111° and 121°, respectively. One- and 2-year results with this larger group of patients were consistent with those of our earlier study. Range of motion at 1- and 2-year follow-up was 125°. The early functional results have been similar to those of the initial 40 patients. However, the operative time has been reduced significantly. The mean tourniquet time is 48 min, which is statistically equivalent to our standard approach. Overall operating time is slightly less than the standard approach due to reduced time for closure. The overall complication rate remains low. There has been a 0.5% incidence of infection and a 0.2% incidence of superficial wound necrosis. Lateral releases were performed in only 2% of cases. There have been no aseptic failures to date (S.B. Haas, unpublished data).

Laskin et al. [14] performed a similar study using cruciate-retaining knees (Genesis II, Smith and Nephew, Memphis, TN). Thirty-two MIS-TKAs were compared with 26 standard TKAs. Preoperative patient demographics, Knee Society Scores, knee flexion, and knee alignment were similar between the two groups.

The patients who underwent an MIS-TKA had a statistically significantly lower amount of pain on a visual analogue scale in the postoperative period. Additionally, the average total dose of morphine sulfate was significantly lower for patients who had had an MIS-TKA (55 mg) than for those who had undergone a standard medial parapatellar arthrotomy (118 mg).

Passive knee flexion was also consistently higher in the MIS-TKA group. On the third postoperative day, 80% of the patients who had had an MIS-TKA were able to achieve knee flexion of greater than 80°, while only 4% of those who had had a medial parapatellar arthrotomy were able to achieve this amount of knee flexion. Also, the average knee flexion at 6 weeks postoperatively was significantly higher in the MIS-TKA group (124°) than in the control group (115°).

There was no statistical difference in either the radiographic position of the components or the postoperative leg alignment. No lateral retinacular releases were performed in either group. The mean tourniquet time in the MIS-TKA group was 58 min, compared with 51 min in the control group. There were no reported skin complications in either group.

Conclusion

The use of the mini-midvastus approach for MIS-TKA allows patients to regain knee flexion faster, and it may lead to a greater ultimate range of motion. It also leads to higher Knee Society Scores and decreases the patients' postoperative pain. Smaller instruments allow the surgeon to decrease the amount of surgical dissection and the size of the incision without excessive soft-tissue retraction or additional complications. By not everting the patella or disrupting the suprapatellar pouch in the MIS-TKA, improvement in patient recovery, as well as an improved cosmetic result, can be achieved without compromising the radiographic positioning of the implants, the clinical results, or surgical exposure.

References

1. Font-Rodriguez DE, Scuderi GR, Insall JN (1997) Survivorship of cemented total knee arthroplasty. Clin Orthop 345:79-86
2. Kelly MA, Clarke HD (2002) Long-term results of posterior cruciate substituting total knee arthroplasty. Clin Orthop 404:51-57
3. Pavone V, Boettner F, Fickert S, et al (2001) Total condylar knee arthroplasty: a long-term follow-up. Clin Orthop 388:18-25
4. Ranawat CS, Flynn WF, Saddler S, et al (1993) Long-term results of the total condylar knee arthroplasty: a 15-year survivorship study. Clin Orthop 286:94-102
5. Hoppenfeld S, deBoer P (1994) The knee. In: Surgical exposures in orthopaedics - the anatomic approach, 2nd edn. JB Lippincott, Philadelphia, pp 429-482
6. Von Langenbeck B (1874) Über die Schussverietzungen [sic] des Hüftgelenks. Arch Klin Chir 16:263
7. Engh GA, Holt BT, Parks NL (1997) A midvastus muscle-splitting approach for total knee arthroplasty. J Arthroplasty 12:322-331
8. Engh GA, Parks NL (1998) Surgical technique of the midvastus arthrotomy. Clin Orthop 351:270-274
9. Dalury DF, Jiranek WA (1999) A comparison of the midvastus and paramedian approaches for total knee arthroplasty. J Arthroplasty 14:33-37
10. White RE, Allman JK, Trauger JA, et al (1999) Clinical comparison of the midvastus and medial parapatellar surgical approaches. Clin Orthop 367:117-122
11. Parentis MA, Rumi MN, Deol GS, et a (1999)l A comparison of the vastus splitting and median parapatellar approaches in total knee arthroplasty. Clin Orthop 367:107-116
12. Cooper RE Jr, Trinidad G, Buck WR (1999) Midvastus approach in total knee arthroplasty: a description and a cadaveric study determining the distance of the popliteal artery from the patellar margin of the incision. J Arthroplasty 14:505-508
13. Haas SB (2005) Minimally invasive total knee arthroplasty: a comparative study. Clin Orthop (in press)
14. Laskin RS, Beksac B, Phongkunakorn A, et al (2005) Minimally invasive total knee replacement through a mini-midvastus incision: an outcome study. Clin Orthop (in press)

45 The Electronic Knee

C. W. Colwell, Jr., D. D. D'Lima

Summary

The knee is a complex joint that is difficult to model accurately. Although significant advances have been made in mathematical modeling, these have yet to be successfully validated in vivo. Direct measurement of knee forces could lead to a better understanding of the stresses seen in total knee arthroplasty. This would enable more accurate mathematical and in vitro modeling of the knee, which could then be used to evaluate and to implement relevant improvements in implant design. An instrumented knee prosthesis was used for wireless measurement of tibial forces. Accurate measurement of these forces can yield insights into the stresses generated during common activities of daily living. The tibiofemoral force data can be used to develop better biomechanical knee models and in vitro wear tests and can be used to evaluate the effect of improvements in implant design and bearing surfaces, rehabilitation protocols, and orthotics. This may lead to refinement of surgical techniques and to enhancement of prosthetic design that will improve the function, quality of life, and longevity of total knee arthroplasty. Given the current increase in the number of older persons who are at higher risk for chronic musculoskeletal disorders, a significant positive impact on clinical outcomes and patient health care could be anticipated.

Introduction

Tibial forces are directly related to the transmission of stresses in the implant. These include contact stresses generated at the bearing surface and subsurface, stresses at the implant-cement-bone interface, and stresses transmitted to underlying bone. Stresses at the bearing surface are a major factor in generating wear and fatigue, which determine the life of the implant. Stresses at the implant-cement interface have been correlated with aseptic loosening, implant migration, and the generation of third-body wear particles. Stresses transmitted to underlying bone affect remodeling, stress shielding, and osteoporosis. Tibial forces, along with the kinematic patterns of the knee, have been shown to have a significant effect on the type and quantity of wear produced [1, 2].

Tibiofemoral forces are therefore highly significant in determining the longevity of total knee arthroplasty. Tibial prostheses have been instrumented with force transducers to measure tibial forces in vitro [3, 4]; however, direct measurement of tibial forces in vivo has not been reported. Telemetry has been shown to be a safe and accurate means of obtaining force data from implanted transducers and has been used to measure in vivo forces in the hip, spine, and femur [5-10]. Hip forces measured through telemetry have typically been lower than those predicted mathematically. The knee is much more complex than the hip, and theoretic estimates of tibiofemoral forces have varied between 3 and 6 times body weight, depending on the mathematical models used and on the type of activity analyzed [11-18]. A major problem with mathematical predictions is the high degree of mechanical redundancy due to the numerous muscles involved in locomotion. Several optimization techniques have been reported to address this problem [13, 15-17, 19-22]; however, laboratory validation has not demonstrated a good agreement between predicted muscle forces and those measured directly [23]. An implantable electronic knee prosthesis with a telemetry system was therefore developed to directly measure tibiofemoral compressive forces in vivo.

History of Tibial Force Measurement

As early as 1975, Perry et al. measured tibial forces in vitro, using a tibial plate connected to an instrumented shaft [4]. They demonstrated an average error of 6% between calculated and measured forces in a two-dimensional static model of the knee. Kaufman et al. [3] reported a tibial prosthesis instrumented with load cells that could measure the magnitude of axial compressive force on the tibia and the center of application in vitro. The prosthesis was subsequently used in cadaver studies that measured the effect of joint-line elevation on tibiofemoral forces after total knee arthroplasty [24]. Singerman et al. reported on a force-transducer design based on two concentric cylinders. The inner cylinder was instrumented with strain gages while the outer cylinder was fixed to bone [25]. This transducer was used to measure tibial forces in normal cadaver knees and was inserted through a 1-cm resection of the proximal tibia. A prototype electronic tibial replacement system was also developed, using radio-frequency transmission of data, which demonstrated comparable accuracy in measuring the location and magnitude of tibiofemoral compressive forces [26]. This telemetry system was found to accurately transmit the signal through bone, cement, and soft tissues with a range of approximately 2 m.

Technical Details

Transducers. A titanium alloy revision tibial prosthesis design was instrumented with force transducers, a microtransmitter, and an antenna. The tibial-force transducers were manufactured by NK Biotechnical and have been described previously [3] and have been used in cadaveric studies [24, 27]. The tibial tray consists of upper and lower halves separated by support posts, below which lie the load cells, located at the four corners of the tibial tray. By measuring the force on each load cell and the total axial load, the location of center of pressure can be determined. In addition, the distribution of forces between the medial and the lateral compartments can be calculated. Figure 45-1 demonstrates the location of the multichannel transmitter and the hermetic feed-through antenna (◘ Fig. 45-1).

Telemetry. The microtransmitter receives the analog signal through leads from the load cells and is connected to the transmitting antenna. The microtransmitter was developed by Microstrain (Burlington, VT) entirely from off-the-shelf surface-mount integrated circuits. The requisite bridge signal conditioning, the multiplexer, the A/D (analog-to-digital) converter, and the programmable gain and filter functions were combined on a single chip (AD7714, Analog Devices, Norwood, MA). The AD7714 features three true differential bridge inputs, five pseudo differential inputs, a maximum resolution of 22 bits, and a software programmable gain of 1-128. The microprocessor (PIC16C, MicroChip Technologies, Chandler Arizona) allows the AD7714 to be reprogrammed through the serial port of a PC. Once programmed, the configuration is stored in nonvolatile, electrically erasable, programmable, read-only memory (EEPROM) on the PIC16C. On power up, the PIC16C reads the EEPROM to configure the AD7714 for the appropriate channel-specific gain, filtering, and sample rate parameters. The microprocessor also performs pulse-code modulation (PCM) of a surface acoustic wave (SAW) radio-frequency (RF) oscillator (RF Monolithics, Dallas, TX). PCM modulation is less prone to interference than pulse-width modulation

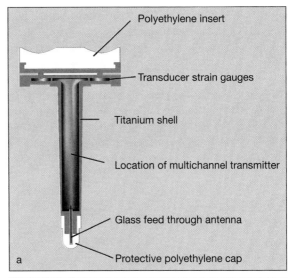

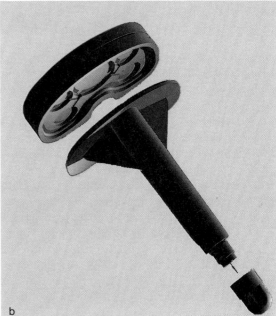

◘ **Fig.45- 1a, b.** *a* Cross-sectional diagram demonstrates the location of the multichannel transmitter and the hermetic feed-through antenna. *b* Exploded view of the tibial tray sections and the polyethylene cap protecting the transmitting antenna

(PWM) and pulse-interval modulation (PIM). Another advantage is the ability for error detection in RF transmission. This is accomplished by sending a checksum byte, which is the sum of the preceding data bytes. A mismatch between the checksum and the number of bytes received generates an error flag in the data.

Transmitting Antenna. Since RF signals do not pass through the sealed titanium shell in the current configuration, a single-pin hermetic feed-through transmitting antenna is located at the distal tip of the stem and is connected to the microtransmitter. The antenna is manufactured by Hermetic Seal Technology (Cincinnati, OH) and is certified medical grade. The feed-through wire is tantalum (ASTM B-365) with a glass insulator (Sandia Cabal-12) and a titanium-retaining ring (Ti-6AL-4V, ASTM F-136).

Receiver. The PCM receiver contains a receiving antenna, a matched RF SAW oscillator, and a level converter to generate RS-232 signals from the incoming data stream. The RS-232 signal is read by custom PC software and can be integrated with data from other instruments.

Power. Powering an implantable system can be demanding. Although batteries have been used in the past, they contain toxic chemicals, have a limited life span, and occupy valuable space. Remote powering can be achieved with the use of magnetic near-field coupling. Briefly, an external coil driven with AC current generates an AC magnetic field, which in turn generates AC voltage in a receiving coil placed within the magnetic field. This voltage is then rectified and filtered to provide the DC power required for the telemetry system. Remote powering through a metallic orthopedic implant presents a further challenge, since the efficiency of coupling is significantly reduced by the presence of metal between the transmitting and receiving coils. Although high frequencies (>125 kHz) increase the coupling efficiency, unacceptable shielding and eddy currents are produced at these frequencies. With the current device the optimum frequency of operation is found to be approximately 3.5 kHz. An external (primary) coil, 7 inches in diameter, is housed in a custom-padded ring that can be contoured to the subject's leg. The external coil has an impedance of 10 Ohms at 1.6 kHz drive frequency. A function generator provides a 3-V AC signal at 3.45 kHz to a 100-W power amplifier, which amplifies the signal and drives the external coil. The implant contains the internal (secondary) coil, which consists of 2000 turns of magnet wire wound on a high-permeability ferrite core. Approximately 40 mW of power can be generated in the internal coil, which is adequate to power the telemetry system.

In Vitro Testing

Following assembly and sealing, the prosthesis was recalibrated and checked for thermal drift between 15° and 45°C. The integrity of the radiofrequency signal was then tested with the prosthesis cemented in five cadaver knees. The device was tested in three knees that were mounted on a dynamic quadriceps-driven knee-extension simulator (Oxford knee rig). The external coil was secured around the upper tibia and the transducer data were measured during knee flexion-extension. The receiving antenna was progressively moved away from the rig, and the range of transmission was measured as the maximum

distance between the transmitter and the antenna without loss of signal.

To test the measurement of the magnitude and the location of applied forces, compressive loads of different magnitudes were applied at various locations. The implant was cemented in a custom fixture and was mounted on a multiaxial testing machine (Force 5, AMTI, Watertown, MA). The machine can apply flexion-extension, axial-tibial rotations, and translations in the anteroposterior direction. Vertical load was applied perpendicular to the tibial tray. To test the effect of the presence of an insert on the tray, loads were applied with and without an 8-mm polyethylene insert that matched the size of the tibial tray (◘ Fig. 45-2). The magnitude and the location of the externally applied loads were compared with those measured by the tibial transducers. In the normal knee, loads are typically bicondylar rather than through a single point. To determine whether the implant could detect bicondylar loading, loads were applied through a femoral prosthesis at different flexion angles and in liftoff. The loads measured by the individual transducers were then analyzed to determine center of contact and load distribution.

In vitro cadaver tests demonstrated that the implant transmitted reliably through bone, cement, and soft tis-

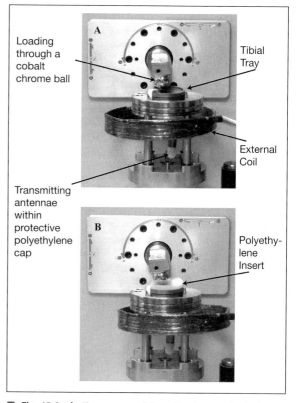

◘ **Fig. 45-2a, b.** The accuracy of the calibration was checked on an AMTI Force 5 multiaxial testing machine. *a* Dynamic loads were applied through *a* cobalt-chrome ball directly to the tibial tray. *b* The same loads were applied through an 8-mm-thick polyethylene insert

sue. After a stable signal was obtained (based on the error detection of the checksum byte), the receiving antenna could be moved between 3 and 5 m before loss of signal was noted.

Accuracy tests were first performed without a polyethylene insert (loads applied directly to the tibial tray). Results comparing the magnitude of externally applied loads with measured loads of up to 2000 N showed close agreement with a mean absolute error of 1.2%. When the location of center of load along the mediolateral direction was considered, the mean absolute error between the applied load location and the measured load location was <1.5 mm for the different locations tested. For location along the anteroposterior direction, the mean absolute error between the applied and the measured location was less than 1 mm.

When loads were applied through an 8-mm polyethylene insert, a small reduction in accuracy was noted. The mean absolute error in total load measurement was 1.5%. The mean absolute error for calculated location was 1.9 mm in the mediolateral direction and 0.7 mm in the anteroposterior direction. During bicondylar loading through a femoral prosthesis, the relative proportion of loads borne by the medial and lateral condyles could be determined by measuring the individual loads acting on the medial versus the lateral transducers. The implant was successful in detecting unicondylar loading in the presence of as little as 1° of mediolateral liftoff. In the presence of liftoff, the center of contact could be calculated to within 2 mm.

The microtransmitter successfully output data through bone, bone cement, and soft tissue. Measurements made by the transducer were highly accurate. A small loss of accuracy was noted when loads were applied through a polyethylene insert as compared with directly loading the tibial tray. The error tended to be highest (1.9 mm mean absolute error) when the location of applied load was calculated in the mediolateral direction. This may be attributed to the generation of shear forces when loads were applied through the curved upper surface of the polyethylene insert. From the loads borne by the individual transducers the distribution of mediolateral loading could be determined. Also encouraging was the fact that the transducer was able to reliably predict unicompartmental loading. This could be a useful validation of the liftoff reported by in vivo fluoroscopic studies [28].

Intraoperative Trial Prosthesis

This system has also been tested intraoperatively as a trial implant (◘ Fig. 45-3). The first intraoperative measurements were made in a patient requiring revision knee arthroplasty for infection [29]. These measurements

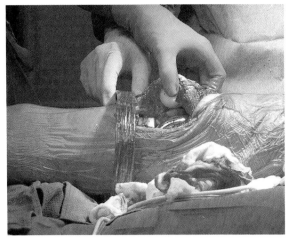

◘ **Fig. 45-3.** The instrumented tibial prosthesis was also used as a trial prosthesis for measuring loads intraoperatively

were made to ensure that the implant could be adequately powered through living tissue (skin, subcutaneous fat, and bone) and could transmit data successfully. In addition, the sensitivity of the implant to intraoperative maneuvers such as passive flexion and extension, varus and valgus angulation, and insert thickness was measured. Subsequently, the implant was used as a trial prosthesis to aid ligament balancing [30]. It was found that the implant sensitive to dynamic imbalance in anteroposterior and mediolateral directions. This was in direct contrast to currently available standard soft-tissue tensioning devices that can measure only static imbalance in the mediolateral direction at 0° and 90° of flexion.

The implant was very sensitive to insert thickness, often recording more than 50% increase in peak axial loads when a trial insert 2 mm thicker than the ideal thickness was used. Determining optimal insert thickness may be a critical factor affecting knee tightness. Even a 2-mm increase in insert thickness resulted in a substantial increase in tibial forces under passive, unloaded knee flexion. This serves to underscore the need for not only balancing the ligaments but also obtaining optimum knee stability. Currently, insert thickness is selected subjectively during surgery, based on the surgeon's "feel" for knee tightness. Precisely measuring forces during surgery may help quantify knee tightness, which can then be correlated with postoperative outcome.

Computer-aided surgical navigation systems have recently gained in popularity. These systems have been reported to increase the precision and accuracy of the bone cuts and the component alignment. However, these systems cannot directly address soft-tissue balance and knee tightness. An instrumented tibial prosthesis could be a valuable adjunct to further enhance the value of such navigation tools.

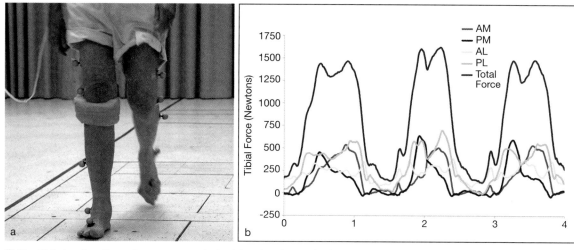

Fig. 45-4a,b. *a* Knee kinematics were measured using infrared markers on the skin. Ground reaction forces and tibial forces were also recorded simultaneously during level walking. *b* Tibial forces during three typical gait cycles are shown. Peak loads were around 2.2 times body weight

In Vivo Implantation

In an attempt to estimate the forces at the knee, an instrumented distal-femoral prosthesis was previously used to measure forces in the femoral shaft [10]. The reported peak femoral shaft axial forces were in the range of 2.2-2.5 times body weight. The estimated tibial axial compressive forces were similar. This represented a significant advance toward directly measuring tibial forces. However, the knee prosthesis used was a tumor replacement design with a rotating hinge, and both heads of the gastrocnemius muscle had been dissected free of the femur. Therefore, these results may not apply to a typical primary total knee arthroplasty.

Clifford Colwell Jr. implanted the first instrumented tibial prosthesis in a patient (J.W.) on Feb 27, 2004. The patient was an 80-year-old man weighing 66 kg with a diagnosis of primary arthritis of the right knee. Preoperative gait analysis and measurements with an ankle accelerometer determined that he walked approximately 1.6 million steps per year. Postoperatively, knee forces were measured during passive and active knee flexion, rehabilitation, rising from a chair, standing, walking, and climbing stairs. ◘ Figure 45-4a shows the patient at 6 weeks postoperatively during a gait analysis session in which lower limb kinematics, ground reaction force, and tibial forces are being measured simultaneously. ◘ Figure 45-4b shows the loads measured during level gait on the 6th postoperative day.

Acknowledgements. We thank Shantanu Patil, MD, Juan Hermida, MD, Pam Pulido, MD, Mary Hardwick RN, Nick Steklov, BS and Bao Nguyen, BS of the Shiley Center for Orthopaedic Research and Education at Scripps Clinic for their contribution to this project.

References

1. Blunn GW et al (1991) The dominance of cyclic sliding in producing wear in total knee replacements. Clin Orthop Rel Res 273:253-260
2. D'Lima DD et al (2001) Polyethylene wear and variations in knee kinematics. Clin Orthop Rel Res 392/124-130
3. Kaufman KR et al (1996) Instrumented implant for measuring tibiofemoral forces. Journal of biomechanics. J Biomech 29:667-671
4. Perry J et al (1975) Analysis of knee-joint forces during flexed-knee stance. J Bone Joint Surg [Am] 57:961-967
5. Bergmann G et al (1993) Hip joint loading during walking and running, measured in two patients. J Biomech 26:969-990
6. Kotzar GM et al (1991) Telemeterized in vivo hip joint force data: a report on two patients after total hip surgery. J Orthop Res 9:621-633
7. Davy DT et al (1988) Telemetric force measurements across the hip after total arthroplasty. J Bone Joint Surg [Am] 70:45-50
8. Hodge WA et al (1989) Contact pressures from an instrumented hip endoprosthesis. J Bone Joint Surg [Am] 71:1378-1386
9. Rohlmann A et al (1995) Telemeterized load measurement using instrumented spinal internal fixators in a patient with degenerative instability. Spine 20:2683-2689
10. Taylor SJ et al (1998) The forces in the distal femur and the knee during walking and other activities measured by telemetry. J Arthroplasty 13/4:428-437
11. Lutz GE et al (1993) Comparison of tibiofemoral joint forces during open-kinetic-chain and closed-kinetic-chain exercises. J Bone Joint Surg [Am] 75:732-739
12. Nisell R et al (1989) Tibiofemoral joint forces during isokinetic knee extension. Am J Sports Med 17:49-54
13. Collins JJ (1995) The redundant nature of locomotor optimization laws. J Biomech 28:251-267
14. Wilk KE et al (1996) A comparison of tibiofemoral joint forces and electromyographic activity during open and closed kinetic chain exercises. Am J Sports Med 24:518-527
15. Li G et al (1998) Prediction of muscle recruitment and its effect on joint reaction forces during knee exercises. Ann Biomed Eng 26:725-733
16. Li G et al (1999) Prediction of antagonistic muscle forces using inverse dynamic optimization during flexion/extension of the knee. J Biomech Eng 121:316-322
17. Seireg A et al (1973) A mathematical model for evaluation of forces in lower extremities of the musculo-skeletal system. J Biomech 6:313-326
18. Ellis MI et al (1984) Forces in the knee joint whilst rising from a seated position. J Biomed Eng 6:113-120
19. Kaufman KR et al (1991) Dynamic joint forces during knee isokinetic exercise. Am J Sports Med 19:305-316

20. An KN et al (1984) Determination of muscle and joint forces: a new technique to solve the indeterminate problem. J Biomech Eng 106:364-367

21. Crowninshield RD et al (1981) A physiologically based criterion of muscle force prediction in locomotion. J Biomech 14:793-801

22. Pedersen DR et al (1987) Direct comparison of muscle force predictions using linear and nonlinear programming. J Biomech Eng 109:192-199

23. Herzog W et al (1991) Validation of optimization models that estimate the forces exerted by synergistic muscles. J Biomech 24 [Suppl 1]:31-39

24. Grady-Benson JC et al (1992) The influence of joint line location on tibiofemoral forces after total knee arthroplasty. Trans Orthop Res Soc 17:324-324

25. Singerman R et al (1999) In vitro forces in the normal and cruciate-deficient knee during simulated squatting motion. J Biomech Eng 121:234-242

26. D'Lima DD et al (1999) An implantable telemetry system to measure intra-articular tibial forces. Trans 45th Orthop Res Soc 24

27. D'Lima DD et al (2005) An implantable telemetry device to measure intra-articular tibial forces. J Biomech 38:299-304

28. Stiehl JB et al (1999) In vivo determination of condylar lift-off and screw-home in a mobile- bearing total knee arthroplasty. J Arthroplasty 14:293-299

29. Morris BA et al (2001) e-Knee: Evolution of the electronic knee prosthesis: Telemetry technology development. J Bone Joint Surg [Am] 83 [Suppl 2]:62-66

30. D'Lima DD et al (2004) In vitro and in vivo measurement of dynamic soft-tissue balance during total knee arthroplasty with an instrumental tibial prosthesis. Trans 50th Orthop Res Society 29:301

VI   Implant Design

46 Bicruciate-Retaining Total Knee Arthroplasty

D. Jacofsky

Summary

Bicruciate ligament retention in total knee arthroplasty has been evaluated since the earliest non-hinged implants were devised in the late 1960s. Retention of the anterior cruciate ligament may theoretically allow for better knee kinematics, improved proprioception, increased maximum flexion, and overall improvement in knee function. The decreased constraint that is permitted with the presence of both cruciate ligaments may decrease implant stresses and potentially improve the longevity of these implants. However, increased technical difficulty and inconclusive clinical benefit regarding ACL preservation have hindered enthusiasm for these designs in total knee arthroplasty. With ongoing critical review of historic and modern clinical studies, and with improvement in implant design, we in the field of orthopedics will anxiously await the ultimate fate of the anterior cruciate ligament in total knee arthroplasty.

Introduction

While debate and research regarding retention, sacrifice, or substitution of the posterior cruciate ligament (PCL) remain intense, questions regarding the benefit of preserving the anterior cruciate ligament (ACL) have received far less attention, both in the literature and in contemporary total knee arthroplasty design. Theoretically, retaining the anterior cruciate ligament may allow for better knee kinematics, improved proprioception [1], increased maximum flexion, and overall improvement in knee function [2]. Additionally, the ability to use less constrained polyethylene tibial components will lessen stresses transmitted to the implant fixation and may potentially improve longevity of the arthroplasty. However, both the purported increased technical difficulty and the inconclusive clinical benefit regarding preservation of the ACL have hindered enthusiasm for these designs in total knee arthroplasty. Retaining both cruciate ligaments by preserving their insertion on the tibial eminence may make exposure, and subsequently the procedure, technically more demanding. The de-

creased surface area of the tibial component may make fixation less predictable. The joint line must be anatomically restored in order to avoid abnormal tensioning or laxity of the retained ligaments. Additionally, correction of deformity may be more difficult when the anterior and posterior cruciates are not excised. Furthermore, one must be able to assess the functional integrity of these ligaments intraoperatively in order to avoid a functionally deficient knee in the face of an unconstrained design. Whether these potential benefits outweigh the drawbacks remains unresolved in the literature.

History

Prosthetic knee arthroplasty utilizing components fixed with acrylic cement was first proposed by Gunston, who developed the polycentric knee (◘ Fig. 46-1a,b) in the late 1960s and reported his findings in the late 1970s [3]. Modifications were soon made by Bryan and Peterson from the Mayo Clinic [4] and Cracchiolo from Los Angeles [5]. Shortly thereafter, the geometric knee prosthesis became available for clinical trials (◘ Fig. 46-2). It was the introduction of these two prostheses that truly began an era of modern management of arthritic knees with non-hinged prosthetic components.

Andrea Cracchiolo reported a prospective comparative clinical analysis of these first-generation knee replacements in 1979. His study of 119 polycentric and 92 geometric knee replacements was performed to determine and compare their clinical effectiveness. These patients were followed for a mean of 3.5 years (2-6 years). Failure occurred in 11% of the polycentric and in 16% of the geometric knees. Both prostheses provided excellent relief of pain [6].

Lewallen et al. reported a 10-year follow-up study of 209 polycentric total knee arthroplasties performed in 159 patients at the Mayo Clinic between July 1970 and November 1971 [7]. The calculated probability of the arthroplasty remaining successful 10 years postoperatively was only 66%. Actual results showed that 42% of the arthroplasties were successful in patients who were

46

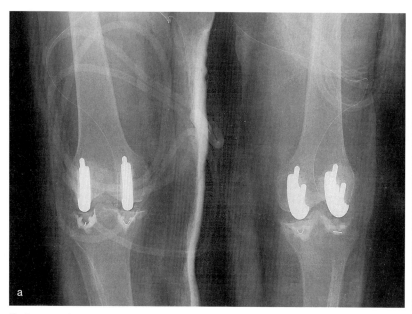
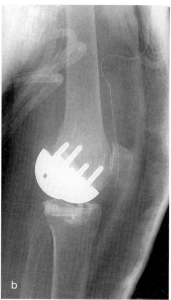

◘ **Fig. 46-1a, b.** Anteroposterior (*a*) and lateral (*b*) radiographs of a polycentric TKA implanted at the Mayo Clinic in 1975

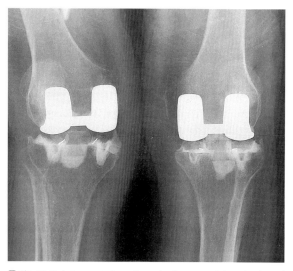

◘ **Fig. 46-2.** Anteroposterior radiograph of a geometric knee implanted at the Mayo Clinic in 1976

still alive at the time of review. The most common causes of failure were instability (13%), component loosening (7%), infection (3%), and extensor mechanism pain (4%).

Although a new era of surgical management for knee arthritis had begun with these implants, by today's standards their reliability and durability were quite poor. Publications reporting the poor long-term survival of the polycentric and geometric knees prompted the introduction of new designs, modification of surgical techniques, and critical investigation into the etiology for each mode of failure seen in these early trials.

Biomechanics and Kinematics

In recent years, evaluation of in vivo kinematics after total knee arthroplasty has gained increased interest for study. During the past decade, fluoroscopy and other modes of dynamic imaging have been used to better define knee kinematics and to determine whether premature polyethylene failure and/or poor operative results could be related to abnormal knee kinematics [8, 9]. In gait studies by Andriacchi et al., the knees in which both cruciate ligaments were retained were the only arthroplasties that had normal flexion when the patient ascended and descended stairs [2, 10]. An in vivo weight-bearing fluoroscopic kinematic analysis comparing subjects with a bicruciate-retaining total knee arthroplasty and a PCL-retaining total knee arthroplasty was published by Stiehl et al. [11]. They found that subjects with a bicruciate-retaining total knee arthroplasty typically experienced posterior femoral roll-back during a deep knee bend. Bicruciate-retaining arthroplasties demonstrated limited anterior-posterior translation and remained posterior to the mid-sagittal line in all positions. The abnormal anteroposterior translation of the medial femoral condyle typically seen in PCL-retaining total knee arthroplasties was not identified in any of the knees with a functioning ACL in this study.

Komistek et al. reported on the in vivo kinematics for 30 patients who received a Hermes anterior cruciate-retaining or posterior-stabilized total knee arthroplasty [12]. Fifteen patients had an anterior cruciate-retaining total knee arthroplasty and 15 had a posterior-substituting design. The two implants had identical frontal and sagittal geometry and were implanted by the same surgeon. Compared with the data for the patients having an anterior cruciate-retaining total knee arthroplasty, the data for patients having a posterior-stabilized total knee arthroplasty were far more variable. Only seven of 15 patients having a posterior-stabilized total knee arthroplasty experienced posterior motion of both condyles from heel-strike to toe-off. Overall, it seemed that the patients with ACL-retaining total knee arthroplasty experienced more normal knee kinematics than patients with a posterior-stabilized total knee arthroplasty. These patients exhibited less variability in their data points, more consistent anteroposterior contact patterns, more normal axial rotational patterns, and posterior femoral roll-back magnitudes that more closely paralleled the normal knee [13].

Modern Series

Buechel and Pappas [14] reported a 91% 12-year survival in bicruciate-retaining, meniscal-bearing prostheses in their cemented cohort of 21 patients. They found these results to be equivalent to those in PCL-only-retaining and bicruciate-substituting prostheses. However, few patients had long-term follow-up.

Cloutier [15] reported the results of 45 patients with total knee arthroplasties 10 years after surgery. He reported a 96% success rate in patients with bicruciate-retaining implants compared with a 75% success rate using the same prosthetic design in knees where the anterior cruciate was not retained. In his series, he deemed it technically possible to retain the ACL in 50% of the knees he replaced. The mean range of flexion was higher for the ACL-retaining prosthesis. However, there are two major weaknesses with this study. No clear survival rate was given, and the tibial design used in these implants was a flat surface with no anterior or posterior lip on the tibial tray. It is now well understood that in an ACL-deficient knee, excessive anterior tibial translation will occur if the geometry of the tibial component does not, at least in part, reconstitute the function of the ACL. This could explain the observed differences between the ACL-retaining and the ACL-sacrificing groups. Cloutier's study also determined that the flexion range, stability, and capacity to climb stairs were significantly better for patients with an ACL-retaining total knee arthroplasty.

Migaud et al. [16] evaluated 68 Cloutier total knee prostheses, 38 ACL-sparing and 30 ACL-sacrificing. They reported no difference in functional score and range of motion between the two groups and noted that the mean anterior tibial translation was not different for either prosthesis unless excessive posterior tibial slope was present.

Jenny and Jenny [17] reported a short-term, prospective study of 32 ACL-retaining and 93 ACL-sacrificing total knee replacements with a minimum follow-up of 2 years. Of note was that the mean operative time, implant positioning radiographically, and revision rates were the same in both groups. Therefore, this particular study did not support the suggestion that technical difficulties may be increased in ACL preservation during total knee arthroplasty. However, the clinical and functional results and range of motion were neither improved nor worsened in the ACL-retaining group. Given the short-term follow-up in this study, it is difficult to say whether a less conforming implant in the ACL-preserving group will lead to improved longevity and decreased loosening rates as compared with the ACL-sacrificing group.

In Cloutier's recent series with 9-11 years follow-up, a total of 163 total knee arthroplasties in 130 patients with cruciate-retaining designs were assessed in a prospective fashion [18]; 107 knees were followed for an average of 10 years. The ACL was considered relatively normal in 96 knees and partly degenerated in 67 knees. The result was good or excellent in 97% of patients and the survival rate, with revision as the end point, was 95% ±2% at an average of 10 years postoperatively. The average knee score was 91 and the average functional score was 82.

Perhaps the most interesting clinical study with regard to the issue of ACL retention in total knee arthroplasty was published by Pritchett [19]. In this study, 50 patients underwent bilateral total knee arthroplasty, bicruciate-retaining on one side and only PCL-retaining on the other. Postoperative flexion averaged 119° in both groups and all patients had full extension. All knees that retained both cruciate ligaments were deemed stable, whereas six knees in the posterior cruciate-only group had sagittal plane instability of more than 1 cm with anterior drawer testing. Most interesting were the patients' opinions regarding their knees: 70% preferred the bicruciate-retaining knee and only 10% preferred the posterior cruciate-only-retaining knee; 20% did not express a preference. Furthermore, 29 of the 50 patients stated that they used their bicruciate-retaining total knee arthroplasty as their lead leg during stair-climbing, compared with only seven for the posterior cruciate-only-retaining knee.

Conclusions

Although regarded by many as technically demanding and of limited clinical value, bicruciate-retaining total knee arthroplasty may hold promise for improved patient satisfaction, improved implant longevity, and improved wear characteristics. As orthopedic surgeons continue to search for designs that will mimic and restore the normal kinematics of the natural knee, the issue of the importance of cruciate ligament retention will continue to raise intense interest. Whether preservation of the ligaments or rather articular geometry that replicates their function will prevail remains to be seen. Nonetheless, we look forward to a future in which patients will feel that their knee replacement is "normal".

References

1. Lew WD, Lewis JL (1982) The effect of knee prosthesis geometry on cruciate ligament mechanics during flexion. J Bone Joint Surg [Am] 64: 734-739
2. Andriacchi TP (1981) In vivo evaluation of patients' function following total knee replacement. Orthop Trans 5:416
3. Gunston FH (1971) Polycentric knee arthroplasty. J Bone Joint Surg [Br] 53:272
4. Bryan RJ, Peterson LFA (1971) The quest for the replacement knee. Orthop Clin North Am 2:715
5. Cracchiolo A (1973) Polycentric knee arthroplasty using tibial prosthetic units of a variable height. Clin Orthop 94:140
6. Cracchiolo A, Benson M, Finerman G, et al (1979) A prospective comparative clinical analysis of the first-generation knee replacements: polycentric versus geometric knee arthroplasty. Clin Orthop 145:37-46
7. Lewallen D, Bryan RS, Peterson LF (1984) Polycentric total knee arthroplasty. J Bone Joint Surg [Am] 66:1211-1218
8. Banks SA, Hodge WA (1996) Accurate measurement of three-dimensional knee replacement kinematics using single plane fluoroscopy. IEEE Trans Biomed Eng 43:638-649
9. Banks SA, Markovich GE, Hodge WA (1997) In vivo kinematics or cruciate retaining and substituting knee arthroplasties. J Arthroplasty 12:297-304
10. Andriacchi TP, Galante JO, Fermier RW (1982) The influence of total knee replacement design on walking and stair climbing. J Bone Joint Surg [Am] 64:1328-1335
11. Stiehl JB, Komistek RD, Cloutier JM (2000) The cruciate ligaments in total knee arthroplasty: a kinematic analysis of two total knee arthroplasties. J Arthroplasty 15:545-550
12. Komistek RD, Allain J, Anderson DT, et al (2002) In vivo kinematics for subjects with and without an anterior cruciate ligament. Clin Orthop 404:315-325
13. Karrholm J, Brandsson S, Freeman MA (2000) Tibial femoral movement. 4: Changes of axial tibial rotation caused by forced rotation at the weight-bearing knee studied by R.S.A. J Bone Joint Surg [Br] 82:1201-1203
14. Buechel FF, Pappas MJ (1990) Long-term survivorship analysis of cruciate sparing versus cruciate sacrificing knee prosthesis with meniscal bearing. Clin Orthop 260:162-169
15. Cloutier JM (1991) Long-term results after nonconstrained total knee arthroplasty. Clin Orthop 274:63-65
16. Migaud H, DeLadoucett A, Dohin B, et al (1996) Influence of posterior tibial slope on anterior tibial translation and mobility after a nonconstrained total knee arthroplasty. Rev Chir Orthop 82:7-13
17. Jenny JY, Jenny G (1998) Preservation of anterior cruciate ligament in total knee arthroplasty. Arch Orthop Trauma Surg 118:145-148
18. Cloutier JM, Sabouret P, Deghrar A (1999) Total knee arthroplasty with retention of both cruciate ligaments: a nine- to eleven-year follow-up study. J Bone Joint Surg [Am] 81:697-702
19. Pritchett JW (1996) Anterior cruciate retaining total knee arthroplasty. J Arthroplasty 11:194-197

47 Bearing Surfaces for Motion Control in Total Knee Arthroplasty

P. S. Walker

Summary

A goal of knee replacement is to achieve normal function and kinematics. One solution is to preserve all of the ligaments and use compartmental components. However, if complete resurfacing is indicated, one or both of the cruciates is usually resected, and dished bearing surfaces are used to replace their function. Intercondylar cams can be added to ensure posterior femoral contacts in high flexion. In this paper, an alternative scheme is presented where the bearing surfaces are not simple combinations of radii but are based on converging or diverging medial-lateral bearing spacing as flexion proceeds. This scheme produces natural roll-back with flexion, more pronounced on the lateral side, while preserving the laxity which is characteristic of the normal knee. It is proposed that this design can produce natural knee kinematics which may result in close to normal function.

Introduction

A frequently stated goal of knee replacement, especially now that increasing numbers of young and active patients are requiring such treatments, is to allow for the restoration of normal function. How to achieve this is a matter of controversy, however. A unicompartmental replacement, performed with a small incision and with the cruciate ligaments preserved, can produce kinematics similar to that of a normal knee. However, when the joint destruction is more generalized and when the cruciates are abnormal, it is not clear which type of total knee will provide the most normal function. The choices of total knees are extensive. The type most commonly used today is the condylar replacement, subdivided into the cruciate-retaining (CR) designs, which usually have bearing surfaces of moderate to low conformity and where the posterior cruciate is preserved, and the posterior-stabilized (PS) designs, which usually have moderate to high conformity and where a cam-post is used to replace the function of the posterior cruciate [14]. There are significant variations in each category, which has been demonstrated by simple laboratory measurements of the AP and rotary

laxity, while both symmetric and asymmetric surface geometries are represented [12]. A recent variant of the surface replacement is the medial pivot knee (Wright Mfg. Co., Memphis, TN), which is an attempt to reproduce the relative stability of the lateral and medial sides. Mobile-bearing knees of the rotating platform type are extensively used, with the rationale of reducing wear and providing additional freedom of motion, which can allow for some surgical error as well as more functional rotation [5]. Some rotating platform designs even provide a medial pivot point, which again is more analogous to normal kinematic behavior.

Determining the outcome of knee designs using the standard evaluation methods [10] has shown that many design types produce similar results in terms of basic function and alignments. Clinical follow-ups have similarly shown that many designs have a similar durability [6]. However, recent evaluation methods which analyzed the expectations and results of different patient groups have shown that, in many cases, the results of total knees are not uniformly satisfactory from a functional point of view [32]. Activities involving the control of motion and position at high flexion angles have been particularly problematic.

What design criteria for a total knee can be formulated which will result in the most successful functional outcome? One possibility is that, 'after implantation, the motion of the knee will be indistinguishable from that of the natural knee in its healthy state'. Taken to its extreme, this criterion would require customizing each patient, but for off-the-shelf knee systems, average natural knee motion would be the criterion. Such motion can be described as follows: As flexion proceeds, there is a progressive posterior displacement of the lateral femoral condyle, the medial femoral condyle moving only a small amount [11, 13, 15, 20, 25]. In rigid body terms, with the origins of femoral and tibial axis systems in the center of the knee, the motion consists of posterior displacement of the femur combined with internal tibial rotation. It is emphasized that the above describes the neutral path of motion. About this neutral path, there is significant anteroposterior and rotational laxity [4].

In this chapter, different design options are discussed with the purpose of identifying what types of design are likely to be most successful in producing natural knee motion. Particular attention is given to designs in which the bearing surfaces themselves are used to guide the motion as well as allowing for laxity and stability.

Designs for Guiding or Controlling the Motion

In a typical surface replacement knee, the femoral bearing surfaces are convex in the frontal and sagittal planes, while the tibial bearing surfaces are concave. With this geometry, if there is a compressive force acting down the tibial axis, the femorotibial contact point (or area) will remain at the 'bottom of the dish' or 'dwell point' of the tibial surface at all angles of flexion. The contact point locations will change, however, if shear forces and torques are applied similar to the way that gives the natural knee laxity about the neutral path. The contact point locations can also be modified by a cam-post mechanism located in the intercondylar area. Usually, the cam-post is used to produce posterior displacement of the contact points in high flexion. Use of a cam-post produces a defined motion, with no laxity. This distinction of laxity or defined motion can be thought of as either guiding or controlling the motion. Different possibilities for producing these two types of motion will now be discussed.

Anatomical Approach

Some of the earlier designs reproduced the shapes of the distal femur and proximal tibia (◘ Fig. 47-1).

The requirement for the Leeds knee of Seedhom [24] was preservation of all of the ligaments and an anatomical surface geometry in relation to the attachment points of the ligaments, so that normal motion and stability could be achieved. In addition, low surface conformity

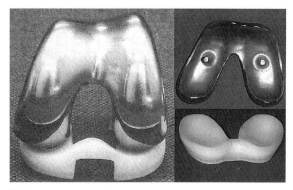

◘ **Fig. 47-1.** Examples of total knees where the bearing surfaces of the femoral component are based on anatomical shapes. *Left*: the tibial surfaces are designed for retention of the cruciates [24]; *right*: the tibial surfaces replace the function of the cruciates and menisci [9]

was required to allow for a high range of flexion. The resulting femoral component was a shell which was made in several sizes, molded from representative examples of knee specimens. The tibial bearing surface was made to be concave in both the ML and AP directions, thus departing somewhat from anatomy, at least on the lateral side. Seedhom also anticipated that laxity of the tibial bearing surfaces would reduce the shear stresses on the fixation, but he was also concerned to minimize the contact stresses on the plastic in order to minimize wear. This is a trade-off which is still a factor in today's designs.

Ewald [9] took a similar approach of reproducing the anatomical bearing surfaces of the distal femur with a metallic shell, not unlike the shape of the MGH (Massachusetts General Hospital) hemiarthroplasty femoral condyle. However, there was one important difference compared with the Seedhom approach. Ewald proposed that because the cruciates and the menisci would not be viable in the arthritic knee, the combination of the femoral and tibial bearing surfaces would have to reproduce their function in terms of providing the necessary laxity and stability. Furthermore, the tibial surfaces should be formed so that the rolling, sliding, and pivoting movements would actually be guided. Ewald proposed not rigid motion, but a guided neutral path with laxity about this path. To achieve this, one of the features of the tibial bearing surface was the divergence of the low points on the tibial surface from anterior to posterior, such that as flexion proceeded, the femoral condyles would locate more posteriorly and also the relative roll-backs of the lateral and medial sides would produce an axial rotation. The only feature that differs from motion data available today was that the medial femoral condyle was said to pivot about the lateral, but that may have reflected early flexion when initial roll-back occurs on the medial side.

Geometrical Approach

In the early 1970s, there were a number of condylar designs which relied on geometrical shapes to control the motion. These approaches ranged from the shallow geometry of Townley to the cylinder-in-trough of Freeman and Swanson, to mention only two [14]. These opposite approaches were intended, as above, to utilize the existing cruciate ligaments as an important part of providing stability, or to eliminate these ligaments and rely on the reproducible geometrical surfaces of the implant for stability. In general, it was found that low inherent stability required accurate balancing of the ligaments; otherwise an incidence of instability and failure would occur, whereas excessive constraint resulted in a high loosening rate, especially when the tibial fixation features were inadequate. An approach to solving these particular problems made use of partially conforming

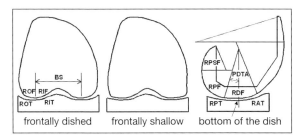

○ **Fig. 47-2.** A parametric description of contemporary total knees with partially conforming bearing surfaces. Varying the radii as shown produces major differences in laxity and stability. BS bearing spacing; *ROF* radius outer femur; *RIF* radius inner femur; *ROT* radius outer tibia; *RIT* radius inner tibia, *RPSF* radius posterior superior femur; *RDF* radius distal femur; *PDTA* posterior-distal transition angle, i.e., angle between the large distal radius and the smaller posterior radius; *RPT* radius posterior tibia; *RAT* radius anterior tibia

bearing surfaces to provide stability but allow laxity [26]. This concept was incorporated into the original total condylar knee, which has been clinically successful over the long term, with few mechanical problems other than a limited range of flexion. The double-dishing of the bearing surfaces in the frontal and sagittal planes provided the required stability and laxity without requiring the cruciate ligaments (○ Fig. 47-2).

It is emphasized that such bearing surfaces were intended to allow the multiplicity of joint motions which occur in vivo, without providing a definite motion path other than containing the femur in the tibial dish within reasonable bounds defined by the amount of tibial dishing. Such bearing surfaces have been used in numerous designs for cruciate resection, for retention of the posterior cruciate, and even for retention of both cruciates. Many refinements have been made to the radii of the bearing surfaces to optimize the constraint characteristics and to minimize the surface and sub-surface contact stresses [23].

Intercondylar Cams and Other Mechanisms

The earliest examples of total knees which achieved guided motion by intercondylar cams were the Kinematic/Kinemax Stabilizer and the Insall-Burstein Posterior Stabilized, designed in the late 1970s [14]. In the former design, the objective was to guide the posterior displacement of the contact points throughout the whole flexion range. This was achieved by a femoral cam whose center was offset from the center of the femoral condylar bearing surfaces. In the PS design, the objective was to produce posterior displacement and to prevent anterior subluxation of the femur in late flexion. To achieve this, the femoral cam had a small radius, located posteriorly at a large eccentricity. Drawbacks of such designs were that the internal-external rotation was limited, and there was no mechanism for roll-forward as the knee was extend-

ed, although the femur would tend to return to the bottom of the tibial dish. Successful long-term results have been achieved with these designs. Recently, the design of intercondylar cams has been systematically analyzed to determine if improvements could be made to the cam-post shapes [29](○ Figs. 47-3 and 47-4).

Figure 47-3 shows a cam design where both roll-back and roll-forward are produced, using a convex tibial cam shape and a shallow femoral housing. Figure 47-4 shows a saddle arrangement on the tibia into which a shallow femoral convex surface is housed [28]. This produces controlled motion throughout the entire range of flexion, including roll-back in flexion and roll-forward in extension. It is noted that the internal-external limitation can be addressed by using rounded cam shapes or by locating the plastic on a rotating platform.

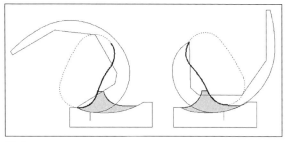

○ **Fig. 47-3.** A computer-generated intercondylar cam where the functions of the anterior cruciate and posterior cruciate are reproduced in early (*right*) and late (*left*) flexion [29]

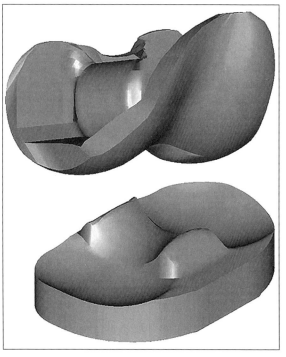

○ **Fig. 47-4.** A computer-generated intercondylar cam which provides anterior-posterior motion control throughout the entire flexion range. There is some posterior displacement of the femoral component with flexion [28]

Recently, two designs have been introduced in which differential contact point locations between extension and flexion have been achieved discretely. The TRAC knee (Biomet, Warsaw, IN), designed by Draganich and Pottenger [8], uses an inner pair of bearing surfaces which contact from 5° hyperextension to 8° of flexion with an anterior dwell point, and an outer pair of bearing surfaces which contact throughout the remaining flexion range, with a more posterior dwell point. The transition from the first pair to the second is obtained by an intercondylar cam. The plastic component itself is pivoted on a smooth metal tibial plate, resembling the LCS rotating platform design. The Kyocera Bi-Surface knee [1] addresses the goal of achieving a very high range of flexion with unrestricted internal tibial rotation. For the major part of the flexion range, the knee behaves as a standard condylar replacement with moderately conforming bearing surfaces. Beyond that, the load is transferred to a spherical surface protruding posteriorly from the femoral intercondylar region, contacting within a spherical depression at the posterior of the plastic tibial component. There is some similarity to the Variable Axis total knee [19]. The Medial Pivot knee (Wright Mfg, Memphis TN) is a slightly different concept, in that there are no guide surfaces or cams per se. Instead, the tibial bearing surfaces are shaped so that normal knee motion is possible; the medial side remains in the same position during flexion but the lateral femoral condyle can displace posteriorly with flexion. However, the design does not actively force this motion to occur, but allows each knee to move individually.

Guiding Surfaces

The concept of guiding surfaces is similar to that advanced by Ewald [9], namely to guide the motion of the knee by interaction of the major bearing surfaces themselves, but allowing for laxity to occur about the guided neutral path. It is possible that the natural knee uses such a strategy to enhance the posterior displacement of the lateral femoral contact area while maintaining an almost constant medial contact area.

Observation shows that the high points of the femoral condyles are almost parallel through most of the range of flexion [27]. However at higher flexion, where most of the internal tibial rotation occurs, the lateral femoral condyle appears to converge inwards (Fig. 47-5) This will assist an inward rotation of the lateral femoral condyle into a lower area of the lateral tibial plateau. Such geometry is not inconsistent with measurements made of the bearings surfaces by Ateshian et al. [2, 3] and by Cohen et al. [7] using stereophotogrammetry. Such features could be reproduced in a total knee replacement.

In a standard condylar replacement, the bearing spacing (Fig. 47-2) of the femoral condyles is constant around

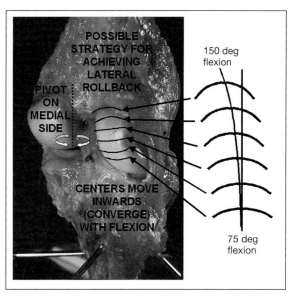

 Fig. 47-5. Mechanisms which may occur in the natural knee for producing internal tibial rotation with flexion, pivoting about the medial condyle, by convergence of the lateral femoral condyle in high flexion, and a decrease in radius of curvature

the sagittal contour, while the tibial surfaces are usually dished in the sagittal plane. In the absence of AP shear and axial torque, the femoral-tibial contact points will be located at the bottom of the tibial dish (dwell points) at all angles of flexion, so as to minimize the potential energy of the system [26]. This is a very important principle of condylar replacement knees where the tibial surfaces are dished. However, if the bearing spacing of the femoral component converges with the flexion angle, a tibial surface can be generated where the low points change in an AP direction with flexion. Such a tibial surface was generated in the computer so that the contact points on both the lateral and medial sides would displace posteriorly with flexion (Fig. 47-6).

The tibial surface was generated by embedding the femoral component into a tibial block in successive positions with progressive roll-back. After successive Boolean operations (subtracting the imprint of the femoral condyles), the tibial surface was generated. Due to the convergence of the bearing spacing of the femoral component, as the femur was progressively flexed, the effective bottom of the tibial dish, or the position of least potential energy, also moved posteriorly with flexion.

To more closely reproduce natural knee motion where there is posterior displacement of the lateral femoral condyle with flexion, equivalent to a pivoting about the medial condyle, a different type of surface was formed [30]. The principle is illustrated in Fig. 47-7.

The femoral condyles are represented by spherical surfaces. On the left is shown a medial pivot knee where the femoral component has been rotated about the medial condyle and an imprint has been formed in the tibial

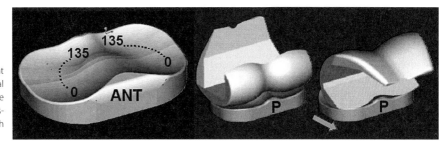

Fig. 47-6. A femoral component with converging lateral and medial condyles has been used to generate a tibial surface which produces posterior femoral displacement with flexion

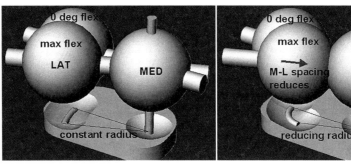

Fig. 47-7. Basic principle of guiding the motion during flexion by the shape of the femoral condyles and a generated tibial surface: *Left*: there is no convergence and the tibial surface is generated by rotation about the medial condyle. There is no fixed neutral motion path. *Right*: convergence occurs by a progressive reduction of the lateral bearing spacing with flexion. This results in a unique neutral motion path consisting of posterior displacement of the lateral femoral condyle and pivoting about the medial side

surface. Such surfaces will allow medial pivoting to occur but will not guide such pivoting. On the right is shown a femoral surface where the bearing spacing moves progressively inwards with flexion. Now, the tibial surface is formed by the femoral imprint with convergence. This means that at any angle of flexion there is a preferred position of the lateral femoral condyle based on the bottom of the dish. In this sense, the motion is guided (**Fig. 47-8 and 47-9**).

Figure 47-8 shows a lateral femoral condyle where there is convergence of the bearing spacing from 75° to 150° of flexion. The imprint of the tibial surface clearly converges inwards with flexion. The medial tibial surface is merely the composite imprint formed from 0° to 150° of flexion, pivoting about the medial side. Figure 47-9 shows a knee replacement designed using this lateral converging geometry. As the femur is flexed, the lateral femoral condyle displaces posteriorly, along with an external rotation (equivalent to an internal tibial rotation).

One factor not taken into consideration in these converging models is the behavior of the contact areas if the femur was displaced from any neutral position. If the tibial surface was generated by the actual femoral component as described, on deviating from the neutral path in either AP displacement or internal-external rotation, edge loading of the plastic would occur. To account for this factor, a 'generating femoral component' needs to be defined which has larger radii of curvature in frontal and sagittal planes than the actual femoral component. This would allow clearance which would then provide laxity about any neutral position without edge loading.

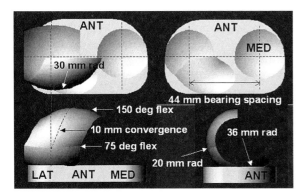

Fig. 47-8. A particular example of a lateral femoral condyle where the bearing surface converges after 75° of flexion. This surface is used to generate a tibial surface. The interaction guides the femur to pivot about the medial condyle as flexion proceeds from 75° to maximum

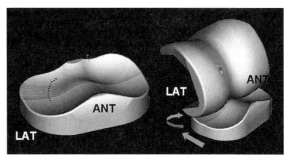

Fig. 47-9. Femoral and tibial surfaces generated using the principle of Fig. 8. The posterior displacement of the lateral femoral condyle and the medial pivoting are indicated by *arrows*

Evaluating Guided-Motion Knee Replacements

Once a knee replacement of any type has been formulated, including a guided-motion knee as described above, the design needs to be evaluated prior to clinical application. What is required are laboratory tests which will predict the behavior in a realistic functional situation. For evaluating a guided-motion knee, the paramount concern is the kinematics. The total knee has been designed to produce a particular type of motion, which will result in proposed functional advantages. An obvious example is a posterior-stabilized knee which is intended to cause the femoral contact points to displace posteriorly in high flexion. This is intended to provide a greater range of flexion by reducing posterior impingements, and by increasing the lever arm of the quadriceps for improved control at those high flexion angles. In general, the evidence is that the goals are realized, although this is not to say that other designs do not provide similar advantages.

However, if a knee replacement is to be designed to reproduce normal function, as far as allowed by the condition of the patient, then a more general design criterion is required which can be tested mechanically. The proposal made in the Introduction is that "after implantation of the knee replacement, the motion of the knee in any activity is indistinguishable from the motion of the knee in its healthy intact state." The motion can be defined as the relative motion of the femur and the tibia, measured with reference to Cartesian coordinate systems in each bone. One inherent requirement is that the muscle activity after rehabilitation will resemble that of the knee in its healthy intact state, because knee motion will depend upon muscle action as well as upon external forces. Furthermore, the criterion would need to be tested in the patient, not in the laboratory.

To consider motion without the effect of muscles, a criterion can be proposed which takes account of only the inherent constraint characteristics of the passive elements of the knee itself, including the implant. In this case the criterion would be that "after implantation of the knee

replacement, the neutral path of motion and the constraint throughout the flexion range is indistinguishable from that of the knee in its healthy intact state." This means that if sets of external forces and moments are applied to an intact knee, and then to the knee after implantation, at a range of flexion angles, the resulting displacements and rotations will be indistinguishable. In order to test such a criterion, one method would be to use a cadaver with all ligaments and menisci preserved, measure the constraint characteristics, then implant the knee replacement and again measure the constraint. This test would use the cadaver as its own control, and would also reproduce the effect of the various passive structures. The test would be applicable to a design where one or both cruciates was preserved, or where both were resected.

Such a test was carried out on a plastic model of a guided-surface knee resembling the design shown in Fig. 47-9. Cadaveric legs were used, and the femur was mounted vertically, with loads applied to the quadriceps and hamstrings, twice the force in the former than in the latter (🔲 Fig. 47-10). The leg was flexed from zero to maximum and fluoroscopic images were taken. Markers in the femoral and tibial components allowed the contact points of the lateral and medial femoral condyles on the tibial plateau to be measured. The guided-surface knee was compared with a standard symmetric posterior cruciate-retaining knee. On average, from six specimens, it was found that the guided surfaces did produce more stability on the medial side and more posterior displacement on the lateral side. These tests were restricted to knee replacements which preserved the posterior cruciate.

Other tests could be carried out which do not require the use of specimens. One of the simplest is constraint testing [31] where a compressive load is applied to the implant components and then a shear force is applied, the shear displacement being measured. Alternatively, a torque can be applied and the rotation measured. These tests are currently required by the FDA for new knee designs, as they provide a basic measure of the constraint [12]. However, the tests do not predict performance, in that the results are independent of whether the cruciates

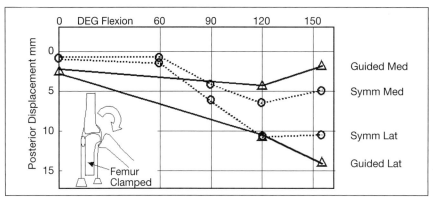

🔲 **Fig. 47-10.** One of the methods that can be used to evaluate a guided-motion knee. Compared with a standard symmetrical knee, the guided-motion knee with a converging lateral femoral condyle has produced increased lateral posterior displacement and reduced medial displacement. (Study coordinated by Mr. Scott Steffensmeier; data reproduced courtesy of Zimmer, Inc., Warsaw, IN, USA)

are preserved or resected, and there is no standard against which to compare the result. For designs such as rotating platforms, for instance, the rotational constraint is zero except for friction. Another test which could be applied is to use a modified Oxford rig, where the lower extremity is loaded with body weight and muscle forces are then used to balance the knee at a required flexion angle [18]. In testing a knee replacement, the criterion here could be to compare the three-dimensional motion of the intact with that of the replaced knee, with particular regard to posterior displacement and internal-external rotation. A robot can also be used with a similar criterion, with the added element of determining ligament forces [16].

From a practical point of view, guided-surface knees must be able to guide the motion in a way similar to that of standard knee replacements which have a distinct bottom of the dish for stability. For example, it would be unsatisfactory if a small amount of deformation or wear were to seriously disrupt the motion the surfaces were intended to provide. This consideration was tested using a computer model which approximated the inherent stability of surface designs by calculating the amount of material displaced from the neutral position, for defined amounts of anterior-posterior displacement or internal-external rotation [30].

Computer modeling of the entire knee assembly should be mentioned here, because it is a method of producing standard tests which are not subject to the variables of cadaveric tests, such as the dependence upon surgical placement and other factors. In principle, computer models can reproduce knees with different bone and ligament geometries and properties, as well as surgical placements, thus providing a parametric evaluation under a range of test conditions. However, one weak link for the intact knee is that modeling the meniscus is problematic. Nevertheless, a validated computer model should be regarded as ultimately the most satisfactory way of evaluating knee replacements for motion characteristics, as well as for other factors.

Finally, on a theoretical basis, can any implanted surfaces satisfy either of the criteria stated above? It may seem self-evident that in a particular knee, if surfaces replicating the natural knee were implanted, and the cruciates and menisci were preserved, the criteria would be satisfied. However, it is not practical at present to retain the menisci and its attachments, in which case their stabilizing function would have to be reproduced in a modification of the tibial bearing surfaces. Likewise, if one or both of the cruciates were resected, the tibial surface would have to be further modified. One factor which would make it difficult to precisely reproduce normal constraint is the friction between the bearing surfaces. In the natural knee the friction is close to zero, whereas in a metal-polyethylene knee the friction is such as to produce considerable modification of contact point locations [17, 22].

In conclusion, while for the older, less active patient standard designs of today may be adequate from a functional point of view, for the more demanding patients, in future it may be shown that functional advantages will be obtained from an approach where normal constraint is reproduced, either by a guided-surface approach or by some other means.

References

1. Akagi M et al (2000) The bisurface total knee replacement: a unique design for flexion. J Bone Joint Surg [Am] 82:1626-1633
2. Ateshian GA et al (1991) Quantitation of articular surface topography and cartilage thickness in knee joints using stereophotogrammetry. J Biomech 24:761-776
3. Ateshian GA (2003) Topography of knee femoral articular surface. (Personal communication)
4. Blankevoort L et al (1988) The envelope of passive knee joint motion. J Biomech 21:705-720
5. Buechel FF (2002) Long-term follow-up after mobile bearing total knee replacement. Clin Orthop 404:40-50
6. Callaghan CM et al (1995) Patient outcomes following unicompartmental or bicompartmental knee arthroplasty: a meta-analysis. J Arthroplasty 10:141-50
7. Cohen ZA et al (2003) Templates of the cartilage layers of the patellofemoral joint and their use in the assessment of osteoarthritic cartilage damage. Osteoarthritis Cartilage 11:569-579
8. Draganich L et al (1998) TRAC PS knee design and clinical outcome. Abstracts Book, Annual Symposium of the Int Soc for Technology in Arthroplasty. Marseille, pp 96-99
9. Ewald FC (1974) Joint prostheses. United States Patent, number 3798679, March
10. Ewald FC (1989) The Knee Society total knee arthroplasty roentgenographic evaluation and scoring system. Clin Orthop 248:9-12
11. Feikes JD et al (1998) The unique track of intact passive knee motion as a kinematic baseline. Trans Orthop Res Soc 23:170
12. Haider H, Walker PS (2005) Measurements of constraint of total knee replacement. J Biomech 38:341-348
13. Hill PF et al (2000) Tibiofemoral movement. II: The loaded and unloaded knee studied by MRI. J Bone Joint Surg [Br] 82:1196-1198
14. Insall JH, Clarke HD (2001) Historic development, classification, and characteristics of knee prostheses. In: Insall JH (ed) Surgery of the knee, 3rd edn. Chap 73, vol 2, pp 1516-1552
15. Iwaki H et al (2000) Tibiofemoral movement. I: The shapes and relative movements of the femur and tibia in the unloaded cadaver knee. J Bone Joint Surg [Br] 82:1189-1195
16. Li G, Zayontz et al (2003) Kinematics of the knee at high flexion angles. J Orthop Res 22:90-95
17. Luger E et al (1997) Inherent differences in the laxity and stability between the intact knee and total knee replacements. Knee 4:7-14
18. MacWilliams BA et al (1999) Hamstrings co-contraction reduces internal rotation, anterior translation, and anterior cruciate ligament load in weight-bearing flexion. J Orthop Res 17:817-822
19. Murray DG et al (1982) The variable axis prosthesis: 2-year follow-up study. J Bone Joint Surg [Am] 63:687-694
20. Nakagawa S et al (2000) Tibiofemoral movement: full flexion in the living knee studied by MRI. J Bone Joint Surg [Br] 82:1199-2000
21. Rovick JS et al (1991) Relation between knee motion and ligament length patterns. Clin Biomech 6:213-220
22. Sathasivam S et al (1997) A computer model with surface friction for the prediction of total knee kinematics. J Biomech 30:177-184
23. Sathasivam S et al (1999) The conflicting requirements of laxity and conformity in total knee replacement. J Biomech 32:239-247
24. Seedhom BB et al (1974) The Leeds knee. Proc Institution of Mechanical Engineers, London, Symposium on Total Knee Replacement. CP16:108-114

25. Thompson WO et al (1991) Tibial meniscus dynamics using three-dimensional reconstruction of the magnetic resonance images. Am J Sports Med 19:210-216

26. Walker PS et al (1974) Proc Institution of Mechanical Engineers, London, Symposium on Total Knee Replacement. CP16: 22-29

27. Walker PS (1991) Design of Kinemax total knee replacement bearing surfaces. Acta Orthop Belg 57:108-113

28. Walker PS et al (1999) The design of guide surfaces for fixed-bearing and mobile- bearing knee replacements. J Biomech 32:27-34

29. Walker PS et al (2000) Controlling the Motion of total knee replacement using intercondylar guide surfaces. J Orthop Res 18:48-55

30. Walker PS (2001) A new concept in guided motion total knee arthroplasty. J Arthroplasty 16:157-163

31. Walker PS et al (2003) Characterising the motion of total knee replacements in laboratory tests. Clin Orthop 410:54-68

32. Weiss JM et al (2002) What functional activities are important to patients with knee replacements? Clin Orthop 404:172-188

47

48 The High-Performance Knee

M. D. Ries, J. Bellemans, J. Victor

Summary

Although total knee arthroplasty is effective in relieving knee pain and improving ambulatory function, the kinematics after knee replacement are quite different from those of the normal knee. During flexion of the normal knee, the lateral femoral condyle moves posteriorly, causing femoral external rotation. After knee replacement "paradoxical" motion typically occurs. The femur is displaced posteriorly during extension and moves anteriorly as the knee flexes. The cam-and-post mechanism of a posterior cruciate-substituting knee design limits anterior femoral translation so that the kinematics are less abnormal than with a posterior cruciate-retaining design. Additional modifications in the conformity of each tibial plateau and the cam-and-post geometry can further guide roll-back of the lateral more than the medial femoral condyle, causing femoral external rotation during knee flexion. Guided motion designs that reproduce more normal knee kinematics may result in improved range of motion and knee function following total knee arthroplasty.

Introduction

Total knee arthroplasty is a very successful treatment for arthrosis of the knee: Pain and function are improved, and most patients resume routine functional activities such as walking, transferring, and stair climbing, as well as low-impact recreational activities including golf, swimming, and use of a bicycle. However, the kinematics of the replaced knee are quite different from those of the normal knee.

The change in kinematics after knee replacement is not unexpected, since many of the anatomical structures present in the normal knee are not retained in the replaced knee. During total knee arthroplasty, one or both cruciate ligaments are removed, both menisci are excised, the orientation of the joint line is changed from approximately 3° of varus to one which is perpendicular to the mechanical axis, and the size and geometry of articulating surfaces are altered. With appropriate surgical tech-

niques, implant design, and rehabilitation, satisfactory range of motion and stability are usually achieved to permit routine functional activities. However, patients who achieve greater range of motion may also have a component of flexion instability. Symptoms of instability include vague pain, intermittent effusions, and occasional giving way or "clunking" sensations. This is more often reported in posterior cruciate-retaining knee designs, particularly those with relatively non-conforming articular surfaces which permit more anteroposterior and rotational movements between the femur and tibia [1].

Kinematics of the Normal Knee

During flexion the lateral femoral condyle moves posteriorly while the position of the medial femoral condyle is relatively stationary. This produces relative internal tibial rotation or external femoral rotation during knee flexion. At high degrees of flexion the lateral femoral condyle may displace posteriorly to the point that it is partially subluxed from the tibial surface. The combined lateral femoral roll-back and femoral external rotation are essential to permit large degrees of knee flexion.

During early flexion (0°-30°) the patella is laterally displaced and tilted relative to the trochlear groove [2,3]. As patellofemoral compressive forces increase during flexion, the patella becomes centralized in the trochlear groove. Also, during flexion, internal tibial rotation causes a relative medialization of the tibial tubercle which may facilitate patellar tracking.

Kinematics of the Replaced Knee

In vivo fluoroscopic studies have consistently demonstrated "paradoxical" motion in which the femur moves anteriorly during flexion and posteriorly during extension [4]. The lack of an anterior cruciate ligament permits relative anterior subluxation of the tibia, when the knee is in an extended position [5]. As the knee flexes, the femur moves "paradoxically" from a posterior to an anterior position on the tibia. Anterior femoral translation may limit knee flexion, since the extensor mechanism must travel a larger distance than in the normal knee. Tibial rotation is variable after total knee arthroplasty, although external tibial rotation is observed more frequently than internal tibial rotation during knee flexion [4]. However, simultaneous MRI images of the tibiofemoral and patellofemoral joints of total knee arthroplasty patients indicate that external tibial rotation is associated with lateral patellar tilt and translation [6]. This suggests that the abnormal tibiofemoral kinematics after total knee arthroplasty may adversely affect patellar tracking, which can contribute to anterior knee pain, patellar subluxation, and wear.

Tibial external rotation may also limit knee flexion, since excursion of the extensor mechanism may not be sufficient to permit full flexion as it does in the normal knee with tibial internal rotation and lateral femoral rollback. Posterior-stabilized total knee arthroplasty patients appear to have less abnormal tibiofemoral kinematics than patients with posterior cruciate-retaining total knee arthroplasties [4]. However, the cam-and-post mechanism does not control rotation. As a result, knee flexion may still be limited and lateral patellar tracking can result if tibial external rotation occurs during knee flexion.

Relationship Between Kinematics and Range of Motion

Although total knee arthroplasty results in predictable pain relief and patient satisfaction, range of motion beyond 120° is not consistently achieved and the kinematic behavior of the knee is markedly altered [4, 6, 7]. The normal knee flexes to over 140°. If the knee functioned as a simple hinge mechanism, flexion to such a high degree would be limited by posterior impingement of the bony or soft-tissue structures (◘ Fig. 48-1). Posterior impingement between the femur and the tibia during high flexion is limited by the amount of posterior offset between the femoral condyles and posterior femoral cortex (◘ Fig. 48-2) [8].

The medial condyle is larger than the lateral condyle. Therefore, the posterior offset of the medial condyle is greater than that of the lateral condyle. During knee flexion the position of the medial condyle on the tibial plateau is relatively constant, similar to a ball-and-socket mechanism. If the same mechanism occurred between the lateral condyle and tibial plateau, posterior impingement between the lateral femur and tibia would occur during knee flexion (◘ Fig. 48-3). However, the lateral condyle moves posteriorly during knee flexion. At high degrees of flexion, the lateral condyle nearly subluxes off the posterior tibial plateau, and posterior impingement between the femur and tibia does not occur (◘ Fig. 48-4). Greater posterior translation of the lateral femoral condyle compared with the medial femoral condyle is associated with

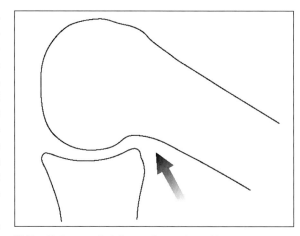

◘ **Fig. 48-1.** Knee in high flexion. Flexion is limited by posterior bony or soft-tissue impingement (*arrow*)

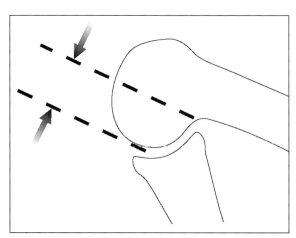

◘ **Fig. 48-2.** Posterior offset is the distance from posterior femoral condyle to femoral cortex (*between arrows*). With larger posterior offset, greater knee flexion can be achieved before posterior impingement occurs

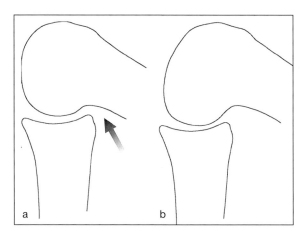

◘ **Fig. 48-3a, b.** *a* Sagittal view of the lateral femoral condyle articulating with the lateral tibial plateau; *b* the medial femoral condyle articulating with the medial tibial plateau. Since the medial femoral condyle is larger than the lateral condyle, posterior offset is greater medially than laterally. If there is no posterior movement of the femur on the tibia during knee flexion, posterior impingement occurs between the lateral femoral cortex and tibial plateau, limiting knee flexion (*arrow*)

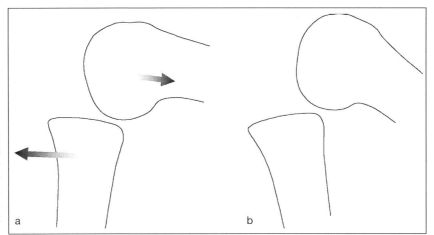

Fig. 48-4a, b. *a* The lateral femoral condyle moves posteriorly relative to the tibia (*arrows*) so that posterior impingement does not occur. *b* As a result of posterior movement of the lateral femoral condyle, flexion is increased until posterior impingement occurs

external rotation of the femur on the tibia. Femoral external rotation during knee flexion, or relative internal tibial rotation, reduces the Q angle, which may also facilitate patellar tracking in deep flexion.

Full flexion is rarely achieved after total knee arthroplasty; this may be related to failure of the replaced knee to reproduce normal knee kinematics. The femoral condyles of the replaced knee are typically posteriorly translated on the tibia during knee extension as a result of absence of the anterior cruciate ligament (◘ Fig. 48-5). During flexion, the femur moves anteriorly on the tibia (paradoxical motion) which causes posterior impingement and limited knee flexion (◘ Fig. 48-6). Knee kinematics are less abnormal with posterior cruciate-substituting than with posterior cruciate-retaining TKA since the cam-and-post mechanism of a posterior cruciate-substituting TKA limits anterior translation of the femur. However, few studies demonstrate significantly better flexion with posterior cruciate-substituting compared with posterior cruciate-retaining knee designs despite the advantage of posterior roll-back caused by the cam-and-post mechanism [9]. This may occur because the cam-and-post mechanism does not control rotation between the femur and tibia.

Combined roll-back and external rotation of the femur on the tibia or posterior translation of the lateral more than the medial femoral condyle, which occurs in the normal knee, may also improve quadriceps efficiency. The anterior translation of the tibia moves the tibial tubercle anteriorly, which increases the quadriceps moment arm in deep flexion. However, most patients with current total knee designs do not typically regain quadriceps strength adequate to get up from a seated position without use of their upper extremities.

Effect of Bearing Surface Geometry on Kinematics

Many tibial component surfaces are dished or concave in order to reduce UHMWPE stresses and provide additional joint stability. However, posterior roll-back of the femoral condyle on a curved tibial surface is limited since the femoral condyle must push against the posterior lip of the tibial insert (◘ Fig. 48-7a). With removal of the posterior lip, posterior roll-back can occur more easily (◘ Fig. 48-7b). In order for the design of the bearing surface to cause guided joint motion, the joint compressive force should be directed to cause femoral roll-back. If the tibial surface is neutrally sloped, the joint compressive force occurs along the axis of the tibia (◘ Fig. 48-7c). However, if the tibial plateau is sloped posteriorly, the joint compressive force is obliquely oriented, which includes a joint compressive force vector along the axis of the tibia as well as a force vector perpendicular to the axis of the tibia (◘ Fig. 48-7d). The latter force vector can drive posterior movement of the femoral condyle.

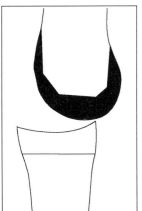
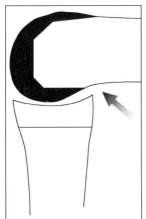

Fig. 48-5. Following total knee arthroplasty, the tibia is subluxed anteriorly during knee extension as a result of absence of the anterior cruciate ligament

Fig. 48-6. During knee flexion, the femur moves anteriorly (paradoxical motion) which limits knee flexion as a result of posterior impingement (*arrow*)

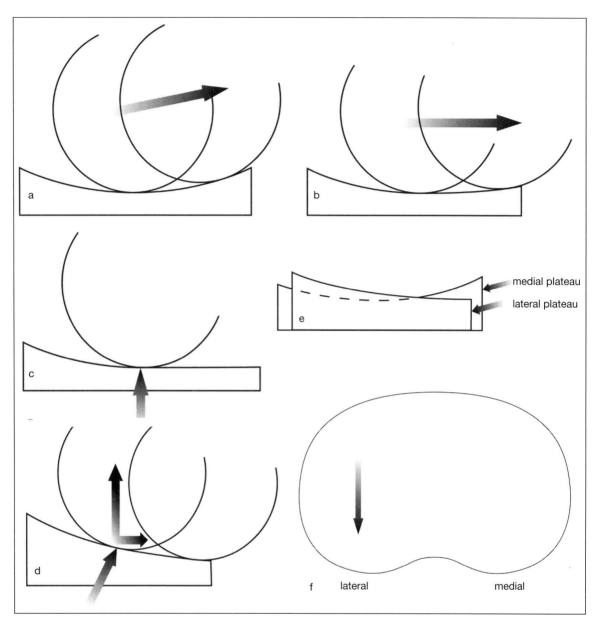

Fig. 48-7a-f. *a* A concave tibial plateau. Posterior roll-back of the femoral condyle requires that the condyle roll uphill. *b* Without the posterior lip, posterior roll-back can occur more easily. *c* Neutrally sloped tibial plateau; joint compressive force is perpendicular to the tibial plateau. *d* Posteriorly sloped tibial plateau surface; joint compressive force is obliquely oriented, which provides a posteriorly directed force vector and drives the femoral condyle posteriorly. *e* Medial tibial plateau shown in a combined with lateral tibial plateau surface shown in d. *f* Guided motion caused by variable slope and conformity of articular surface shown in e. The lateral femoral condyle moves posteriorly as the knee flexes, while the medial femoral condyle position remains relatively stationary

Using differential geometries of the medial and lateral tibial plateau surfaces, selective guided posterior roll-back of the lateral plateau can be achieved (▣ Fig. 48-7e). If the medial plateau is dished or concave and the lateral plateau is posteriorly sloped and without a posterior lip, the medial femoral condyle will be relatively constrained in the tibial plateau while the lateral femoral condyle will move posteriorly during knee flexion (▣ Fig. 48-7f).

Guided motion of a posterior-stabilized knee can also be influenced by the design of the cam-and-post mechanism. Conventional cam-and-post designs are symmetric

in cross-section and intended to allow unrestricted rotation between the femoral and tibial surfaces while still providing posterior roll-back of the femoral condyles (▣ Fig. 48-8a). However, a conical cam or post can force more roll-back of one condyle than the other. For a conical cam-and-post mechanism which is wider laterally than medially, more roll-back of the lateral than the medial plateau occurs (▣ Fig. 48-8b).

In order to achieve the goal of relatively normal kinematic function after total knee arthroplasty, designs and surgical techniques must produce greater posterior trans-

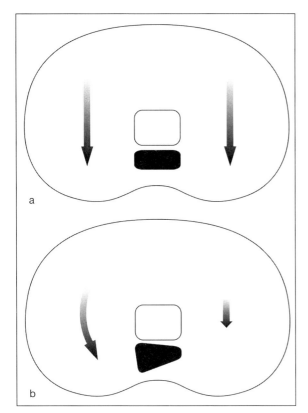

☐ **Fig. 48-8a, b.** *a* Rectangular cam and post causes similar medial and lateral femoral roll-back. *b* Conical cam causes more lateral than medial femoral roll-back

lation of the lateral than the medial femoral condyle during knee flexion in a controlled manner. This may be accomplished by use of an obliquely oriented cam-and-post mechanism and a more posterior slope of the lateral than of the medial tibial plateau. The greater slope of the lateral plateau allows the femoral condyle to roll down the posterior lateral slope during knee flexion.

Design of a High-Performance Knee Using a Virtual Knee Computer Model

One great benefit of using an analytical model to evaluate the functional performance of a total knee design is that the test conditions do not change between experiments. Therefore, the functional behavior of a new design feature may be isolated by simulating subsequent design trials.

The method utilizes three-dimensional computer modeling of a lower limb mounted to a virtual Oxford knee testing rig in a physics-based dynamic software program. The Oxford rig is a modified slider crank mechanism where the hip is analogous to the slider, the femur is the connecting rod, and the tibia is the crank. The knee is then simulated by the joint between the crank and the connecting rod. This type of setup allows the experi-

menter to simulate different activities on the virtual Oxford rig - stair climbing, deep knee bend, gait, etc. – and to validate the results by comparison with empirical laboratory data from a physical Oxford rig.

In the virtual simulation, anatomically accurate femur, tibia, and patella 3-D bone models with the desired anthropometrics are integrated with the model of the Oxford rig and serve as guides for joint line position, scale, and virtual ligament/muscle attachment points. The bone models also serve as geometric references for the virtual implantation of patellar, tibial, and femoral prosthesis 3-D models. Attached to the bone models are virtual muscles and ligaments that serve to drive and constrain the model during simulation.

The constraints imparted on the simulation include hip/ankle joint, ligament/capsule tissue, and the intrinsic constraints imparted by the geometric conformity of the TKA models and their respective stick/slip friction and stiffness characteristics. The hip joint is modeled as a revolute joint with 1° of rotational freedom that is parallel to the flexion axis of the knee. The ankle joint is modeled as a combination of several joints that combine to allow free translation in the M/L direction, as well as internal-external rotation (along axis of tibia), flexion, and varus/valgus rotations. All other degrees of freedom in the ankle are fixed. The ligament constraints are modeled as spring/damper elements and are attached to the virtual bones at their respective anatomical locations with the aid of the information derived from Blankevoort and Huskins [10]. The mechanical properties of the tissues were obtained from Woo et al. [11]. The LCL is simulated with a single constraint element, and the MCL is modeled with two separate constraint elements to simulate the anterior and posterior fibers. For cruciate-retaining knees, a PCL element is added and attached at the respective anatomical locations. The final soft-tissue constraint is the general capsule force, which simulates the general soft-tissue reactions of the knee capsule. This force is directed such that it draws the femur and tibia together in a similar manner to the capsular tissues in the actual knee.

The constraint characteristics imparted by the conforming geometry of the TKA models vary with each design. This is a variable that can be modified by the experimenter to assess the stability imparted by different geometric conformities. Other contact-oriented constraints include stick/slip friction and local deformation of the bearing surfaces. These friction and deformation constraints are determined with an algorithm that models the polyethylene surfaces as a bed of springs with the stiffness characteristics of the polyethylene bearing material. The method allows for intermittent contact, contact pressure, and center of pressure determination. The algorithm is used to model the patellofemoral contact, the tibiofemoral contact, and quadriceps tendon femoral conformity.

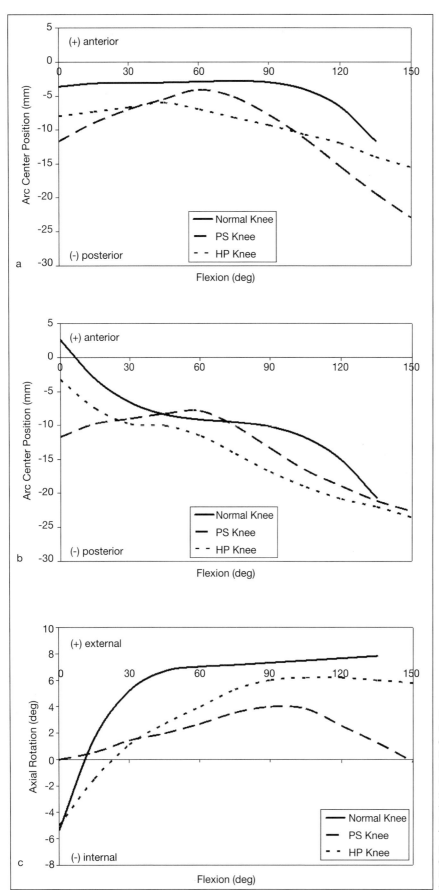

■ **Fig. 48-9a-c.** *a* Position of the medial femoral condyle arc center during knee flexion for the normal knee, conventional posterior-stabilized (*PS*) TKA, and high-performance (HP) TKA obtained from computer simulation. *b* Position of the lateral femoral condyle arc center during knee flexion for the normal knee, PS TKA, and HP TKA obtained from computer simulation. *c* Femoral rotation during knee flexion for the normal knee, PS TKA, and HP TKA obtained from computer simulation

The driving elements in the model are the quadriceps and hamstrings muscle forces. The quadriceps muscle attaches to the quadriceps tendon and is discretized into six components which conform to the distal head of the femur or anterior flange of the TKA, permitting proper force transmission to the femur and patella. The patella is attached to the tibia tubercle through a patellar tendon force which conforms to the tubercle and TKA insert component. The simulation is driven by a controlled actuator arrangement similar to the physical machine. A closed-loop controller is used to apply a tension to the quadriceps and hamstring muscles to match a prescribed knee flexion vs. time profile. No large antagonistic forces are modeled. Ground reaction forces are applied as varus/valgus forces and internal/external torques during the cycle using time history data derived from force plate experiments [12].

In the functional evaluation of a new implant design, two main activities are simulated: a complete cycle gait, and a 0° – 160° – 0° – 160° double deep knee bend cycle. The double cycle is performed so as to capture the inertial loading conditions at full flexion (the second 0°). Data are reported via graphical animations and numerical results. Usually, only the TKA components and soft tissues are displayed during the animations. Scaled force vectors for each tissue force are displayed on the model during animation, as are center-of-pressure locators (with scaling force vectors) for each tibiofemoral and patellofemoral contact zone. Eighty-four data time-histories are reported for each simulation. These include patellofemoral kinematics, tibiofemoral kinematics, tissue loads and locations, actuator loads and locations, contact forces, center-of-pressure locations and contact area, interface forces and locations, and all applied forces and locations. Three different reference frames are utilized for the reporting of the kinematic and kinetic data. These reference frames are rigidly attached to the femur, tibia, and patella, respectively, at the interface where the implant models meet the bone models. This is done so that interface forces can be easily obtained by resolving all forces acting on an implant component to the corresponding reference frame located at the interface. In the simulation, kinematic and kinetic data are typically reported relative to the reference frame fixed in the tibia. Kinematic and kinetic data for the patella can also be reported from the reference frame in the femur. Component orientation is reported using a three-cylindric model of knee motion similar to Hefzy and Grood [13] or a variety of other methods.

The computer model of the Oxford rig has been validated in a variety of ways including mechanical tests, cadaver tests, and live subject tests. Mechanical tests have been used to tune the performance of the contact force algorithm for both the shear component (friction/stiction) of the force and the normal component of the force. The shear component of the contact force was tuned by comparing the Instron test machine results for the ASTM 1223 component laxity test with a virtual model of the laxity test. The normal component of the forces was tuned by comparing the resulting contact area of virtual compression tests with the contact areas reported from Instron-Fuji film tests. With the current set of contact parameters, the algorithm has consistently delivered results within 10% of mechanical tests [14]. Cadaver tests have been used to tune the soft tissues (attachment locations and mechanical properties) and the system controller function comparing the virtual Oxford rig results with the results of the physical machine.

Results obtained with the computer model are similar to the kinematic patterns observed after TKA with fluoroscopic studies. For a posterior-stabilized knee, the femur moves anteriorly during knee flexion (paradoxical motion) until the cam-and-post mechanism engages. Following cam-and-post engagement, the femur moves posteriorly. However, with the modifications introduced into the HP bearing surface and cam-and-post mechanism shown in Figs. 48-7 and 48-8, a much more normal kinematic pattern occurs. The position of the medial femoral condyle is relatively stationary during knee flexion while the lateral femoral condyle moves posteriorly, very similar to the normal knee (◘ Fig. 48-9a and b). The differential positions of the femoral condyles are associated with femoral external rotation during knee flexion which follows the pattern of the normal knee (◘ Fig. 48-9c). The computer simulation indicates that by modifications in the articular geometry and cam-post mechanism, guided motion can be achieved to more closely reproduce normal kinematics after TKA.

References

1. Pagnano MW, Hanssen AD, Lewallen DG, Stuart MJ (1998) Flexion instability after primary posterior cruciate retaining total knee arthroplasty. Clin Orthop 356:39-46
2. Patel VV, Hall K, Ries M, Lindsey C, Ozhinsky E, Lu Y, Majumdar S (2003) Magnetic resonance imaging of patellofemoral kinematics with weight-bearing. J Bone Joint Surg [Am] 85:2419-2424
3. Tennant S, Williams A, Vedi V, Kinmont C, Gedroyc W, Hunt DM (2001) Patello-femoral tracking in the weight-bearing knee: a study of asymptomatic volunteers utilizing dynamic magnetic resonance imaging: a preliminary report. Knee Surg Sports Traumatol Arthrosc 9:155-162
4. Dennis DA, Komistek RD, Mahfouz MR, Haas BD, Steihl JB (2003) Multi-center determination of in vivo kinematics after total knee arthroplasty. Clin Orthop 416:37-57
5. Logan M, Dunstan E, Robinson J, Williams A, Gedroye W, Freeman M (2004) Tibiofemoral kinematics of the anterior cruciate (ACL)-deficient weight bearing, living knee employing vertical access open "interventional" multiple resonance imaging. Am J Sports Med 32:720-726
6. Lee K-Y, Slavinsky JP, Ries MD, Blumenkrantz G, Majumdar S (2004) Magnetic resonance imaging of in vivo kinematics after total knee arthroplasty. Program of the Assoc Bone Joint Surgeons Annual Meeting, Nashville, TN, June 16-19
7. Banks SA, Harman MK, Bellemans J, Hodge WA (2003) Making sense of knee arthroplasty kinematics: news you can use. J Bone Joint Surg [Am] 85 [Suppl 4]:64-72

8. Bellemans J, Banks S, Victor J, Vandenneucker H, Moermans A (2002) Fluoroscopic analysis of the kinematics of deep flexion in total knee arthroplasty. Influence of posterior condylar offset. J Bone Joint Surg [Br] 84:50-53

9. Victor J, Banks S, Bellemans J (2005) Posterior stabilized knee replacements have more natural kinematics than cruciate retaining knee replacements: A prospective randomised outcome and in-vivo kinematic analysis. J Bone Joint Surg [Br] (in press)

10. Blankevoort L, Huskins R (1991) Ligament-bone interaction in a three-dimensional model of the knee. J Mech Eng 113:263-269

11. Woo SL, Hollis JM, Adams OJ, Lyon RM, Takai S (1991) Tensile properties of the human femur-anterior cruciate ligament-tibia complex. Am J Sports Med 19:217-225

12. Winter DA (1990) Biomechanics and motor control of human movement, 2nd edn. Wiley-Interscience, p 277

13. Hefzy MS, Grood E (1988) Review of knee models. Appl Mech Rev 41:1-23

14. Masson M, McGuan SP, Bushelow M, Dumbleton J, et al (1993) Computer modeling of articular contact for assessing total knee replacement constraint criteria. 10th Eur. Conf. on Biomaterials, Davos, August 28-31

48

49 Deep Knee Flexion in the Asian Population

M. Akagi

Summary

The design of a high-flexion prosthesis should allow deep knee flexion after total knee arthroplasty "without affecting the durability and stability of the prosthesis." Although it is not impossible to design a knee prosthesis that provides full flexion, the task is difficult. There is always a trade-off between the range of flexion possible with the prosthetic design, the intrinsic stability provided by the articular geometry, and the durability of the prosthesis. The high-flexion knee has to balance these three factors to a fine degree. Until now this has been a new frontier and a great challenge in the world of TKA. Surgeons must be meticulous in their selection of patients and prostheses. Furthermore, appropriate education and careful long-term follow-up are necessary for the patients.

Introduction

Total knee arthroplasty (TKA) is a common procedure with established outcomes [1]. In general, modern TKA designs produce satisfactory pain relief and improvement in walking ability. However, one major problem that has not been fully resolved is that patients usually do not regain deep flexion over 120° after TKA [2].

In the traditional Japanese life style, as well in some other countries such as Korea, India, China, and Muslim countries, deep flexion of the knee is necessary for daily activities such as eating, socializing, and religious or traditional ceremonies. Even in non-traditional Japanese houses many people continue to sit down on a tatami mat and adopt a posture of either cross-legged sitting or full squatting, and sometimes sit with one knee down and one up (◘ Fig. 49-1) [3].

When people practice flower arranging at school or in public, or participate in the tea ceremony, they are supposed to sit in a full squatting position (Fig. 49-1b). Even patients with a good preoperative range of motion (ROM) often lose deep flexion after TKA. Gross loss of flexion can result in patient dissatisfaction with the operation, and therefore the surgical indications for TKA have tended to

be limited to patients with poor preoperative ROM. When TKA is indicated for a patient with good ROM but severe disability due to knee pain, the surgeons must inform the patient of the probable postoperative loss of deep flexion – with the possible consequence that the patient will adopt a Western lifestyle using a bed, a Western-style toilet, tables, and chairs – and must obtain informed consent on this point. Many elderly Japanese patients follow a traditional lifestyle in a Japanese-style house, which they have to modify to accommodate a Western lifestyle suitable for their knee function after surgery. In this chapter, the author discusses the challenges in Japan to achieving high flexion in total knee design and a worldwide trend towards developing posterior-stabilized prostheses that can achieve deep flexion.

Although the task is difficult, it is not impossible to design a knee prosthesis that provides full flexion reaching 155°. An enlarged posterior femoral condyle with smaller radii of curvature can reduce contact stress in the polyethylene of the tibial insert [4]. A number of knee implant manufacturers in the US and Europe have developed, or are in the process of developing, total knee prostheses aimed at full flexion reaching 155°. However, it is important to recognize that full flexion of the knee is achievable even using some conventional knee prostheses in patients with full preoperative ROM if the surgery is technically appropriate, if there is a high degree of motivation to regain deep flexion, and if the patients cooperate fully with postoperative rehabilitation [5]. If this is

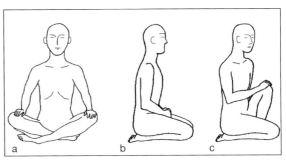

◘ **Fig. 49-1.** Sitting postures on a tatami mat. (*a*) Cross-legged position; (*b*) sitting in full squatting position, called seiza in Japanese, which means "formal sitting" in English; (*c*) sitting with one knee down and one up

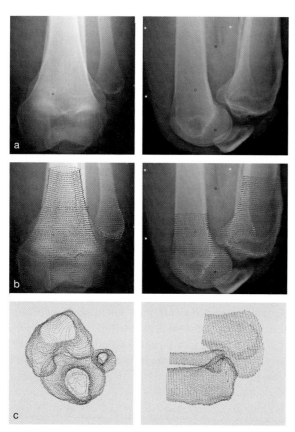

Fig. 49-2a-c. Biplanar image matching to observe the relationship between the femur and the tibia in a full squatting position. (*a*) Anteroposterior and lateral radiographs of the knee taken during full squatting. The bi-directional radiographs were taken almost simultaneously. (*b*) Projection image of a three-dimensional knee model was matched onto both radiographs. (*c*) The position of six degrees of freedom was determined and the knee was observed axially (*right*) and laterally (*left*). The femur is subdislocated on the tibia posteriorly because of the large roll-back and axial rotation

the case, how does the design of a high-flexion knee prosthesis differ from that of a conventional prosthesis?

A high-flexion prosthesis should not interfere with deep knee flexion after total knee arthroplasty "without affecting the durability and stability of the prosthesis" [6]. There is always a trade-off between the range of flexion allowed by the prosthetic design, the intrinsic stability provided by the articular geometry, and the durability of the prosthesis. The high-flexion knee has to balance these three factors to a fine degree. Furthermore, the knee with an ordinary condylar-type prosthesis has never managed to restore normal knee kinematics of deep flexion. The author, in collaboration with Dr. Taiyo Asano, is investigating the three-dimensional relationship between the femur and tibia of the normal knee in the full squatting position using the biplanar image-matching technique [7]. It has been demonstrated that the femur can be subdislocated on the tibia posteriorly in full flexion because of a large roll-back and axial rotation (Fig. 49-2). It seems impossible for the artificial knee prosthesis to

simulate such normal kinematics without compromising its durability and intrinsic stability.

Development of a High-flexion Knee in Japan

The background material mentioned above has created strong interest among Japanese knee surgeons in the restoration of deep flexion after total knee arthroplasty since the early days of TKA introduction to Japan. In 1984, Dr. Shinichi Yoshino, in collaboration with Dr. Hiromu Shoji, developed the Y/S total knee system (Biomet Inc., Warsaw, IN, USA), aimed at postoperative high flexion [8]. The Y/S knee system, which is a predecessor of the Hy-flex II knee (Depuy International Inc., Leeds, UK) [9], incorporates several design parameters aimed at high flexion following TKA. The specific features of the design and instrumentation system include: (a) gradually reduced radius of curvature in the posterior femoral condyles; (b) flat posterior articular surface of the tibial component to allow a sliding and rolling motion of the femoral condyles and to provide free axial rotation in deep flexion; (c) a 4° posterior slope for the tibial articular surface; and (d) a ligament tensor for equal medial and lateral ligament balance in both flexion and extension. In one study of 39 patients, this prosthesis was implanted in 50 knees. The average follow-up period was 2.1 years (1.5-2.5 years) and the maximum flexion averaged 124.0° ±19.9° (preoperative motion arc had been 104.7° ±32.9°). In 90% of these patients, the arc of knee motion was better than before surgery. Full flexion necessary to perform full squatting was achieved in 12% of operated knees [8].

In December 1989, the Bisurface knee prosthesis (Kyocera Inc., Kyoto, Japan) was developed, with the aim of achieving sufficient improvement in knee flexion after TKA without affecting the durability of the prosthesis. This prosthesis had been originally used by Dr. Toyoji Ueo, the head doctor of the development team, in the Department of Orthopedic Surgery at Kyoto University Hospital, and was released for general use in 1992. The prosthesis incorporates one design-specific feature aimed at improving knee flexion: The knee is a PCL-substituting prosthesis and has a unique ball-and-socket joint in the mid-posterior portion of the femoral and tibial component. This secondary joint functions as a posterior-stabilizing cam and, as a load-bearing surface in deep flexion, causes femoral roll-back, which prevents posterior tibiofemoral impingement [6]. In a new version of the prosthesis (Type 3 Plus and Type 4), the femoral ball comes into contact with the tibial socket at around 60° of flexion. Therefore, the prosthesis has three contact areas on the tibial articular surface at more than 60° of flexion: the medial and lateral condylar surfaces and the ball-and-socket joint [10]. The posterior condylar part of

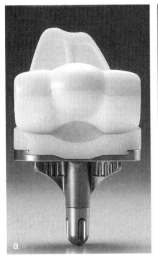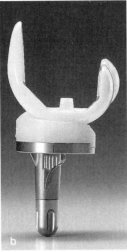

◘ **Fig. 49-3a, b.** The Bisurface knee prosthesis (Type 4): (*a*) posterior view, (*b*) lateral view. Note the ball-and-socket joint in the mid-posterior portion of the femoral (composed of zirconia ceramics) and tibial component. Although this prosthesis is classified as a posterior-stabilized knee, the box-cut in the intercondylar part for the cam mechanism is not necessary and the bone loss for implantation is comparable to that with PCL-retaining prostheses

the tibial articular surface is flattened in the anterior-posterior direction to provide freedom of axial rotation around the ball-and-socket joint. Although this prosthesis is classified as a posterior-stabilized knee, the box-cut in the intercondylar part for the cam mechanism is not necessary, and the bone loss for implantation is comparable to that with PCL-retaining prostheses. The author reviewed the clinical results of the first 223 arthroplasties performed with this prosthesis. The follow-up period averaged 6 years (3.9-9.0 years). The mean postoperative range of flexion was 124°, and there were no failures attributable to wear or breakage of the tibial polyethylene insert. Ten percent of the patients achieved full squatting. However, 20% of these patients felt mild looseness in their knee [6]. These results prompted the author to improve the intrinsic stability of the prosthesis by improving the congruity of the ball-and-socket joint. This new prosthesis is called Type 3 Plus and has been used since July 1998. This modification of the ball-and-socket joint associated with the proper ligament balancing technique has drastically reduced the prevalence of knee looseness to less than 1%(◘ Fig. 49-3).

Design Requirements in Total Knee Prostheses Aiming at Full Flexion

There are three requirements for the design of a total knee prosthesis. First, it must continue to be serviceable for a sufficient period after implantation. The minimum longevity should be more than 10-15 years if the prosthesis has been implanted with appropriate alignment, fixa-

tion, and ligament balance [11]. Second, the knee with the prosthesis should have adequate stability for the activities of daily life, such as walking on flat surfaces, going up and down slopes, negotiating stairs, and standing up from a low chair. In the traditional Japanese lifestyle, patients with knee prostheses have to sit down on, and stand up from, the floor and a 20- to 25-cm-high bathroom chair. Knee stability after TKA depends not only on the prosthetic design but also on the surgical technique, including ligament balance adjustment and alignment of the prosthesis. However, some allowance for technical variations should be built into the prosthetic design. Third, the knee implanted with the prosthesis should simulate natural knee kinematics as far as possible. In particular, in deep flexion over 135°, large roll-back and internal rotation of the tibia occur simultaneously, resulting in subluxation of the knee, which causes a space to be made in the popliteal region, avoiding posterior tibiofemoral impingement. A knee with a prosthesis cannot mimic this motion in extreme deep flexion. It is difficult for the prosthetic designer to balance these three factors to a fine degree. The wide variety of knee prosthesis designs currently on the market means that a consensus regarding the effects of articular geometry on longevity, stability, and kinematics has not been obtained among knee prosthesis designers [12].

Longevity in High-flexion Knees

When a high-flexion knee is designed, it is important that the articular surface maintains an area of contact between femur and tibia to 135° or more of flexion. There are several ways to solve this problem. One is to extend the articular surface in the posterior condyles with smaller radii of curvature. Without the extension of the posterior condylar surface, the edges of the femoral posterior flange can dig into the polyethylene tibial insert in deep flexion, resulting in premature polyethylene damage. One solution is to thicken the posterior femoral flange with an additional posterior condylar resection of about 2-4 mm [13]. However, reduction of bone stock due to additional bone resection may produce problems requiring revision surgery [14]. The other method is to cover the articular surfaces of the posterior femoral condyles completely with flexed posterior flanges, which fit obliquely into the cut surfaces of the posterior condyles. Because the anterior and posterior cut surfaces are not parallel in this design, a special method of assembly would be necessary to attach the femoral component to the femur. Although additional bone resection is not necessary, retrieval of the femoral component may be difficult during revision surgery. Another way to avoid digging into the tibial insert with the sharp edge of the posterior flanges is to shorten and round the edges of the femoral flanges. However, the contact area between the rounded tips of the posterior flange and the tibial polyethylene may be insufficient, leading to premature polyethylene wear attributable to the high forces exerted during deep squatting. In the Bisurface knee, the major bearing surface between the femur and the tibia is the ball-and-socket joint installed in the mid-posterior portion of the tibiofemoral joint in deep flexion [15]. Therefore, in this prosthesis, the area of contact at the articular surface is not disrupted insofar as the posterior impingement occurs in deep flexion.

The next point to consider regarding the longevity of the high-flexion knee is wear and fracture of the tibial post in the posterior-stabilized knee [16-19]. The posterior-stabilized knee has a post-cam mechanism facilitating the predictable femoral roll-back, which is advantageous to achieving high flexion. However, it has been indicated that the cam mechanism may be another source of wear debris, resulting in osteolysis [16, 17]. Furthermore, considering the high load bearing on the tibial post during deep squatting [20], further attention to the strength and the design of the post is needed [19]. The cam mechanism should be designed to work not only as a femoral roll-back provider and a posterior stabilizer but also as a weight-bearing articular surface, particularly during deep flexion. To prevent the fracture of the post and dislocation of the cam, the femoral cam should be designed to engage as near the base of the post as possible during deep flexion. The thickness and mechanical strength of the post should be sufficient to bear the large load during deep flexion. However, this cam design may cause the timing of the cam engagement to occur later in the range of flexion, and the knee may not have posterior stability during early and mid flexion. Anterior wear of the tibial post attributable to impingement between the edge of the femoral box and the base of the tibial post at hyperextension may not only be a source of polyethylene debris but may also cause post fracture. Some new prostheses addressing this problem have an anterior femoral cam to prevent anterior damage to the post at hyperextension. In the Bisurface knee, the need for revision due to wear or breakage of the tibial insert has not been reported so far, although the follow-up period is still short (the maximum is 14 years). One concern about wear in the Bisurface knee is the thickness of the polyethylene in the socket. The thickness of the thinnest tibial component available is 9 mm and the polyethylene thickness at the lowest point of the socket is 4 mm. The contact area appears to be the anterior half of the socket, and the ball does not contact the lowest point of the socket during deep flexion. The size of wear debris produced by the ball-and-socket joint may be as small as has been reported in total hip arthroplasty. This smaller size of particulate wear debris might cause periprosthetic osteolysis.

Stability in High-flexion Knees

Prostheses aiming at high flexion usually have low intrinsic stability due to their articular geometry. The posterior flat surface of the tibia is necessary for large femoral roll-back on the tibia, for freedom of axial rotation, and to decrease posterior bony and soft-tissue impingement. Contact areas between the femur and tibia during deep flexion should be small because the posterior femoral condyle has a small radius on the flat surface of the tibial insert. Again, the small contact area must bear a large load transmitted through the knee during deep flexion. This can affect the durability of the tibial polyethylene insert.

The height of the tibial post in a high-flexion knee prosthesis may be relatively low to avoid patellar-post impingement in the deep patellar groove, which can decrease tension in the quadriceps and provide an increase in the range of postoperative flexion [21]. The knee prosthesis with the low post is designed to engage the tibial post at the base of the post with the femoral cam during deep flexion. Therefore, the dislocation safety factor (DSF, the so-called jumping distance) [22] is estimated to be

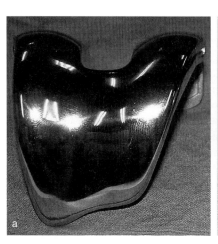 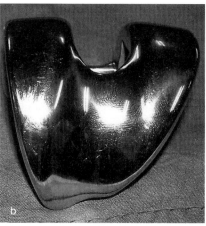

◘ Fig. 49-4a, b. Tangential views of the patellar groove in deep flexion. (*a*) A prosthesis with a deep patellar groove; a high tibial post may impinge a patella during deep flexion. (*b*) A prosthesis with a shallow patellar groove; the quadriceps tension seems to be high during deep flexion with this design

large during deep flexion despite the low post. In early to mid flexion, however, the cam mechanism does not engage and does not provide posterior stability in this cam design. Correct ligament balance and alignment of the knee in the frontal, sagittal, and axial planes may be essential to prevent cam dislocation in such prostheses. A prosthesis with a high post and a deep patellar groove has a risk of patellar-post impingement in deep flexion because the position of the tibial post relative to the femoral articular surface is anterior due to the large roll-back during deep flexion (◘ Fig. 49-4a) [21].

A prosthesis with a high post and a shallow patellar groove cannot loosen the high tension of the contracted quadriceps during deep flexion. Therefore, a prosthesis with a shallow patellar groove is somewhat disadvantageous for achieving deep flexion, although the patellar-post impingement can be avoided (◘ Fig. 49-4b). In the Bisurface knee, the posterior half of the intercondylar eminence is replaced with the socket. Therefore, the medial-lateral intrinsic stability is as small as in the the cruciate-retention prosthesis. Correct ligament balancing and component setting are as important for postoperative knee stability as in the low-post design. The patello-femoral joint congruity between the patella and the patellar groove may be disrupted in full flexion because of anterior protrusion of the femoral ball.

In general, the intrinsic stability of a high-flexion posterior-stabilized knee may be low compared with that of a conventional posterior-stabilized knee. Appropriate surgical technique is necessary to obtain both deep flexion and stability. Design features of the high-flexion knee prosthesis should be sufficiently examined preoperatively in each patient, with each deformity, contracture, and laxity of the knee requiring assessment.

Kinematics of High-flexion Knees

In normal knees, the knee can flex fully until the heel touches the buttock. In full squatting, the lateral condyle of the femur rolls back extremely on the tibia, resulting in subluxation. The medial condyle also rolls back greatly, but maintains the articulation with the femur (see Fig. 49-2). This alignment of the femur and tibia in the squatting position seems to provide enough room for the soft tissue and neurovascular bundles posterior to the knee joint, and reduces tension in the soft tissue. No knee prosthesis can mimic this kinematic (relative position between the femur and tibia) during deep flexion. A post-cam mechanism or a ball-and-socket joint is installed in the middle of the knee in a medial and lateral direction. Therefore, axial rotation during deep flexion results in posterior translation of the contact point in one compartment with anterior translation of the contact point in the other (the so-called center pivot motion). Because the anterior translation of the femoral

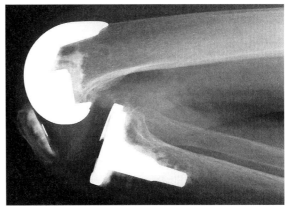

◘ **Fig. 49-5.** Lateral radiograph in full squatting position. Note the condylar liftoff, suggesting posterior soft-tissue impingement. This patient complains of abnormal compressive sensation in the popliteal region when squatting fully and cannot maintain the position for a long time

condyle on the tibia might pinch the posterior soft tissues with the posterior edge of the tibial insert during deep flexion, it may be difficult for the knee to rotate freely. A lateral plain X-ray of the knee with a prosthesis during full squatting demonstrates condylar liftoff, suggesting the posterior soft-tissue impingement (◘ Fig. 49-5). Actually, my observation shows that patients who can squat fully after TKA often complain of an abnormal compressive sensation in the popliteal region when squatting fully and cannot maintain the position for a long time.

Consideration of the Knee with a High-flexion Prosthesis

The knee prostheses aiming at full flexion that have been presented to the market recently involve many new ideas for achieving their design objectives: namely, longevity, stability, and kinematics. If a patient with a good preoperative range of flexion undergoes a technically good operation, maintains a high degree of motivation to obtain full flexion, and endures vigorous postoperative rehabilitation, he or she will end up with a knee having almost the full range of motion and good stability postoperatively. However, we surgeons cannot be overjoyed by such wonderful results. There are no long-term follow-up data available on patients with high-flexion knees after TKA. It has been demonstrated that the prosthetic knee with full flexion cannot achieve normal knee kinematics, and a very high load is transmitted to the knee when a person is standing up from the squatting position [20]. I consider it very important to educate patients with high-flexion knees. They need to learn how to use their knee safely in their daily activities to obtain sufficient longevity. For example, standing up from the squatting position and squatting down without aids should be prohibited. When

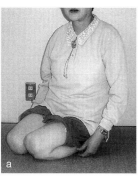
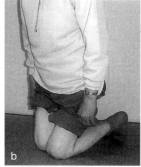
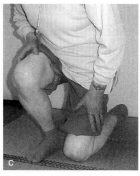
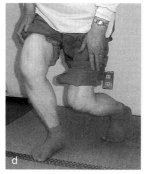

■ **Fig. 49-6a-d.** A safe way to stand up from a full squatting position: (*a*) Sitting in a full squatting position on the tatami; (*b*) kneeling on the mat; (*c*) placing one leg prior to standing up; (*d*) standing up using both legs

49

standing up from a full squatting position on the floor, the patient should keel at first, next place one leg to stand up, and then stand up using both legs (■ Fig. 49-6).

It is possible for high-flexion knee prostheses to function quite adequately and for patients to be completely satisfied with them. However, until now this has been a new frontier and a great challenge in the world of TKA. Surgeons must be meticulous in their selection of patients and prostheses and must perform technically good surgery. Furthermore, appropriate education and careful long-term follow-up are necessary for the patients, and doctors must report the outcomes (knee function, longevity, stability, and patient satisfaction) of high-flexion prostheses.

References

1. Callahan CM et al (1994) Patient outcomes following tricompartmental total knee replacement. A meta-analysis. JAMA 271:1349-1357
2. Anouchi YS et al (1996) Range of motion in total knee replacement. Clin Orthop 331:87-92
3. Mulholland SJ et al (2001) Activities of daily living in non-Western cultures: range of motion requirements for hip and knee joint implants. Int J Rehabil Res 24:191-198
4. Sathasivam S et al (1994) Optimization of the bearing surface geometry of total knees. J Biomech 27:255-264
5. Kim JM et al (1995) Squatting following total knee arthroplasty. Clin Orthop 313:177-186
6. Akagi M et al (2000) The Bisurface total knee replacement: a unique design for flexion. Four- to nine-year follow-up study. J Bone Joint Surg [Am] 82:1626-1633
7. Asano T et al (2001) In vivo three-dimensional knee kinematics using a biplanar image-matching technique. Clin Orthop 388:157-166
8. Shoji H et al (1987) Improved range of motion with the Y/S total knee arthroplasty system. Clin Orthop 218:150-163
9. Yamazaki J et al (2002) Hy-Flex II total knee system and range of motion. Arch Orthop Trauma Surg 122:156-160
10. Akagi M et al (2002) Functional analysis of the effect of the posterior stabilising cam in two total knee replacements. A comparison of the Insall/Burstein and Bisurface prostheses. J Bone Joint Surg [Br] 84:561-565
11. Gill GS et al (1999) Total condylar knee arthroplasty. 16- to 21-year results. Clin Orthop 367:210-215
12. Sathasivam S et al (1999) The conflicting requirements of laxity and conformity in total knee replacement. J Biomech 32:239-247
13. Sultan PG et al (2003) Optimizing flexion after total knee arthroplasty: advances in prosthetic design. Clin Orthop 416:167-173
14. Ranawat CS (2003) Design may be counterproductive for optimizing flexion after TKR. Clin Orthop 416:174-176
15. Akagi M et al (2002) A mechanical comparison of 2 posterior-stabilizing designs: Insall/Burstein 2 knee and Bisurface knee. J Arthroplasty 17:627-634
16. Puloski SK et al (2001) Tibial post wear in posterior stabilized total knee arthroplasty. An unrecognized source of polyethylene debris. J Bone Joint Surg [Am] 83:390-397
17. O'Rourke MR et al (2002) Osteolysis associated with a cemented modular posterior-cruciate-substituting total knee design: five- to eight-year follow-up. J Bone Joint Surg [Am] 84:1362-1371
18. Mestha P et al (2000) Fracture of the polyethylene tibial post in posterior stabilized (Insall-Burstein II) total knee arthroplasty. J Arthroplasty 15:814-815
19. Mauerhan DR (2003) Fracture of the polyethylene tibial post in a posterior cruciate-substituting total knee arthroplasty mimicking patellar clunk syndrome: a report of 5 cases. J Arthroplasty 18:942-945
20. Nagura T et al (2002) Mechanical loads at the knee joint during deep flexion. J Orthop Res 20:881-886
21. Verborgt O et al (2004) Post impingement in posterior stabilised total knee arthroplasty. Acta Orthop Belg 70:46-50
22. 0Delp SL et al (1995) Tradeoffs between motion and stability in posterior substituting knee arthroplasty design. J Biomech 28:1155-1166

50 Fixed-bearing Unicompartmental Knee Arthroplasty

P. Cartier, A. Khefacha

Summary

After using the Marmor implant for 10 years we improved the design, introducing the Mod III knee in 1984 and later the Genesis uni system in 1994. The aims of the corresponding changes were to improve the implant press-fit and the fixation strength for the cemented and cementless versions and also to decrease polyethylene wear. Cobalt-chrome was replaced by titanium at the tibial level and by oxynium for the condyle. Nevertheless, thorough knowledge of uni basic principles and specific rules represents the best guarantee of a better future in unicompartmental knee arthroplasty.

Introduction

Since 1974 we have – taught by Leonard Marmor – defended the concept of the unicompartimental prosthesis. Improving the design, the biomechanical quality of the implants, and the accuracy of their fitting has always been our aim and that of the bioengineering research team with whom we collaborate. This evolution in successive steps from the Marmor to the Mod III prosthesis and to the Genesis unicompartimental knee and the development of ancillary instrumentation has allowed us to improve reliability of fitting and considerably reduce the phenomena of polyethylene wear and loosening. Consequently, the operation can be performed in younger and more active patients. This study represents our experience and the outcome of 2024 implanted unicompartimental knees with a fixed bearing.

The Past

The Marmor Prosthesis

The pure resurfacing nature of this implant is represented by a minimal posterior condylar resection, the femoral support on the resistant subchondral underlying bone, and the limited condylar width. Our concept was that a unicompartimental knee was not half a total knee [1].

The main problem posed by this type of prosthesis was the great poverty of the initial ancillary instrumentation available for fitting it. This invited us to complete the pre-existing system with a pretibial jig and trial femoral implants, condyles with pegs, which allowed us to perform as many trials as necessary until an ideal positioning and autostability of the implants was obtained without weakening the adjacent subchondral bone. The anchoring holes for the final femoral implants were drilled only when the quality of the positioning was guaranteed. For these reasons, our long-term results have been more favorable than those published by the inventor, reflected in survivalship of 92% stable implants at 12 years' follow-up [2].

The Mod III Prosthesis

Encouraged by the previous results, we decided to make some improvements to the Marmor implant:

- At the femoral level, by improving the original curvature and using a central peg to obtain a "press-fit" effect and avoid the introduction of cement in the central implantation hole, in order to simplify any later revision with a total knee replacement.
- At the tibial level, by using a cobalt-chrome metal-backed support, stronger fixation was obtained. The thickness of the bone resection was reduced by using a 7.5-mm implant, without falling into the pitfall of the Marmor 6-mm plateaus.

The Mod III prosthesis used between 1984 and 1994 represented the outcome of all these modifications (◘ Fig. 50-1), allowing the prosthesis to be used in younger and more active patients.

However, the results obtained did not live up to our expectations. Of 790 implants of this type, a failure rate of 6% was noted in a series. The real rate could be considered close to double, given the information from other centers. The main causes of these failures were:

- The excessive rigidity of the chrome-cobalt on these necessarily undercorrected knees

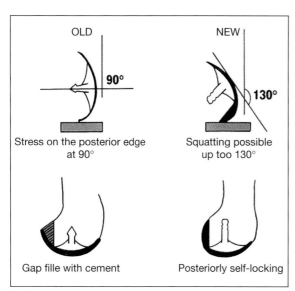

Fig. 50-1. Design improvements from Marmor to Mod III knee

bone to severe osteosclerosis or to a morphotypical anomaly such as lateral condylar dysplasia.

This system therefore offers a higher level of modularity than the pre-existing systems, ethylene oxide sterilization again being used. The differences with the Mod III at the femoral level are basically:

- A proportional increase in each size between the width and the length of the implant
- A tapered and contoured femoral aspect to minimize patellar impingement
- A large choice of sizes, offering seven possibilities, and the existence of two thicknesses of femoral implants, standard 4 mm and 7.5 mm for lateral condylar dysplasias or post-traumatic reconstruction

Differences at the tibial level are:

- The possibility of a complete cortical rim support
- The use of titanium for metal-backed prostheses with the advantages over chrome-cobalt of more strength and less rigidity and the possibility of limiting the thickness of the metal back in favor of the polyethylene

- The insufficient thickness of the polyethylene (7.5-mm plateaus)
- The method of sterilization, gamma irradiation having replaced ethylene oxide, leading to rapid delamination of the polyethylene

The Genesis Uni System

The experience with the two previous implants allowed the development of the Genesis Uni system. It includes a choice of implants, allowing us to deal with the different situations encountered in unicompartimental surgery (◘ Fig. 50-2). These range from poor-quality cancellous

Regarding instrumentation, at the tibial level the previous extramedullary guide has been improved through replacement of the fixed horizontal part by an adjustable and mobile part with a goniometer. This system allows us to obtain a tibial resection parallel to the healthy cartilage, the best guarantee in tibial varus bows of maintaining the alignment of the implants in the long term.

At the femoral level, free-hand femoral resurfacing is replaced by automatic resurfacing with a reaming and bushing system, which allows resurfacing to be stopped when the subchondral bone is reached.

The limits of this instrumentation, in spite of the improvement it brought, were essentially the arbitrary nature of the thickness of the initial tibial resection, and equally so in the posterior part of the femur. Very frequently, this led to recutting being necessary during the delicate procedure for surgeons unaccustomed to this type of implant. Moreover, the dimensions of the femoral resurfacing system did not allow a minimally invasive approach.

The Present

The present situation must be appreciated by taking into account the results of the Genesis Unis and essentially the analysis of the series' complications, and by bearing in mind the improvement in surgical techniques with the recent introduction of the Accuris system (Leo Pinczewski).

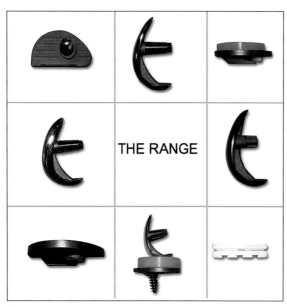

THE RANGE

Fig. 50-2. The Genesis Uni knee system

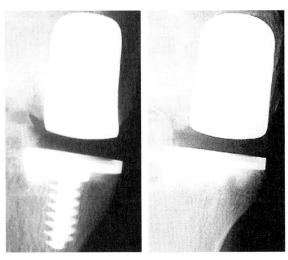

Fig. 50-3. Polyethylene wear in two middle-aged patients at 8 and 9 years of follow-up

Analysis of the Results

A total of 944 knees were operated on between 1991 and 2003. In order to evaluate the functional performance of the system, the results of patients younger than 60 at the time of the operation were analyzed. The analysis of the complications concerned all patients in the series, whatever their age, operated on between 1991 and 2003.

Results in Middle-aged Patients

The results in 94 patients from a series of 96 operated on before the age of 60, with a minimum follow-up period of 5 years and a maximum of 10 years [3], reveal the quality of resistance of the Genesis implant to wear at a high level of activity. The quality of the clinical result with an ISK score (pre-operation 96.11 against 188.4 post-operation) corresponded with the virtual absence of wear. The mean linear wear was 0.5 mm (■ Fig. 50-3). Thirty-seven patients with a level of activity higher than the average – strenuous work (*n*=18), sport activity (*n*=19) – before the dete-

rioration of their knee returned to their pre-disease functional level.

Overall Complications

In a series of 944 Genesis Unis fitted between 1991 and 2003, 26 complications (2.75%) were observed. Some of them correspond to rare phenomena: Three cases of loosening were post-traumatic in origin, and there was one deterioration of the opposite compartment and one case of unexplained pain. The other complications may be divided into two main categories: problems of a technical origin and inappropriate surgical indications. The study of polyethylene wear, on the other hand, has been quite reassuring, with wear in no case exceeding a thickness of 1 mm.

Technical Problems

Nine problems due to a technical mistake were noted, mainly at the tibial level having led to a loosening, and only one at the femoral level. The encouraging nature of this parameter is due essentially to the improvement in the ancillary instrumentation, but also, and above all, to increased knowledge of the tips and tricks of unicompartimental surgery, acquired as our experience has grown.

Inappropriate Indications

Twelve patients illustrate the main cause of failure observed in our series. The failure mechanism is predominately increased laxity due to wear and true front soft-tissue laxity leading to a subluxation of the implant in a load-bearing situation. It may also be due to an incorrect judgement of the quality of the anterior cruciate ligament, which may appear to be continuous but is functionally insufficient. This has previously been described by Deschamps et al. [4] (■ Fig. 50-4). The indication error may also concern the type of implant chosen, as the met-

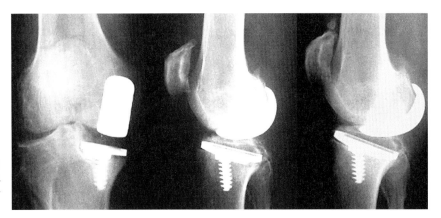

Fig. 50-4. Progressive sagittal femorotibial subluxation due to ACL deficiency in conjunction with excessive posterior tibial slope

al-backed implant should be discarded in favor of full poly implants in women with poor-quality underlying bone and whenever the width of the plateau is less than size medium.

All these complications have the simplicity of their revision in common, contrary to the opinion expressed by Douglas, Padgett, and Stern [5]. This favorable difference is due (a) to the use of a resurfacing implant, (b) to the very small quantity of cement used, indeed even its absence at the tibial level, and (c) to the early diagnosis of loosening at follow-up, which must be annual and systematic in patients who have received unicompartimental prostheses.

The Accuris Knee System

The Accuris knee system developed by Leo Pinczewski constitutes considerable progress in the technical reproducibility of the implantation of unicompartimental prostheses. As John Goodfellow has noted [6], more than for total knee replacements, the learning curve is essential in unicompartimental knee replacement. Even allowing for the fact that more and more orthopedic surgeons are performing unicompartimentals, the number carried out each year by the majority makes it difficult to respect the learning curve. The use of the Accuris system considerably simplifies the reproducibility of this operation.

This system has the following notable advantages over the previous system:

- Prebalancing of the knee joint is done prior to bone cuts using intra-articular shims.
- Tibial and posterior femoral resection are performed at the same time and at the ideal level.
- The parallelism between the tibial cutting surface and the femoral resurfacing level is respected, thanks to the use of a power femoral resurfacing drill adaptable to the trial tibial base plate.

The Accuris ancillary is suited to minimally invasive approaches; still, it by no means eliminates the need for knowing the rules of the unicompartimental implant, even if it does minimize the causes of error compared with the earlier techniques. These uni rules [7, 8] must be systematically applied and controlled by the operator during the final checks using non-fixed trial implants. Any residual abnormality must be corrected prior to the final implantation.

The Future

Future developments must be considered in the light of recent improvements in technique, materials, and indications.

Minimally Invasive Technique in Unicompartimental Arthroplasty

The minimally invasive surgical technique (MIS), as promoted by Repicci [9], undoubtedly represents a formal evolution concerning the rapidity of functional recovery and the shortening of the hospital stay. The problem posed by the strict minimally invasive technique, limited to the opening of only the medial or the lateral retinaculum, is the absence of sufficient visualization of the operation area while the trials are being done. Repeating the fitting errors of the past is a risk.

Though we may hope that computer-assisted surgery will be able to prevent this in the future, this is not yet the case for the uni prosthesis. One way of getting around this problem is to perform a very moderate extension of the exposure, not exceeding two finger widths from the upper pole of the patella (less-invasive surgical arthroplasty, LISA). In our experience, the rapidity of postoperative recovery has not been affected by this procedure and the visualization of the operation area during the trial checks has been just as reassuring as with conventional parapatellar approaches.

New Materials

At the tibial level, the polyethylene currently used has not shown any worrying tendency to wear, even for active subjects. Perhaps we can hope for even better wear characteristics with changes to the femoral bearing surface.

The use of oxidized zirconium femoral components seems to be the most appropriate solution, as has been shown by Myron Spector and colleagues [10], as it gives an 85% lower polyethylene wear rate than cobalt-chrome. The reduction of UHMWPE wear is basically due to the superior lubricity and abrasion resistance of the oxidized zirconium.

Indications for Unicompartimental Surgery

The indications have been codified by Deschamps, Epinette, and Hernigou [7] and by the authors. As long as we remain within the proposed framework, the risk of error at this level is minimial.

Some difficult problems remain, however: namely, the delicate differentiation between osteoarthitis that is purely mechanical in origin and inflammatory monoarthritis, particularly in chondrocalcinosis-type disorders. The problem of the patient age limit has not been resolved to date.

High tibial osteotomy is often proposed as a surgical alternative for young patients. However, in case of an incorrect clinical indication for HTO, this procedure has a short life span and requires revision to TKR at a young age. This is, in our view, worse than a well-performed unicompartimental replacement that has a better chance of a long survival.

Conclusion

The design of unicompartimental prostheses, as well as the quality of their ancillary instrumentation, has considerably improved since they were first invented. The basic concept of resurfacing advocated by Marmor has been shown in long-term follow-up to be perfectly reliable. The majority of modern implants, including the Genesis Uni system, are derived from it.

If the quality of the results obtained in active middle-aged subjects convinces us to maintain our confidence in the Genesis system, the recent improvements in the accuracy of fitting (Accuris technique) and the new materials (oxidized zirconium) will allow us to restore people to a level of functional activity that corresponds to "real life" and does not confine them to a reduction in the level of activity, as imposed by difficult osteotomies performed at indication stages that have gone by, or to TKRs with an indication unjustified by unicompartimental degenerative changes.

References

1. Grelsamer RP, Cartier P (1992) A unicompartmental knee replacement is not "half a total knee": five major differences. Orthop Rev 21:1952-1356
2. Cartier P et al (1996) Unicompartmental knee arthroplasty surgery. 10-years minimum follow-up period. J Arthroplasty 11:782-788
3. Cartier P (2002) U.K.A. benefits and pitfalls. AAOS Dallas Symposium
4. Deschamps G, Lapeyre B (1987) La rupture du ligament croisé antérieur: une cause d'échec souvent méconnue des prothèses unicompartimentales du genou. A propos d'une série de 79 prothèses Lotus revues au-delà de 5 ans. Rev Chir Orthop 73:544-551
5. Padgett D et al (1991) Revision total knee arthroplasty for failed unicompartmental replacement. J Bone Joint Surg [Am] 73:186-190
6. Goodfellow J et al (1990) The anterior cruciate ligament in knee arthroplasty: a risk-factor with unconstrained meniscal prostheses. Clin Orthop 276:245-252
7. Cartier P et al (1997) Unicompartmental knee arthroplasty. Paris, Expansion Scientifique Française
8. Cartier P (2000) Unicompartmental prosthetic replacement. In: Surgical techniques in orthopaedics and traumatology. Editions Scientifiques et Médicales Elsevier SAS, Paris, 55-570-A-10
9. Repicci JA (1999) Minimally invasive surgical technique for unicondylar knee arthroscopy. J South Orthop Assoc 8:1
10. Myron Spector et al (2001) UHMWPE wear performance of oxidized zirconium total knee femoral components. Scientific Exhibit SE034, American Academy of Orthopedic Surgeons, San Francisco

51 Mobile-Bearing Unicompartmental Knee Arthroplasty

D. G. Murray

Summary

Medial unicompartmental knee arthroplasty (UKA) has many advantages over total arthroplasty (TKA) including better function and less morbidity. However, the long-term failure rates of many designs of fixed-bearing UKA are high because of polyethylene wear, lack of sophisticated instrumentation, and imprecise patient selection.

Introduction

The fully congruent mobile bearing of the Oxford UKA exhibits minimal polyethylene wear, and failure from this cause does not occur. The instrumentation allows precise implantation to restore isometric function to the ligaments. During its 20-year development, the limits of usefulness of the implant have been established and found to include about one in three knees requiring replacement. There are now a number of published series, using these selection criteria, which have achieved very high survival rates at 10 and 15 years.

Since 1998, the phase-3 implant has been used with modified instruments through a small incision, avoiding damage to the extensor mechanism. Patients now recover substantially faster than after TKA or traditional open UKA and regain better function with no compromise in their survival rate. We believe that minimally invasive Oxford UKA is the treatment of choice for medial compartment osteoarthritis, provided the correct indications are applied and the appropriate surgical expertise is available.

Advantages

Medial unicompartmental knee arthroplasty (UKA) preserves all the undamaged structures of the joint, in particular the cruciate ligaments, and can therefore restore knee function nearly to normal. After UKA the range of movement is better than after TKA, the knee feels more natural, and pain relief is as good or better [1-3]. In terms of morbidity, operative blood loss is less and transfusion unnecessary; complications are less frequent and less serious, and recovery is more rapid. However, UKA has the disadvantage that the medium and long-term revision rates are generally higher than for TKA. The reasons for this include:

1. The high polyethylene wear rate of thin tibial components subjected to incongruous loading
2. Imprecise (and inappropriate) limits for patient selection
3. Lack of instruments to accurately implant the device

Over the years we have addressed these points and have developed a unicompartmental system that should have a long-term survival similar to that of TKA.

Material

The Oxford UKA has spherical femoral and flat tibial components, both made of cobalt chrome. Between them lies an unconstrained mobile bearing, the upper surface of which is spherically concave and the lower surface flat, so that it is fully congruent with both metal components in all positions. The contact area is large (about 6 cm²) and the contact pressure is therefore low. This form of articulation, while imposing no constraints upon movement, diminishes polyethylene wear to very low values. Measurement of retrieved bearings has shown a mean linear wear rate (combining both articular surfaces) of 0.03 mm/year, and even less (0.01 mm/year) if the knee had been functioning normally with no impingement [4, 5]. Furthermore, the rate of wear is no more rapid in thin components (i.e., 3.5 mm) than in thicker ones. The use of thin polyethylene is advantageous, as bone stock is preserved.

Indications and Contraindications

The main indication for UKA is medial compartment osteoarthritis [6]. The anterior cruciate ligament should be functionally intact [7]. We believe this requirement to be paramount. It will be found that, if the ACL is intact, the other requirements for success are also usually present

[8]. The fixed flexion deformity should be less than 15°. The intra-articular varus deformity should be correctable, indicating that the medial collateral ligament is not shortened. There should be full-thickness cartilage in the lateral compartment (best demonstrated by valgus stress X-rays taken with the knee in 20° of flexion) [9]. At operation, a full-thickness ulcer is often seen in the cartilage on the medial side of the lateral femoral condyle from impingement on the tibial spine; this is not a contraindication.

We have shown that many of the contraindications proposed for fixed-bearing UKA are unnecessary for the mobile-bearing device [6]. In our practice, no knee is excluded because of patellofemoral disease, except for the very rare case in which there is gross eburnation and grooving. In medial unicompartmental arthritis, extensive fibrillation and erosions are commonly found in the patellofemoral joint. We have found no correlation between the state of the patellofemoral joint or the presence of anterior knee pain and the clinical outcome [10,11], and we have not had to revise a knee for patellofemoral pain. Furthermore, we have shown by radiographic comparison at an interval of 10 years that arthritis does not progress in the patellofemoral joint after UKA [11]. Nor is age a contraindication. The low morbidity of UKA is a clear advantage over TKA in elderly patients. In younger subjects, UKA can be recommended as no more likely to fail at 10-15 years than TKA and with the advantage that, should failure occur, revision to TKA is simple and has good results [13,14]. We have shown that patients in their 50s have a 10-year survival rate better than 90% and that this is not significantly different from older subjects [13]. Moderate obesity and the presence of chondrocalcinosis have both been shown to be without adverse effect on long-term survival [15].

Avascular necrosis (AVN) is also an appropriate indication [16] and, although the numbers are small, the long-term results of medial UKA for AVN are similar to those for osteoarthritis. Currently, we do not recommend the use of a mobile-bearing UKA in the lateral compartment because of the high dislocation rate [17]. However, we do believe that in the future there will be a role for a mobile-bearing UKA with a modified design and surgical technique. Similarly, we do not recommend UKA after failed high tibial osteotomy (HTO), as the survival is about 66% at 10 years [18]. Inflammatory arthritis is a definite contraindication. Using our indications, about one in three knees needing replacement are suitable for UKA.

Instrumentation and Technique

Instrumentation and surgical technique are very important in unicompartmental replacement, the object of which is to restore the kinematics of the damaged com-

partment so that it functions in compliance with the retained articular surfaces and ligaments of the undamaged compartment. Using a mobile-bearing implant ensures that the prosthesis itself imposes no artificial constraints, but the stability of such a device depends upon restoring ligament tension isometrically throughout the range of movement. In TKA, ligament balancing is achieved by ligament release; in UKA it is attained by placement of the artificial articular surfaces to match the anatomy of the ligaments which are never released.

In the first design of the Oxford Knee (phase 1), the femur was prepared with a saw. Precise ligament balance was difficult to achieve, and the bearings occasionally dislocated. Since 1985, using the phase-2 and phase-3 instruments, the femur has been prepared with a guided power mill which can remove bone from the inferior surface of the femoral condyle in 1-mm increments, gradually increasing the gap between the articular surfaces in extension until it is the same as the gap in flexion. When the gap is filled with a bearing of the right thickness, the ligaments are restored to their normal tension and remain so throughout the range of movement. This results in normal ligament function and a very low incidence of dislocation: The in vivo kinematics of the Oxford Knee, assessed fluoroscopically, were found to be identical to those of normal knees and substantially better than those after TKA [19]. A meta-analysis of published results of the phase-2 implant, used for appropriate indications in the medial compartment, revealed a dislocation rate of 0.4% (two of 551 UKA) [20].

Results

The designer's own series of primary medial unicompartmental arthroplasty (phase 1 and phase 2) for anteromedial osteoarthritis consisted of 144 knees (patients aged 35-90), one of which was lost to follow-up [6]. The 10-year survival was 98% [95% confidence limits (CI) 93%-100%]. The designer's own results may need to be treated with caution as susceptible to bias; however, there are now a number of published independent series of 10 years or more with a similar survival rate. For example, Svard and Price [21] reported a series of 420 medial UKA with none lost to follow-up treated by three surgeons at a non-teaching hospital in Sweden [22]. The 15-year survival was 94% (CI 86%-100%). One hundred twenty-two of these had a follow-up of 10 years or more and were reviewed clinically; 92% had good or excellent results. In Smith's series of 135 medial UKA with none lost to follow-up the 10-year survival was 94% (CI 84%-98%) [23]. In Keyes' series of 40 medial UKA with none lost to follow-up the 10-year survival was 100% [24]. In these survival studies revision for any cause was considered to be a failure. The results from these series are therefore as good as the published results of TKA and better than the published results of fixed-bearing UKA [6].

By contrast, a survival of only 90% at 5 years was reported in 1995 for the phase-1 and phase-2 Oxford UKA enrolled in the Swedish Knee Arthroplasty Register (SKAR) [25]. There were 699 knees from 19 surgical centers and they included medial and lateral replacements. We were able to obtain data from 13 of these 19 centers and found 944 Oxford UKA, suggesting that the Register failed to recruit at least 25% of the knees. We found that the failure rate varied from center to center, from 0% to as high as 30%, and that centers implanting greater numbers had lower failure rates. About 70% of the failures were in the first 2 years, and dislocation of a bearing was the most common cause. As the same implant was used in all cases, the poor early results must be attributed to wrong indications and/or inappropriate technique, occasioned, perhaps, by the effect of at least 19 "learning curves". The 2001 report from the SKAR [26] confirms our observation that a surgeon needs to perform a reasonable number of Oxford UKA to be proficient. It also revealed that, in centers doing at least two UKAs per month, the 8-year survival of the Oxford UKA was 93%, marginally higher than that achieved by other UKA.

In 1998 the phase-3 implant was introduced, partly to address the problem of inconsistent results by making the operation simpler, and partly to facilitate a minimally invasive approach. The operation is now performed through a short incision from the medial pole of the patella to the tibial tuberosity. There is minimal damage to the extensor mechanism, the patella is not dislocated, and the suprapatellar synovial pouch remains intact. As a result, patients recover much more rapidly. We have found that knee flexion, straight leg raising, and independent stair climbing are achieved three times faster after this procedure than after TKA and twice as fast as after open UKA [27]. With appropriate pain control the procedure can be done safely as a day case with substantial cost savings, and patients report less pain during the postoperative period than they suffered preoperatively [28, 29].

Conclusions

A study of postoperative radiographs has shown that the Oxford components can be implanted equally precisely through the limited approach and through the traditional open incision [27], suggesting that the long-term results of the minimally invasive phase 3 should be as good as those of the phase 2. With the first 500 phase-3 Oxford UKAs implanted by two surgeons in Oxford the 5-year survival was 98% [30]. This demonstrates that at least at 5 years the survival of the phase 2 and phase 3 are similar. The functional results of the minimally invasive phase-3 UKA are better than those of the phase 2, how-

ever [31]. The greatest difference is in range of movement: With the phase 3 the average postoperative flexion (:130°) is about 10° higher than the preoperative flexion, whereas with phase 2 they are similar. We attribute the excellent functional results of both phase 2 and phase 3 to the accurate restoration of function in all the ligaments, particularly the cruciate mechanism, and the additional improvement in phase 3 to the avoidance of damage to the extensor mechanism and the suprapatellar pouch.

We believe we have shown that, when the indications are met, the Oxford UKA is the treatment of choice for medial osteoarthritis of the knee. It provides the patient with the many advantages of UKA over TKA without increasing the risk of failure, at least in the first 15 years.

References

1. Laurencin CT, Zelicof SB, Scott RD, Ewald FC (1991) Unicompartmental versus total knee replacement in the same patient: a comparative study. Clin Orthop 273:151-156
2. Rougraff BT, Heck DA, Gibson AE (1991) A comparison of tricompartmental and unicompartmental arthroplasty for the treatment of gonarthrosis. Clin Orthop 273:157-164
3. Newman JH, Ackroyd CE, Shah NA (1998) Unicompartmental or total knee replacement? Five-year results of a prospective randomised trial of 102 osteoarthritic knees with unicompartmental arthritis. J Bone Joint Surg [Br] 80:862-865
4. Argenson JN, O'Connor JJ (1992) Polyethylene wear in meniscal knee replacement: a one- to nine-year retrieval analysis of the Oxford knee. J Bone Joint Surg [Br] 74:228-232
5. Psychoyios V, Crawford RW, Murray DW, O'Connor JJ (1998) Wear of congruent mensal bearings in unicompartmental knee replacement. J Bone Joint Surg [Br] 80:976-982
6. Murray DW, Goodfellow JW, O'Connor JJ (1998) The Oxford medial unicompartmental arthroplasty: a ten-year survival study. J Bone Joint Surg [Br] 80:983-989
7. Goodfellow JW, O'Connor JJ (1992) The anterior cruciate ligament in knee arthroplasty. A risk factor with unconstrained meniscal prostheses. Clin Orthop 276:245-252
8. White S, Ludkowski PF, Goodfellow JW (1991) Anteromedial osteoarthritis of the knee. J Bone Joint Surg [Br] 73:582-586
9. Gibson P, Goodfellow JW (1986) Stress radiography in degenerative arthritis of the knee. J Bone Joint Surg [Br] 68:608-609
10. Goodfellow JW, Kershaw CJ, Benson MKD, O'Connor JJ (1988) The Oxford knee for unicompartmental osteoarthritis. J Bone Joint Surg [Br] 70:692-701
11. Hollinghurst D, Pandit H, Beard D, Ostlere S Dodd C. Murray D (2005) Is patellofemoral osteoarthritis a contraindication to unicompartmental knee arthroplasty? J Bone Joint Surg [Br] Abstract (in press)
12. Weale A, Murray DW, Crawford R, Psychoyios V, Bonomo A, Howell G, O'Connor J, Goodfellow JW (1999) Does arthritis progress in the retained compartments after "Oxford" medial unicompartmental arthroplasty? J Bone Joint Surg [Br] 81:783-789
13. Price AJ, Svard U, Dodd C, Goodfellow JW, O'Connor J, Murray DW (2000) The Oxford medial unicompartmental knee arthroplasty in patients under 60. ESSKA, London, September
14. Martin J, Wallace D, Woods D, Carr A, Murray DW (1995) Revision of unicompartmental knee replacement to total knee replacement. Knee 2:121-125
15. Woods D, Wallace D, Woods C, McLardy-Smith P, Carr A, Murray D, Martin J, Gunther T (1995) Chondrocalcinosis and medial unicompartmental knee arthroplasty. Knee 2:117-120

16. Langdown A, Pandit H, Price A, Dodd C, Murray D, Svard U, Gibbons C (2005) Oxford medial unicomparmental arthroplasty for focal spontaneous osteonecrosis of the knee. Acta Orthop Scand (in press)

17. Gunther T, Murray DW, Miller R, Wallace D, Carr A, O'Connor J, McLardy-Smith P (1996) Lateral unicompartmental arthroplasty with the Oxford meniscal knee replacement. Knee 3:33-39

18. Rees JL, Price AJ, Lynskey TG, Svard UCG, Dodd CAF, Murray DW (2001) Medial unicompartmental arthroplasty after failed high tibial osteotomy. J Bone Joint Surg [Br] 83:1034-1036

19. Price AJ, Rees J, Beard D, Gill H, Dodd C, Murray D (2004) Sagittal plane kinematics of a mobile-bearing unicompartmental knee arthroplasty at 10 years. A comparative in vivo fluoroscopic analysis. J Arthroplasty 19:590-597

20. Price AJ, Svard U, Murray D (2000) Bearing dislocation in the Oxford medial unicompartmental knee arthroplasty. ESSKA, London, September

21. Svard U, Price AJ (2001) Oxford unicompartmental knee arthroplasty. J Bone Joint Surg [Br] 83:191-194

22. Price AJ, Waite J, Svard U (2005) Long-term clinical results of the Oxford unicompartmental knee replacement. Clin Orthop (in press)

23. Rajasekhar C, Das WS, Smith A (2004) Unicompartmental knee arthroplasty. 2- to 12-year results in a community hospital J Bone Joint Surg [Br] 86:983-985

24. Keys GW, UL-Abiddin Z, Toh EM (2004) Analysis of first forty Oxford medial unicompartmental replacements from a small district hospital in UK. Knee 11:375-378

25. Lewold S, Goodman S, Knutson K, Robertsson O, Lidgren L (1995) Oxford meniscal-bearing knee versus the Marmor knee in unicompartmental arthroplasty for arthrosis: a Swedish multi-centre survival study. J Arthroplasty 10:722-731

26. Robertsson O, Knutson K, Lewold S, Lidgren L (2001) The routine of surgical management reduces failure after unicompartmental knee arthroplasty. J Bone Joint Surg [Br] 83:45-49

27. Price AJ, Webb J, Topf H, Dodd C, Goodfellow JW, Murray DW (2001) Rapid recovery after Oxford unicompartmental knee arthroplasty through a short incision. J Arthroplasty 16:970-976

28. Beard DJ, Rees JL, Price AJ, Dodd CAF, Murray DW (2002) Accelerated recovery for unicompartmental knee replacement - a feasibility study. Knee 9:221-224

29. Reilly K, D Beard, K Barker, C Dodd, A Price, D Murray (2005) Efficacy of an accelerated recovery protocol for Oxford unicompartmental knee arthroplasty. Knee (in press)

52 Metallic Hemiarthroplasty of the Knee

R. D. Scott, R. D. Deshmukh

Summary

Metallic hemiarthroplasty may continue to have a very selective, limited role in the treatment of unicompartmental osteoarthritis. Fewer than 1% of patients with OA should be appropriate candidates. Indications might include a young osteoarthritic patient with unicompartmental arthritis in whom an osteotomy is contraindicated, but who is considered too young, heavy, and/or active for total knee arthroplasty. Advantages include the conservative nature of the operation and permission for the patients to engage in activity to tolerance. Disadvantages are the possibility of incomplete pain relief and the fact that the procedure is technically demanding and sensitive.

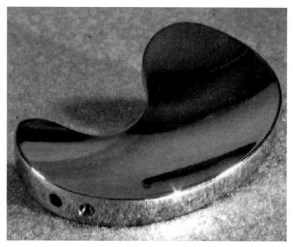

◨ **Fig. 52-2.** Unispacer metallic hemiarthroplasty

Introduction

Surgical options for the treatment of unicompartmental osteoarthritis include osteotomy, unicompartmental arthroplasty, and total knee arthroplasty [3]. Osteotomy is favored for young, heavy, and active patients, especially men, whose opposite compartment is free of significant disease. Unicompartmental metal-to-plastic arthroplasty is recommended for older or more sedentary patients as

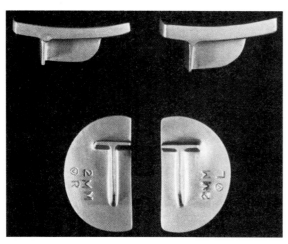

◨ **Fig. 52-1.** McKeever metallic hemiarthroplasty

a conservative procedure that spares both cruciate ligaments and preserves bone stock for future revision [5, 6, 12]. Total knee arthroplasty often is favored over unicompartmental arthroplasty for elderly patients because revision is less likely in the second postoperative decade for the patient who has less than two full decades of life expectancy [1].

A fourth alternative, metallic hemiarthroplasty, was introduced in the 1950s by MacIntosh and McKeever (MacIntosh and McKeever prostheses, Howmedica, Inc. Rutherford, N.J.; ◨ Fig. 52-1) with limited popularity [7, 8]. This alternative was all but forgotten until recently, when the concept was re-introduced with a prosthetic device called the UniSpacer,[11] (Centerpulse Inc., Austin, Texas; ◨ Fig. 52-2).

Past Experience

Both MacIntosh and McKeever published their early experience in the late 1950s [7, 8]. MacIntosh reported good initial results in 72 of 103 knees with a minimum 6-month follow-up [7]. McKeever claimed good initial results with a slightly different prosthesis in 39 of 40 knees [8]. Potter et al. followed up 19 knees in patients with OA who had either a McKeever or a MacIntosh prosthesis for an average of 3 years (range 1-9 years) and reported good to excellent results in 17 of the 19 knees [9].

The most recent reports of metallic hemiarthroplasty were both published in 1985. Scott et al. reported on 40 patients with 44 unicompartmental McKeever arthroplasties followed up for 5-13 years (average 8 years). At final follow-up, 70% of the knees were rated as good or excellent [10]. Also in 1985, Emerson and Potter published the results of 61 unicompartmental McKeever arthroplasties in patients followed up for 2-13 years (average 5 years), with a similar number (72%) rated as good or excellent [2]. Despite these results, metallic hemiarthroplasty never became popular, possibly because of the advent of cemented metal-to-plastic total knee arthroplasty with its better initial and long-term results.

Current Role of Metallic Hemiarthroplasty

Certain patients, however, may still qualify for metallic unicompartmental hemiarthroplasty as an alternative to high tibial osteotomy (HTO) or metal-to-plastic unicompartmental (UKA) or total knee arthroplasty (TKA). Indications would include a young osteoarthritic patient with unicompartmental arthritis of either the medial or the lateral side, in whom an osteotomy is contraindicated by early opposite compartment disease or poor range of motion and who is considered too young, heavy, or active for TKA. It is estimated that approximately 1% of osteoarthritic patients would be candidates. Another relative indication involves a patient with a past history of sepsis at the knee joint because of the minimally invasive nature of metallic hemiarthroplasty.

The senior author has continued to use McKeever hemiarthroplasty for highly selected patients over the past three decades. An unpublished series of 24 knees in

patients under the age of 60 years has shown that excellent clinical results can be long lasting and allow a high level of activity. After 10 years, some patients have continued to participate in activities such as downhill skiing and competitive ice hockey (Fig. 52-3). At an average 14 years of follow-up, half of the knees are still in situ, with Knee Society knee scores [4] averaging 93 and function scores averaging 98. The longest successful result is at 28 years after implantation.

The UniSpacer

The UniSpacer can be thought of as a "mobile" McKeever or MacIntosh hemiarthroplasty [11]. Rather than attempting fixation to the tibial plateau via a keel or roughened undersurface, it is designed to translate freely on the tibial plateau as determined by the conforming articulation of its top surface with the femoral condyle. This mobility makes it inappropriate for use in the lateral compartment, where the femoral roll-back could cause prosthetic dislocation and/or soft-tissue impingement.

In the only report published to date, Dr. Richard Hallock reported in 2003 on 71 knees in 67 patients with a minimum 1-year follow-up [3]. Five (7%) had been revised to a TKA and an additional ten (14%) had their UniSpacer exchanged for either dislocation (6) or pain (4). The overall 1-year revision rate, therefore, was 21%. Among the 66 knees that retained a UniSpacer, the average flexion was 117°, with an average knee score of 78 and a function score of 72. Additionally, 17 patients (24%) had arthrofibrosis requiring manipulation under anesthesia for flexion ranging from 60° to 100°. The authors maintain that this problem has been reduced by beginning early ROM rather than a period of immobilization for 2 weeks as had been the initial protocol.

These results would appear to be inferior to those published for McKeever hemiarthroplasty by Scott et al. [10], except for a slightly higher flexion arc of 117° vs. 110°. The revision rate was 50% higher for the UniSpacer at 1 year (21%) vs. the McKeever at 8 years (14%). It must be conceded, however, that the UniSpacer does have the advantage of possible insertion through a minimally invasive approach, whereas the McKeever arthroplasty requires a larger exposure for contouring the femur and tibia and for insertion of the prosthesis.

References

1. Deshmukh RV, Scott RD (2002) Unicompartmental knee arthroplasty for young patients. Clin Orthop 404:108-112
2. Emerson R, Potter T (1985) The use of the McKeever metallic hemi-arthroplasty for unicompartmental arthritis. J Bone Joint Surg [Am] 67:208-212
3. Hallock RH, Fell BM (2003) Unicompartmental tibial hemiarthroplasty: early results of the UniSpacer knee. Clin Orthop 416: 154-163

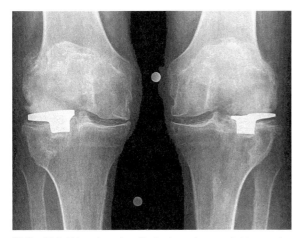

 Fig. 52-3. This patient played ice hockey twice a week, 11 years after undergoing bilateral McKeever hemiarthroplasty

4. Hanssen AD, Stuart MJ, Scott RD, Scuderi GR (2000) Surgical options for the middle-aged patient with osteoarthritis of the knee joint. J Bone Joint Surg [Am] 82:1768-1781
5. Insall JN, Dorr LD, Scott RD, Scott WN (1989) Rationale of The Knee Society clinical rating system. Clin Orthop 248:13-14
6. Karpman RR, Volz RG (1982) Osteotomy versus unicompartmental prosthetic replacement in the treatment of unicompartmental arthritis of the knee. Orthopedics 5:989-991
7. Kozinn SC, Scott R (1989) Unicondylar knee arthroplasty. J Bone Joint Surg [Am] 71:145-150
8. MacIntosh DL (1958) Hemi-arthroplasty of the knee using a space-occupying prosthesis for painful varus and valgus deformities. Proceedings of the joint meeting of the orthopaedic associations of the English speaking world. J Bone Joint Surg [Am] 40:1431
9. McKeever DC (1960) Tibial plateau prosthesis. Clin Orthop 18:86-95
10. Potter TA, Weinfeld MS, Thomas WH (1972) Arthroplasty of the knee in rheumatoid arthritis and osteoarthritis. A follow-up study and implantation of the McKeever and MacIntosh prosthesis. J Bone Joint Surg [Am] 54:1-24
11. Scott RD (2003) Unispacer: insufficient data to support its widespread use. Clin Orthop 416:164-166
12. Scott RD, Joyce MS, Ewald FC, Thomas WH (1985) McKeever metallic hemi-arthroplasty of the knee in unicompartmental degenerative arthritis. J Bone Joint Surg [Am] 67:203-207
13. Weale AE, Newman JH (1994) Unicompartmental arthroplasty and high tibial osteotomy for osteoarthritis of the knee: a comparative study with a 12- to 17-year follow-up period. Clin Orthop 302:134-137

53 Patellofemoral Arthroplasty

M. M. Glasgow, S. T. Donell

Summary

Isolated patellofemoral osteoarthritis is present in approximately 10% of patients presenting with symptomatic degenerative knee joint disease. The current gold standard for treatment of end-stage disease after failure of conservative measures is total knee arthroplasty. The early results of isolated patellofemoral arthroplasty have been disappointing, but newer designs and an appreciation of the need to balance the soft tissues hold out the hope that a less invasive procedure may achieve results that match those of total knee arthroplasty. Concerns remain about progression of disease to the medial tibiofemoral compartment.

Introduction

Approximately half of patients with degenerative arthritis of the knee have involvement of the patellofemoral joint. Given the female predilection for patellofemoral maltracking and the known association with premature patellofemoral osteoarthritis, it is perhaps surprising that Davies et al. noted in a population of symptomatic osteoarthritic knees presenting over the age of 60 that 18.5% of men and 17.1% of women had isolated patellofemoral disease as compared with 4.5% of men and 10% of women between the ages of 40 and 60 [1]. There is no doubt that isolated patellofemoral disease is a more common phenomenon than many clinicians realise and that it occurs more frequently than isolated lateral tibiofemoral disease. This review looks at the various arthroplasty options for isolated patellofemoral osteoarthritis.

Anatomy

The patellofemoral joint includes the trochlear groove and the entire extensor mechanism of the knee, namely the quadriceps tendon, patella, and patellar ligament. The patella is a sesamoid bone that acts as a marker for the alignment of the extensor mechanism. The trochlear groove and an arch of articular cartilage around the intercondylar notch make up the femoral side of the joint.

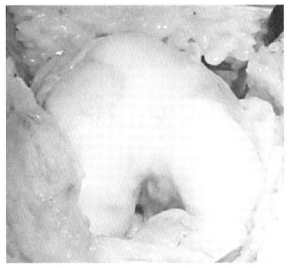

Fig. 53-1. Severe trochlear dysplasia

Except in deep flexion, the tibial articular surface comes into contact with a different part of the femur than the patella does, and the majority of intercondylar notch osteophytes result from patellofemoral disease. In many patients with patellofemoral osteoarthritis the problem is secondary to trochlear dysplasia (Fig. 53-1). This may vary from a slightly shallow groove to an actual dome. This will inevitably distort the anatomy and kinematics to a significant degree [2].

Kinematics

The movements of the patellofemoral joint are complex and have been reported by Goodfellow et al. [3]. In full extension only the distal part of the patella articular surface is in contact with the femoral groove, and as flexion proceeds the contact area on the patella sweeps proximally until 90° of flexion, when the proximal part is in contact with the distal groove. From 90° of flexion the odd facet articulates with the lateral edge of the medial femoral condyle, and the lateral facet articulates with the medial edge of the lateral femoral condyle. The medial facet lies in contact with the synovium overlying the anterior cru-

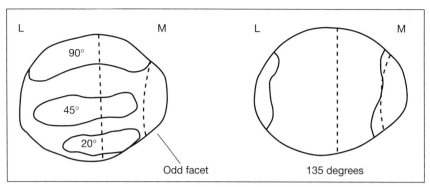

Fig. 53-2. Contact area of patellar surface at varying angles of knee flexion. (After [3])

Odd facet   135 degrees

ciate ligament. In deep flexion the patella effectively bridges the intercondylar notch, and at 135° of flexion the patella articulates with parts of both the medial and lateral femoral articular surfaces that also come into contact with the anterior meniscal horns (Fig. 53-2).

Indications for Patellofemoral Arthroplasty

Patellofemoral arthroplasty should be considered for patients with isolated patellofemoral arthritis who have anterior knee pain uncontrolled by conservative and medical measures. It is very important to exclude tibiofemoral disease, inflammatory disorders, and referred pain (especially from the hip). There is no firm evidence base in the literature to support or refute inclusion or exclusion on the grounds of age or weight. It is important for patients to understand that isolated patellofemoral replacement is experimental, and not the "gold standard" operation, i.e., total knee arthroplasty. In our practice we have treated patients as young as 45 years of age with patellofemoral replacement as an alternative to patellectomy with success. In this young age-group it is essential that the patients show a positive attitude to treatment. The results are predictably bad in patients who have a significant psychological component to their pain. We emphasize that the operation may require revision to a total knee arthroplasty in the future. Usually, the patients are in the same age range for total knee replacement, but the isolated replacement preserves the anterior cruciate ligament and allows for full flexion. Its success postoperatively depends on building up the quadriceps muscle.

Arthroplasty

The patellofemoral joint has been the 'Cinderella' of knee arthroplasty. It is obvious from a glance at some of the early total knee implants that no real consideration was given to the patellofemoral joint. The Freeman-Samuelson implant had no trochlear groove. The Attenborough

had a very short anterior femoral flange, and the spherocentric implant completely disregarded the patellofemoral joint. Arthroplasty options for isolated patellofemoral arthritis are:
1. Total knee arthroplasty with patella resurfacing
2. Total knee arthroplasty without patella resurfacing
3. Isolated hemiarthroplasty patella resurfacing
4. Patellofemoral replacement

Total knee arthroplasty with patella resurfacing has, in effect, created the gold standard [4, 5], with good or excellent results that match those of total knee arthroplasty for tibiofemoral disease. There are, however, persisting concerns about the scale of surgery to deal with what is, in effect, an osteoarthritic process confined to the anterior compartment. One novel approach has been to reduce the morbidity of surgery by leaving the patella unresurfaced in total knee arthroplasty for isolated patellofemoral disease, as an extrapolation of the as yet unresolved and long-running debate about patella resurfacing in total knee arthroplasty for tibiofemoral disease. Beverland has shown good results using the LCS mobile-bearing total knee implant with simple patella débridement, but leaving the patella unresurfaced [6].

Whilst the concept of unicompartmental replacement has recently gained considerable popularity following publication of excellent 10-year results for the treatment of isolated medial tibiofemoral disease, there remains a considerable degree of scepticism about the advantages of isolated patellofemoral joint arthroplasty, for a variety of reasons:
1. The already established excellent long-term results both in terms of quality of pain relief and long-term survival for conventional total knee replacement
2. Concern about progression of the osteoarthritic process to the tibiofemoral joint - particularly the medial compartment
3. Concerns about persisting extensor mechanism instability, given that a large majority of patients who will be eligible for isolated patellofemoral replacement present with end-stage extensor mechanism malalignment and maltracking

4. The extensor mechanism, and in particular the patellofemoral joint, has consistently been the largest single cause of problems and failure following total knee replacement.

5. Amis [7] has pointed out that the implant companies have been reluctant to put large investments into the development of isolated patellofemoral implants, because they perceive isolated patellofemoral disease as an uncommon phenomenon. It is to be hoped that this will change as clinicians become aware of the need to perform axial radiographs in patients presenting over the age of 40.

Biomechanics

The patellofemoral joint has to withstand very considerable contact forces with increasing knee flexion. Huberti and Hayes [8] noted that in extension the patella was subjected to 1.5 times body weight, and this increased to 7 times body weight in deep flexion. The contact pressure was further increased by a larger Q-angle, which tended to cause skewing of the patella. There is a part of both the medial and lateral femoral condyle which comes into contact both with the anterior horn of the relevant meniscus in extension of the knee and with the odd and lateral facets of the patella in deep flexion. As it is not possible to resurface the whole of the trochlear area which comes into contact with the patella in deep flexion, it is therefore imperative that any implant at least match the normal femoral geometry at the distal end of the femoral component, to allow a smooth transition from bearing surface to articular surface, as the patella will effectively transfer on to the articular cartilage of the femoral condyles. The component will also require smooth radiused edges that can be fitted flush with the femur to prevent meniscal 'catching' and inevitably pain. The transition from implant to articular surface is aided by soft-tissue infill - particularly on the patellar component, as described by Cameron [9].

Particularly with an all-polyethylene component, the significant loading on the patella in flexion may result in bending in deep flexion when bridging the intercondylar notch, thus increasing the potential for loosening and dislocation.

In addition to high contact stresses, the relative lack of congruency of the normal patellofemoral joint results in relatively low stability, and it is essential that any trochlear component is properly aligned in the vertical orientation and that appropriate soft-tissue balancing is performed to ensure satisfactory tracking of the patella [10-12].

One way to reduce potential patellar instability would be to increase the depth of the trochlea, with consequent reduction in the facet angle of the patella. This produces

a more 'captive' design, as was advocated by Renard and Blazina [13, 17]. In this situation, however, it is even more incumbent upon the surgeon to ensure satisfactory alignment and soft-tissue balance to avoid the potential risk of significant increase in mediolateral sheer stresses and articular contact pressure on, predominantly, the lateral facet, which might lead to premature component loosening. In essence, the surgeon should not rely on the constraint of the implant to ensure satisfactory patellar tracking.

Patellar Hemiarthroplasty

The first recognized patella resurfacing device was introduced by McKeever in 1949 [14]. This consisted of a metal anatomical shell with slightly concave medial and lateral articular facets, which were asymmetric. Fixation was achieved with a single screw. The prosthesis was not sided but was merely turned upside down depending on whether the right or the left knee was being operated on.

McKeever reported his early results in 1955, but interpretation of data was complicated by the wide indications for surgery; e.g., six patients had rheumatoid arthritis, and additional surgical procedures including meniscectomy and synovectomy were included.

In 1992, Harrington [15] reported use of the implant "as a salvage procedure for severe chondromalacia," indicating reasonable long-term results with a mean follow-up of 8.1 years. There was no evidence of patellofemoral instability or prosthetic loosening.

A new patella prosthesis based on anatomical dimensional studies was reported by Aglietti [16]. For the first time his group considered cement fixation and also the option of a plastic component for use with conventional total condylar knee replacement. Their results using a metallic patella hemiarthroplasty were disappointing at medium term follow-up, however, probably on account of the dome shape, which was not congruent with the unresurfaced trochlea and resulted in high contact pressure. Patellar hemiarthroplasty has now fallen into disrepute.

If the ongoing debate about resurfacing of the patella at the time of total knee arthroplasty continues unresolved, then it is interesting to speculate as to whether later advocates of patellofemoral arthroplasty may suggest that the patella component be left unresurfaced after appropriate débridement.

Patellofemoral Arthroplasty

Concern about the use of patellar hemiarthroplasty in patients with trochlea changes led to the development of patellofemoral arthroplasty. The ideal features of a patellofemoral replacement are:

1. The patella button should be compatible with other total joint replacement systems.
2. The trochlear component should not encroach on the intercondylar notch, which could result in injury to the anterior cruciate ligament.
3. There should be a smooth anatomical transition from the distal part of the trochlear component onto the articular cartilage of the two femoral condyles, to permit movement of the patellar component from the distal part of the trochlear prosthesis onto the articular cartilage of the femoral condyles in deep flexion.
4. It should be possible to achieve minimal femoral bone resection to allow the implant to sit flush on the anterior femoral cortex.
5. It should be possible to determine correct rotation of the femoral trochlear component, as well as vertical alignment.

The Bechtol patella I system was introduced by the then Richards medical company in 1974, and the modified type II system was introduced in 1976 [17]. This was a very constrained prosthesis with a deep metal trochlear groove that tapered to a point at the apex of the intercondylar notch, and a matching patella implant (◘ Figs. 53-3, 53-4). In 1975 Lubinus introduced his own patellofemoral endoprosthesis, which was more anatomical and attempted to reproduce the shape of the anterior aspect of the distal femur [18]. Unlike the Richards patella mod I, II, and III systems, this involved the use of a sided trochlear implant. Several patellofemoral prostheses have been developed in France, perhaps the best-known being the autocentric prosthesis [14].

The initial reviews were not encouraging. Study numbers were small with short follow-up and the results did not come close to matching those of total knee arthroplasty [12, 17, 19-23]. Of the larger series, Cartier reported on 72 arthroplasties, reviewed at between 2 and 12 years following implantation with a relatively short average follow-up of 4 years [11]. The use of Smith and Nephew mod III prostheses demonstrated good or excellent results in 85% of cases. Interpretation of the results was rendered difficult, however, because in 36 of the cases a concomitant unicompartmental tibiofemoral replacement was also performed. Cartier emphasized that extensor mechanism realignment should be carried out at the time of arthroplasty surgery. It is of note that he performed 27 lateral retinacular releases and 34 tibial tubercle transpositions, utilizing a very constrained prosthesis, but persisting lateral subluxation was noted in only two patients following surgery. This was in contrast to the original review by Blazina et al. of 57 implants, 20 of which had to undergo revision procedures to correct lateral patellar maltracking [17].

In 2001 the Bristol group in the UK presented a prospective review of the outcome of 76 Lubinus arthroplasties with a mean follow-up of 7.5 years [24]. The clini-

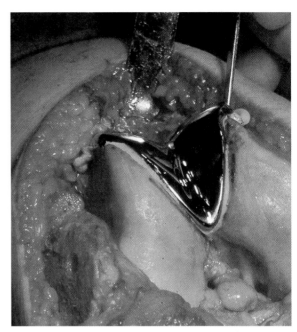

◘ **Fig. 53-3.** Femoral component Smith & Nephew Mod III arthroplasty in situ

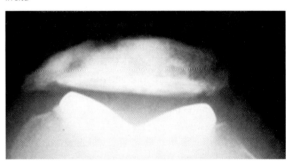

◘ **Fig. 53-4.** Postoperative skyline view of Smith & Nephew Mod III arthroplasty

cal outcome was satisfactory in only 45% of cases using the Bristol knee scoring system. Interpretation of the results is confused by virtue of the fact that in the majority of cases the sided femoral trochlear component was reversed, so that a left-sided component was used on the right side and vice versa. This was stated by the authors to have optimized patellofemoral tracking. Again, meticulous attention was paid to patellar tracking at the time of surgery, with a secondary procedure (usually a lateral retinacular release) being performed in 4% of cases. At the time of review patellar malalignment was noted in 32% of patients and was the most common complication. Some concern was also expressed about the possibility of progression of medial tibiofemoral disease. Following publication of these results they abandoned the procedure.

Argenson reported a medium-term follow-up of 183 patellofemoral arthroplasties in 1994 [10]. However, as 104 of these patients also underwent concomitant unicompartmental tibiofemoral arthroplasty, only 79 implants were available for study at an average follow-up of 5.5

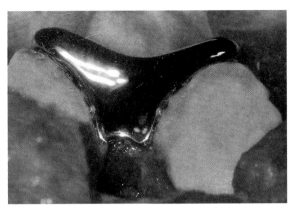

Fig. 53-5. Intraoperative view of Avon patellofemoral joint replacement

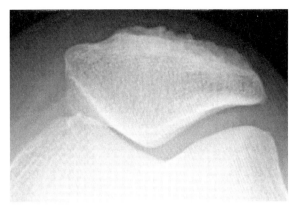

Fig. 53-6. Medial patellofemoral osteoarthritis

years. They identified a bias in favor of patients with osteoarthritis secondary to extensor mechanism dysplasia and fracture, and recorded a much higher failure rate in patients treated with primary patellofemoral osteoarthritis. As a consequence they recommended patellofemoral arthroplasty for patients with secondary patellofemoral osteoarthritis.

As a result of dissatisfaction with the Lubinus implant, Ackroyd and the Bristol group developed the Avon implant, which was based on the anterior compartment of the Kinemax total knee implant [25] (◘ Fig. 53-5). Instrumentation was devised to enable the surgeon to implant the prosthesis with a greater degree of accuracy, in terms of both anterior positioning, to avoid "overstuffing" the anterior compartment, and femoral rotation. The first was implanted in September 1996, and they recently reported on their experience with 360 implants, 59 of which have been in place for 5 years [26]. The incidence of patellar maltracking was only 4% and disease progression to the tibiofemoral joint 7%. The functional result matched those of current total knee arthroplasty designs. The most common complication was progression to symptomatic medial tibiofemoral disease, noted in 6% of cases. They also reported on a subgroup of 63 arthroplasties in younger patients under the age of 55, admittedly with a very short follow-up (mean 24 months). The early results matched those seen in older patients. This is the authors' current preferred implant in cases of isolated patellofemoral osteoarthritis.

The dramatic increase in the use of unicompartmental tibiofemoral implants, fuelled partly by long-term reviews suggesting results that match the best of total knee arthroplasty results with a much more conservative procedure, have resulted in a rekindled interest in the concept of isolated patellofemoral arthroplasty. Long-term non-inventor reviews are awaited with interest, but it would appear that with the newer designs it is possible to achieve short- to medium-term results that match those of established total knee arthroplasty designs, with a less morbid

surgical procedure and a more rapid recovery. To put it into context, it is important to record that the total UK sales of the Avon implant in 2003 amounted to only 603 implants. It would appear that earlier concerns about the high level of residual patellar instability following use of these implants have been resolved, largely as a result of careful attention to extensor mechanism balancing at the time of the primary procedure. As with all unicompartmental replacements, there are persisting concerns about progression of disease to other compartments in the knee, and there does appear to be an increased liability to progression of medial tibiofemoral disease. Given the Oxford unicompartmental knee replacement group's data, which suggest a link between medial patellofemoral facet osteoarthritic change and medial tibiofemoral unicompartmental disease, caution is perhaps appropriate when one is confronted with a patient who has isolated medial patellofemoral osteoarthritis (◘ Fig. 53-6).

There are no hard data with regard to ease of revision and conversion to total knee replacement, but there is evidence [22] to suggest that revision of the femoral component presents little difficulty and that revision of the patellar component presents no additional difficulties over and above those of total knee arthroplasty. The recent development of minimally invasive surgical techniques may ultimately offer reduced morbidity when a patellofemoral prosthesis is implanted, but the need to access both the trochlear and the retropatellar surfaces without the ability to "decompress" the extensor mechanism by resection of distal, femoral, and proximal tibial bone leaves little scope for significant developments in minimally invasive access.

References

1. Davies AP et al (2002) The radiological prevalence of patellofemoral osteoarthritis. Clin Orthop 402:206-212
2. Dejour H et al (1990) La dysplasie de la trochlée fémorale. Rev Chir Orthop 76:45-54

3. Goodfellow J et al (1976) Patello-femoral joint mechanics and pathology. Functional anatomy of the patello-femoral joint. J Bone Joint Surg [Br] 58:287-290
4. Laskin RS, van Steijn M (1999) Total knee replacement for patients with patellofemoral arthritis. Clin Orthop 367:89-95
5. Mont MA et al (2002) Total knee arthroplasty for patellofemoral arthritis. J Bone Joint Surg [Am] 84:1977-1981
6. Thompson NW et al (2002) Knee arthroplasty without patellar resurfacing as an option in the management of patients with isoloated patellofemoral osteoarthritis. J Bone Joint Surg [Br] 84:157
7. Amis AA (1999) Patello-femoral joint replacement. Curr Orthop 13:64-70
8. Huberti HH, Hayes WC (1984) Patellofemoral contact pressures. The influence of the Q-angle and tendofemoral contact. J Bone Joint Surg [Am] 66:715-724
9. Cameron HU, Cameron GM (1987) The patellar meniscus in total knee replacement. Orthop Rev 16:170-172
10. Argenson JNA et al (1995) Is there a place for patellofemoral arthroplasty? Clin Orthop 321:162-167
11. Cartier P, Sanouiller JL (1990) Patellofemoral arthroplasty: 2- to 12-year follow-up study. J Arthroplasty 5:49-55
12. Thiess SM et al (1996) Component design affecting patellofemoral complications after total knee arthroplasty. Clin Orthop 326:183-187
13. Renard JF (1986) Prothèses autocentriques de rotule. Thesis, Dijon
14. McKeever DC (1955) Patellar prosthesis. J Bone Joint Surg [Am] 37:1074-1084
15. Harrington KD (1992) Long-term results for the McKeever patellar resurfacing used as a salvage procedure for severe chondromalacia patellae. Clin Orthop 279:201-213
16. Aglietti R (1975) A new patella prosthesis - design and application. Clin Orthop 107:175-187
17. Blazina ME et al (1979) Patellofemoral replacement. Clin Orthop 144:98-102
18. Lubinus HH (1979) Patella glide bearing total replacement. Orthopedics 2:119-127
19. Arciero RA et al (1988) Patellofemoral arthroplasty. A three-to-nine year follow-up study. Clin Orthop 236:60
20. de Winter WE et al (2001) The Richards type 11 patellofemoral arthroplasty: 26 cases followed for 1-20 years. Acta Orthop Scand 72: 487-490
21. Kooijman HJ et al (2003) Long-term results of patellofemoral arthroplasty. A report of 56 arthroplasties with 17 years of follow-up. J Bone Joint Surg [Br] 85:836-840
22. Krajca-Radcliffe, JB Coker TP (1996) Patellofemoral arthroplasty. A 2- to 19-year follow-up study. Clin Orthop 330:143-151
23. Levitt RL (1973) A long-term evaluation of patellar prostheses. Clin Orthop 97:153
24. Tauro B et al (2001) The Lubinus patellofemoral arthroplasty. A five- to ten-year prospective study. J Bone Joint Surg [Br] 83:696-701
25. Ackroyd CE, Newman JH (2001) The Avon patello-femoral arthroplasty - development and early results. J Bone Joint Surg [Br] 83 [Suppl 11]:146
26. Ackroyd CE (2004) Patello-femoral arthroplasty. Fifteen years experience with 436 cases. Combined Orthopaedic Associations Meeting, Sydney

54 Current Role of Hinged Implants
H. Reichel

Summary

This chapter will review hinged knee designs, describe the correct indications for using them, and discuss the advantages and disadvantages of this type of implant especially in revision surgery. The new modular rotating-hinge prostheses provide better knee kinematics than older rigid-hinge devices and offer many modular options. Modular rotating hinges, however, are rarely indicated. They may be considered in salvage situations with massive bone loss and soft-tissue deficiencies which cannot be treated sufficiently by posterior-stabilized or condylar-constrained implants. To determine long-term success of these components, further follow-up studies are necessary.

Introduction

The goals of total knee arthroplasty (TKA) in primary and in revision surgery are the relief of pain and the restoration of function and stability. To accomplish these goals, the least amount of prosthetic constraint should be used.

All designs of TKA can be divided into three groups, considering the kind of internal mechanical link and the residual ligament function:

I. Minimum constraint (MC): TKA with a congruent design which preserves one or both cruciate ligaments

II. Intermediate constraint (IC): TKA with a central post-and-cam mechanism replacing the posterior cruciate ligament

III. Total constraint (TC): TKA with an intrinsic biplanar stability which substitutes for all ligaments, like condylar-constrained or hinged designs

Evolution of Hinged Knees

A review of the literature defines a distinct path of evolution for the hinged knee designs. The first generation of hinged devices (e.g., Walldius, Stanmore, Guepar) pro-

vided excellent stability but only one degree of freedom. These rigid hinges securely linked the femoral and the tibial component and restricted motion in the knee to flexion and extension. Because of the rigid constraint, stress from shear and torsional loading was transferred directly to the metal hinged articulation and to the bone-cement interfaces, leading to metal debris and component loosening [1, 5, 9]. Due to the linked mechanism between the femoral and tibial component, distraction of the joint during gait or sitting created additional tensile stress on the bone-cement interfaces [7]. Rigid hinged prostheses were associated with high rates of aseptic loosening, infections, and other complications and thus had high failure rates. In a multicenter study, Knutson et al. [12] reported a cumulative survival rate of 65% at 6 years for rigid hinged knees in patients with primary osteoarthritis. Poor survival rates were also attributed to metal-on-metal bearing surfaces, large implant sizes requiring significant bone removal, and insufficient medullary canal fill (◘ Table 54-1).

With the second-generation of hinged prostheses (e.g., St. Georg Rotation Knee, Endo-model Rotating Hinge, Kinematic Rotating Hinge), another degree of freedom, the rotation ability around a vertical axis, was introduced. With metal-on-polyethylene bearing surfaces that allowed axial rotation, better results were achieved (◘ Table 54-2). Some of these designs are still in use [16]. However, the main drawback to these hinged devices was the lack of modularity. The variety of implant sizes was rather small, large bone resections were necessary, and there was almost no opportunity to alter the stem length and style during surgery or to treat bone defects with metal augments. Again, there was a significant incidence of complications with second-generation hinges. Rand et al. [17] reported the results of 38 Kinematic Rotating Hinges with a 16% incidence of septic complications, 22% incidence of patellar instability, and 6% incidence of component breakage at 55 months average follow-up. Shindell et al. [18] reported a 56% failure rate in an average of 32 months using the Noiles Rotating Hinge Knee. Failures occurred mostly in patients who weighed over 90 kg (approximately 198 lbs) and in revision cases.

▫ Table 54-1. Results of first-generation rigid-hinge devices

Reference	Component	n	Follow-up (years)	Results (%) Good to excellent	Fair	Poor	Survival (%)
Primary							
Freeman [4]	Walldius	80	–	78	16	6	88
Jones et al. [9]	GUEPAR	108	1-3	61	10	29	89
Bargar et al. [1	GUEPAR	39	2-4				87
Grimer et al. [5	Stanmore	81	7 (max.)				80
Insall [8	GUEPAR	45	2-3.5	69	22	9	96
Oglesby and Wilson [15]	Walldius	90	6				91
Revision							
Bargar et al. [1]	GUEPAR	17	2-4				76
Karpinski and Grimer [11]	Stanmore	52	4	23	48	29	90

▫ Table 54-2. Results of rotating-hinge devices (second- and third-generation hinges)

Reference	Component	n	Follow-up (years)	Results (%) Good to excellent	Fair	Poor	Survival (%)
Primary							
Rand et al. [17	Kinematic	15	2-6	33			80
Finn et al. [3]	Finn	25	1	–			92
Petrou et al. [16]	ENDO Model	100	7-15	91			96
Revision							
Rand et al. [17]	Kinematic	23	2-3	70			57
Barrack et al. [2	S-ROM	14	2-6				100
Westrich et al. [22]	Finn	15	2-5				100
Jones et al. [10]	S-ROM	30	2-6				100
Springer et al. [20]	Kinematic segmental	22	2-11				91

In the GSB prosthesis, another representative of this generation which was used extensively in German-speaking countries, a different second degree of freedom was added, allowing for some anterior-posterior translation between the tibial metal post and the femoral polyethylene cam. The polyethylene in the femoral cam as well as the tibial polyethylene inserts were non-modular. This often led to extensive wear, and the entire prosthesis had to be exchanged. Therefore, the mid-term results of the GSB prosthesis were also not acceptable [19].

The third generation, the modular rotating-hinge prostheses (e.g., S-ROM Modular Knee, NexGen RHK, Stryker MRH), provides better knee kinematics with a rotation ability throughout the flexion-extension range. These modern designs are not linked in the same fashion as the rigid hinged implants. Usually, the hinge is secured only to the femoral component, and is inserted freely into the tibial component using a long hinge post extension. Because of this mechanism, and due to the rotating articulating surface, the stress on the cement interfaces is reduced and can be transferred in parts to the soft tissue. Modular canal-filling stems provide additional fixation

and more reliable alignment. Compared with previous designs, the amount of bone resection required has been reduced. In modern designs standard bone cuts are used to conserve condylar bone. Additionally, the intercondylar box dimensions have been optimized to provide a secure hinge mechanism while minimizing bone removal. Modular augments and an improved patellofemoral articulation are additional features not found in earlier rotating hinges. Although there are only limited data on newer-generation rotating hinges [2, 10, 22] and long-term data are not yet available, good survival rates can be expected.

Technical Issues of Third-generation Hinged Prostheses

Third-generation hinged designs allow the femoral condyles to interact with the tibial plateau as the main articulating surface. Varus-valgus, anterior-posterior, and medial-lateral loads are only partially transferred to the tibial stem through the hinge post extension. Due to the highly conforming articular surfaces, stability is achieved not only with the constraint mechanism but also by means of the direct condylar contact, and shear stress on the hinge is thus minimized. Patellar tracking has been improved by an anatomical patellar groove, a roll-back mechanism of the femur during flexion, and by the rotation around a vertical axis allowing the screw-home phenomenon in extension. The femoral roll-back in particular may decrease the pressures at the patellofemoral joint during flexion.

Nevertheless, the stress at the bone-cement interfaces remains an important issue in rotating-hinge knees. Although modern rotating hinged designs represent a significant progress in reducing the rotational load, some of the shear and tensile stress is still transferred to the bone-cement interfaces. Therefore, these implants should be used with long intramedullary stems and cement fixation only. The core prosthesis, i.e., the condylar surfaces of the femoral and tibial components, has to be fixed with cement. Whether the intramedullary stems should be also cemented or used uncemented as press-fit or porous stems is under discussion. As the remaining stress is high but reasonable, a strong endosteal fixation of the stems should be achieved.

Another issue is the load on the hinge mechanism. If a rotating hinged knee design uses a posteriorly located hinge mechanism that links the femoral component directly to the tibial component or to a secondary platform that inserts into the tibial component, the hinge bears the majority of weight throughout the full range of motion. This can create a significant stress on the hinge and may lead to high wear of the polyethylene bushings. The result can be an early failure and/or the need for polyethylene bushing exchange. From a biomechanical point of view, a hinge design in which the femoral condyles articulate with a highly conforming rotating polyethylene insert and which uses a hinge-post extension has two main advantages. First, the majority of weight-bearing loads are transferred to the tibial component through the condyles rather than the hinge mechanism. In laboratory testing, more than 95% of compressive weight-bearing loading was on the condyles (NexGen RHK, data by Zimmer, Inc.). Second, as the hinge-post extension is inserted freely into the tibial component, varus-valgus, anterior-posterior, and medio-lateral axial movements are secured but their resulting loads are partially transferred through the long hinge-post extension to the tibial stem (◻ Fig. 54-1). There are no reported data on the amount of reduction in stresses that may occur with these designs compared with previous ones. However, if the stresses are reduced by some amount such as 10% or 15%, this might have a substantial effect on reducing the mechanical failure rate.

The length and the geometry of the hinge-post extension are important to avoid an implant dislocation. If the laxity, especially in flexion, exceeds the jumping

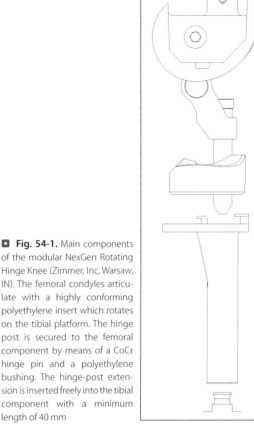

◻ **Fig. 54-1.** Main components of the modular NexGen Rotating Hinge Knee (Zimmer, Inc, Warsaw, IN). The femoral condyles articulate with a highly conforming polyethylene insert which rotates on the tibial platform. The hinge post is secured to the femoral component by means of a CoCr hinge pin and a polyethylene bushing. The hinge-post extension is inserted freely into the tibial component with a minimum length of 40 mm

height of the hinge mechanism, a separation of the post from the tibial component is possible. Therefore, the minimum length of the hinge-post extension should be greater than the amount of laxity that would normally occur in a knee joint where the ligaments have been removed. Studies in adult cadavers showed that without cruciate or collateral ligaments the remaining soft tissues will stretch to allow the knee joint to be distracted 20-32 mm [13]. In a biomechanical study by Ward et al. [21], the stem length and tapers of rotating hinged knees made by seven manufacturers were measured. The Howmedica, Techmedica, Intermedics/Sulzer Medica, and Wright Medical Technology/Dow Corning Wright designs required a minimal distraction of 39 mm before they dislocated. The Biomet knee prosthesis required 33 or 44 mm of distraction to dislocate, depending on the polyethylene thickness. The S-ROM knee required only 26 mm of distraction [21]. The hinge-post extension of the NexGen RHK is designed to provide a minimum length of 40 mm.

Indications for Modular Rotating-Hinge Prostheses

Generally, a rotating-hinge prosthesis is rarely indicated. In each revision, ligament balancing and bone reconstruction should be performed first using the prosthesis with the least constraint that provides sufficient stability. However, a rotating hinge may be considered in the following cases:

1. Massive bone loss, especially if the insertions of collateral ligaments are involved

2. Extreme imbalance of flexion-extension gaps
3. Complete loss of the medial collateral ligament
4. Chronic rotational dislocation between femur and tibia
5. Chronic extensor mechanism disruption or deficiency

These indications are more common in post-infection revisions, after multiple revision arthroplasties, ankyloses, periprosthetic fractures, in rheumatoid arthritis, in Charcot-like arthropathy, and after tumor resection. If an older hinged knee has to be revised, where all ligaments were resected at the time of the arthroplasty, it may be necessary to use a hinged implant again (◘ Fig. 54-2). Sometimes a rotating hinge is also indicated in difficult primary arthroplasties when bone, ligaments, or both are severely damaged.

Role of Modular Rotating Hinges in Revision

Revision TKA is often characterized by bone loss and ligament laxity. This necessitates the use of components with a higher degree of constraint. In many revisions, an upgrading of prosthesis constraint is necessary. Surgeons today often address knees requiring extensive revision with stabilizer and superstabilizer implants. Many revision arthroplasties can be performed using a posterior-stabilized prosthesis to substitute the posterior cruciate ligament. Collateral ligament insufficiency can be addressed by a condylar constrained prosthesis which provides good varus-valgus stability when soft tissues are present but attenuated and alignment is achieved. If this type of implant is used, however, in a case with extensive flexion-extension gap mismatch or complete loss of the medial collateral ligament, the consequence could be a remaining varus-valgus instability, a marked hyperextension in the knee, the risk of peg dislocation (◘ Fig. 54-3), or even fracture of the overloaded central polyethylene peg [6, 14]. Therefore, in a patient with a grossly unstable TKA, with ligament damage and bone destruction, a modular rotating-hinge prosthesis that substitutes for the articular surface of the knee as well as for the ligament function may be the better solution. Due to the large amount of bone loss, however, it must be taken into account that only few viable options exist should this rotating hinge have to be revised again. The options remaining in those cases are custom-made devices, tumor prostheses, or a large amount of bone grafting. In view of these limited options, a restricted use of modular rotating hinges even in revision surgeries is recommended.

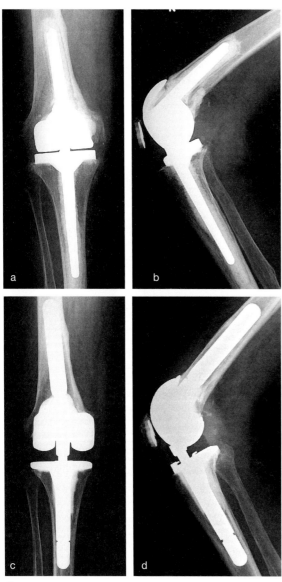

◘ Fig. 54-2a-d. *a, b* Anteroposterior and lateral radiographs show aseptic loosening of a GSB prosthesis in a 73-year-old woman. Note the significant proximal migration of the femoral component. The non-modular polyethylene inlays on the tibial component were completely worn out. During the arthroplasty 9 years earlier the collateral and cruciate ligaments were resected. *c, d* Two years following implantation of a NexGen Rotating Hinge Knee. The femoral and tibial components were cemented; the rather short diaphyseal press-fit stems remained uncemented. The patellar component showed no polyethylene wear and was retained

54

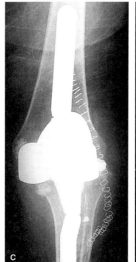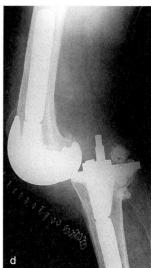

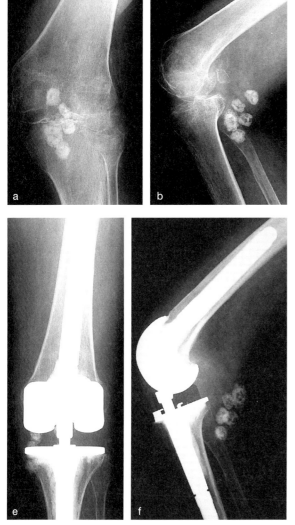

Fig. 54-3a-f. *a, b* Preoperative radiographs of a 79-year-old woman with a grossly unstable valgus knee and an extension lack of 20°. A patellectomy had been done 13 years earlier, following a traffic accident. *c, d* Radiographs made 10 days after implantation of a condylar constrained knee prosthesis (NexGen LCCK). Due to the deficiency of the extensor mechanism and a remained flexion-extension gap mismatch, the knee dislocated during a fall on the ward. *e, f* One year after revision with a Nex-Gen Rotating Hinge Knee using long diaphyseal fluted stems the knee joint is stable. The patient walks without crutches and is able to actively extend the knee up to a lack of 10°. The loose bodies in the popliteal region were not removed because they are extra-articularly located

3. Different stem lengths and styles to be altered during surgery
4. Different stem offsets to match anatomical variations
5. Variety of augments to be added if there is severe bone loss
6. Wide range of implant sizes to reduce the bone resection if the implant is used in difficult primary arthroplasty
7. Opportunity to be built up to a tumor resection-style prosthesis in severe cases

The results of short- and medium-term studies show that rotating hinges of the current designs can be successful when used for specific indications. Longer follow-up studies will be necessary to better define the role of modern rotating hinges for total knee arthroplasty. Due to the increasing number of revisions which must be expected in the future, the role of hinged implants in revision total knee arthroplasty will probably be expanded.

Conclusions

A modern hinged implant needs to be a modular rotating-hinge design that fulfills the following demands:
1. Complete and immediate varus-valgus, anterior-posterior, and medio-lateral stability
2. Rotational component to avoid torsional stress being transmitted through the implant-bone interfaces

References

1. Bargar WL, Cracchiolo A, Amstutz HC (1980) Results with the constrained total knee prosthesis in treating severely disabled patients and patients with failed total knee replacements. J Bone Joint Surg [Am] 62:504-512
2. Barrack RL, Lyons TR, Ingraham RQ, Johnson JC (2000) The use of a modular rotating hinge component in salvage revision total knee arthroplasty. J Arthroplasty 15:858-866
3. Finn HA, Kneisl JS, Kane LA, Simon MA (1991) Constrained endoprosthetic replacement of the knee. Abstracts of the 6th Int. Symposium on Limb Salvage, Montreal, Canada, September 10
4. Freeman PA (1973) Walldius arthroplasty: a review of 80 cases. Clin Orthop 94:85-91
5. Grimer RJ, Karpinski MRK, Edwards AN (1984) The long-term results of Stanmore total knee replacements. J Bone Joint Surg [Br] 66:55-62
6. Hendel D, Garti A, Weisbort M (2003) Fracture of the central polyethylene tibial spine in posterior stabilized total knee arthroplasty. J Arthroplasty 18:672-674

7. Inglis AE, Walker PS (1991) Revision of failed knee replacements using fixed-axis hinges. J Bone Joint Surg [Br] 73:757-761
8. Insall JN (1984) Total knee replacement. In: Insall JN (ed) Surgery of the knee. Churchill Livingstone, New York, pp 587-695
9. Jones EC, Insall JN, Inglis AE, Ranawat CS (1979) GUEPAR knee arthroplasty - results and late complications. Clin Orthop 140:146-152
10. Jones RE, Barrack RL, Skedros J (2001) Modular, mobile-bearing hinge total knee arthroplasty. Clin Orthop 392:306-314
11. Karpinski MRK, Grimer RJ (1987) Hinged knee replacement in revision arthroplasty. Clin Orthop 220:185-191
12. Knutson K, Lindstrand A, Lidgren L (1986) Survival of knee arthroplasties: a nation-wide multicentre investigation of 8000 cases. J Bone Joint Surg [Br] 68:795-803
13. Krackow KA, Mihalko WM (2001) The effect of severe femoral bone loss on the flexion-extension joint space in revision total knee arthroplasty: a cadaveric analysis and clinical consequences. Orthopedics 24:121-126
14. Krüger T, Reichel H, Decker T, Hein W (2000) Arthroscopy of the dysfunctional total knee arthroplasty: Two cases with peg fracture of the polyethylene insert. Arthroscopy 16:E21
15. Oglesby JW, Wilson FC (1984) The evolution of knee arthroplasty. Clin Orthop 186:96-103
16. Petrou G, Petrou H, Tilkeridis C, Stavrakis T, Kapetsis T, Kremmidas N, Gavras M (2004) Medium-term results with a primary cemented rotating-hinge total knee replacement: a 7- to 15-year follow-up. J Bone Joint Surg [Br] 86:813-817
17. Rand JA, Chao EYS, Stauffer RN (1987) Kinematic rotating-hinge total knee arthroplasty. J Bone Joint Surg [Am] 69:489-497
18. Shindell R, Neumann R, Connolly JF, Jardon OM (1986) Evaluation of the Noiles hinged knee prosthesis: a five-year study of seventeen knees. J Bone Joint Surg [Am] 68:579-585
19. Sprenger TR, Doerzbacher JF (2002) Long-term follow-up of the GSB II total knee used in primary total knee arthroplasty. J Arthroplasty 17:176-183
20. Springer BD, Sim FH, Hanssen AD, Lewallen DG (2004) The Modular Segmental Kinematic Rotating Hinge for non-neoplastic limb salvage. Clin Orthop 421:181-187
21. Ward WG, Haight D, Ritchie P, Gordon S, Eckardt JJ (2003) Dislocation of rotating hinge total knee prosthesis: a biomechanical analysis. J Bone Joint Surg [Am] 85:448-453
22. Westrich GH, Mollano AV, Sculco TP, Buly RL, Laskin RS, Windsor R (2000) Rotating hinge total knee arthroplasty in severely affected knees. Clin Orthop 379:195-208

54

VII Materials

55 Biology of Foreign Bodies: Tolerance, Osteolysis, and Allergy

S. Nasser

Summary

In most individuals implanting the polymers and metals used in contemporary knee replacement surgery results in little or no reaction from the immune system. These materials are described as biologically tolerated or bioinert. However, as the functioning joint begins to wear, generating primarily polymer debris, the immune system commonly mounts an aggressive, macrophage-mediated response. This becomes evident after several years, both clinically and radiographically, as osteolysis [1, 2]. In a much smaller percentage of individuals, a second type of reaction, a very rapid, T-cell-mediated, "allergic" response, usually to metal, may be identified [3]. While the underlying processes are quite different, both reactions may ultimately lead to implant failure.

Introduction

All materials implanted within the human body degrade, the rate and method of degradation varying with the material involved. Materials that degrade very slowly are usually well tolerated by the body, while those that degrade rapidly cause a more intense response [4]. With regard to what are commonly termed orthopedic biomaterials, the usual degradation products include particulate debris, organo-particulate complexes and oxidative products of the various materials. In addition, metals may form insoluble salts as well as free metal ions [5]. The response of the immune system to these degradation products is often far different than the reaction to the bulk material [6-8].

Tolerance to Biomaterials

The success of modern knee arthroplasty is due, in no small part, to the biocompatible materials used to manufacture the various types of prosthetic implants and fix them permanently to the surrounding osseous structures. Early attempts at arthroplasty surgery using such materials as ivory, leather, wood, metal foils of various types, and even fascia soaked in chromium salts were doomed to failure, even if aseptic surgical techniques and contemporary implant designs had been widely available [9-12]. The use of naturally occurring materials and reactive metals to repair or replace human joints remained largely a matter of trial and error, and almost universally unsuccessful, well into the twentieth century. These materials were simply not tolerated by the body.

The first attempts at an organized, rational analysis of the in vivo effects of implanted materials were carried out shortly after World War I. Zierold's studies on metals, for example, identified adverse tissue reactions to iron, steel, and nickel-plated steel, the materials most commonly used for orthopedic devices at that time [13]. These were noted to corrode rapidly, with associated erosion of the adjacent bone. Significant reactions were also noted in the soft tissues surrounding implants made of nickel, copper, zinc, and magnesium, while gold, silver, and even lead were "tolerated" by the body. Obviously the usefulness of these soft (and even toxic) metals in joint arthroplasty was limited, but the foundation for identifying appropriate materials had been laid.

The anti-corrosive properties of high concentrations (greater than 12%) of chromium in steel alloys were first identified in 1913, during work to make gun barrels more resistant to deterioration. These alloys were protected by a thin layer of chromium (III) oxide (Cr_2O_3) that formed spontaneously on the surface of the metal by the process of auto-passivation. Within a few years, stainless steels such as "18/8" (72% Fe, 18% Cr, 8% Ni, still the most commonly used alloy for cooking utensils) were introduced for orthopedic applications. Several studies noted the usefulness of these alloys in fracture fixation. However, early stainless steels were found to be reactive with the surrounding bone and soft tissues in the long term, and were also vulnerable to fatigue fracture, limiting their usefulness for permanent implantation. Fortunately, an alternative was found in the first non-ferrous, cobalt-chromium-based alloy, Vitallium (Austentel Laboratories, Chicago, IL).

Vitallium was introduced for dental applications in 1932, and by 1936 was being used experimentally for orthopedic devices [14]. Vitallium was described as "completely inert in the body," and additionally showed great strength and resistance to fatigue fracture as both a cast and a forged material. The alloy was rapidly adopted for a variety of implant uses, including interposition arthroplasty of the hip. The first use of Vitallium in knee arthroplasty, the Carrell-Virgin Knee Cap, came just 2 years later in 1939, and cobalt-chromium alloys have been used in nearly every knee design, both successful and un-successful, since that time [12, 15, 16].

The earliest knee arthroplasty prostheses employed metal-on-metal articulations, the majority being constrained hinge designs such as the Walldius and GUEPAR Knees. The use of these implants gave what can generously be described as "mixed results". The prostheses loosened quickly, and the articulating surfaces wore rapidly, often filling the knee joint with metal debris (■ Fig. 55-1) However, in almost all retrieval analyses, the metal particles were described as "well tolerated" and inflammation was described as "minimal". These results, although nearly 40 years old, compare favorably with analysis of many contemporary metal-on-metal hip replacement designs, in that cobalt-chromium-based alloys, both in bulk and in particulate form, appear to be well tolerated by the vast majority of patients undergoing joint replacement surgery [17, 18]. This biocompatibility also appears to be due to the development of the same type of stable chromium oxide layer, similar to but stronger than stainless steel, which shields the underlying metal from the saline environment of the body.

The application of two additional materials has led to the successful knee arthroplasty implants currently in use. Polymethylmethacrylate (PMMA) was first introduced to orthopedic surgery by the Judet brothers in the form of hip hemiarthroplasty components [19], and was subsequently used experimentally as a fixation material in 1953 [20]. Charnley's seminal work on cement fixation for his Low Friction Arthroplasty of the hip led to the widespread use of cold-curing acrylic cement for a

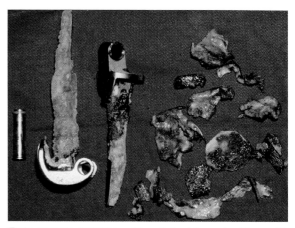

■ **Fig. 55-2.** This GUEPAR-type hinge design (Zimmer, Inc., Warsaw, IN), implanted with cement, was revised after it began to squeak during normal use. Even though metal wear was significant, the implants were well fixed

variety of applications, including fixation of knee replacement prostheses [21, 22]. Cement was used to stabilize both older hinge designs (■ Fig. 55-2) and newer implants specifically designed to use PMMA for permanent attachment to bone [23-25].

In addition to acrylic bone cement, the use of a second biomaterial, ultra-high-molecular-weight polyethylene (UHMWPE), was pioneered by Charnley [6] and first adapted for use as a bearing surface in total knee arthroplasty (the "Polycentric Knee") by Gunston [26]. Fortunately, the disastrous results related to the use of polytetrafluoroethene (Teflon) bearings in hip replacements were avoided, and the early results of the Polycentric Knee were relatively good, and certainly far superior to the hinge designs available at that time [27]. In fact, the bearing surface combination of cobalt-chrome alloy and UHMWPE fixed with PMMA remains the gold standard for knee replacement arthroplasty today.

The bioinert nature of both PMMA and UHMWPE in bulk form has been known for some time [6]. Stable implants of both materials are generally described as provoking a "minimal inflammatory response" and large pieces of both polymers rapidly become encased in a "fibrous tissue pseudocapsule". Implants of both materials not subjected to movement or wear appear to maintain this inert status almost indefinitely. Unfortunately, such conditions are rarely, if ever, encountered in the normally functioning knee replacement.

Osteolysis

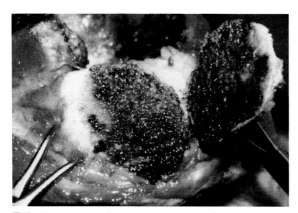

■ **Fig. 55-1.** Gross metallosis is obvious at revision of an early, metal-on-metal, hinged knee implanted without cement. Even though metal debris was found deep within the patella, the immune response in the absence of polymer debris was very limited

Wear occurs when there is relative motion between two surfaces in contact. Debris is generated as a result, made up of particles of material from one or both surfaces. In total knee replacements wear debris can be generated at any interface: at the articular surfaces, at the cement interfaces with both bone and implant, and at the junctions between any modular features such as stems or tibial tray inserts and the main implant. In practical terms, however, well over 90% of wear debris in current prosthetic designs is generated at the articular surfaces during normal motion of the knee and consists almost entirely of microscopic and submicroscopic UHMWPE particles [28, 29].

If polymer wear were solely a mechanical problem, the treatment would be straightforward. The worn polyethylene would be replaced at the point where instability became clinically evident, and the prosthetic knee would return to normal function. Unfortunately, the most important clinical manifestations of wear have much more to do with the body's response to the particulate material generated by the wear process than with loss of mechanical integrity. These particulates induce a foreign-body inflammatory response which may result in the development of inflammatory bone reabsorption, or osteolysis [30].

At the present time the most common cause of failure of joint replacement arthroplasty is this periprosthetic osteolysis [31-33]. The condition was initially termed "cement disease," reflecting an early misunderstanding of the etiology of the process [34-36]. It is now understood that "cement disease" also occurs in cementless joint replacements [37], both hips and knees (◘ Fig. 55-3), as well as in association with upper-limb arthroplasty procedures. Some estimates suggest that over 25% of all knee replacements will show radiographic features of the condition, and it will lead to revision surgery in roughly half of these cases (◘ Fig. 55-4a and b). In fact, it is generally agreed that osteolysis is the limiting factor in the long-term performance of contemporary joint replacements.

Exactly how wear particulates initiate the process that results in clinically significant bone loss remains some-

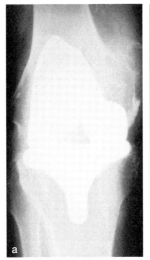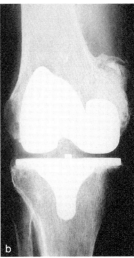

◘ **Fig. 55-4a,b.** An 82-year-old patient presented with massive osteolysis of the distal femur (a) 9 years following placement of this hybrid PCA knee (Howmedica, Inc., Rutherford, NJ). Extension of the granuloma into the soft tissues is seen proximal to the medial epicondyle. Despite the massive bone loss, the implants were well fixed and supported by healthy bone. The revision procedure consisted of thorough débridement, allograft impaction grafting, and replacement of the heat-pressed polyethylene. Seven years later, the grafted bone is radiographically incorporated (b)

what of a mystery. However, some features of osteolysis appear to be relatively consistent, and the process is well described in the literature. Retrieval analyses of periprosthetic tissues reveal a synovial-like membrane containing a variety of cellular elements including fibroblasts, macrophages, plasma cells, lymphocytes, neutrophils, and fibroblastic giant cells invading the adjacent bone and soft tissues [38]. In general, macrophages predominate, comprising 60%-80% of the cellular population, followed by fibroblasts (15%-30%) and T-lymphocytes (<10%), with considerable individual variation. As its numbers indicate, the macrophage is considered to be primarily responsible for the activation and maintenance of the aggressive local environment leading to bone loss [39, 40].

Most studies suggest that the inability of the macrophage to enzymatically digest wear debris particulates is the crucial factor involved in the runaway process that leads to clinically significant osteolysis (◘ Fig. 55-5). Since the debris cannot be digested, it is released back into the surrounding extracellular environment, along with nitric oxide (NO), free radicals, and proteolytic enzymes which cause local tissue destruction [41-43]. The debris may then be re-ingested by the same macrophage, if it remains viable, or by a neighboring macrophage, continuing the cycle of activation and destruction [44].

In addition to free radicals and enzymes, activated macrophages secrete a complex mixture of cytokines containing IL-1β, TNF-α, and IL-6 [45-49]. These cytokines recruit and maintain the presence of activated macrophages in the region of osteolysis. In addition, these

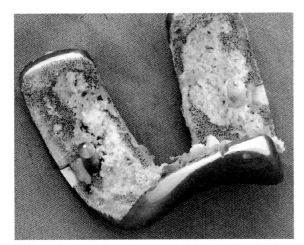

◘ **Fig. 55-3.** This AMK femoral component (DePuy, Inc. Warsaw, IN) from a cementless total knee failed when the supporting bone, weakened by osteolysis, fractured at 8 years. Osteolytic granuloma is visible in direct contact with healthy bone

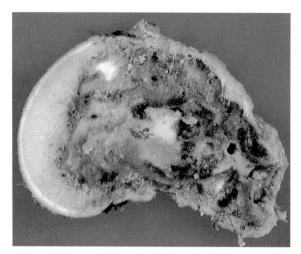

◻ Fig. 55-5. Osteolysis of the proximal tibia under a failed cementless implant. Note the direct apposition of healthy bone with the infiltrating osteolytic membrane

same intercellular mediators are known to promote osteoclast differentiation, proliferation, and activation, leading to bone reabsorption at the cellular level [50, 51] (◻ Fig. 55-6). However, even though the osteoclast is thought to be the cell type predominantly responsible for direct bone reabsorption, there is substantial evidence to suggest that debris-activated macrophages are also at least partially responsible for bone destruction [52, 53].

In order to identify the characteristics of wear debris that are responsible for the adverse cellular reactions leading to osteolysis, a number of parameters have been investigated [54, 55]. For example, it was initially suggested that the aggressive granulomatous response to Teflon debris, described as consisting of "ragged particles" of up to 500 μm, was due to the large size of the particles, which prevented phagocytosis [22]. More recently, several authors have suggested that the most reactive UHMWPE

particles are actually the smallest, less than 0.5-1 μm [56-59]. Interestingly, metal debris of the same size may be much more benignly addressed by the macrophage [60]. Obviously, particle size alone is not the only factor involved in initiation of the osteolytic process [61].

In addition to size, other factors that may determine the reactivity of debris are particle composition, shape, surface charge and energy, and the character of the surface proteins bound to particles comprised of different materials [62]. This may also explain, in part, the differences in an individual patient's response to wear debris as well as the differences in the reaction induced by polymers, metals, and ceramics [63].

Unfortunately, it is difficult to identify specific characteristics of individual materials, especially in vivo, as at least two different materials are involved, and each material produces debris of a different size and shape, depending on the manner in which the wear particles are generated [64]. For example, UHMWPE debris produced by knee replacement prostheses tends to be larger than that produced by hip replacements (some studies indicate an average of three times to an order of magnitude larger) indicating a likely difference in the mechanism of debris production [65, 66]. One possible explanation for this particular dissimilarity is that in the conforming hip joint adhesive/abrasive wear predominates, while in the less conforming knee a sliding motion generates debris by delamination at the polymer surface [67-69] (◻ Fig. 55-7). Whatever the cause, the difference in size may be one important reason for the difference in the rate that osteolysis occurs in knees versus hips [70]. Clinically, osteolytic membranes around hips often tend to be characterized as more inflammatory in nature, while those from prosthetic knees are more fibrous. It is therefore difficult, and possibly misleading, to combine the results of studies involving these different types of joint replace-

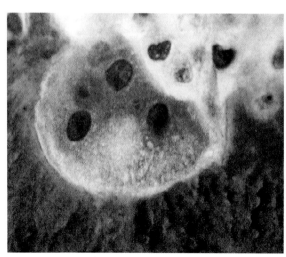

◻ Fig. 55-6. Microscopic analysis of the tibial bone stock seen in Fig. 55-5 shows a front of bone destruction caused by osteoclastic reabsorption

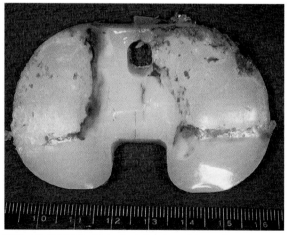

◻ Fig. 55-7. This PCA tibial polyethylene insert (Howmedica, Inc, Rutherford, NJ) shows a combination of adhesive/abrasive wear and delamination. Both types of damage were accelerated by malposition of the implants as well as by heat-pressing of the implant surface

ments. To further complicate matters, UHMWPE hip debris tends to be spherical, while that from knees appears more flattened or fibrillar [67, 71]. These differences in aspect ratio and surface texture appear to have a profound influence on the ability of the macrophage to ingest the particles and, hence, on their ultimate effects [68, 72].

Two further complicating factors also emerge regarding investigations of osteolysis. First, *in vivo*, all debris is a mixture of elements from all the different materials involved. It is not uncommon to see particles of PMMA, UHWMPE, cobalt-chromium alloy, and bone debris, all of different sizes and shapes, all in the same tissue, and all under the hydrostatic pressure fluctuations generated as the joint moves [73]. Second, at present there is no good animal model for osteolysis that addresses all the factors involved in the process of debris generation. Large animal studies are expensive and time consuming and lack a true bipedal representation of human gait. Studies with smaller animals such as mice are reliant on "pre-formed" debris. Unfortunately, there is as yet no way to produce in quantity debris that accurately resembles the particles generated by normally functioning joints. Debris produced by joint simulators tends to be relatively uniform in character [74], while that retrieved from periprosthetic tissues shows considerable variability on electron-microscopic analysis. Commercially available polymer "debris" tends to be much larger than retrieved samples. The use of retrieved particulates harvested from human joint replacement periprosthetic tissues necessitates isolation by chemical means, such as NaOH digestion of the tissue, which may alter the surface properties of the debris.

What is clear is that the volume of debris and the number of debris particles produced by a joint replacement have a direct correlation with the development of osteolysis [30]. The concentrations of debris particles that have been found in osteolytic tissues have been measured at 8×10^8 to as high as 6×10^{11} particles per gram of tissue, related to numerous variables including the age of the implant [36]. It is generally agreed that any factor that contributes to the generation of debris will increase the rate of periprosthetic bone loss [49]. For example, many attempts to "improve" the properties of UHMWPE have resulted in rapid wear and resulted in increased osteolysis. The use of graphite fibers (Poly II, Zimmer, Inc, Warsaw, IN) to limit the creep and cold flow of the material resulted in massive third-body wear and rapid prosthetic failure. Increased crystallinity (Duracon, DePuy, Inc. Warsaw, IN) led to an increase in brittleness, a decrease in fatigue strength, and excessive fragmentation. Heat-pressed polyethylene was found to be more prone to delamination and often provoked a very intense osteolytic reaction, while titanium bearing surfaces, even when ion-hardened, proved prone to accelerated wear and a combined polymer-metal-induced osteolysis [70].

If factors that increase debris generation lead to osteolysis, it is logical to assume that a decrease in the rate of wear should lower the rate of osteolysis. Several hip arthroplasty studies have shown the use of cross-linked UHMWPE, and ceramic bearings on UHMWPE may decrease adhesive/abrasive wear by 50% or more, while bearing combinations such as alumina/alumina and CoCr/CoCr reduce particulates by at least one order of magnitude. Unfortunately, "hard-on-hard" bearings are not available for the knee, and while the use of ceramics, ceramic-metal composites, and advanced UHMWPE holds promise, the advantages seen in the hip are not likely to be realized in the knee. Only time will tell.

Immune Hypersensitivity

Allergy, or, more correctly, immune hypersensitivity to biomaterials, is a much different phenomenon than osteolysis. While osteolysis is visible on radiographs and easily identified during revision surgery, hypersensitivity to biomaterials is often described in terms of "vague pain", "skin rashes", and even more general signs such as fatigue and malaise [75, 76]. Rather than being a local reaction like osteolysis, immune sensitivity may manifest some distance from the implant, and may even demonstrate systemic reactions [77, 78]. As a result, the symptoms of immune hypersensitivity may go unnoticed or be incorrectly interpreted even when present.

At a recent international knee surgery symposium, the attendees were polled to identify those surgeons who had seen an "allergic reaction" in *any* of their arthroplasty patients. The result was an unimpressive 11% positive response [79]. At the same time, one North American prosthesis manufacturer that specializes in ceramic knee implants has suggested that over half of all total knee arthroplasty revisions are due to hypersensitivity to the cobalt-chromium alloy used in the femoral components of the failed knee implants. The difference is substantial, and suggests the controversy that exists regarding biomaterial allergy. With regard to joint arthroplasty in general and total knee arthroplasty in particular, five questions must be considered with regard to material immune hypersensitivity. First, does immune hypersensitivity to contemporary biomaterials actually exist? Second, is it a significant problem? Third, if it does exist, can it be tested for in a reliable manner? Fourth, are there any treatments for the condition? Finally, are there alternative materials which will not cause immune hypersensitivity reactions?

Part of the confusion and controversy involving immune hypersensitivity to orthopedic biomaterials relates to older ideas about the nature of "allergic reactions". Adverse cardiovascular reactions to methacrylate monomer, for example, were mistakenly referred to as allergic reactions to the cement [22]. However, such reactions are toxic in nature, not immune related. Hypersensitivity reactions are related to the normal immune responses to foreign substances, such as bacteria, that might be harmful. These processes may also, for example, be turned against the host organism itself in a pathological manner, causing autoimmune conditions such as rheumatoid arthritis.

Hypersensitivity reactions have been divided into four types depending on the kind of response involved. The first three types of reaction involve an antibody-mediated response and are often termed "humeral responses". Type I reactions involve the interactions of the antigenic material with immunoglobulins of the class IgE. The antibodies then attach to a variety of host cells, releasing several vasoactive agents such as histamine and serotonin. The reaction generally requires some form of previous exposure to the antigen to sensitize the host and is rapid, manifesting symptoms within a few minutes to a few hours. Allergic rhinitis, "hay fever," is a typical type I reaction. With regard to biomaterials, documented type I reactions are rare, with the exception of some cases of dermal sensitivity to metals such as nickel that may be used in some alloys such as 316L stainless steel, or as unwanted trace elements in Ti-6Al-4V alloy. Type I reactions to silicone plastics have been reported but are controversial for a variety of economic and medico-legal reasons. Type II reactions are similar to type I but involve IgG or IgM as the mediator. This type of reaction to orthopedic biomaterials has never been fully documented and needs little additional discussion. Type III reactions are commonly termed "immune complex diseases" and occur when quantities of antigen and antibody are in circulation together. These form large complexes of material that lodge in vessel walls, leading to further damage. As with type II reactions, this type of response has not been shown in relation to orthopedic biomaterials.

Type IV reactions are the type generally associated with material hypersensitivity and involve a complex series of steps that elicit a T-cell response to the antigen, rather than an antibody response, hence the term "cellular response". The classic example of this form of hypersensitivity is contact dermatitis.

Type IV reactions to orthopedic materials including metals, acrylics, and silicones are well documented in the literature [3, 80]. As these materials degrade, the reaction products: particulates, oxides, insoluble salts, and free metal ions, rapidly interact with host proteins in a process known as haptenization. The combination of protein and degradation product may become immunogenic, eliciting a type IV, T-cell-mediated response. These reactions vary significantly from individual to individual as well as from one material to another.

Nickel has long been known as a cause of allergic dermatitis, with approximately 11%-14% of individuals in the

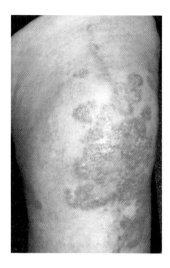

Fig. 55-8. Shortly after surgery for rheumatoid arthritis, a 56-year-old secretary began to show changes in the skin over her knee. Three years later, a skin biopsy was required to distinguish this case of immune hypersensitivity to the cobalt in her prostheses from psoriatic arthritis

U.S. and Canada demonstrating sensitivity [81]. Anecdotally, the problem seems to be more common in women and in industrial areas, possibly indicating some form of sensitization. Cobalt sensitivity has been shown in approximately 1%-2% of the same population, with a significant degree of cross-reactivity between the two metals [82]. There have also been reports of dermal sensitivity to many other metals including chromium, beryllium, and vanadium [83, 84].

The first report of such a reaction to an orthopedic implant was published in 1966 and described an eczematous rash over a stainless steel fracture plate [85]. The rash resolved only after the fracture healed and the plate was removed. Since that time numerous reports have documented similar observations, with symptoms of discomfort, erythema, swelling, and skin changes in the general area of the implant [86]. In addition, some patients report a general malaise, fatigue, or weakness. While such findings have been described in association with polymers, particularly acrylics and silicones, the majority are related to metal implants, and in particular, those of the "reactive metals" nickel and cobalt [87] (Fig. 55-8).

On the other hand, three "orthopedic metals" in particular appear to be nearly inert, with regard to both dermal and implant reactivity. Titanium (Fig. 55-9) has a very low incidence of immune hypersensitivity, and the cases that have been reported have almost always described either alloys containing vanadium, a relatively high concentration of nickel contaminates, or both [88]. Tantalum has been reported only once as the cause of an allergic response [89], and the surgical clips suspected of causing the symptoms were not analyzed after removal for the presence of nickel or other reactive metals. Finally, zirconium has never been reported to induce immune reactions.

Accepting the existence of immune hypersensitivity to implanted orthopedic materials, the surgeon must consider whether the problem is of clinical significance.

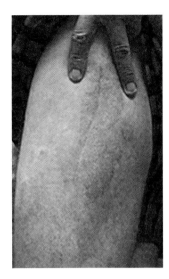

◘ Fig. 55-9. This 53-year-old telephone lineman sustained a hip fracture in a 6-m fall. The fracture was fixed with a titanium screw and side plate. Within a week he began to show skin changes consisting of a weeping, erythematous rash and extreme pruritis. After the fracture healed the plate and screws were removed, and analysis showed a nickel content at the upper limit of the A.S.T.M. standard. His symptoms resolved within days of implant removal

Certainly the incidence of reactions to implanted materials does not match the 11% rate of dermal sensitivity to nickel, possibly approaching just 1% of the population, but several other factors must be considered. First, most individuals who complain of nickel allergy relate the manifestations to "cheap jewelry," and orthopedic devices certainly do not fit this description. Second, implants such as fracture fixation devices can be removed once their job is done. In such cases the small risk of sensitivity is far outweighed by the benefits of surgery. However, the risk must be considered seriously for individuals with a strong history of dermal sensitivity undergoing permanent placement of orthopedic implants such as knee arthroplasty components. If such a risk to a patient exists, can it be identified preoperatively in a reliable manner? The simple answer is, "Not yet."

Skin testing as currently performed is unreliable for several reasons. Usually, the patient is asked to wear a small billet of metal against the skin for a few days to a week, and the test is positive if the area becomes erythematous. However, the conditions under a skin patch are very different from that inside the body. In addition, the skin is an excellent barrier, effectively sealing the immune system from contact with the outside world. A much better surface for allergy testing would be the use of a mucous membrane such as the oral cavity [90-94], but placement and maintenance of test samples would be difficult, and they would still not have the same environment of proteins, cellular elements, and pH of the knee joint. Lacking the ability to actually implant a piece of the test material on the joint surface, recent studies have centered on the development of in vitro testing methods [95-98].

In a recent, comprehensive review, Hallab and his colleagues described four different in vitro tests for metal sensitivity, all based on inhibition of leukocyte migration [3]. Unfortunately, all were investigational with, as yet, limited clinical application, and none were termed reli-

able. In the author's institution a different in vitro method based on leukocyte stimulation and proliferation remains investigational but promising. Unfortunately, the issue of material hypersensitivity is most often addressed retrospectively, after the patient has already manifested symptoms of an immune response. With regard to knee arthroplasty, these symptoms often resemble infection with peri-incisional erythema, urticaria, effusion, and pain. However, the infection workup is negative, with the joint fluid showing few white cell elements. The diagnosis then becomes one of exclusion, usually with a disgruntled patient and a very frustrated surgeon.

Short of revision surgery, totally removing the insulting materials, there are few options. Allergy medications are ineffective in relieving symptoms as they are directed at treating a type I reaction, such as preventing histamine release, not T-cell responses. Low-dose corticosteroids may be used in making the diagnosis as an immune suppressive but have too many side effects for long-term use. Fortunately, there are biomaterial options that exist for the knee arthroplasty patient that may make it possible for most patients with material hypersensitivity to benefit from knee arthroplasty.

If the adverse reaction is to acrylic, the obvious solution is to choose a prosthesis which uses biological fixation [99]. Such implants experienced considerable popularity in the 1990s and are still available from many manufacturers. Options also exist for the metal allergy patient. Ceramics are among the least reactive biomaterials, and ceramic femoral components for knee replacement surgery have been available for some time in Europe and Japan. Some designs are currently under evaluation by the Food and Drug Administration and may soon be available in the United States. When combined with "all-polyethylene" tibial and patellar components, metal can be totally eliminated from the knee replacement.

To further increase the options available to the surgeon, a new material, Oxinium (Smith and Nephew, Memphis, TN), has been introduced which has the hypoallergenic properties of ceramics without their adverse material properties and high cost. Oxinium is a very interesting material in which a base of 97.5% zirconium/2.5% niobium is surface-oxidized, forming a metal/ceramic composite. A recent comparison of femoral implants of Oxinium with those of alumina and zirconia ceramics (◘ Fig. 55-10a and b) showed no difference in immune response, including revision cases in which the Oxinium implants replaced ceramic components originally placed for reasons of metal allergy [100].

Finally, several studies have shown that immune hypersensitivity to implanted biomaterials is higher in individuals with failed joint prostheses than those with stable implants [101-108]. The obvious question, then, is do failing or loose implants stimulate the immune system to generate this response, or do some patients have a pre-

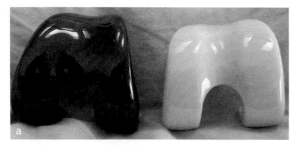
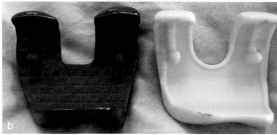

■ **Fig. 55-10a,b.** An Oxinium (Smith and Nephew, Memphis, TN) and custom alumina ceramic (Kyocera, Inc., Kyoto, Japan) femoral component used for total knee replacement in patients with immune hypersensitivity to more conventional materials (*a*). Design limitations (lack of interior texture, need for buttressing of the lugs) imposed by the material properties of the ceramic are clearly visible (*b*)

existing sensitivity that leads to implant failure? If the first is the case, it may soon be possible to modify the immune response by the use of medications, gene therapy, or other means, so that such processes as osteolysis and material hypersensitivity can be limited [109]. On the other hand, it may also be possible in the near future to determine which materials are appropriate for each individual patient so that the immune response is never provoked. Such an integration of material science with immunology can only serve to improve knee arthroplasty surgery in the years to come.

References

1. Bauer TW, Schils J (1999) The pathology of total joint arthroplasty. II. Mechanisms of implant failure. Skeletal Radiol 28:483-497
2. Jacobs JJ, Roebuck KA, Archibeck M, Hallab NJ, Glant TT (2001) Osteolysis: basic science. Clin Orthop 393:71-77
3. Hallab N, Jacobs JJ, Black (2000)J Hypersensitivity to metallic biomaterials: a review of leukocyte migration inhibition assays. Biomaterials 21:1301-1314
4. Coury J, Levy RJ, McMillin, et al (1996) Degradation of materials in the biological environment. In: Ratner BD, Hoffman AS, Schoen FJ, Lemons JE (eds) Biomaterials science, an introduction to materials in medicine. Academic, San Diego, CA, pp 243-281
5. Merritt K, Brown SA, Sharkey NA (1984) The binding of metal salts and corrosion products to cells and proteins in vitro. J Biomed Mater Res 18:1005-1015
6. Charnley J (1979) Low friction arthroplasty of the hip. Springer-Verlag, Berlin Heidelberg New York
7. Black J (1984) Systemic effects of biomaterials. Biomaterials 5:11-18
8. Boynton EL, Henry M, Morton J, Waddell JP (1995) The inflammatory response to particulate wear debris in total hip Arthroplasty. Can J Surg 38:507-515
9. Ollier LEX (1872) Greffes cutanees ou autoplastiques. Bull Acad de Med Paris 2:1, R413
10. Hey-Groves EW (1923) Arthroplasty. Br J Surg 11:234
11. Hey-Groves EW (1927) Some contributions to the reconstructive surgery of the hip. Br J Surg 14:486
12. LeVay D (1990) Implants in orthopaedic surgery. In: LeVay D (ed) The history of orthopaedics. Parthenon, Park Ridge, IL
13. Zierold AA (1924) Reaction of bone to various metals. Arch Surg 9:365
14. Howmedica, Inc. (1995) Strength for life: the Vitallium alloy story (monograph) . Pfizer Hospital Products Group, Rutherford, N.J.
15. Walker PS (1977) Historical development of artificial joints. In: Walker PS (ed) Human joints and their artificial replacements. Charles C. Thomas, Springfield, IL
16. Williams DF, Roaf R (1973) Implants in surgery. W.B. Saunders, London
17. Donati ME, Savarino L, Granachi D, Ciapetti G, Cervallati M, Rotini R, Rizzoferrato A (1998) The effects of metal corrosion debris on immune system cells. Chir Organi Mov 83:387-393
18. Doorn P, Campbell P, Worral J, et al (1998) Metal wear particle characterization from metal on metal total hip replacements: transmission electron microscopy study of periprosthetic tissues and isolated particles. J Biomed Mater Res 42:103-111
19. Judet J, Judt R, Legrange L, Dunoyer J (1954) Resection reconstruction of the hip. Arthroplasty with acrylic prosthesis. E. & S. Livingstone, Edinburgh
20. Harboush EJ (1953) A new operation for arthroplasty of the hip. Bull Hosp Joint Dis NY 14:242
21. Charnley J (1964) Bonding of prostheses to bone by cement. J Bone Joint Surg [Br] 46:518
22. Charnley J (1970) Acrylic cement in orthopaedic surgery. William and Wilkins, Baltimore
23. Bain AM (1973) Replacement of the knee joint with the Walldius prosthesis using cement fixation. Clin Orthop 94:65-71
24. Convery FR, Beber CA (1973) Total knee arthroplasty. Clin Orthop 94:42-49
25. Girzadas DV, Geens S, Clayton ML, Leidholt JD (1968) Performance of a hiinged metal knee prosthesis. J Bone Joint Surg [Am] 50:355-364
26. Gunston FH (1971) Polycentric knee arthroplasty. Prosthetic simulation of normal knee movement. J Bone Joint Surg [Am] 53:272-277
27. Gunston FH, MacKenzie RI (1976) Complications of polycentric knee arthroplasty. Clin Orthop 120:11-17
28. Campbell P, Ma S, Yeom B, et al (1995) Isolation of predominantly submicron-sized UHMWPE wear particles from periprosthetic tissues. J Biomed Mater Res 29:127-131
29. Jacobs JJ, Shanbhag A, Glant TT, Black J, Galante JO (1994) Wear debris in total joint replacements. J Am Acad Orthop Surg 2:212-220
30. Margevicius KJ, Bauer TW, McMahon JT, Brown SA, Merritt K (1994) Isolation and characterization of debris in membranes around total joint prostheses. J. Bone Joint Surg [Am] 76:1664-1675
31. Amstutz HCA, Campbell P, Kossovsky N, Clarke IC (1992) Mechanisms and clinical significance of wear debris-induced osteolysis. Clin Orthop 276:7-18
32. Aspenberg P, Van der Vis H (1998) Migration, particles and fluid pressure: a discussion of causes of prosthetic loosening. Clin Orthop 352:75-80
33. Aspenberg P (1998) Wear and osteolysis in total joint replacements. Acta Orthop Scand 69:435-436
34. Harris WH (1995) The problem is osteolysis. Clin Orthop 311:46
35. Jasty MJ, Floyd WE III, Schiller AL, Goldring SR, Harris WH (1986) Localized osteolysis in stable, non-septic total hip replacement. J Bone Joint Surg [Am] 68:912-919
36. Maloney WJ, Smith RL, Schmalzried TP, Chiba J, Huene D, Rubash H (1995) Isolation and characterization of wear particles generated in patients who have had failure of a hip arthroplasty without cement. J Bone Joint Surg [Am] 77:1301-1310
37. Zicat B, Engh CA, Gokcen E (1995) Patterns of osteolysis around total hip components inserted with and without cement. J Bone Joint Surg [Am] 77:432-439
38. Goodman SB, Huie P, Song Y, Schurman D, Malondy W, Woolson S, Sibley R (1998) Cellular profile and cytokine production at prosthetic interfaces. Study of tissues retrieved from revised hip and knee replacements. J Bone Joint Surg [Br] 80:531-539

55

39. Lind M, Trindade MC, Yaszay B, Goodman SB, Smith RL (1998) Effects of particulate debris on macrophage-dependent fibroblast stimulation in coculture. J Bone Joint Surg [Br] 80:924-930

40. Maloney WJ, Smith RL, Castro F, Schurman DJ (1993) Fibroblast response to metallic debris in vitro: enzyme induction, cell proliferation, and toxicity. J Bone Joint Surg [Am] 75:835-844

41. Shanbhag AS, Macaulay W, Stefanovic-Racic M, Rubash HE (1998) Nitric oxide release by macrophages in response to particulate wear debris. J Biomed Mater Res 41:497-503

42. Watkins SC, Macaulay W, Turner D, Kang R, Rubash HE, Evans CH (1997) Identification of inducible nitric oxide synthase in human macrophages surrounding loosened hip prostheses. Am J Pathol 150:1199-1206

43. Wooley PH, Nasser S, Fitzgerald RH Jr (1996) The immune response to implant materials in humans. Clin Orthop 326:63-70

44. Vronov I, Santerre JP, Hinek A, Callahan JW, Sandhu J, Boynton EL (1998) Macrophage phagocytosis of polyethylene particulate in vitro. J Biomed Mater Res 39:40-51

45. Cardona MA, Simmons RL, Kaplan SS (1992) TNF and IL-1 generation by human monocytes in response to biomaterials. J Biomed Mater Res 26:851-859

46. Ingham E, Green TR, Stone MH, Kowalski R, Watkins N, Fisher J (2000) Production of TNF-alpha and bone resorbing activity by macrophages in response to different types of bone cement particles. Biomaterials 21:1005-1013

47. Nathan CF (1987) Secretory products of macrophages. J Clin Invest 79:319-326

48. Nakashima Y, Sun DH, Trindade MC, Maloney WJ, Goodman SB, Schurman DJ, Smith RL (1999) Signaling pathways for tumor necrosis factor-alpha and interleukin-6 expression in human macrophages exposed to titanium-alloy particulate debris in vitro. J Bone Joint Surg [Am] 81:603-615

49. Jiranek WA, Machado M, Jasty M, Jevsevar D, Wolfe HJ, Goldring SR, Goldberg MJ, Harris WH (1993) Production of cytokines around loosened cemented acetabular components. Analysis with immunohistochemical techniques and in situ hybridization. J Bone Joint Surg [Am] 75:863-879

50. Baron R, Raves J, Ravesloot L, Neff M, Chakraborty D, Chatterjee A, Lomri A, Horne W (1993) Cellular and molecular biology of the osteoclast. In: Noda M (ed) Cellular and molecular biology of bone. Academic, New York, pp 446-484

51. Rifas L (1999) Bone and cytokines: beyond IL-1, IL-6 and TNF-alpha. Calcif Tissue Int 64:1-7

52. Kurosaka K, Watanabe N, Kobayashi Y (2001) Production of proinflammatory cytokines by resident tissue macrophages after phagocytosis of apoptotic cells. Cell Immunol 211:1-7

53. Pandey R, Quinn J, Joyner C, Murray DW, Triffitt JT, Athanasou NA (1996) Arthroplasty implant biomaterial particle associated macrophages differentiate into lacunar bone resorbing cells. Ann Rheum Dis 55:388-395

54. Shanbhag AS, Jacobs JJ, Black J, Galante JO, Glant TT (1994) Macrophage/particle interactions: effect on size, composition and surface area. J Biomed Mater Res 28:81-90

55. Yang SY, Ren W, Park Y, Sieving A, Hsu S, Nasser S, Wooley PH (2002) Diverse cellular and apoptopic responses to variant shapes of UHMWPE particles in a murine model of inflmmation. Biomaterials 23:3535-3543

56. Gelb H, Schumacher HR, Cuckler J, Ducheyne R, Baker DG (1994) In vivo inflammatory response to polymethylmethacrylate particulate debris: effect of size, morphology, and surface area. J Orthop Res 12:83-92

57. Green TR, Fisher J, Stone M, Wroblewski BM, Ingham E (1998) Polyethylene particles of a "critical size" are necessary for the induction of cytokines by macrophages in vitro. Biomaterials 19:2297-2302

58. Rao SK, Shirata KS, Furukawa T, Ushida T, Tateishi T, Kanazawa M, Katsube S, Janna S (1999) Evaluation of cytotoxicity of UHMWPE wear debris. Biomed Mater Eng 9:209-217

59. Santavirta S, Nordstrom D, Metsarinne K, et al (1993) Biocompatibility of polyethylene and host response to loosening of cementless total hip replacement. Clin Orthop 297:100-110

60. Horowitz SM, Luchetti WT, Gonzales JB, Ritchie CK (1998) The effects of cobalt chromium upon macrophages. J Biomed Mater Res 41:468-473

61. Shanbhag AS, Jacobs JJ, Black J, Galante JO, Glant TT (1995) Human monocyte response to particulate biomaterials generated in vivo and in vitro. J Orthop Res 13:792-801

62. Gonzalez O, Smith RL, Goodman SB (1996) Effect of size, concentration, surface area, and volume of polymethylmethacrylate particles on human macrophages in vitro. J Biomed Mater Res 30:463-473

63. Lee SH, Brennan FR Jacobs JJ, Urban RM, Ragasa DR, Glant TT (1997) Human monocyte/macrophage response to cobalt-chromium corrosion products and titanium particles in patients with total joint replacements. J Orthop Res 15:40-49

64. Shanbhag AS, Jacobs JJ, Glant TT, Gilbert JL, Black JM, Galante JO (1994) Composition and morphology of wear debris in failed uncemented total hip replacement. J Bone Joint Surg [Am] 76:60-67

65. Howling GI, Barnett PI, Tipper JL, Stone MH, Fisher J, Ingham E (2001) Quantitative characterization of polyethylenbe debris isolated from periprosthetic tissue in early failure knee implants and early and late failure Charnley hip implants. J Biomed Mater Res 58:415-420

66. Shanbhag AS, Bailey HO, Hwang S, Cha CW, Eror NG, Rubash HE (2000) Quantitative analysis of ultrahigh molecular weight polyethylene (UHMWPE) wear debris associated with total knee replacements. J Biomed Mater Res 53:100-110

67. Hirakawa K, Bauer TW, Stulberg BM, Wilde AH, Borden LS (1996) Characterization of debris adjacent to failed knee implants of 3 different designs. Clin Orthop 331:151-158

68. Kadoya Y, Kobayashi A, Ohashi H (1998) Wear and osteolysis in total joint replacements. Acta Orthop Scand [Suppl] 278:1-16

69. Magnissalis EA, Eliades G, Eliades T (1999) Multitechnique characterization of articular surface of retrieved ultra high molecular weight polyethylene acetabular sockets. J Biomed Mater Res 48:365-373

70. Nasser S, Campbell PA, Kilgus DJ, Kossovsky N, Amstutz HC (1990) Cementless total joint arthroplasty prostheses with titanium alloy articular surfaces: a human retrieval analysis. Clinical Orthop 261:171-185

71. McKellop H, Park SH, Chiesa R, Doorn P, Lu B, Normand P, Grigoris P, Amstutz HC (1996) In vivo wear of three types of metal on metal hip prostheses during two decades of use. Clin Orthop 329 [Suppl]: S128-S140

72. Kadoya Y, Revell PA, Kabayashi A, al Saffar N, Scott G, Freeman MA (1997) Wear particulate species and bone loss in failed total joint arthroplasties. Clin Orthop 340:118-129

73. Van der Vis HM, Aspenberg P, Marti RK, et al (1998) Fluid pressure causes bone resorption in a rabbit model of prosthetic loosening. Clin Orthop 350:201-208

74. Niedzwiecki S, Klapperich C, Short J, Jani S, Pruitt L (2001) Comparison of three joint simulator wear debris isolation techniques: acid digestion, base digestion, and enzyme cleavage. J Biomed Mater Res 56:245-249

75. Merle C, Vigan M, Devred D, Girardin P, Adessi B, Laurent R (1992) Generalized eczema from vitallium osteosynthesis material. Contact Dermatitis 27:257-258

76. Mayor MB, Merritt K, Brown SA (1980) Metal allergy and the surgical patient. Am J Surg 139:477-479

77. Merritt K (1996) Systemic toxicity and hypersensitivity in biomaterials science. In: Ratner BD, Hoffman AS, Schoen FJ, Lemons JE (eds) Biomaterials science, an introduction to materials in medicine. Academic, San Diego, CA, pp 188-193

78. Merritt K, Brown SA (1996) Distribution of cobalt chromium wear and corrosion products and biologic reactions. Clin Orthop 329:S233-S243

79. Nasser S (2002) Immune hypersensitivity to orthopaedic biomaterials. Proc. of the Smith and Nephew 12th Annual International Knee Meeting, Rome, October 2-6, 2002. Smith & Nephew, Memphis, TN

80. Allardice JT (1967) Dermatitis due to an acrylic resin sealer. Trans A Rep St. John's Hosp Derm Soc Lond 53:86

81. Gawkrodger DJ (1993) Nickel sensitivity and the implantation of orthopaedic prostheses. Contact Dermatitis 28:257-259

82. Griem P, von Vultee C, Panthel K, Best SL, Sadler PJ, Shaw CF 3rd (1998) T cell cross-reactivity to heavy metals: identical cryptic peptides may be presented from protein exposed to different metals. Eur J Immunol 28:1941-1947

83. Hallab NJ, Jacobs JJ, Skipor A, Black J, Mikecz K, Galante J (2000) Systemic metal-protein binding associated with total joint replacement arthroplasty. J Biomed Mater Res 49:353-361

84. Jacobs JJ, Gilbert JL, Urban RM (1994) Corrosion of metallic implants. In: Stauffer RM (ed) Advances in operative orthopedics, vol 2. Mosby, St. Louis, pp 279-319

85. Foussereau J, Laugier P (1966) Allergic eczemas from metallic foreign bodies. Trans St. Johns Hosp Derm Soc 52:220-225

86. Halpin DS (1975) An unusual reaction in muscle in association with a Vitallium plate: a report of possible metal hypersensitivity. J Bone Joint Surg [Br] 57:451-453

87. Rooker GD, Wilkinson JD (1980) Metal sensitivity in patients undergoing hip replacement: a prospective study. J Bone Joint Surg [Br] 62:502-505

88. Moulon C, Vollmer J, Weltzien HU (1995) Characterization of processing requirements and metal cross-reactivities in T-cell clones from patients with allergic contact dermatitis to nickel. Eur J Immunol 25:3308-3315

89. King I Jr, Fransway A, Adkins RB (1993) Chronic urticaria due to surgical clips [letter]. N Engl J Med 329:1583-1584

90. Fisher AA (1956) Allergic sensitization of the skin and oral mucosa to acrylic denture materials. J Prosthet Dent 6:593

91. Velen NK, Svejaard E, Menne T (1979) In vitro lymphocyte transformation to nickel: a study of nickel-sensitive patients before and after epicutaneous and oral challenge with nickel. Acta Derm Venereol 59:447-451

92. Spiechowicz E, Glantz PO, Axell R, Chmielewski W (1984) Oral exposure to a nickel-containing dental alloy of persons with hypersensitive skin reactions to nickel. Contact Dermatitis 10:206-211

93. Hubler WR Jr, Hubler WR Sr (1983) Dermatitis from a chromium dental plate. Contact Dermatitis 9:377-383

94. Vilaplana J, Romaguera C, Cornellana F (1994) Contact dermatitis and adverse oral mucus membrane reactions related to the use of dental prostheses. Contact Dermatitis 30:80-84

95. Schor SL, Allen TD, Winn B (1983) Lymphocyte migration into three-dimensional collagen matrices: a quantitative study. J Cell Biol 96:1089-1096

96. Nelson RD, Quie PG, Simmons RL (1975) Chemotaxis under agarose: a new and simple method for measuring chemotaxis and spontaneous migraton of human polymorphonuclear leukocytes and monocytes. J Immunol 115:1650-1656

97. Soborg M, Bendixen G (1967) Human lymphocyte migration as a parameter of hypersensitivity. Acta Med Scand 181:247-256

98. Pizzoferrato A, Ciapetti, G, Stea S, Cenni E, Arciola CR, Granchi D, Savarino L (1994) Cell culture methods for testing biocompatibility. Clin Mater 15:173-190

99. Chadha HS, Wooley PH, Sud S, Fitzgerald RH Jr (1995) Cellular proliferation and cytokine responses to polymethylmethacrylate particles in patients with a cemented total joint arthroplasty. Inflamm Res 44:145-151

100. Nasser S, Wooley PA (2005) Comparison of ceramic and oxinium total knee femoral components in patients with cobalt-chrome hypersensitivity. Proc. of the Mid-America Orthopaedic Society 23rd Annual Meeting, Amelia Island, FL, April 20-24, 2005 (to be published)

101. Brown GC, Lockshin MD, Salvati EA, Bullough PG (1977) Sensitivity to metal as a possible cause of sterile loosening after cobalt-chromium total hip replacement arthroplasty. J Bone Joint Surg [Am] 59:164-168

102. Deutman R, Mulder TJ, Brian R, Nater JP (1977) Metal sensitivity before and after total hip arthroplasty. J Bone Joint Surg [Am] 59:862-865

103. Elves MW, Wilson JN, Scales JT, Kemp HB (1975) Incidence of metal sensitivity in patients with total joint replacements. Br Med J 4:376-378

104. Granchi D, Ciapett G, Stea S, Cavedagna D, Bettini N, Blanco T, Fontanesi G, Pizzoferrato A (1995) Evaluation of several immunological parameters in patients with aseptic loosening of hip arthroplasty. Chir Organi Mov 80:399-408

105. Merritt K, Rodrigo JJ (1996) Immune response to synthetic materials: sensitization of patients receiving orthopaedic implants. Clin Orthop 326:71-79

106. Wooley PH, Fitzgerald RH, Song Z, Davis P, Whalen JD, Trumble S, Nasser S (1999) Antibodies to implant-bound proteins in patients with aseptic loosening of total joint arthroplasty: a preliminary report. J Bone Joint Surg [Am] 81: 616-621

107. Wooley PH, Petersen S, Song S, Nasser S (1997) Cellular immune responses to orthopaedic implant material following cemented total joint replacement. J Orthop Res 15:874-880

108. Yang J, Merritt K (1994) Detection of antibodies against corrosion products in patients after CoCr total joint replacements. J Biomed Mater Res 28:1249-1258

109. Horowitz SM, Alkgan SA, Purdon MA (1996) Pharmacologic inhibition of particulate induced bone resorption. J Biomed Mater Res 31:9196

56   Conventional and Cross-Linked Polyethylene Properties

L. A. Pruitt

Summary

Highly cross-linked ultra high-molecular-weight polyethylene has shown great promise as an orthopedic bearing in total hip replacements. However, the enhanced resistance to plastic deformation that benefits wear behavior comes at the expense of other mechanical properties.
Ultimate tensile strength, ductility, modulus, toughness,
and crack propagation resistance are degraded at high
cross-linking doses. The degradation in fracture properties indicates that highly cross-linked polyethylene
should not be used in applications where high stresses are
expected. Lower degrees of cross-linking may be more
appropriate when designing for both wear and fatigue in
total joint replacements.

Table 56-1. Physical properties of conventional (unirradiated) GUR 1050. Mechanical properties are taken from engineering stress-strain plots. (Adapted from [1])

Physical property	GUR 1050
Molecular weight	3-6 million g/mol
Crystallinity	45-50%
Density	0.93-0.935
Ultimate tensile strength (21°C)	42-44 MPa
Ultimate tensile strength (37°C)	36 MPa
Yield strength (21°C)	20-23 MPa
Yield strength (37°C)	21 MPa
Elastic modulus (21°C)	1.0-1.39 GPa
Elastic modulus (37°C)	0.67 GPa
Elongation at break (21°C)	330%
Elongation at Break (37°C)	375%
Shore D Hardness (21°C)	60-65

Introduction

Ultra high-molecular-weight polyethylene (UHMWPE) has been used as the bearing surface in total joint arthro-plasty for over four decades. UHMWPE was originally chosen for this application because it offers unique prop-erties including exceptional toughness, good wear resis-tance, a low friction coefficient, and biocompatibility. These properties are a result of the molecular structure of UHMWPE. In its conventional form the material is not cross-linked, but the polymer has exceptional mechani-cal integrity owing to its chain entanglements, high tie molecule density, moderate crystallinity, and very high molecular weight [1]. A summary of the physical proper-ties of conventional UHMWPE is provided in Table 56-1. Surface damage resulting from articulation and high con-tact stresses of UHWMPE remains the limiting factor for the longevity of the joint replacement. Over time in vivo, accumulated damage to the polymer implant results in debris formation. This polymer debris can lead to in-flammation, foreign-body response, and the need for re-vision surgery.

Conventional UHMWPE is generated from the poly-merization of ethylene gas into a fine powder that is con-solidated under elevated pressure and above its melt tem-perature, using compression molding or ram-extrusion processes. Orthopedic components such as tibial plateaus or acetabular cups are typically machined from this stock material or molded directly into the final shape and subse-quently sterilized prior to implantation. Sterilization of conventional polyethylene is typically done with ethylene oxide gas, ionizing irradiation, or plasma treatment. Until 1995, the majority of orthopedic companies sterilized their devices with gamma irradiation in the presence of air at a dose of 25-40 kGy. By 1998, sterilization had shifted to non-ionizing techniques or irradiation in low oxygen environ-ments This change was prompted by scientific evidence that ionizing irradiation in the presence of oxygen results in a time-dependent process known as shelf aging that is accompanied by chain scission, loss of molecular weight, increased crystallinity, oxidation, and a concomitant de-crease in mechanical properties [2]. This shelf-aging prob-lem plagued the orthopedics community for a number years. Retrieved devices that had been sterilized by gamma irradiation in air showed evidence of pitting, delamina-tion, subsurface oxidation, and fatigue cracking. However, gamma-sterilized UHMWPE was used for many years and a plethora of literature is available for UHMWPE sterilized with ionizing irradiation; thus it remains a "gold standard" for comparison to material improvements to this polymer [3]. "Conventional" UHMWPE can refer to UHMWPE sterilized by non-ionizing treatments such as EtO or gas plasma, or it can refer to UHMWPE sterilized via low doses of gamma irradiation. In general, "conventional" polyethylene refers to this polymer in the non-cross-linked form.

Recent advances improving the performance of this polymer have focused around creating a highly cross-linked structure to improve its wear resistance in total joint replacements [4-6]. Cross-linking is obtained by exposing the polymer to high doses of gamma irradiation or e-beam irradiation along with a thermal treatment that can be done below or above the melt temperature. Commercially, cross-linked UHMWPE materials range in doses of 40-100 kGy, and these treatments can be followed by heating the material above its melt temperature (135°C) or annealing the polymer below its melt temperature. The thermal processing annihilates free radicals and completes the cross-linking step to prevent time-dependent oxidation of the polymer. The coupled effects of cross-linking and thermal treatments can have considerably different effects on the polymer microstructure and mechanical properties [7, 8].

Cross-linking of the molecular chains in UHMWPE has been shown to dramatically reduce the abrasive and adhesive wear in several in vitro joint simulator studies [4-6]. It has been speculated that cross-linking the polymer enhances the resistance to plastic flow and lamellae alignment at the articulating surface, resulting in better resistance to wear [9,10]. Muratoglu et al. [4] and McKellop et al. [5] have shown that wear rates decrease dramatically with irradiation dose and begin to saturate at a dose of about 150 kGy. However, cross-linking procedures inherently alter the polymer structure and the mechanical properties of UHMWPE. Recent studies [11-20] have shown that high degrees of cross-linking in UHMWPE result in a reduction of several important mechanical properties including strength, ductility, elastic modulus, toughness, and crack propagation resistance. The long-term clinical implications of such changes for mechanical properties remain unknown. The aim of this chapter is to provide a comparison of mechanical properties for conventional and highly cross-linked polyethylene. The mechanical properties discussed include the quasi-static tensile and compressive properties, fracture toughness, and fatigue resistance. The findings in this review will be discussed in the context of total joint replacement.

Mechanical Properties of Conventional and Cross-linked Polyethylene

Quasi-Static Tensile and Compressive Properties

Uniaxial quasi-static mechanical properties are important parameters for UHMWPE. These properties are the basis of comparison for UHMWPE materials with various process conditions, cross-link dosages, thermal treatments, and sterilization protocols. All UHMWPE materials used in total joint replacements must adhere to strict national (ASTM) and international (ISO) requirements, which designate acceptable ranges of yield strength, elastic modulus, ultimate strength, ductility, and impact resistance [3]. A complicating factor in such evaluations is that many researchers utilize engineering stress-strain behavior to assess such mechanical properties. While such measurements are easily obtained, the engineering stress-strain curves do not fully capture the yielding and plastic flow behavior of UHMWPE. Kurtz and co-workers [8, 9, 11] have been instrumental in establishing formal protocols for assessing true stress-strain curves in UHMWPE. Not only are these measured properties more appropriate for comparison purposes; they are also critical for the development of accurate constitutive models.

Kurtz et al. [8] recently examined the role of coupled cross-linking and thermal processing on the uniaxial tensile and compressive properties of UHMWPE. ◘ Table 56-2 summarizes their findings. In this study, two conventional and two highly cross-linked UHMWPE materials were examined. Mechanical properties were assessed at room temperature and at body temperature (37°C). A standard non-irradiated GUR 1050 material represented conventional polyethylene, and that same material subjected to a 30 kGy gamma irradiation dose in an inert (nitrogen) environment represented a sterile version. The two highly cross-linked groups were both irradiated to 100 kGy using gamma irradiation but were post-processed with different thermal treatments. One highly cross-linked group was annealed at 110°C, which is below the melt transition temperature (135°C), and the other group was remelted above the melt transition temperature at 150°C. This enabled the researchers to look at the effects of crystallinity and irradiation dose on mechanical properties. These four groups were tested under uniaxial conditions (in both compression and tension) and over a range of strain rates and temperatures. Their findings revealed that thermal treatment affected crystallinity of the polymer, and that this morphological change affected yielding, flow, and fracture properties of the polymer.

Engineering stress-strain behavior was measured using a nominal reference to the original (undeformed) gauge length and cross-section of the specimen. The equations for engineering stress and engineering strain are as follows:

$$\sigma_e = P/A_o$$
$$\varepsilon_e = (l-l_o)/l_o$$

where P is the uniaxial load, A_o is the original cross-sectional area of the specimen, and l_o and l are the undeformed and final gauge lengths of the specimen. In or-

Table 56-2. Physical properties of conventional and highly-cross-linked GUR 1050. Mechanical properties are taken from engineering and true stress-strain plots. (Adapted from [8])

Property	GUR 1050	30 kGy (N$_2$)	100 kGy (110°C)	100 kGy (150°C)
Crystallinity (%)	50.4 ±3.3	51.3 ±1.0	60.8 ±0.9	45.7 ±0.3
Tensile properties (20°C, 30 mm/min)				
Yield strength (MPa)	23.5 ±0.3	24.1 ±0.14	24.79 ±0.12	21.36 ±0.13
Yield strain (%)	14.4 ±0.6	13.4 ±0.6	12.7 ±0.6	14.5 ±0.9
Ultimate strength (MPa)	50.2 ±1.6	47.1 ±4.2	46.4 ±3.4	37.1 ±3.2
Ultimate strain (%)	421 ±11	373 ±8	248 ±11	232 ±8
True yield stress (MPa)	26.9 ±0.4	27.35 ±0.24	27.94 ±0.10	24.47 ±0.24
True yield strain (%)	0.134 ±0.005	0.126 ±0.005	0.120 ±0.005	0.136 ±0.008
True ultimate stress (MPa)	262 ±12	223 ±22	162 ±16	123 ±13
True ultimate strain (%)	1.65 ±0.02	1.55 ±0.02	1.25 ±0.03	1.20 ±0.02
Compressive properties (20°C, 0.021/s)				
Elastic modulus (MPa)	833.0 ±9.1	932.1 ±21.2	994.3 ±29.2	778.9 ±6.8
Offset yield (MPa)	12.0 ±0.2	12.8 ±0.1	13.2 ±0.1	11.6 ±0.1
Maximum true stress (MPa)	39.6 ±0.1	39.8 ±0.1	40.3 ±0.1	37.2 ±0.1
Maximum true strain (MPa)	0.446 ±0.002	0.444 ±0.003	0.431 ±0.002	0.507 ±0.004
Compressive properties (37°C, 0.021/s)				
Elastic modulus (MPa)	648.2 ±23.5	737.2 ±15.8	771.4 ±30.6	570.0 ±15.2
Offset yield (MPa)	9.7 ±0.2	10.3 ±0.1	10.8 ±0.2	8.8 ±0.1
Maximum true stress (MPa)	35.7 ±0.1	35.6 ±0.4	36.4 ±0.2	32.7 ±0.3
Maximum true strain (MPa)	0.548 ±0.002	0.552 ±0.011	0.529 ±0.051	0.631 ±0.006

der to measure true stress-strain behavior, the current deformed condition must be continually monitored throughout the test. Using assumptions of conservation of volume (incompressibility) the equations for true stress and true strain are given as:

$$\sigma_t = P/A$$
$$\varepsilon_t = \ln(1 + \varepsilon n)$$

where A is the current (deformed) cross-sectional area of the specimen.

Kurtz and co-workers found that under uniaxial tension the highly cross-linked groups exhibited decreases in ultimate strength and strain, ultimate true stress, and ultimate true strain (Table 56-2). They found that enhanced crystallinity brought about through thermal processing increased the yield strength and modulus of the material. Their compression studies revealed that increased temperature resulted in a decrease in elastic modulus, yield strength, and ultimate true stress, and this trend was captured by an Arrhenius model. Their study provided evidence that thermal treatments alter the crystallinity and mechanical behavior of UHMWPE, and that irradiation dose and crystallinity dictate yielding, plastic flow, and ultimate properties of conventional and cross-linked polyethylene.

A recent study by Gomoll et al. investigated the effect of cross-link dose on the mechanical properties of

UHMWPE. In their analysis, they investigated four gamma irradiation dosages (25 kGy, 50 kGy, 100 kGy, and 200 kGy) along with conventional UHMWPE. In their study, all cross-linked materials were subjected to a remelting treatment at 138°C following irradiation (in nitrogen). Uniaxial tests of these materials were performed at room temperature. They found that elastic modulus, ultimate true stress, and ultimate true strain decreased monotonically with irradiation dose. The physical properties of UHMWPE materials as a function of irradiation dose are summarized in Table 56-3. In their study, very little change was noted in crystallinity for the various cross-link dosages. Gomoll et al. attribute the monotonic reduction in elastic modulus with changes in microstructure brought about through cross-linking. They postulate that the reduction in elastic modulus is due to a higher number of smaller fragmented lamellae. The fragmentation of lamellae is believed to reduce the tensile modulus of UHMWPE. This theory is supported by other morphological studies in which transmission electron microscopy of conventional and highly cross-linked UHMWPE showed smaller lamellae with shorter lengths in highly cross-linked materials [11]. In the study by Gomoll et al., the greatest reduction in mechanical properties was found in strain-to-break and ultimate tensile strength properties. These findings indicate that for a given crystallinity, cross-linking results in loss of modulus, strength, and ductility.

Table 56-3. Physical properties of UHMWPE as a function of irirradiation dose. Mechanical properties are taken from true stress-strain plots. Fracture toughness is determined from Rice and Sorenson J-integral method. (Adapted from [14])

Property	GUR 1050	25 kGy	50 kGy	100 kGy	200 kGy
Crystallinity (%)	50.7 ±0.5	45.4 (0.7	46.2 ±0.7	46.9 ±0.8	47.7 ±0.4
Yield stress (MPa)	20.2 ±1.0	19.0 ±0.4	19.9 ±0.8	18.9 ±0.7	21.2 ±1.0
Modulus (MPa)	495 ±56	433 ±14	412 ±50	386 ±23	266 ±30
True stress at break (MPa)	315.5 ±31.6	284.8 ±18	237.6 ±12.3	185.7 ±7.5	126.0 ±14
True strain at break	1.82 ±0.01	1.74 ±0.03	1.59 ±0.01	1.50 ±0.02	1.37 ±0.06
Fracture toughness (J_{IC}, kJ/m^2)	2.1	23.8	76.2	$= J_{SS}$	$= J_{SS}$
Steady-state fracture toughness (J_{SS}, kJ/m^2)	116.9 ±0.1	101.2 ±0.1	98.5 ±0.2	87.6 ±0.1	79.3 ±1.9

Fracture Toughness

Fracture toughness is a mechanical property that describes a material's intrinsic resistance to fracture. There are two basic parameters used to describe fracture toughness: K_{IC} and J_{IC}. The first of these parameters, K_{IC}, is known as the plane strain mode I fracture toughness. The plane strain condition assures that the fracture toughness is independent of material thickness, and mode I refers to a tensile "opening" mode of fracture. K_{IC} is based on a stress intensity factor, K, derived from linear elastic fracture mechanics. This parameter is used to describe the magnitude of the stresses, strains, and displacements in the region ahead of the crack tip. The stress intensity factor can be found for a wide range of specimen types and is used to scale the effect of the far-field load, crack length, and geometry of the flawed component. The basic form of this material property is:

$$K_{IC} = \sigma^\infty \sqrt{a} \cdot Y(a/W)$$

where σ^∞ is the far-field stress, a is the flaw size, and $Y(a/W)$ is the geometric factor for the specimen. When the value of K_I attains a critical value (K_{IC}) unstable crack growth ensues and fast fracture occurs. Thus materials with higher fracture toughness are able to sustain higher stresses for a given flaw size than materials with lower fracture toughness.

The other parameter used to describe fracture toughness is J_{IC}. This parameter utilizes non-linear fracture mechanics (J-integral) to measure the change in energy per unit area of new crack surface for a tensile (mode I) mode of fracture. The J-integral describes the stresses and strains ahead of the crack tip under elastic-plastic conditions. J_{IC} captures the initial crack driving force needed to initiate crack growth (resistance to crack initiation), while a steady-state value of J-integral, J_{SS}, is used to assess the resistance to propagation of the crack. Using a Rice and Sorenson model [14], the J-integral takes the form:

$$J = \alpha \varepsilon_o \sigma_o c h_1(a/b, n)(P/P_o)^m$$

where ε_o and σ_o represent the strain and stress from a power-law fit, strain hardening expression $\varepsilon_o = \alpha \varepsilon_o (\sigma_e/\sigma_o)^n$, with a fitting constant $\alpha \varepsilon_o$. The tensile yield stress is used for σ_o, a is the crack length, b is the distance from the loading line to the free end of the specimen, and c is the uncracked ligament length (b-a). n is the strain hardening exponent, $m = 1/n$, and h_1 is a tabulated function of a/b and n. P is the maximum pin load per unit specimen thickness and P_o is $1.455 \eta c \sigma_o$ where η is a polynomial function of a and c.

As stated above, cross-linking of UHMWPE results in a loss in ultimate strength and ductility. Thus it is expected that cross-linking will also degrade the fracture toughness of UHMWPE. Studies have shown that in conventional polyethylene subjected to uniaxial tensile loading, fracture originates at a single defect [12]. The defect first coalesces in a stable manner and then grows unstably once it attains a critical length. Linear elastic fracture mechanics (LEFM) is utilized to estimate fracture toughness of UHWMPE based on the size of the flaw, location (surface or embedded), and the true ultimate strength of the material. These LEFM concepts have also been used to characterize fracture toughness in highly cross-linked UHMWPE. In this work, Gencur et al. [12] found that the region of stable crack growth was enhanced in the conventional polyethylene. Critical flaws were observed to be circular in cross-section when embedded and semicircular in form when they had initiated at the surface. The same mechanism of fracture, microvoid nucleation, and coalescence was observed in all groups, but the resistance to unstable crack growth was found to be superior in the conventional polyethylene. Their work demonstrated that irradiation dose was linearly related to fracture toughness. A summary of their findings is shown in Table 56-4.

Duus et al. [21] utilized the J integral approach to quantify fracture toughness as a function of irradiation dose. They found a 50% decrease in the J-resistance curve for the highly cross-linked polyethylene (100 kGy) as compared with conventional (25 kGy) polyethylene. Gillis et al. [13] also found a reduction in J-integral fracture toughness with irradiation dose. Similarly Gomoll et al.

□ **Table 56-4.** Fracture properties of conventional and highly-cross-linked GUR 1050. Fracture toughness is calculated using LEFM. (Adapted from [12])

Property	GUR 1050	30 kGy (N2)	100 kGy (110°C)	100 kGy (150°C)
Crystallinity (%)	50.4 ±3.3	51.3±1.0	60.8 ±0.9	45.7 ±0.3
True ultimate stress (MPa)	262 ±12	223 ±22	162 ±16	123 ±13
True ultimate strain (%)	1.65 ±0.02	1.55 ±0.02	1.25 ±0.03	1.20 ±0.02
Fracture toughness K_C (MPa√m)	4.0 ±0.5	4.5 ±0.02	2.8 ±0.4	3.0 ±0.6

[14] utilized the Rice and Sorenson model to measure JIC and JSS for a range of dosages (0 kGy, 25 kGy, 50 kGy, 100 kGy, and 200 kGy). They found that for low dosages (up to 50 kGy) cross-linking benefited JIC and provided more resistance to crack initiation, while steady-state values, JSS, decreased monotonically with irradiation dose. They observed that for 0-50 kGy, UHMWPE exhibited a ductile tearing behavior with stable crack growth, while highly cross-linked polyethylene exhibited spontaneous unstable fracture once JIC was attained. These findings are consistent with the fracture studies performed by Gencur et al. [12]. A summary of the J-integral fracture toughness as a function of irradiation dose is provided in Table 56-3.

Fatigue Resistance

Fatigue resistance of conventional and highly cross-linked polyethylene used in orthopedics is important due to the cyclic nature of the physiological loading and the large values of contact stresses acting along the articulating surface. This is especially important in total knee replacements, where cyclic contact stresses can range from 1-15 MPa in tension to -40 MPa in compression [22]. A complicating factor in the assessment of the fatigue resistance of conventional and cross-linked polyethylene lies in the apparent dichotomy of the results reported in the literature [16-20]. For example, O'Connor et al. reported that no failures were observed in their cross-linked specimens after 20 million fatigue cycles [17], while Baker et al. reported that cross-linking resulted in a significant decrease in the resistance to fatigue crack propagation [20]. The conflicting results from these two studies are due to differences in testing methodology and design philosophy. The O'Connor study utilized a total-life philosophy premised on no initial flaws in the un-notched samples, while the Baker study utilized a defect-tolerant philosophy and notched specimens to measure the material's resistance to fatigue crack propagation. Both studies contribute to our understanding of the material fatigue resistance; however, the philosophical difference between them is critical to the design and prediction of the performance of the orthopedic device. Life predictions based on the results of a total-life study are based on the

assumption that an orthopedic device is initially defect free or that it contains flaws that will spend the majority of their life in the initiation process. A more conservative life prediction is based on a fracture mechanics philosophy that assumes the device contains defects or flaws that are capable of propagation under cyclic loading.

In the total-life philosophy, it is assumed that no flaws pre-exist in the polyethylene materials and that the majority of the fatigue life will be spent in the initiation phase. In total life stress-based fatigue testing, the applied stress, (a, is typically described by the stress amplitude of the loading cycle and is defined as:

$$\sigma_a = \frac{\sigma_{max} - \sigma_{min}}{2}$$

where σ_{max} is the maximum stress and σ_{min} is the minimum stress of the fatigue cycle. The stress amplitude is generally plotted against the number of cycles to failure on a linear-log scale. This plot is termed the S-N plot where S represents the stress amplitude and N denotes the cycles to failure. This process is continued at increasingly smaller values of stress amplitude until an endurance limit is reached. An endurance limit is defined as the stress level that results in 10 million cycles without failure. The assumption is that if the device is exposed to stress values below the endurance limit then the device is safe from fatigue failure. S-N curves enable life to be predicted based on the stress amplitude or range of stress amplitudes that the device is expected to encounter.

In contrast, the defect-tolerant philosophy is based on the implicit assumption that structural components are intrinsically flawed and that the fatigue life is based on propagation of an initial flaw to a critical size. Fracture mechanics is used to characterize the propagation of fatigue cracks in these materials. The stress intensity factor, *K*, derived from linear elastic fracture mechanics, is the parameter used to describe the magnitude of the stresses, strains, and displacements ahead of the crack tip. There are three distinct regimes of crack propagation under constant amplitude cyclic loading conditions (□ Fig. 56-1).

Figure 56-1 schematically illustrates the sigmoidal curve that captures the crack growth rate as a function of

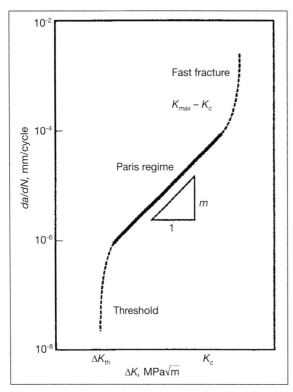

Fig. 56-1. Sigmoidal plot used to measure fatigue crack propagation resistance. Note three regimes (near-threshold, Paris, and fast-fracture) associated with fatigue crack propagation

imentally generated curves where a is plotted as a function of N. The stress intensity factor range, $\Delta K = K_{max} - K_{min}$, which itself captures the far-field stress, crack length, and geometry, is the characteristic driving parameter for fatigue crack propagation. This is known as the Paris law, and it states that da/dN scales with ΔK through the power-law relationship:

$$\frac{da}{dN} = C \cdot \Delta K^m$$

where C and m are material constants. While this linear regime is most often used for life prediction, the fatigue threshold is key for designing against the inception of crack growth.

The Paris law is commonly employed for fatigue life prediction of polymer components that have known stress concentrations or safety-critical applications. It is implied in this defect-tolerant approach that the device or component contains an initial defect or crack size, a_i. Assuming that the fatigue loading is performed under constant stress amplitude conditions, that the geometric factor, $f(\alpha)$, does not change within the limits of integration, and that fracture occurs when the crack reaches a critical value, a_c, one can integrate the Paris equation in order to predict the fatigue life of the component:

$$N_f = \frac{2}{(m-2)C_f(\alpha)^m(\Delta\sigma)^m\pi^{m/2}} \cdot \left[\frac{1}{a_i^{(m-2)/2}} - \frac{1}{a_c^{(m-2)/2}} \right] \text{ for m} \neq 2.$$

stress intensity range (illustrated on log-log scale). The plot captures three distinct regions: the slow crack growth or threshold-regime, the intermediate crack growth or Paris regime, and the rapid crack growth or fast-fracture regime. The velocity of moving fatigue crack subjected to a constant stress amplitude loading is determined from the change in crack length, a, as a function of the number of loading cycles, N. This velocity represents the fatigue crack growth per loading cycle, da/dN, and is found from exper-

Recent work by Baker et al. [20] examined both the fatigue initiation and propagation resistance of irradiation cross-linked orthopedic-grade UHMWPE at varying cross-link doses. The cross-linking was performed with three different dosages of gamma irradiation followed by a thermal treatment above the melt. A stress-based total-life and a fracture mechanics approach were used to de-

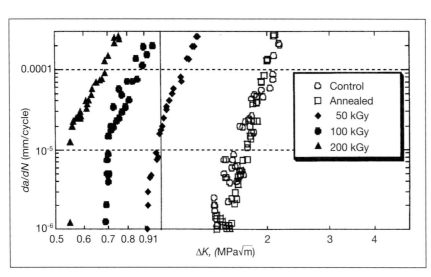

Fig. 56-2. Plot of crack propagation rate as a function of stress intensity for a range of cross-link doses

■ **Table 56-5.** Summary of fatigue crack propagation data. Fatigue crack inception and propagation data for the cross-linked materials and their control groups. (Adapted from [19, 20])

Paris Regime Fatigue $da/dN = C(\Delta K)^m$	GUR 1050	GUR 1050 (150°C)	50 kGy	100 kGy	200 kGy
ΔK_{incep} (MPa√m)	1.41	1.43	0.91	0.69	0.55
Decrease in Δ_{Kincep}	—	—	35%	51%	61%
Slope, m	11.74	19.40	10.77	9.07	8.92

termine the effect of irradiation dose (cross-linking) on the fatigue crack initiation and propagation resistance of polyethylene. Three doses of gamma irradiation (50 kGy, 100 kGy, and 200 kGy) were used. Additionally, two conventional groups were examined and included an untreated GUR 1050 rod stock and a rod stock with the same thermal treatment as the cross-linked groups. Fatigue crack propagation results for this study are presented in ■ Fig. 56-2.

It is apparent that irradiation cross-linking results in a monotonic decrease in crack propagation resistance. A summary of these fatigue crack inception values is given in Tables ■ 56-5 and 56-6. The thermally treated UHMW-PE exhibited a fatigue inception value similar to that of the control group. However, cross-linking resulted in a decreased value in fatigue crack inception. This degradation scaled with irradiation dose. For clinical comparison, the fatigue crack inception values and crack propagation slopes, m, for gamma-air sterilized and accelerated aging conditions for GUR 1050 are also included in Table 56-6 [19]. Note the similar relative decreases in the crack growth inception values for the gamma-sterilized and gamma-sterilized, aged conditions as compared with the highly cross-linked groups. The stress-life results from this study indicate that cross-linking is beneficial to fatigue initiation. Cross-linking resulted in an increased resistance to cyclic yield for any given stress range. The results of this study indicate that the high degree of cross-linking is detrimental to fatigue propagation resistance but not flaw initiation resistance. This trend is consistent with monotonic fracture studies [12, 14]. The in vivo fatigue and fracture resistance of highly cross-linked poly-

ethylene may therefore be dependent on the relative absence of manufacturing flaws, sharp locking mechanism edges, or other defects within the material that could act as crack initiation sites.

References

1. Li S, Burstein AH (1994) Ultra-high molecular weight polyethylene. The material and its use in total joint implants. J Bone Joint Surg [Am] 76:1080-1090
2. Premnath V, Harris WH, Jasty M, Merrill EW (1996) Gamma sterilization of UHMWPE articular implants: an analysis of the oxidation problem. Biomaterials 17:1741-1753
3. Kurtz SM, Muratoglu OK, Evans M, Edidin AA (1999) Advances in the processing, sterilization, and cross-linking of ultra-high molecular weight polyethylene for total joint arthroplasty. Biomaterials 20:1659-1688
4. Muratoglu OK, Bragdon CR, O'Connor DO, Jasty M, Harris WH, Gul R, McGarry F (1999) Unified wear model for highly crosslinked ultra-high molecular weight polyethylenes (UHMWPE). Biomaterials 20:1463-1470
5. McKellop H, Shen FW, Lu B, Campbell P, Salovey R (1999) Development of an extremely wear-resistant ultra high molecular weight polyethylene for total hip replacements. J Orthop Res 17:157-167
6. Jasty M, Bragdon CR, O'Connor DO, Muratoglu OK, Premnath V, Merrill EW, Harris WH (1997) Marked improvement in the wear resistance of a new form of UHMWPE in a physiologic hip simulator. Trans. 43rd Annual Meeting Orthop Res Soc, San Francisco, 1:785
7. Sun DC, Wang A, Stark C, Dumbleton JH (1996) The concept of stabilization in UHMWPE. Trans. 5th World Biomaterials Congress 1:195
8. Kurtz SM, Villarraga ML, Herr MP, Bergstrom JS, Rimnac CM, Edidin AA (2002) Thermomechanical behavior of virgin and highly cross-linked ultra-high molecular weight polyethylene used in total joint replacements. Biomaterials 23:3681-3697
9. Edidin AA, Pruitt L, Jewett CW, Crane DJ, Roberts D, Kurtz SM (1999) Plasticity-induced damage layer is a precursor to wear in radiation-cross-linked UHMWPE acetabular components for total hip replacement. J Arthroplasty 14:616-627
10. Wang A, Sun DC, Yau SS, Edwards B, Sokol M, Essner A, Polineni VK, Stark C, Dumbleton JH (1997) Orientation softening in the deformation and wear of ultra-high molecular weight polyethylene. Wear 203:230-241
11. Kurtz SM, Pruitt LA, Jewett CW, Foulds JR, Edidin AA (1999) Radiation and chemical cross-linking promote strain hardening behavior and molecular alignment in ultra high molecular weight polyethylene during multiaxial loading conditions. Biomaterials 20:1449-1462
12. Gencur SJ, Rimnac CM, Kurtz SM (2003) Failure micromechanisms during uniaxial tensile fracture of conventional and highly cross-linked ultra-high molecular weight polyethylenes used in total joint replacements. Biomaterials 24:3947-3954
13. Gillis AM, Schmiegg JJ, Bhattacharyya S, Li S (1999) An independent evaluation of the mechanical, chemical and fracture properties of UHMWPE cross-linked by 34 different conditions. Proc. 45th Annual Meeting Orthop Res Soc, Anaheim, 24:908

■ **Table 56-6.** Summary of fatigue crack propagation data. Fatigue crack inception data for gamma irradiation-sterilized GUR 1050, gamma irradiated GUR 1050 subjected to accelerated aging, and non-sterile 1050 control. (Adapted from [19, 20])

Paris Regime Fatigue $da/dN = C(\Delta K)^m$	Control	25 kGy air	25 kGy aged
ΔK_{incep} (MPa√m)	2.01	1.51	0.90
Decrease in ΔK_{incep}	—	24%	55%
Slope, m	21.4	24.3	—

14. Gomoll A, Wanich T, Bellare A (2002) J-Integral fracture toughness and tearing modulus measurement of radiation cross-linked UHMWPE. J Orthop Res 20:1152-1156

15. Greenwald AS, Bauer TW, Ries MD (2001) New polys for old: contribution or caveat. Trans Am Acad Orthop Surg, San Francisco, p 68

16. Baker DA, Hastings RS, Pruitt L (1999) Study of fatigue resistance of chemical and radiation cross-linked medical grade ultrahigh molecular weight polyethylene. J Biomed Mater Res 46:573-581

17. O'Connor DO, Muratoglu OK, Bragdon CR, Lowenstein J, Jasty M, Harris WH (1999) Wear and high cycle fatigue of highly crosslinked UHMWPE. Trans. 44th Annual Meeting Orthop Res Soc, Anaheim, p 816

18. Krzypow DJ, Bensusan J, Sevo K, Haggard W, Parr J, Goldberg V, Rimnac C (2000) The fatigue crack propagation resistance of gamma radiation or peroxide cross-linked UHMW polyethylene. Trans Sixth World Biomaterials Congress, Hawaii, p 382

19. Baker DA, Hastings RS, Pruitt L (2000) Compression and tension fatigue resistance of medical grade ultra high molecular weight polyethylene: the effect of morphology, sterilization, aging and temperature. Polymer 41:795-808

20. Baker DA, Bellare A, Pruitt L (2003) The effects of degree of cross-linking on the fatigue crack initiation and propagation resistance of orthopedic grade polyethylene. J Biomed Mater Res 66A:146-154

21. Duus LC, Walsh HA, Gillis AM, Noisiez E, Li S (2000) The effect of resin grade, manufacturing method, and cross-linking on the fracture toughness of commercially available UHMWPE. Trans Orthop Res Soc 25:544

22. Bartel DL, Bicknell VL, Wright TM (1986) The effect of conformity, thickness, and material on stresses in ultra-high molecular weight components for total joint replacement. J Bone Joint Surg [Am] 68:1041-1051

57 Wear in Conventional and Highly Cross-Linked Polyethylene

M. D. Ries

Summary

Ultra-high-molecular-weight polyethylene (UHMWPE) has been used successfully as a bearing surface in total knee arthroplasty for over 30 years, although material failures have typically resulted from gamma irradiation-induced oxidative degradation and the high cyclic stress environment of the knee. Since conversion to non-gamma irradiation sterilization methods, the failure mechanisms that were observed with gamma irradiation in air-sterilized UHMWPE have not occurred. Highly cross-linked UHMWPE has been developed in an effort to further reduce wear in total joint arthroplasty. However, cross-linking reduces the mechanical properties of UHMWPE, including fatigue crack propagation resistance, which may limit its application in total knee arthroplasty.

Relationship Between Contact Stress and Wear Mechanisms

As a result of the different loading conditions and contact stresses in the hip and knee, the wear mechanisms that occur in total hip and total knee arthroplasties are different (◘ Fig. 57-1).

The hip is a congruent ball-and-socket joint with a relatively large contact area at the bearing surface. The larger contact area of the hip results in lower contact stress. At low contact stress, surface wear mechanisms (abrasion and adhesion) predominate. However, the contact stresses in the knee are typically an order of magnitude higher than in the hip [1]. As a result of the lower conformity and contact area in total knee tibial components, the yield stress of UHMWPE is exceeded in most designs [2]. In a tibial insert with relatively high contact stresses and moving contact area, alternating tensile and compressive stresses are created which can lead to fatigue (delamination and pitting) wear mechanisms [3, 4]. Surface-wear mechanisms produce relatively small particles, typically less than 1 μm in size, while fatigue-wear mechanisms produce larger particles. The smaller particles can elicit more of an osteolytic response than the larger par-

ticles [5]. Wear particles are generally smaller in total hip compared with total knee arthroplasty, and osteolysis appears to be more common in total hips than in total knees [6]. However, osteolysis does occur in total knee replacements, particularly in those which have large contact ar-

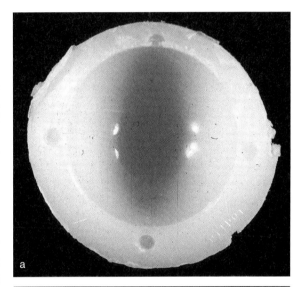

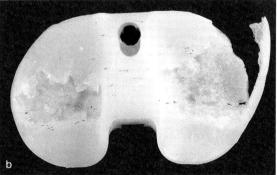

◘ **Fig. 57-1a, b.** *a* A clinically retrieved total hip acetabular component which had failed as a result of wear and osteolysis. The articulating surface appears smooth, consistent with surface-wear mechanisms (abrasion and adhesion), which produce relatively small, submicron particles. *b* A clinically retrieved total knee tibial insert which failed as a result of UHMWPE wear. The surface is delaminated and fragmented, consistent with fatigue-wear mechanisms (delamination and pitting), which occur at high contact stress and usually produce particles that are larger than those retrieved form total hip components. (Reproduced with permission from [10])

eas and low contact stresses, such as mobile-bearing de-signs [7].

Conventional UHMWPE

Total knee arthroplasty with the use of extruded or mold-ed UHMWPE which is sterilized by gamma irradiation in air has been reported to have survivorship rates of 90%-95% after 10 years [8, 9]. Failures are typically associated with UHMWPE fatigue damage and wear is associated with oxidative degradation. Oxidative degradation occurs after gamma irradiation sterilization and exposure to air [10]. Gamma irradiation causes polymer chain scission and the formation of chemically unstable free radicals. The free radicals can react with oxygen to form a chemi-cally stable carbonyl group. This process results in oxida-tive degradation. The free radicals can also remain pre-sent for long periods of time after gamma irradiation. As oxygen diffuses into the UHMWPE implant more oxida-tive degradation occurs, as oxygen reacts with remaining free radicals. The fatigue strength and wear resistance of UHMWPE are both reduced by oxidative degradation [11, 12]. Components which are shelf-aged and then implant-ed have a higher failure rate than those which are stored for shorter periods of time [13]. Since oxidative degrada-tion requires both gamma irradiation sterilization and exposure to oxygen, the process can be avoided by using either non-irradiation sterilization (ethylene oxide or gas plasma) or an inert environment during and after irradi-ation (vacuum, argon, or nitrogen) which eliminates oxy-gen exposure.

Molded components, made from Himont 1900 resin, are particularly resistant to oxidative degradation even after gamma irradiation sterilization and exposure to air [14]. The reason for this resistance to oxidative degrada-tion is not clear, but it may be related to better consolida-tion of the resin material which limits oxygen diffusion into the polymer. However, since UHMWPE total knee tibial inserts are no longer sterilized by gamma irradia-tion in air, the potential benefit of a material with greater resistance to gamma irradiation-induced oxidative degradation is not clear.

In the past, conventional UHMWPE could be consid-ered to be gamma-irradiated UHMWPE, which is steril-ized and stored in air. However, this material is no longer manufactured for use in total knee tibial components. Cur-rent conventional UHMWPE may be defined as either non-gamma-irradiation sterilized (ethylene oxide or gas plasma) or gamma-irradiation sterilized and stored in an inert (vacuum, nitrogen, or argon gas) environment. Both of the current methods used to sterilize UHMWPE elimi-nate or minimize the potential for oxidative degradation compared with materials which have been used in the past and on which most long-term clinical studies are based.

Effect of Current Sterilization Methods

UHMWPE implants are currently sterilized by either a non-irradiation method (gas plasma or ethylene oxide) or gamma irradiation and storage in an inert atmosphere without oxygen. Gas sterilization methods eliminate ox-idative degradation since free radicals, formed by gam-ma irradiation, are not present. Gamma irradiation in an inert environment reduces oxidative degradation since free radicals are still present after sterilization, but oxy-gen is not available in the atmosphere to react with the free radicals. However, some in vivo oxidative degrada-tion may occur, since oxygen can be present in the joint fluid.

The mechanical properties of UHPMWPE, including fatigue strength, are not affected by gas sterilization since there is no chemical change in the polymer structure [11]. The fatigue crack propagation resistance is reduced by gamma-irradiation sterilization, although abrasive wear resistance is improved as a result of cross-linking caused by irradiation. To the author's knowledge, the failures typ-ically observed with gamma-irradiated in air UHMWPE have not been reported with the use of current gas, or gamma irradiation in an inert atmosphere, sterilization methods.

Highly Cross-linked UHMWPE

Highly cross-linked UHMWPE has been developed in an effort to reduce the abrasive and adhesive wear which oc-curs in total hip arthroplasty. In total hip simulators, vol-umetric wear is dramatically reduced after cross-linking [15, 16]. However, the mechanical properties, including fa-tigue crack propagation resistance, tensile strength, yield strength, and elongation, are also reduced. The reduced mechanical properties, particularly fatigue crack propa-gation resistance, may lead to problems of fatigue wear after cross-linking.

Fatigue crack development can be separated into phases of crack initiation and crack propagation. Crack initiation requires a defect in the material, which may be present from manufacturing flaws or may occur sponta-neously due to in vivo loading (◘ Fig. 57-2).

Crack propagation, or the rate at which the defect en-larges, is dependent on the material properties. After cross-linking, fatigue crack propagation resistance is re-duced, indicating that a crack would be expected to trav-el through highly cross-linked UHMWPE more rapidly than non-cross-linked UHMWPE [17]. If cracks are not initiated in highly cross-linked UHMWPE, then fatigue failures would not be expected to occur. However, early clinical retrieval studies of highly cross-linked UHMW-PE demonstrate a high rate of surface defects which could lead to further fatigue wear mechanisms [14].

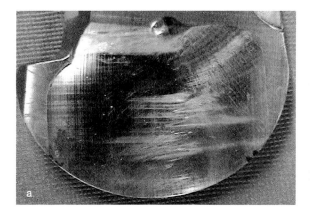

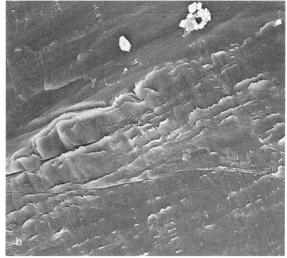

◨ **Fig. 57-2a, b.** *a* A clinically retrieved e-beam highly cross-linked tibial insert removed after only 3 months in vivo, demonstrating abrasive scratches. *b* Scanning electron micrograph of the highly cross-linked tibial plateau demonstrating abrasive sratches in line with the flexion axis and cracks in the surface perpendicular to scratches

Despite the reduction in material properties, knee wear simulator studies demonstrate less volumetric wear of highly cross-linked than of non-cross-linked UHMWPE under clean conditions [18]. Although fatigue wear mechanisms occur more commonly in total knee tibial components than in total hip acetabular components, surface wear mechanisms (abrasive and adhesive wear) do occur in total knee arthroplasty. Wear simulators which test total knee components under ideal conditions may evaluate only abrasive and adhesive wear mechanisms and thus can be expected to show an apparent benefit to using highly cross-linked UHMWPE. However, fatigue wear as well as wear caused by counterface roughening commonly occurs in vivo and may not be represented by wear simulations under clean conditions. Roughening of a total knee femoral component in vivo may occur as a result of third-body abrasives (such as cement or bone particles) or oxidative wear of the metal [19]. In order to predict the effects of counterface roughening on wear in vivo, wear simulator studies with artificially roughened femoral

components have been performed. One method of in vitro roughening has been produced by tumbling the femoral component in alumina particles prior to wear testing [20]. The roughness of the components was similar to that of in vivo retrieved femoral components. The roughened implants were then articulated with highly cross-linked and non-cross-linked UHMWPE in a knee simulator. Wear was increased by counterface roughening for both highly cross-linked and non-cross-linked UHMWPE [21]. These findings indicate that highly cross-linked UHMWPE can reduce surface wear mechanisms in a knee simulator. However, if in vivo roughening of the femoral counterface occurs, wear may be increased.

Clinical studies will be necessary to determine the safety and efficacy of highly cross-linked UHMWPE in total knee arthroplasty. However, because of the reduction in fatigue crack propagation resistance caused by cross-linking and sensitivity to counterface roughening, currently available highly cross-linked polyethylenes may not to be beneficial for use in fixed-bearing total knee arthroplasty.

Effect of Counterface Roughness

Although fatigue wear mechanisms are more common in total knee than in total hip UHMWPE components, both fatigue and abrasive wear occur in total knee tibial components. The roughness of the femoral component surface can have an effect on UHMWPE abrasive wear. A single scratch in the metallic counterface articulating with UHMPWE can significantly increase wear [22]. Total knee femoral components, which are typically made from cast cobalt chrome, roughen in vivo [19]. In vivo roughening can occur from third-body abrasives such as cement, bone, or metal particles. Wear of UHMWPE in total knee arthroplasty is increased after counterface roughening [20]. However, wear is reduced by the use of a scratch-resistant femoral component under both clean and abrasive conditions [20, 23]. Use of a scratch-resistant femoral component, such as oxidized zirconium, subjected to roughening with alumina particles produces wear similar to a cobalt-chrome femoral component under clean conditions. These observations imply that the use of a scratch-resistant counterface rather than highly cross-linked UHMWPE may be more effective in reducing abrasive wear in total knee arthroplasty without compromising the mechanical properties of the UHMWPE tibial insert.

References

1. Bartel DL, Bicknell VL, Wright TM (1986) The effect of conformity, thickness, and material on stresses in ultra-high molecular weight components for total joint replacement. J Bone Joint Surg [Am] 68:1041-1051

2. Wrona FG, Mayor MB, Collier JP, Jensen RE (1994) The correlation between fusion defects and damage in tibial polyethylene bearings. Clin Orthop 299:92-103

3. Blunn GW, Walker PS, Joshi A, Hardinge K (1991) The dominance of cyclic sliing in producing wear in total knee replacements. Clin Orthop 273:253-260

4. Blunn GW, Joshi AB, Minns RJ, Lidgren L, Lilley P, Ryd L, Engelbrecht E, Walker PS (1997) Wear in retrieved condylar knee arthroplasties. J Arthroplasty 12:281-290

5. Green TR, Fischer J, Matthews LB, Stone MH, Ingham E (2000) Effect of size and dose on bone resorption activity of macrophages by in vitro clinically relevant ultra high molecular weight polyethylene particles. J Biomed Mater Res 53:490-497

6. Schmalzried TP, Jasty M, Rosenberg A, Harris WH (1994) Polyethylene wear debris and tissue reactions in knee as compared to hip replacement prostheses. J Appl Biomater 5:185-190

7. Huang CH, Ma HM, Liau JJ, Ho FY, Cheng CK (2002) Abstract osteolysis in failed total knee arthroplasty: a comparison of mobile-bearing and fixed-bearing knees. J Bone Joint Surg [Am] 84:2224—2229

8. Rand JA, Trousdale RT, Ilstrup DM, Harmsen WS (2003) Factors affecting the durability of primary total knee prostheses. J Bone Joint Surg [Am] 85:259-265

9. Ranawat CS, Hansraj KK (1989) Effect of posterior cruciate sacrificing on durability of the cement-bone interface: a nine-year survivorship study of 100 total condylar knee arthroplasties. Orthop Clin North Am 20:63-39

10. Greenwald AS, Bauer TW, Ries MD (2001) New polys for old: contribution or caveat? J Bone Joint Surg [Am] 83:S27-S31

11. Ries MD, Weaver K, Rose RM, Greer J, Sauer W, Beals N (1996) Fatigue strength of polyethylene after sterilization by gamma irradiation or ethylene oxide. Clin Orthop 333:87-95

12. Sutula LS, Collier JP, Saum KA et al (1995) Impact of gamma sterilization on clinical performance of polyethylene in the hip. Clin Orthop 319:28-40

13. Bohl JR, Bohl WR, Postak PD, Greenwald AS (1999) The Coventry Award. The effects of shelf life on clinical outcome for gamma sterilized polyethylene tibial components. Clin Orthop 367:28-38

14. Bradford-Collons L, Baker DA, Graham J, Chawan A, Ries MD, Pruitt L (2005) Wear and surface cracking in early retrieved highly crosslinked Durasul acetabular liners. J Bone Joint Surg (in press)

15. McKellop H, Shen FW, Lu B, Campbell P, Salovey R (1999) Development of an extremely wear-resistant ultra high molecular weight polyethylene for total hip replacements. J Orthop Res 17:157-167

16. Muratoglu O K, Bragdon CR, O'Connor DO, Jasty M, Harris WH (2001) A novel method of cross-linking ultra-high-molecular-weight polyethylene to improve wear, reduce oxidation, and retain mechanical properties. Recipient of the 1999 HAP Paul Award. J Arthroplasty 16:149-160

17. Baker D, Bellare A, L Pruitt (2003) The effects of degree of crosslinking on the fatigue crack initiation and propagation resistance of orthopedic grade polyethlene. J Biomed Mater Res 66:146-154

18. Muratoglu OK, Mark A, Vittetoe DA, Harris WH, Rubash HE (2003) No abstract Polyethylene damage in total knees and use of highly crosslinked polyethylene. J Bone Joint Surg [Am] 85:S7-S13

19. Levesque M, Livingston BJ, Jones WM, Spector M (1998) Scratches on condyles in normal functioning total knee arthroplasty. Trans Orthop Res Soc 23:247

20. Ries MD, Salehi A, Widding K, Hunter G (2002) Polyethylene wear performance of oxidized zirconium and cobalt-chromium knee components under abrasive conditions. J Bone Joint Surg [Am] 84:S129-S135

21. Widding K, Scott M, Jani S, Good V (2003) Crosslinked UHMWPE in knees: clean versus abrasive conditions. Trans Orthop Res Soc 28:1427

22. Dowson D, Taheri S, Wallbridge N (1987) The role of counterface imperfections in the wear of polyethylene. Wear 119:277-293

23. Spector M, Ries MD, Bourne RB, Sauer WL, Long M, Hunter GB (2001) Wear performance of ultra high molecular weight polyethylene on oxidized zirconium total knee femoral components. J Bone Joint Surg [Am] 83 S80-S86

57

58 Modular UHMWPE Insert Design Characteristics

A. S. Greenwald, C. S. Heim

Summary

The evolution of knee implant design reflects recognition of the principle that implant geometry, acting in concert with surrounding soft-tissue structures, determines joint stability, range of motion, interface forces, and material stresses. Interchangeable plateau geometries associated with modular knee designs permit the orthopedic surgeon to optimize the articulation for a patient's presenting pathology within a single system. This chapter presents performance characteristics for contemporary knee designs including intrinsic stability and surface stress distributions.

Introduction

The introduction of modular total knee designs in the late 1980s addressed several contemporary concerns, both clinical and economic. With regard to the former, modularity has proved successful, as the orthopedic surgeon can address a variety of presenting soft-tissue inadequacies and bony pathologies with the use of a single knee system. Further, in revision situations where the tibial insert has failed but the femoral component and tibial tray are well fixed and their surfaces not damaged, an easier revision procedure involving only polymer component exchange is an option. Optimization of system instrumentation has facilitated an overall improvement in technical proficiency and clinical outcome. Finally, hospitals were able to virtually eliminate their stock of multiple knee designs and abandon this cost-prohibitive practice.

However, there were unforeseen circumstances associated with the implementation of the process, including shelf storage of ultra-high-molecular-weight polyethylene (UHMWPE) tibial insert components gamma irradiated in an air environment [1], material selection [2, 3], component finishing, component sizing, fixation methodology [4, 5], and device design. This chapter focuses on the tibial-femoral articulating interface particular to intrinsic stability and surface stress distributions for contemporary modular total knee systems.

Intrinsic Stability

Restoration of normal knee joint function through surgical reconstruction is dependent upon load sharing between the implant, surrounding ligaments, and other supporting soft-tissue structures. Excision, surgical release and progressive pathological weakening of ligamentous structures will result in an increased dependency upon the implant system for stability.

Stability is achieved in non-hinged total knee replacements through geometric variation of the tibial-femoral condylar surfaces. The capacity of an implant to resist rotational, anterior-posterior, and medial-lateral displacement during physiological loading defines its intrinsic stability [6].

Rotational Stability

Figures 58-1 and 58-2 present the rotational stability for contemporary modular knee systems at 15° of flexion under 1900 N [4.45 N = 1 pound force (lbf)] axial compressive load [7-9]. Low-torque designs are characterized by flat tibial plateau surfaces whose resistance to rotation is due primarily to frictional forces between the metal and the UHMWPE bearing surfaces. Higher torques are noted in designs with either marked geometric congruity or a prominent intercondylar eminence, which abuts in rotation (◘ Fig. 58-1, 58-2).

Torques generated by rotation of implant systems under axial load are, of necessity, dissipated by transfer to both fixation interfaces and soft tissues. Excessive torque experienced at fixation interfaces may accelerate cement fixation failure or compromise bone ingrowth on porous surfaces. Despite a clinical demand for increasing anterior-posterior and medial-lateral constraint in modular knee designs, rotational constraint should be kept to a minimum to reduce the potential for loosening.

Posterior Stability

Figures 58-3 and 58-4 present the posterior stability for contemporary modular knee systems at 0° and 90° of flex-

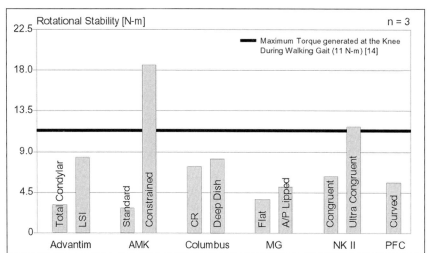

Fig. 58-1. Rotational stability of contemporary primary modular total knee systems. The loading conditions are 15° of flexion with an applied compressive axial load of 1900 N. Three tibial inserts were evaluated for each design (n=3), and the average at ±15° is presented. Advantim (Wright Medical Technology, Inc., Arlington, TN, USA), AMK (DePuy Orthopedics, Warsaw, IN, USA), Columbus (Aesculap, Center Valley, PA, USA), MG (Zimmer, Inc., Warsaw, IN, USA), NK II (Sulzer Orthopedics, Austin, TX, USA), PFC (Johnson & Johnson Orthopedics, Raynham, MA, USA)

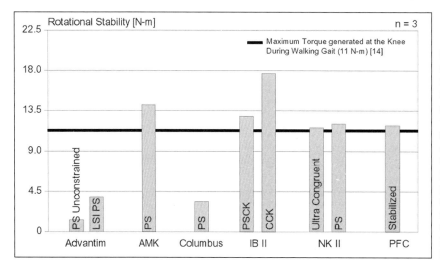

Fig. 58-2. Rotational stability of contemporary posterior-stabilized modular total knee systems. The loading conditions are 15° of flexion with an applied compressive axial load of 1900 N. Three tibial inserts were evaluated for each design (n=3), and the average at ±15° is presented. Advantim (Wright Medical Technology, Inc., Arlington, TN, USA), AMK (DePuy Orthopedics, Warsaw, IN, USA), Columbus (Aesculap, Center Valley, PA, USA), IB II (Zimmer, Inc., Warsaw, IN, USA), NK II (Sulzer Orthopedics, Austin, TX, USA), PFC (Johnson & Johnson Orthopedics, Raynham, MA, USA)

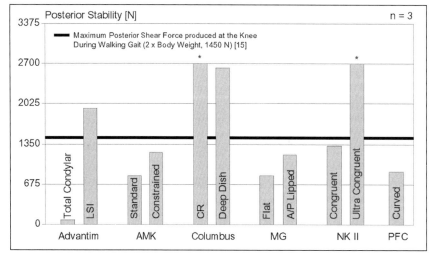

Fig. 58-3. Posterior stability of contemporary primary modular total knee systems. The loading conditions are 0° extension with an applied compressive axial load of 2900 N. Three tibial inserts were evaluated for each design (n=3), and the average is presented. Advantim (Wright Medical Technology, Inc., Arlington, TN, USA), AMK (DePuy Orthopaedics, Warsaw, IN, USA), Columbus (Aesculap, Center Valley, PA, USA), MG (Zimmer, Inc., Warsaw, IN, USA), NK II (Sulzer Orthopedics, Austin, TX, USA), PFC (Johnson & Johnson Orthopaedics, Raynham, MA, USA). Testing was stopped at 2700 N, as this force represents an excessive stability when compared with values reported by Seireg et al. [15]

ion [7, 8]. A major part of the posterior stability generated at the normal knee is attributed to the posterior cruciate ligament (PCL). In the absence of a PCL, the intrinsic stability of the tibial-femoral articulation must play a significantly more prominent role in resisting posterior dislocation, particularly for the posteriorly unstable knee at 90° of flexion. For systems demonstrating intrinsic constraint below the shear forces estimated for the normal knee [10], competent soft tissues are mandated for functional stability (**Fig. 58-3, 58-4**).

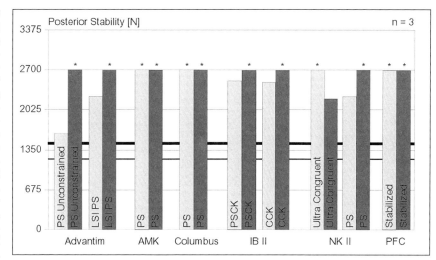

Fig. 58-4. Posterior stability of contemporary posterior stabilized modular total knee systems. The two loading conditions are 0° extension with an applied compressive axial load of 2900 N and 90° of flexion with an applied compressive axial load of 1780 N. Three tibial inserts were evaluated for each design (n=3) at each loading condition and the averages are presented. Advantim (Wright Medical Technology, Inc., Arlington, TN, USA), AMK (DePuy Orthopaedics, Warsaw, IN, USA), Columbus (Aesculap, Center Valley, PA, USA), IB II (Zimmer, Inc., Warsaw, IN, USA), NK II (Sulzer Orthopedics, Austin, TX, USA), PFC (Johnson & Johnson Orthopaedics, Raynham, MA, USA). Testing was stopped at 2700 N, as this force represents an excessive stability when compared with values reported by Morrison [10]

Clinical longevity of primary and revision knee arthroplasty is enhanced by attaining the correct balance between the intrinsic stability provided by the tibial-femoral articulating interface and the patient's presenting pathology. In general, soft-tissue involvement should be encouraged to decrease dependency on the intrinsic constraints afforded by condylar geometry for a particular knee design. This load sharing will reduce the stresses transferred to the implant-bone interface, which is important for promoting the longevity of the fixation surface.

Surface Stress Distributions

While modularity expanded the armamentarium of the orthopedic surgeon, it also increased the variables affecting the longevity of the tibial-femoral articulating interface, which was not fully appreciated at the outset [11]. Surface deterioration characterized by material removal as a result of the relative motion between opposing surfaces defines wear. And while component wear is an inevitable consequence of in vivo articulation, optimization of design and material variables should seek to minimize regions of high surface stresses.

Condylar Conformity

One of the advantages of modularity in knee systems is that several UHMWPE tibial components with differing intrinsic stabilities articulate with a single femoral component and tibial tray. However, **Fig. 58-5** demonstrates the influence of flexion on the surface stress distributions, which should be taken into consideration when evaluating additional patient factors inclusive of body weight and activity level.

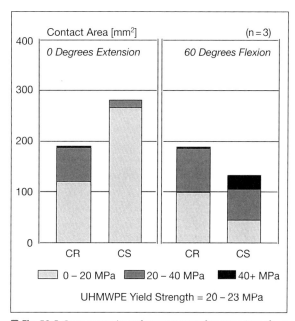

Fig. 58-5. Contact areas by surface stress range for comparison of two contemporary tibial-femoral conformal geometries (n=3 for each condition). CR, Cruciate retaining; CS, cruciate substituting

When comparing a tibial design with minimal constraint (CR) with one that provides joint stability through increased curvature in anterior and posterior elevations (CS), it is apparent that positional changes associated with gait dramatically affect the resulting surface stress distributions. At 0° extension, the more conforming design has less potential for polymer damage due to the small amount of contact area in the surface stress ranges exceeding the UHMWPE yield strength. However, with increasing flexion, this same articulating geometry looses conformity more rapidly and results in a higher potential for polymer damage.

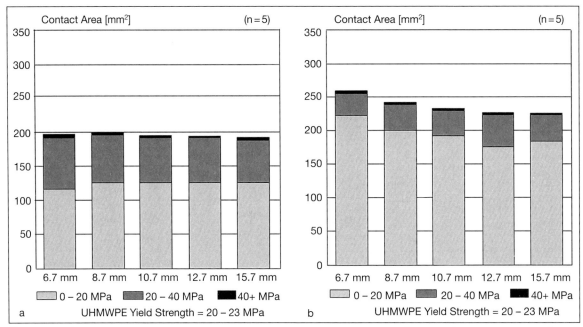

Fig. 58-6a, b. Contact areas by surface stress range for comparison of two contemporary tibial-femoral conformal geometries (*n*=3 for each condition). (*a*) Cruciate retaining, (*b*) cruciate substituting

Tibial Plateau Thickness

Figure 58-6 presents surface stress distributions for two insert designs mated with a common femoral component and tibial tray at varying UHMWPE thicknesses under a single loading condition (10° of flexion and 2900 N). The cruciate-retaining tibial insert consistently produced higher surface stresses than did the cruciate-substituting design for all of the insert thicknesses evaluated. However, within each design, thickness did not significantly ($p>0.05$) influence the potential for polymer damage as measured by peak surface stress for the thicknesses measured, which is in contrast to an earlier analytical paper [16]. Therefore, clinical decisions pertaining to joint line restoration and preservation of bone stock should be the

primary considerations in determining the thickness of the UHMWPE tibial components utilized in knee arthroplasty procedures. Patient age and anticipated activity level are further considerations that should be evaluated by the reconstructive surgeon.

The process of UHMWPE damage is multifactorial, and an appreciation of all variables is necessary to meet the increasing service life requirements of contemporary knee designs (◘ Fig. 58-6a, b).

Tibial Tray Design

Modularity in knee arthroplasty was introduced through the application of metal-backed UHMWPE tibial compo-

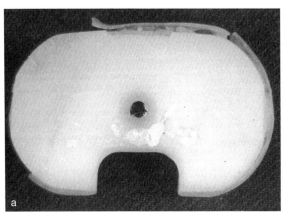
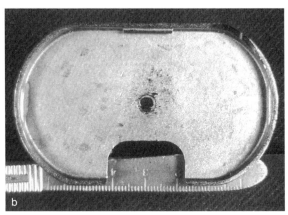

◘ **Fig. 58-7a, b.** Retrieved Synatomic modular knee replacement. (*a*) Distal UHMWPE surface indicates failure of the capture mechanism and wear. (*b*) Mating tibial tray demonstrates UHMWPE film transfer indicative of component motion

nents. This stiffer substrate was designed to attenuate and distribute the stresses transferred to the implant-bone interface while providing off-the-shelf flexibility to address a variety of knee pathologies including tissue incompetence, skeletal deformity, and bone loss.

There are an increasing number of citations in the clinical literature pertaining to the onset of tibial osteolysis as a result of UHMWPE wear debris coincident with tibial tray design in modular knee systems [12, 13]. One of the most influential variables in this equation is the UHMWPE capture mechanism utilized on the tibial tray. It has been well documented that most modular tibial inserts displace during in vivo articulation (◘Fig. 58-7). Therefore, all efforts should be applied to decreasing the potential for backside wear of these components, including polishing the proximal metal surface of the tibial tray, fully seating the screws (if utilized), and filling unused screw holes with a spacer. In this regard, cobalt-chrome-molybdenum as a tray metal has distinct advantages over titanium alloy.

Discussion

The evolution of total knee systems over the past two decades has resulted in contemporary design configurations which have been influenced by mid- to long-term clinical reports as well as an appreciation of component retrieval. Material factors which contribute to long-term in vivo durability include polymer selection, the sterilization process, and the articulating counterface. Ongoing optimization of design variables such as tibial plateau capture mechanisms, articulation conformities, and intrinsic stability will continue to help shape future knee systems. In the years ahead, with a growing interest in small-incision surgery, both knee instrumentation and design alteration of proven knee systems will offer a challenge to the designer and reconstructive surgeon. Finally, improved technical surgical proficiency in conjunction with appropriate patient and knee system selection define a triad which assures clinical in vivo longevity. In the former regard, the emerging interest in computer-assisted knee surgery will play a role.

References

1. Bohl JR et al (1999) The effects of shelf life on clinical outcome for gamma sterilized polyethylene tibial components. Clin Orthop 267:28-38
2. Busanelli L et al (1996) Wear in carbon fiber-reinforced polyethylene (poly-two) knee prostheses. Chir Organi Mov 81:263-267
3. Wright TM et al (1992) Wear of polyethylene in total joint replacements. Observations from retrieved PCA knee implants. Clin Orthop 276:126-134
4. Collier JP et al (1991) Analysis of the failure of 122 polyethylene inserts from uncemented tibial knee components. Clin Orthop 273:232-242
5. Peters PC et al (1992) Osteolysis after total knee arthroplasty without cement. J Bone Joint Surg [Am] 74:864-876
6. Greenwald AS et al (1981) Total knee replacement. American Academy of Orthopedic Surgeons Instructional Course Lectures 30:301-312
7. Heim CS et al (1996) Stability characteristics of Posterior Stabilized Total Knee Systems. Scientific Exhibit at the 63rd Annual Meeting of the American Academy of Orthopedic Surgeons
8. Postak PD et al (1991) Performance characteristics of modular total knee systems. Scientific Exhibit at the 58th Annual Meeting of the American Academy of Orthopedic Surgeons
9. Postak PD et al (1992) Performance characteristics of primary modular total knee systems. Scientific Exhibit at the 59th Annual Meeting of the American Academy of Orthopedic Surgeons
10. Morrison JB (1969) Function of the knee joint in various activities. Biomed Eng 4:573-580
11. Heim CM et al (1996) Factors influencing the longevity of UHMWPE tibial components. American Academy of Orthopedic Surgeons Instructional Course Lectures 45:303-314
12. Berger RA et al (2001) Problems with cementless total knee arthroplasty at 11 years follow-up. Clin Orthop 392:196-207
13. Engh GA et al (1994) Tibial osteolysis in cementless total knee arthroplasty. A review of 25 cases treated with and without tibial component revision. Clin Orthop 309:33-43
14. Morrison JB (1970) The mechanics of the knee joint in relation to normal walking. J Biomech 3:51-61
15. Seireg A et al (1975) The prediction of muscular load sharing and joint forces in the lower extremities during walking. J Biomech 8:89-102
16. Bartel DL et al (1985) The effect of conformity and plastic thickness on contact stresses in metal-backed plastic implants. J Biomech Eng 107:193-199

59 Oxidized Zirconium

G. Hunter, W. M. Jones, M. Spector

Summary

The advantages of oxide ceramic materials as articulating surfaces for total knee arthroplasty (TKA) and hemiarthroplasty devices include their greater lubricity and abrasion resistance. Unfortunately, the benefits of ceramics cannot often be accessed because of their brittle character and the difficulty of fabricating them into the necessary prosthetic shapes. There are advantages to a substance that would allow the benefits of ceramic materials to be wedded to the mechanical resiliency of a metallic substrate. With only its metallic surface transformed by oxidation into ceramic oxide, oxidized zirconium (OxZr) alloy is such a substance. The oxidized surface of the zirconium alloy has the characteristics of zirconia ceramic for reducing wear when articulating against UHMWPE or cartilage. In addition, the oxide is very durable and adherent to the underlying metal substrate. Based on laboratory investigations and early clinical results, it appears that this combination of properties may contribute to the reduction of wear-related complications in arthroplasty. Prior work indicates that OxZr would be an appropriate bearing surface for total joint arthroplasty and for hemiarthroplasty and that it may have meaningful advantages over CoCr alloys.

Introduction

The materials employed for the fabrication of total knee replacement prostheses need to meet an array of specifications related to their mechanical performance and biocompatibility. Interrelationships among properties further challenge the selection and development of biomaterials for this application. For example, all of the materials employed in TKA are biocompatible in bulk form but, when present as particular debris, can provoke an inflammatory response driven by macrophages that may result in degradation of tissue surrounding the implant, including bone (osteolysis). The tribological performance (i.e., lubrication, friction, and wear) of biomaterials used for articulating applications, such as TKA, is of paramount importance. In his original work, Sir John Charnley recognized the value of low-friction arthroplasty associated with the lubrication and friction of the articulating couple. Once long-term follow-up studies of total joint arthroplasty became available it was clear that the wear of the articulating materials was of even greater importance. Wear debris was found to lead to osteolysis and aseptic loosening.

Efforts to reduce wear in TKA have focused primarily on improving implant design and ultra-high-molecular-weight polyethylene (UHMWPE) quality. Although these address issues related to fatigue wear of the UHMWPE component, concerns remain about adhesive and abrasive wear caused by the hard counterface of the femoral component. Previous studies have shown that roughening of the condyles occurs clinically, and that many observed scratches have a shape and orientation that can increase polyethylene wear [13, 16. 30, 41]. Not only does volumetric wear of polyethylene increase with increasing counterface roughness; it also has been found that increasingly sharp peaks associated with counterface scratches increase the tendency for the production of

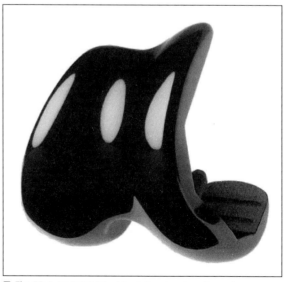

Fig. 59-1. An OXINIUM oxidized zirconium knee femoral component (Smith & Nephew, Inc., Memphis, TN) combines the abrasion resistance and lubricity of ceramics with the toughness of metals

submicron debris that may be related to osteolysis. These findings suggest that a hard counterface that resists roughening and provides low friction with UHMWPE should reduce abrasive and adhesive wear and thereby prolong survivorship of TKA. This same analysis applies to the use of hard counterfaces for hemiarthroplasty (e.g., hip hemiarthroplasty and the metal-cartilage articulation following TKA with an unresurfaced patella).

A metallic cobalt-chromium (CoCr) alloy (Co-28% Cr-6%Mo) is the standard material for femoral components. In recent years, OxZr was developed as an alternative bearing material for orthopedic prostheses (◘ Fig. 59-1) to provide an improvement over CoCr in resistance to roughening, frictional behavior, and biocompatibility. The objective of this chapter is to provide a framework for the rationale of using an abrasion-resistant counterface for TKA and hemiarthroplasty applications, and to introduce a novel biomaterial for these applications.

The Role of a Scratched Metal Counterface in Wear of Polyethylene and Articular Cartilage

Metal-Polyethylene Articulation

In vivo scratching of the metallic femoral condylar components of total knee prostheses can occur as a result of three-body wear related to the action of bone cement and bone particles, or fragments of coatings from non-cemented components. These scratches, even if few in number, may lead to an increased rate of wear of the UHMWPE tibial component.

The few studies that have determined the prevalence of scratches on femoral components or characterized their profiles have used the average roughness, R_a, as the principal parameter to describe the topography. R_a is the arithmetic average of vertical deviations from the mean surface calculated over the entire surface that is evaluated [44]. Hailey et al. [18] measured the R_a values of femoral components from 11 Accord TKAs (six revised for femoral loosening and five revised for sepsis) using a profilometer and found little wear of the devices. That study did not give any description of the scratches observed other than the fact that they ran in the direction of articulation. Que et al. [41] analyzed the surface roughness of PCA knee prostheses grouped into three categories, based on the presence of embedded particles in the polyethylene inserts and whether the condylar component had worn through the UHMWPE insert to the metal tray. The R_a value and the sum of the peak height and valley depth (peak to valley roughness, R_{pv}) of the wear regions were measured. As might have been expected, components that had worn through the polyethylene insert and that were articulating with the metal tray had the greatest surface

roughness. No meaningful correlations among patient age, duration of implantation, or patient weight and the surface roughness were found. In another study, Dwyer et al. [14] examined the wear regions of 42 femoral components revised for aseptic loosening and UHMWPE wear using a scanning electron microscope. In addition, they performed topographical analysis (R_a and R_{pv}) by optical interferometry on seven of the failed components and three controls. Their study noted scratches, in varying directions, on all components. No detailed evaluation of the profiles of the scratches was provided, however.

In contrast to the few papers investigating scratches on femoral components in TKA, several studies have evaluated the surface roughness of the femoral heads of total hip arthroplasty (THA). These investigators have linked the presence of scratches to cement and metal particles embedded in the acetabular liners. One THA retrieval study [52] correlated three-body wear and osteolysis by noting that all of the patients in the study who exhibited bone loss radiographically had an abundance of metallic and hydroxyapatite particles in the articulating surfaces of the retrieved polyethylene liners. Another study [3] correlated the surface roughness, UHMWPE wear rate, and incidence of osteolysis, thereby linking rougher surfaces with an increase in osteolysis.

Laboratory studies have shown that an increase in the metal counterface roughness can lead to an increase in polyethylene wear. One such study [13] showed that even a single scratch of a certain size on a metal counterface could have a significant effect on polyethylene wear. The pile-up of metal bordering a scratch reflected in the surface parameter R_p, and not in the depth of the scratch which contributes to R_a, was the primary factor in the increasing polyethylene wear. R_p is the maximum profile peak height, i.e., the distance between the highest point of the surface and the mean surface, and Rpm is the average profile peak height [44]. Scratches with features known to

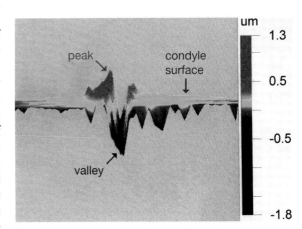

◘ **Fig. 59-2.** Hard particles scratch CoCr surfaces and can increase polyethylene wear by plowing up adjacent peaks that can increase abrasive wear of polyethylene, as seen on this interferometer image of a retrieved clinical specimen

affect polyethylene wear rates (■ Fig. 59-2) have been observed on clinically retrieved TKA femoral condyles [30].

Metal-Articular Cartilage Articulation

Factors contributing to wear of acetabular tissue in hemiarthroplasty include roughness of the head (associated with scratching) as well as lubricity. That there can be an increase in the roughness of prosthetic heads in hemiarthroplasty is being demonstrated by an ongoing investigation of retrieved bipolar prostheses in our laboratory. Scratches of varying depth and orientation have been found on the surface of retrieved bipolar devices. The pattern of scratches on many devices was typical of that found on worn femoral components of total joint replacement prostheses. The profile of many of the scratches was typical of that produced by three-body wear. Some components displayed a matte finish suggestive of a corrosion process or plating with another material. Optical interferometry revealed a roughness (R_a) exceeding 0.2 µm for certain devices. The scratches could have been produced by bone cement or bone fragments or fragments from the surface of the stem entrapped in the articular cartilage or between the head and bone (after erosion of articular cartilage has occurred). These results demonstrate that the CoCr alloy surface of hemiarthroplasty devices is susceptible to wear processes that could produce a topography that might accelerate the breakdown of opposing tissue.

Composition and Microstructure of Oxidized Zirconium

Observations of metal component roughening and its effects on wear of the counterface suggest that a more abrasion-resistant surface can prolong the survival of a joint replacement. Oxide ceramics, such as alumina and zirconia, have demonstrated improved wear performance over metal surfaces in numerous investigations [8]. The use of monolithic ceramics has been restricted because their brittle nature has limited implant designs and created concerns for component fracture. The desired alternative would combine the fracture toughness of metals with the wear performance of ceramics.

OxZr was developed for orthopedic applications to address these desires and provide improvements over CoCr alloy for resistance to roughening, frictional behavior, and biocompatibility [9, 22]. Prosthetic components are produced from a wrought zirconium alloy (Zr-2.5%Nb) that is oxidized by thermal diffusion in heated air to create a zirconia surface about 5 µm thick (■ Fig. 59-3). The oxide is not an externally applied coating, but rather a trans-

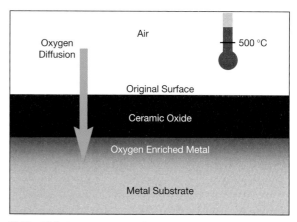

■ Fig. 59-3. Oxygen naturally diffuses into the zirconium alloy when it is heated in air, causing the original metal surface to transform to zirconium oxide (zirconia) ceramic

formation of the original metal surface into zirconium-oxide ceramic. The oxidized component is then burnished to produce an articular surface at least as smooth as that of a CoCr component.

A small amount of niobium is alloyed with the zirconium metal to create a two-phase microstructure with sufficient strength and other mechanical properties for use as an orthopedic prosthesis. Like titanium, the metallic elements of zirconium and niobium are very biocompatible, with minimum biological availability and electrocatalytic activity due to their passive oxide layers with extremely low solubility and excellent protective ability [25]. The biocompatibility of the alloy both with and without an oxide was found to be at least equivalent to that of titanium alloy (Ti-6%Al-4%V) and CoCr [9]. All results were negative, indicating excellent biocompatibility, in the following tests:

- Cytotoxicity: L929 MEM Mouse Fibroblast Test
- Sensitization: Kligman Guinea Pig Maximization Test
- Intracutaneous Reactivity: USP XXII Class VI Rabbit Injection Test
- Systemic Toxicity: USP XXII Class VI Mouse Injection Test
- Hemolysis: Autian Method Rabbit Blood Contact Test
- Pyrogenicity: USP XXII Rabbit Injection Test
- Intramuscular Implantation: USP XXII Class VI and 90-Day Rabbit Tests
- Genotoxicity: Ames Mutagenicity and Mouse Bone Marrow Micronucleus Tests

Although poorly understood, implant-related metal sensitivity has been found to be a concern for a small number of TKA patients [19]. All metals in contact with biological systems undergo corrosion and release metal ions, a process that is accelerated on articular surfaces [8]. Adverse reactions ranging from mild rashes to severe pain have been linked to allergic responses to these ions, particularly from metals known as sensitizers such as nickel, cobalt, and chromium. In comparison to CoCr, OxZr minimizes these concerns because the oxide surface inhibits release of metal ions and because residual levels of metal sensitizers in the alloy are undetectable. As a result, OxZr femoral components have been used clinically in cases where metal sensitivity is a concern [48].

During the oxidation process, the metallic surface transforms into a dense ceramic that is predominantly monoclinic zirconia [4]. Components are made from wrought alloy because the local rate of oxide growth and the resulting oxide microstructure are affected by the metallic microstructure. Thus, the refined metallic microstructure produces a fine-grained (almost nanostructural) oxide of uniform thickness. This oxide is comprised primarily of a staggered columnar microstructure oriented perpendicular to the outer surface (■ Fig. 59-4). It is left in a compressive stress state without pores or voids internally or at the interface. All of these microstructural features inhibit crack propagation and intra-oxide spallation under shear, contributing to the excellent integrity observed for this material.

Nano-hardness testing indicated that the OxZr is more than twice as hard as CoCr on the articular surface, but this alone does not mean that it is more abrasion resistant [24, 33]. The hard surface also must be durable during articulation, so a series of laboratory tests were devised in order to demonstrate the mechanical integrity of the oxidized surface [10, 36]. In one test, the abrasive effect of third-body debris on the hard

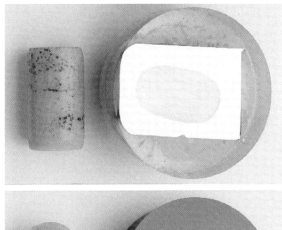

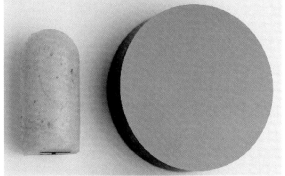

■ **Fig. 59-5.** An OxZr disk (*below right*) exhibits 4900 times less volumetric loss than a CoCr disk (*top right*) when abraded by spherical-tipped bone cement pins (*remains on left*, respectively) for 10 million cycles

counterface of the joint prosthesis was approximated by rubbing bone cement against flat plates [23]. Cylindrical pins with spherical tips were made of bone cement and then articulated against linearly reciprocating plates for 10 million cycles with an initial contact stress of 82 MPa. This simulated a severe instance of debris embedded in the polyethylene rubbing against the counterface for approximately 10 years. OxZr plates exhibited over 4900 times less volumetric wear loss and over 160 times less roughness than CoCr alloy plates in this test (■ Fig. 59-5). The oxidized surface did not chip off or wear away even when a strip of oxide was removed perpendicularly across the wear track before testing [21]. Not only did this demonstrate that OxZr is much more abrasion resistant than CoCr; it also indicated that the oxide could tolerate localized damage or loss without catastrophic failure.

Mechanical testing and finite element analysis indicated that knee femoral components made from OxZr and CoCr have equivalent device fatigue strength, with both exceeding a strength of 450 MPa for 10 million cycles [47]. In contrast to the limitations exhibited by monolithic ceramics such as alumina and zirconia, OxZr does not exhibit brittle fracture during crush tests [46]. Continuous loading of a single OxZr condyle up to 20 kN can cause it to bend to an angle of 45°, but the condyle does not break and the oxide remains attached and functional

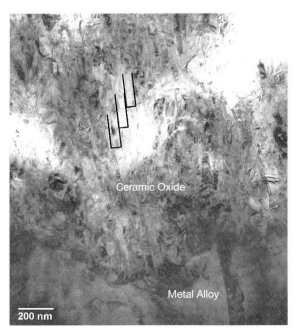

■ **Fig. 59-4.** The oxide exhibits excellent integrity, which is due in part to grains (*three examples outlined*) that are columnar, staggered, almost nano-structural, and generally perpendicular to the surface (transmission electron microscope image at the ceramic-metal interface)

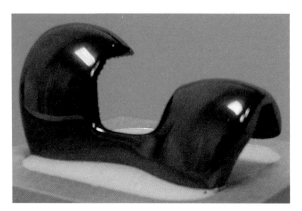

Fig. 59-6. The OxZr component bent but did not shatter, and the oxide remain attached and functional, when one condyle (*right*) was loaded continuously to 20 kN

(■ Fig. 59-6). In addition, the monoclinic crystal structure of the oxide on OxZr is not affected by repeated autoclave sterilization exposures [46]. The same autoclave exposures can produce significant roughening and weakening of yttria-stabilized zirconia with a tetragonal crystal structure. Because of the strength, toughness, and stability of OxZr, it can be used in components that duplicate the design of CoCr and other metal parts. This allows the flexibility of offering the advantages of a ceramic component interchangeably with metallic component designs and without the requirement of unique surgical procedures and associated training.

Tribology of Oxidized Zirconium – Polyethylene Articulation

Wear of the polyethylene components is often cited as a reason for knee replacement complications and failure. Delamination, pitting, and cracking of the polyethylene caused by fatigue wear are readily apparent to the eye and have been the historic concern for knee failure. Improvements in the polyethylene material and component designs have minimized these features. Gas sterilization (fumigation in ethylene oxide, hydrogen peroxide, or gas-plasma) to avoid gamma irradiation prevents embrittlement of the polyethylene. Elimination of fusion defects and calcium stearate inclusions removes initiation sites for fatigue wear. More conforming articular shapes minimize contact stresses that drive fatigue mechanisms. Nevertheless, less-apparent wear mechanisms still produce microscopic wear particles that are of concern for periprosthetic osteolysis. Adhesive wear is caused by frictional shear as the polyethylene surface articulates against the hard counterface. Abrasive wear is caused as hard counterface asperities scrape against the polyethylene surface. Improving lubrication and maintaining smooth counterfaces can reduce small particle generation from these two wear mechanisms, so OxZr was developed with these features in mind.

Oxide ceramic surfaces can reduce friction (and thereby adhesive wear of polyethylene) relative to that of metal surfaces by roughening less and better maintaining a lubricating film [8]. In the joint, lubrication is provided by synovial fluid wetting the counterfaces. A recent study showed that the lubricating quality of synovial fluid can vary greatly among individuals, placing the prostheses at greater risk for wear in certain patients [34]. OxZr was found to be less sensitive than CoCr to these variations and maintained a lower coefficient of friction when articulated with UHMWPE, even in poor lubricants. Other pin-on-disk studies also have shown that OxZr is more wettable and produces less friction and UHMWPE wear than CoCr [40, 43, 49].

Knee simulator tests have been used to help understand how OxZr counterfaces compare with the standard CoCr counterfaces for wear of the polyethylene components. The pioneering study was conducted using a simulator that mimics the rolling and plowing motions of knee prosthesis kinematics [50]. Early OxZr prototypes made from castings were used in this study, and the oxide was thinner and had less integrity than was later developed. In addition, the polyethylene liners were gamma-irradiated in air. Despite these material limitations, the OxZr components produced significantly fewer wear features and none of the macroscopic polyethylene delamination observed in the tests with CoCr components. It also was noted that the CoCr surfaces roughened during testing, while the OxZr surfaces were not affected.

After full development of the manufacturing processes, a study was conducted using a four-axis, displacement-controlled, physiological knee simulator [45]. Components were tested for 6 million cycles of 90% walking-gait and 10% stair-climbing activity, and polyethylene wear was measured periodically during the test by weight loss and by wear particle characterization. In comparison to CoCr, OxZr produced an aggregate wear rate of polyethylene that was 85% less. This comparison had a 90% confidence level because the test parameters generated lower wear rates and more measurement variability than desired. It was noted that all of the OxZr components generated lower polyethylene wear rates and produced less burnishing of the inserts. In contrast to the OxZr surfaces, the CoCr surfaces were found to have roughened during testing even though the lubricant was filtered before testing (■ Fig. 59-7). Analysis of the wear debris also indicated that OxZr produced fewer small polyethylene particles and less total volume of particles, but the sample size was too limited for statistical significance.

A separate study was conducted on a different component design in the same type of simulator, but the test parameters were modified to produce greater wear rates and less measurement variability using just a walking-gait motion [20]. In comparison to CoCr, OxZr produced a mean wear rate that was 42% less when measured either

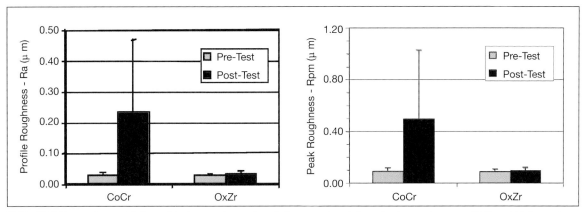

■ **Fig. 59-7.** The roughness of CoCr condyles increased approximately five to ten times in knee simulator testing even with filtered lubricant, whereas OxZr condyles remained smooth

gravimetrically or volumetrically. This reduction is substantial, although less than the 85% comparison of the previous study. The later study may be more representative of the "normal" performance advantage of OxZr knees because it achieved a 95% confidence limit and the relative performance is similar to that found with hip simulators [17]. This study continued, however, to show that the knee wear rates were sensitive to test conditions. The wear rate using OxZr was 62% less than that using CoCr under conditions of greater rotation and an additional varus moment. This indicated that the performance advantage for OxZr might increase for conditions associated with "more demanding" patient kinematics.

Besides kinematics, another "more demanding" condition occurs commonly as the femoral component surface roughens. CoCr femoral components were tumbled in an abrasive alumina powder before simulator testing [42]. The resulting roughness values were within the clinically relevant range. The components were tested for 5 million cycles using the same displacement-controlled simulator protocol as the first test series. OxZr components tumbled using the same procedure roughened less and produced an aggregate wear rate of polyethylene that was 89% less ($p<0.05$). Because the components were pre-roughened, particle analysis was conducted on the wear debris without the complicating presence of numerous abrasive particles in the test lubricant. In comparison to CoCr, OxZr produced 44% fewer polyethylene particles ($p<0.05$). A separate test with pre-roughened components was conducted for 5 million cycles using a force-controlled simulator [11]. Compared with CoCr in this test, OxZr produced an average wear rate that was 82% less ($p<0.001$).

Collectively, these knee simulator tests indicate that OxZr components can reduce wear of the polyethylene counterface by 40%-90% depending on test conditions. Similar wear reductions have been found for monolithic ceramic femoral components in knee simulator tests [1, 37]. These results indicate that OxZr may contribute to

reducing wear-related clinical complications such as debris-induced osteolysis. It is interesting to note that the performance advantage for OxZr relative to CoCr seems to increase as the testing conditions become more demanding. This trend indicates that OxZr may be of particular help to "high-demand" patients who are most in need of assistance to prolong the survival of their prostheses.

Over 50 000 total knee replacements were performed using OxZr femoral components from the first surgery in 1997 to the middle of 2004. Over 15 000 total hip replacements have been performed using OxZr femoral heads since the first surgery in 2002. Numerous clinical studies are being organized to compare the performance of OxZr and CoCr components. The first study to be published involved knee patients, and no adverse effects had been observed at the 2-year evaluation [28]. In the randomized prospective portion of this study, the OxZr patients experienced a more rapid return of flexion and regaining of functional milestones. A much longer time period will be required to measure differences in polyethylene wear and implant survivorship.

Tribology of Oxidized Zirconium – Cartilage Articulation

Concern about the longevity of total joint replacement has renewed interest in hemiarthroplasty as a treatment for certain hip disorders and TKA without patella resurfacing. Hemiarthroplasty has been well established as a practical and beneficial treatment for elderly patients with femoral neck fractures because of it entails low morbidity and allows an expedient return to independence [7,12,15,29]. Young patients with avascular necrosis of the femoral head have also been considered to be good candidates for conservative reconstructive surgical procedures involving hemiarthroplasty. However, reports of relatively early failure [2,7,12,29,31] have made this indication for the prosthesis questionable.

Causes of failure of hemiarthroplasty prostheses include pain and the erosion (i.e., wear) of acetabular articular cartilage and bone. A critical element of the hemiarthroplasty prosthesis is the material from which the head is produced and its topography. Previous laboratory studies have revealed some of the determinants of wear of articular cartilage when it is articulated with metal counterfaces. Lipshitz and Glimcher [32] developed a laboratory test apparatus to rub articulate cartilage against a stainless steel counterface. They found that the wear rate of cartilage increased with roughness of the metal and that the presence of a third body greatly increased wear. In these experiments, calcium phosphate particles were employed as the third bodies in order to simulate the conditions when bone fragments or mineral deposits are introduced between the articulating components. Also of note was the finding that there was no correlation between the orientation of the cartilage plug, relative to the direction of sliding, and wear rate.

CoCr alloy is the primary material employed as the bearing surface for the hemiarthroplasty device. However, both animal [6] and the aforementioned human studies have documented the degradative changes in articular cartilage associated with the use of this material for hemiarthroplasty prostheses. Moreover, comparable findings were reported in an investigation employing CoCr alloy devices to resurface the trochlea of the dog knee [26]. The study documented the degradative changes in the articular cartilage of the opposing patella 3 months after implantation of the hemiarthroplasty device. The investigation also demonstrated the increase in wear rate with roughness of the metallic surface.

In an attempt to develop prostheses with improved tribological performance, several investigators have studied the effects of the material of fabrication of the hemiarthroplasty device on the wear of the opposing articular cartilage using canine models for hemiarthroplasty of the hip. Mendes et al. [35], demonstrated the unsuitability of high-density polyethylene (HDPE) as the material for the hemiarthroplasty head. Significant wear of articular cartilage and the HDPE was found with these devices. Investigation of similar devices employed in human studies yielded similar findings [51]. Canine studies employing alumina heads identified some erosion through the articular cartilage to bone after 2 years [27]. These studies demonstrated, however, that despite the articulation of the head with bone, there was no scratching of the ceramic. This finding led the investigators to recommend ceramic for hemiarthroplasty devices. A more recent study showed that there was less wear of articular cartilage with carbon heads than with CoCr alloy or titanium alloy devices [5]. In summary, results of previous animal investigations have suggested that some materials might be superior to CoCr alloy for hemiarthroplasty. These studies have confirmed laboratory experiments that showed that the wear rate of cartilage increases with the roughness of the metal counterface. Benefits have been demonstrated with the use of scratch-resistant ceramic materials. Moreover, there has been some evidence that certain materials, perhaps by virtue of their lubricity, yield less wear of articular cartilage than CoCr alloy.

Results of a prior study showed that the coefficient of friction of articular cartilage rubbed against an OxZr counterface was significantly lower than with the CoCr control [38, 39]. The results also indicated a trend (but no statistically significant difference) toward less wear of adult bovine articular cartilage articulated with OxZr, when compared with the CoCr alloy control. At higher load, shear failure of the calf osteochondral plugs occurred only one of four times when articulated with OxZr, in comparison to six of eight times with the CoCr alloys, associated with the higher frictional force generated with the latter. The fact that shear failure of articular cartilage occurred under a load that was at the low end of the physiological range was probably related to the conditions of the laboratory test, which included continuous unidirectional motion and constant load. Shear failure of the immature (i.e., calf) specimens could also reflect an incompletely developed attachment of collagen to the calcified cartilage zone.

Acknowledgments. M. Spector, Director, Tissue Engineering, VA Boston Healthcare System, was supported by the Department of Veterans Affairs, Veterans Health Administration, Rehabilitation Research and Development Service; M. Spector is a Research Career Scientist.

References

1. Alberts LR, Neff JR, Webb JD (2001) Wear simulation comparison of a zirconia and a cobalt chrome femoral knee implant. Trans Orthop Res Soc 26:1101
2. Amstutz HC, Grigoris P, Safran MR, Grecula MJ, Campbell PA, Shmalzried TP (1994) Precision-fit surface hemiarthroplasty for femoral head osteonecrosis. J Bone Joint Surg [Br] 76:423-427
3. Barrack RL, Castro Jr. FP, Szuszczewicz ES, Schmalzried TP (2002) Analysis of retrieved uncemented porous-coated acetabular components in patients with and without pelvic osteolysis. Orthopedics 25:1-6
4. Benezra V, Mangin S, Treska M, Spector M, Hunter G, Hobbs LW (1999) Microstructural investigation of the oxide scale on Zr-2.5Nb and its interface with the alloy substrate. In: Neenan T, Marcolongo M, Valentini RF (eds) Biomedical materials. MRS Symposium Proc. 550. Materials Research Society, Warrendale, PA, pp 337-342
5. Cook SD, Thomas KA, Kester MA (1989) Wear characteristics of the canine acetabulum against different femoral prostheses. J Bone Joint Surg [Br] 71:189-197
6. Cruess RL, Kwok DC, Duc PN, Lecavalier MA, Dang GT (1984) The response of articular cartilage to weight-bearing against metal. A study of hemiarthroplasty of the hip in the dog. J Bone Joint Surg [Br] 66:592-597
7. D'arcy J, Devas M (1976) Treatment of fractures of the femoral neck by replacement with the Thompson prosthesis. J Bone Joint Surg [Br] 58:279-286
8. Davidson JA (1993) Characteristics of metal and ceramic total hip bearing surfaces and their effect on long-term ultra high molecular weight polyethylene wear. Clin Orthop 294:361-378

9. Davidson JA, Asgian CM, Mishra AK, Kovacs P (1992) Zirconia (ZrO2)-coated zirconium-2.5Nb alloy for prosthetic knee bearing applications. In: Yamamuro T, Kokubo T, Nakamura T (eds) Bioceramics, vol 5. pp 389-401. Kobunshi Kankokai, Kyoto

10. Davidson JA, Poggie RA, Mishra AK (1994) Abrasive wear of ceramic, metal, and UHMWPE bearing surfaces from third-body bone, PMMA bone cement and titanium debris. Biomed Mater Eng 4:213-229

11. DesJardins JD, LaBerge M (2003) UHMWPE in-vitro wear performance under roughened oxidized zirconium and CoCr femoral knee components. Trans Soc Biomaterials 26:364

12. Devas M, Hinves B (1983) Prevention of acetabular erosion after hemiarthroplasty for fractured neck of femur. J Bone Joint Surg [Br] 65:548-551

13. Dowson D, Taheri S, Wallbridge NC (1987) The role of counterface imperfections in the wear of polyethylene. Wear 119:277-293

14. Dwyer KA, Topoleski LDT, Bauk DJ, Nakielny R, Engh GA (1993) The neglected side of the wear couple: analysis of surface morphology of retrieved femoral components. Trans Orthop Res Soc 18:82

15. Eiskjaer S, Ostgard SE (1993) Survivorship analysis of hemiarthroplasties. Clin Orthop 286:206-211

16. Fisher J, Firkins P, Reeves EA, Hailey JL, Isaac GH (1995) The influence of scratches to metallic counterfaces on the wear of ultra-high molecular weight polyethylene. Proc Instn Mech Engrs 209-H:263-264

17. Good V, Ries M, Barrack RL, Widding K, Hunter G, Heuer D (2003) Reduced wear with oxidized zirconium femoral heads. J Bone Joint Surg [Am] 85 [Suppl 4]:105-110

18. Hailey JL, Ingham E, Stone M, Wroblewski BM, Fisher J (1996) Ultra-high molecular weight polyethylene wear debris generated in vivo and in laboratory tests; the influence of counterface roughness. Proc Instn Mech Engrs 210-H:3-10

19. Hallab N, Merritt K, Jacobs JJ (2001) Metal sensitivity in patients with orthopaedic implants. J Bone Joint Surg [Am] 83:428-436

20. Hermida JC, Patil S, D'Lima DD, Colwell CW Jr, Ezzet KA (2004) Polyethylene wear against metal-ceramic composite femoral components. Am Acad Orthop Surg Ann Mtg Proc 5:449

21. Hunter G (2001) Adhesion testing of oxidized zirconium. Trans Soc Biomaterials 24:540

22. Hunter G, Dickinson J, Herb B, Graham R (2005) Creation of oxidized zirconium orthopaedic implants. J ASTM International

23. Hunter G, Long M (2000) Abrasive wear of oxidized Zr-2.5Nb, CoCrMo, and Ti-6Al-4V against bone cement. In: Sixth World Biomaterials Congress Transactions, Society For Biomaterials, Minneapolis, MN, p 835

24. Hunter G, Pawar V, Salehi A, Long M (2004) Abrasive wear of modified CoCr and Ti-6Al-4V surfaces against bone cement. In: Shrivatsava S (ed) Medical device materials. Materials Park, OH, ASM International pp 91-97

25. Kovacs P, Davidson JA (1996) Chemical and electrochemical aspects of the biocompatibility of titanium and its alloys. In: Brown SA, Lemons JE (eds) Medical Applications of Titanium and Its Alloys, ASTM STP 1272. American Society for Testing and Materials, West Conshohocken, PA, pp 163-178

26. LaBerge M, Bobyn JD, Drouin G, Rivard CH (1992) Evaluation of metallic personalized hemiarthroplasty: a canine patellofemoral model. J Biomed Mater Res 26:239-254

27. Lade R, Sauer B, Doerre E (1983) Long-term performance of high-purity aluminium oxide ceramic heads in canine endoprosthetic hip replacement. In: Vincenzini P (ed) Ceramics in surgery. Elsevier, Amsterdam, pp 277-286

28. Laskin RS (2003) An oxidized Zr ceramic surfaced femoral component for total knee arthroplasty. Clin Orthop 416:191-196

29. Lestrange NR (1990) Bipolar arthroplasty for 496 hip fractures. Clin Orthop 251:7-19

30. Levesque M, Livingston BJ, Jones WM, Spector M (1998) Scratches on condyles in normal functioning total knee arthroplasty. Trans Orthop Res Soc 23:247

31. Leyshon RL, Matthews JP (1984) Acetabular erosion and the Monk "hard top" hip prosthesis. J Bone Joint Surg [Br] 66:172-174

32. Lipshitz H, Glimcher MJ (1979) In vitro studies of the wear of articular cartilage. II: Characteristics of the wear of cartilage when worn against stainless steel plates having characterized surfaces. Wear 52:297-339

33. Long M, Riester L, Hunter G (1998) Nano-hardness measurements of oxidized Zr-2.5Nb and various orthopaedic materials. Trans Soc Biomaterials 21:528

34. Mazzucco D, Spector M (2004) Friction of oxidized zirconium versus cobalt-chromium alloy against polyethylene. Trans Orthop Res Soc 29:1460

35. Mendes DG, Figarola F, Bullough PG, Loudis P (1975) High-density polyethylene prosthetic femoral head replacement in the dog. Clin Orthop 111:274-283

36. Mishra AK, Davidson JA (1993) Zirconia/zirconium: a new, abrasion resistant material for orthopaedic applications. Mater Tech 8:16-21

37. Oonishi H, Hanatate Y, Tsuji E, Yunoki H (1989) Comparisons of wear of UHMW polyethylene sliding against metal and alumina in total knee prostheses. In: Oonishi H, Aoki H, Sawai K (eds) Bioceramics, vol 1. Ishiyaku EuroAmerica, Tokyo, pp 219-224

38. Patel AM, Spector M (1995) Oxidized zirconium for hemiarthroplasty: an in vitro assessment. In: Wilson J, Hench LL, Greenspan D (eds) Bioceramics, vol 8. Elsevier, Tarrytown, NY, pp 169-175

39. Patel AM, Spector M (1997) Tribological evaluation of oxidized zirconium using an articular cartilage counterface: a novel material for potential use in hemiarthroplasty. Biomaterials 18:441-447

40. Poggie RA, Wert JJ, Mishra AK, Davidson JA (1992) Friction and wear characterization of UHMWPE in reciprocating sliding contact with Co-Cr, Ti-6Al-4V and zirconia implant bearing surfaces. In: Denton R, Keshavan MK (eds) Wear and friction of elastomers, ASTM STP 1145. American Society for Testing and Materials, Philadelphia, pp 65-81

41. Que L, Topoleski LD (2000) Third-body wear of cobalt-chromium-molybdenum implant alloys initiated by bone and poly(methyl methacrylate) particles. J Biomed Mater Res 50:322-330

42. Ries MD, Salehi A, Widding K, Hunter G (2002) Polyethylene wear performance of oxidized zirconium and cobalt-chromium knee components under abrasive conditions. J Bone Joint Surg [Am] 84 [Suppl 2]:129-135

43. Salehi A, Aldinger P, Sprague J, Hunter G, Bateni A, Tavana H, Neumann AW (2004) Dynamic contact angle measurements on orthopaedic ceramics and metals. In: Shrivatstava S (ed) Medical Device Materials. ASM International, Materials Park, OH, pp 98-102

44. Sherrington I, Smith EH (1987) Parameters for characterizing the surface topography of engineering components. Proc Instn Mech Engrs. 201-C:297-306

45. Spector M, Ries MD, Bourne RB, Sauer WS, Long M, Hunter G (2001) Wear performance of ultra-high molecular weight polyethylene on oxidized zirconium total knee femoral components. J Bone Joint Surg [Am] 83 [Suppl 2]:80-86

46. Sprague J, Salehi A, Tsai S, Pawar V, Thomas R, Hunter G (2004) Mechanical behavior of zirconia, alumina, and oxidized zirconium modular heads. In: Brown S, Clarke IC, Gustafson A (eds) ISTA 2003, vol 2. International Society for Technology in Arthroplasty, Birmingham, AL, pp 31-36

47. Tsai S, Sprague J, Hunter G, Thomas R, Salehi A (2001) Mechanical testing and finite element analysis of oxidized zirconium femoral components. Trans Soc Biomaterials 24:163

48. Vittetoe DA, Rubash HE (2002) Strategies for reducing ultra-high molecular weight polyethylene wear and osteolysis in total knee arthroplasty. Semin Arthroplasty 13:344-349

49. Walker PS, Blunn GW, Lilley PA (1996) Wear testing of materials and surfaces for total knee replacement. J Biomed Mater Res 33:159-175

50. White SE, Whiteside LA, McCarthy DS, Anthony M, Poggie RA (1994) Simulated knee wear with cobalt chromium and oxidized zirconium knee femoral components. Clin Orthop 309:176-184

51. Wroblewski BM (1979) Wear of high-density polyethylene on bone and cartilage. J Bone Joint Surg [Br] 61:498-500

52. Zou L, Bloebaum RD, Shea KG, Hofmann AA, Dunn HK (1996) Presence of third-body particulate in acetabular components retrieved from patients with osteolysis. Trans Orthop Res Soc 21:454

VIII The Wider Scope

60 Patient Selection and Counseling
C. Mahoney, K. L. Garvin

Summary

When selecting patients for total knee replacement, it is important to assess both the chronological and the physiological patient age to gage longevity of the implant as well as perioperative co-morbidity risk. The severity of clinical and radiographic disease can factor into postoperative functional status and can also direct the surgeons in their implant selection. The number of potential complications has been reduced in recent years by optimizing the patient's health prior to surgery. Interventions such as preoperative antibiotics and aggressive postoperative DVT prophylaxis have also reduced the risk of complication. The surgeon considering total knee replacement in a patient needs to spend time with that patient to let him or her know about the expectations postoperatively as well as to summarize the risks of surgery.

Introduction

Total knee arthroplasty (TKA) is one of the most successful interventions in the treatment of patients with significant osteoarthritis of the knee. Criteria used by the surgeon to select patients for this operation significantly affect the success and longevity of the surgery. Factors that affect the success and durability of the implant include the patient's age, activity level, size, medical comorbidities, and severity of clinical and radiographic arthritis.

At the time of selection for surgery, patients should be made aware of potential medical complications that can occur both during and after TKA. The most common and serious complications include perioperative mortality, infection, and deep venous thrombosis (DVT).

This chapter outlines criteria used to aid the surgeon in selecting appropriate candidates for TKA and also discusses the counseling of patients regarding possible complications that can occur around the time of surgery.

Patient Selection

The average age of patients in the United States receiving primary TKA for the treatment of arthritis of the knee is 69 years [1]. Despite different activity levels corresponding with different ages, no consistent correlation has been found between patient satisfaction and patient age [2]. While the average age is 69 years, the percentage of patients having primary total knee arthroplasty under the age of 60 is actually rising [1]. When age is considered, both the very young and very old require special attention.

Younger patients require special attention because they tend to show earlier wear and joint failure when compared with age-adjusted counterparts. The most likely reason for this is the higher activity level of younger patients. Younger patients have higher levels of expectation and are usually healthier than older patients, which contributes to greater wear. When weighing surgical intervention in a patient under the age of 60, both osteotomy and unicompartmental arthroplasty should be considered.

When examining younger patients, special attention should be given to the patient's range of motion, history of previous surgery, varus or valgus malalignment, ligamentous stability, and to assessing all three compartments of the knee for both symptoms and radiographic evidence of arthrosis. Patients with flexion contractures greater than 15°, patients with greater than 10° of varus or 15° of valgus, and those with ligamentously deficient knees have historically not done well with unicompartmental arthroplasty [3]. In the osteotomy patient, the presence of significant degenerative changes in the opposite compartment may lead to less than satisfactory results [4].

The results of TKA in patients under the age of 55 are encouraging and in most studies exceed the results of those patients who have had osteotomy or unicompartmental arthroplasty. Three studies of young patients with an age range of 36-51 show good to excellent results in anywhere from 93% to 100% [5-8]. Survivorship in two of these studies was greater than 90% at a minimum of 10 years [5, 8]. Based on these data, TKA can currently be safely considered for patients under the age of 55 as long as they accept the risk of increased wear and earlier failure rates.

While there is no true minimum age for doing a total knee replacement, there is certainly no maximum age after which patients should be excluded. There are a number of studies that show that mortalities do rise among older patients; however, there is a high correlation between the number of medical co-morbidities and mortality [9]. Accepting that, there is no correlation between age and patient satisfaction, and therefore, healthy patients into their 90s can be considered reasonable candidates for TKA.

The severity of preoperative arthritis in the knee does affect the long-term outcome of TKA. One of the most important factors in postoperative satisfaction is the level of preoperative functional loss. Patients who have severe clinical and radiographic arthritis typically are more satisfied after TKA compared with patients who are less affected both radiographically and clinically [10]. However, it is accepted that preoperative range of motion correlates relatively highly with postoperative range of motion, so those patients who do have severe disease and preoperative stiffness, while achieving high levels of satisfaction, may experience a postoperative range of motion which does not equal that of patients who are less affected with severe clinical arthrosis and stiffness.

In severely deformed patients, there has been a higher rate of success using a posterior-stabilized prosthesis. Booth [11] has reported increased range of motion, greater stability, equal survival rates, and greater accommodations for joint line alterations using a posterior-stabilized implant compared with a cruciate-retaining implant. Based on these factors, we typically select a posterior-stabilized implant for all patients, but specifically for those who have severe radiographic and clinical arthrosis.

Postoperative medical complications are correlated with preoperative medical conditions [10]. Medical complications that can occur after TKA include DVT, superficial or deep wound infection, seroma or hematoma formation, fat embolism, and numbness around the wound. Patients should be advised that pre-existing medical conditions can be worsened by the procedure. Whether a clinical condition will become significantly worse depends on the preoperative status, the age of the patient, the skill of the surgeon, the anesthetic, and the preoperative medical workup. Only those patients who have had a full medical workup and for whom all medical issues have been completely addressed preoperatively should be considered for total knee replacement [12-15].

Counseling

Prior to surgery, the patient and physician should discuss complications that may arise as a result of total knee replacement. Those complications include death, venous thromboembolism, and infection [16]. A complete understanding of the potential complication achieves two goals. Initially, it allows the patient to make an informed decision about whether to have surgery. An open discussion will allow patients to feel that they are deciding along with the surgeon that total knee replacement is both a correct and a safe decision. Later, in the event of a complication, the patients and their families will have been prepared for the possibility that complications do occur despite our best efforts.

The most serious complication that occurs is death. The overall 30-day mortality after total knee replacement is 0.21% [9]; the 90-day mortality is 0.46% [17]. Patients under the age of 65 have a significantly reduced mortality compared with those older than 85 years. The under-65 rate is 0.13%, while those over the age of 85 have an approximately 4.65% 90-day mortality [17]. Significant pre-existing co-morbidities do result in higher mortality. This has been estimated to be as high as 16 times greater than for patients without medical co-morbidities. As discussed above, older patients typically have more medical problems and, therefore, the morbidities themselves are likely the cause of most deaths.

The most common complication experienced in total knee replacement is venous thromboembolism [18]. The prevalence of DVT without prophylaxis in TKA has been estimated anywhere from 40% to 84%, with symptomatic pulmonary emboli ranging from 1.8% to 7%. Based on these percentages, most surgeons take preventive measures that can include blood thinners, pressure stockings, early motion after surgery, or compression devices. Patients should be counseled that the risk of having a clot can be dramatically reduced with a combination of the interventions listed above. Regardless of the type, this risk can be reduced, but not eliminated.

Aside from death, deep infection after TKA is the most serious and debilitating complication that can occur. With standard prophylaxis, including perioperative antibiotics, laminar air flow, and body exhaust suits, infection rates should not exceed 2%. Patients with rheumatoid arthritis, previous open surgeries, immunosuppressive therapy, poor nutrition, diabetes, renal failure, and alcohol abuse have all been shown to have higher infection rates. Patients with psoriatic arthritis also have higher rates of infection; psoriatic lesions should be avoided if possible when making incisions. When counseling patients regarding the risk of infection, the hospital's surgical infection rate is a useful number for the patient. Again, patients should be counseled that while the chance of infection cannot be eliminated, it can be reduced with careful attention to detail and state-of-the-art surgical practice. The surgeon can also lower the risk by completing the surgery in an expedient fashion that minimizes soft-tissue trauma.

The operating time, amount of dissection, and rehabilitation potential are all affected by the patient's habitus. Obese patients require more dissection and extra re-traction during surgery. This leads to increased operating time. The mobility of the adipose tissue should be assessed preoperatively. Patients with loose or mobile fat are much easier to operate on, as their soft tissue can be retracted very readily. Patients with body mass indices (BMIs) that are equal but who have tight fat require more dissection and retraction. Obese patients also have an increased risk of wound-healing problems. All these issues should be addressed preoperatively with the patient.

References

1. National Center for Health Statistics (1997) Nationwide Inpatient Survey: Osteoarthritis of the knee group defined as individuals who had an ICD-9 CM diagnosis that was classified as osteoarthritis and any listed diagnosis that was classified as applying to the knee region. In: AAOS Manual (2002) Osteoarthritis of the Knee: a Compendium of Evidence-based Information and Resources
2. Robertsson O, Dunbar M, Pehrsson T, Knutson K, Lidgren L (2000) Patient satisfaction after knee arthroplasty: a report on 27,372 knees operated on between 1981 and 1995 in Sweden. Acta Orthop Scand 71:262-267
3. Tria AJ (2004) Unicondylar knee arthroplasty - the MIS technique. American Academy of Orthopedic Surgeons Annual Meeting, San Francisco, March 10-14
4. Hanssen AD (2001) Osteotomy about the knee: American perspective. In: Insall JN, Scott WN (eds) Surgery of the knee, 3rd edn. Churchill Livingstone, New York, pp 1447-1464
5. Diduch DR, Insall JN, Scott WN, Scuderi GR, Font-Rodriguez D (1997) Total knee replacement in young, active patients. Long-term follow-up and functional outcome. J Bone Joint Surg [Am] 79:575-582
6. Dalury DF, Ewald FC, Christie MJ, Scott RD (1995) Total knee arthroplasty in a group of patients less than 45 years of age. J Arthroplasty 10:598-602
7. Mont MA, Lee CW, Sheldon M, Lennon WC, Hungerford DS (2002) Total knee arthroplasty in patients ≤50 years old. J Arthroplasty 17:538-543
8. Ranawat CS, Padgett DE, Ohashi Y (1989) Total knee arthroplasty for patients younger than 55 years. Clin Orthop 248:27-33
9. Parvizi J, Sullivan TA, Trousdale RT, Lewallen DG (2001) Thirty-day mortality after total knee arthroplasty. J Bone Joint Surg [Am] 83:1157-1161
10. Heck DA, Robinson RL, Partridge CM, Lubitz RM, Freund DA (1998) Patient outcomes after knee replacement. Clin Orthop 356:93-110
11. Booth RE (2001) The posterior stabilized: a knee for all seasons. Orthopedics 24:887-888
12. Ansari S, Warwick D, Ackroyd CE, Newman JH (1997) Incidence of fatal pulmonary embolism after 1,390 knee arthroplasties without routine prophylactic anticoagulation, except in high-risk cases. J Arthroplasty 12:599-602
13. Sharrock NE, Cazan MG, Hargett MJ, Williams-Russo P, Wilson PD Jr (1995) Changes in mortality after total hip and knee arthroplasty over a ten-year period. Anesth Analg 80:242-248
14. Frostick SP (2000) Death after joint replacement. Haemostasis 30 [Suppl 2]:84-87; discussion pp 82-83
15. Mantilla CB, Horlocker TT, Schroeder DR, Berry DJ, Brown DL (2002) Frequency of myocardial infarction, pulmonary embolism, deep venous thrombosis, and death following primary hip or knee arthroplasty. Anesthesiology 96:1140-1146
16. Callahan CM, Drake BG, Heck DA, Dittus RS (1995) Patient outcomes following unicompartmental or bicompartmental knee arthroplasty. A meta-analysis. J Arthroplasty 10:141-150
17. Gill GS, Mills D, Joshi AB (2003) Mortality following primary total knee arthroplasty. J Bone Joint Surg [Am] 85:432-435
18. Colwell CW (2004) Low molecular weight heparins. American Academy of Orthopedic Surgeons Annual Meeting, San Francisco, March 10-14

61   Pain Management

T. Deckmyn

Summary

Many patients experience severe pain after total knee arthroplasty (TKA) which can lead to several pathophysiological responses, increasing morbidity and delaying prompt rehabilitation. Analgesic regimens, based on a multimodal approach including preemptive NSAIDs and opioids, neuraxial or regional peripheral nerve blockade, and patient-controlled opioid infusions, not only provide effective pain relief and high patient satisfaction but also result in improved functionality, decreased recovery time, and shortened hospital stay. Though epidural techniques provide the best results, use of this method is limited by increased risk of serious complications due to combination with thromboembolism prophylaxis, and femoral three-in-one or lumbar plexus blocks may be preferable.

Introduction

Pain is a significant component of patients' experience after total knee arthroplasty (TKA). It is severe in 60% of patients and moderate in 30%, which may hinder early physical therapy [1]. The average worst pain during the 48 h before discharge was found to be moderate to severe, supporting the existence of an "analgesic gap" [2,3]. Even treated with on-demand doses of narcotics, patients may experience severe pain as a result of delays, improper route of administration, underestimation of effective dose ranges, or overestimation of analgesic duration [3]. Acute pain, limiting mobility, may contribute to complications such as pulmonary or urinary problems, thromboembolism, hyperdynamic circulation, and increased oxygen consumption, through pathophysiological responses including peripheral sensitization and neuroendocrine and sympathoadrenal activation. It can also develop into chronic pain. Lack of pain control results in anxiety, sleeplessness, intensified reflex responses, and release of catecholamines, as well as inhibiting early mobilization of the knee, possibly leading to arthrofibrosis [3]. Pain assessment has also become a new standard implemented by the Joint Commission on Accreditation of Healthcare Organizations [2]. This emphasizes the importance of recognizing recent therapeutic advancements, including the introduction of potent analgesics and more efficient and safe methods of administration.

Oral Analgesics: Oral Opioids

To achieve adequate pain control, an individualized prescription is needed, taking into account the physiological and psychological condition of the patient, the pathophysiological alterations resulting from surgery, and the technical and economic resources available. Oral administration of opioids and non-steroidal anti-inflammatory drugs (NSAIDs) should always be considered first, because of their safety. However, despite their ease of use and combination, which reduces opioid consumption and related side effects, postoperative pain often remains severe [4]. The choice of oral analgesics is very wide, but alterations in gastrointestinal function after general anesthesia may reduce efficacy. Orally administered morphine and meperidine undergo substantial enterohepatic metabolism, have late onset and duration, and may require high doses. Therefore, the sustained-release oxycodone is a better choice and can be used as a transition analgesic after discontinuation of epidural analgesics [3]. The sustained-release preparations provide superior pain control and reduce opioid-related side effects, but the risk of constipation or ileus is higher. Tramadol is a less potent analgesic but does not cause respiratory depression, so it may be a better choice for elderly or very young patients.

Oral Analgesics: Oral NSAIDs

NSAIDs are often prescribed for patients with painful osteoarthritis, many of whom subsequently require total joint arthroplasty. Because of the increased risk of perioperative bleeding, wound hematoma, and hemarthrosis, NSAIDs should be discontinued 7-10 days before surgery. However, NSAID cessation can result in an arthritic flare-up, leading to increased preoperative pain. The severity of preoperative pain correlates directly with postoperative pain and with the amount of opioid analgesic required

[5]. The arthritic flare in other joints may interfere with postoperative physical therapy and rehabilitation. The concomitant use of NSAIDs with warfarin or low-molecular-weight heparin (LMWH) can lead to increased bleeding complications. However, the new COX-2 selective inhibitors maintain platelet function and gastric mucosal integrity. Rueben et al. concluded that rofecoxib 50 mg or celecoxib 200 mg daily, can be used safely in TKA patients in combination with warfarin 5 mg daily without an increase in the INR [5,6]. The preoperative use of rofecoxib did not alter blood loss during surgery. Other COX-1 NSAIDs, such as ketoprofen (100 mg twice daily), indomethacin (100 mg twice daily), ibuprofen (600 mg every 8 h), diclofenac (50-100 mg), or ketorolac (30 mg every 6 h) are still used [4,7-9]. However, concerns remain about the possible impairment of bone growth and higher non-union rates (in spine fusion) [3].

Parenteral Analgesics

Morphine (0.1 mg/kg every 4 h) is still commonly used for severe pain, although the relatively slow onset after intramuscular or subcutaneous injection and side effects (nausea, pruritus, histamine release, and biliary colic) make it less favorable than meperidine, hydromorphone, or piritramide [3]. Ketorolac is a potent NSAID available for parenteral use but also carries an increased risk of causing hemorrhage, gastric ulcer, and renal toxicity. Parenteral selective COX-2 inhibitors would be expected to be safer.

Infusion devices allow the patient to receive small doses of parenteral medication without delay, within prescribed limits and lockout intervals. Patients' control of frequency adjusts the total dose to meet the individual needs, differences in pain perception, and variability in pharmacokinetics. By minimizing the bolus amount and extending the lockout interval sufficiently, the technique avoids cycles of excessive sedation and ineffective pain control. Another advantage is the option of controlling the variations of analgesic requirements during day and night, or during physical therapy [10]. A loading dose should be titrated to achieve a baseline plasma concentration. Patients must be trained to treat pain before the stimulus becomes overwhelming and should understand that their pain will not be completely eliminated.

Epidural and Intrathecal Analgesia

Many studies confirm the superior efficacy of postoperative analgesia and accelerated rehabilitation with epidural and intrathecal analgesia [1, 6, 7]. Single intrathecal boluses of opioids such as morphine (0.3 mg) provide an analgesic effect superior to i.v. patient-controlled analgesia (PCA) with morphine but also have a high incidence of adverse effects, including late onset respiratory depression due to rostral cerebral spinal fluid spread [3]. These problems have been overcome with the use of continuous epidural infusion, avoiding high peak cerebral fluid concentrations. Continuous epidural infusion of local anesthetics offers reliable segmental analgesia and reduced opioid related side effects, but causes more hypotension and urinary retention. The use of low-dose bupivacaine (0.125%) or ropivacaine (0.2%) at rates of 5-12 ml/h prevents motor block. The association of lipophilic opioids with fast onset and short duration has a synergistic effect and seems to further reduce the side effects of both opioids and local anesthetics. The introduction of patient-controlled epidural analgesia has improved the efficacy, tolerability, and comfort and satisfaction of the patient. Despite the fact that patient-controlled epidural analgesia provides the best pain scores and better revalidation, some patients prefer i.v. PCA. Probably they favor a classical maintained, well-tolerated pain level, and they maintain control through self-administration with fewer side effects [3, 7]. To reduce these side effects, present research is focused on the addition of adjuvant drugs. In Europe, the α2-agonist clonidine (1-2 µg/ml) is added to obtain a longer duration of analgesia. It is known to block conduction in C-fibers and provides better control of dynamic pain [1, 7, 8]. Activation of the NMDA receptors within the spinal cord is considered to be central to the development of acute and chronic pain. Ketamine may inhibit a facilitated state of excitability by suppressing the progressive nociceptive response caused by wind-up phenomena and long-term potentiation (anti-hyperalgesic action). Once pain sensitization from incisional and inflammatory injury is established, ketamine reduces NMDA-receptor related altered pain transmission and thus hyperalgesia. Small doses of ketamine (0.25 mg/kg epidural) efficiently block injury-induced pain sensitization without any side effects and provide supplemental pain relief for an extended period of time [9]. Despite the better pain relief and faster rehabilitation [7,11], reduction in blood loss and deep vein thrombosis [6], and good blockade of the 'hidden' endocrine response [12], some occasionally serious side effects can occur. Clinically relevant respiratory compromise is reported to occur in between 0.1% and 0.4% of patients, and can be of late onset (after 8-12 h). It may develop slowly, often preceded by nausea and sedation, and can be treated with naloxone infusions (400 µg/l at 100 ml/h) [3]. Epidural analgesia can mediate hypotension that is not always well tolerated. Bilateral motor block and urinary retention impede functional recovery and may increase the risk of infection arising from urinary catheters. The risk for epidural hematoma is a major concern in TKA patients who receive LMWH for deep venous thrombosis prophylaxis [6,11,13]. The present guidelines do not guarantee against the occurrence of epidural hematoma [6,13].

61

Regional Blocks

Regional block techniques can provide analgesia equal to or better than epidural analgesia without the risk of epidural hematoma [1, 6, 7, 8]. The use of postoperative continuous femoral infusion is associated with a decrease in morphine consumption by up to 70%. This technique permits more rapid postoperative functional recovery [1], better immediate and secondary functional outcomes, and a reduction in length of hospital stay [6, 7]. However, the best technique for establishing blockade of the lumbar plexus is not clear. The knee joint is supplied by the femoral, obturator, and sciatic nerves, and some cutaneous areas of surgical incision with the lateral femoral cutaneous nerve. The osteotomal segments of the femur and tibia at the knee are supplied by the sciatic nerve from the S1 root. Singelyn et al. reported excellent results with a three-in-one approach, first described by Winnie et al. in which after neurostimulation, a catheter is inserted under the inguinal ligament 1.5 cm lateral to the femoral artery and then advanced proximally (12-20 cm) in the sheath of the femoral nerve alongside the psoas muscle, blocking the femoral, obturator, and lateral femoral cutaneous nerves [14]. Because of the variable blockade of the obturator nerve (and the S1 root), Ganapathy et al. proposed a modification placing the catheter under the fascia lata and the fascia iliaca (double-pop technique) [8]. The most reliable method of accessing the lumbar plexus is through the posterior paravertebral approach. However, because of the increased risks of bleeding at the puncture site, psoas hematoma, renal subcapsular hematoma, and lumbar plexopathy, Bogoch et al. found insufficient justification for its use [14,15]. Since the sciatic nerve supplies the posterior region of the knee joint, the combination with a sciatic nerve block may be necessary [14]. Others have noted that a single femoral block provides pain relief as satisfactory as that from a combined femoral and sciatic block, suggesting that the sciatic nerve provides a minor contribution to postoperative pain [4]. When concentrations of local anesthetic are high enough (bupivacaine and ropivacaine 0.2% or lidocaine 1% at rates of 10 ml/h) obturator and lateral femoral cutaneous nerve block can be achieved in 80% of patients [1, 7, 8]. Plasma levels remain below the toxic range, so even higher doses can be used [8]. With the admixture of clonidine (1-2 µg/ml) and/or opioids (sufentanil 0.1 µg/ml, morphine 0.03 mg/ml) pain relief can be further improved.

Regional blocks may also help reduce blood loss and subsequent transfusion requirements [14]. Two mechanisms can influence blood loss: a direct effect on vasoconstrictive sympathetic fibers contained in peripheral nerves (resulting in vasodilation in small and medium vessels, leading to reduced arterial and venous pressure), and an indirect effect mediated by antinociception and reduced systemic blood pressure [6].

The augmented analgesic effects of the regional techniques on pain permit early mobilization with continuous passive motion (CPM) [6, 7]. Pain after knee surgery can be associated with severe spasm of the quadriceps muscle, causing further pain, impaired muscle function, and hindering early rehabilitation. Regional anesthesia may block the massive afferent nociceptive input thought to trigger the increased excitability of the peripheral nociceptors, as well as the dorsal horn neurons. Muscle relaxation can be enhanced by use of a local anesthetic such as lidocaine 1%, which offers greater motor blockade than bupivacaine 0.25% or ropivacaine 0.2%.

The control of postoperative pain may also indirectly influence the risk of wound infection. Patients with a continuous femoral infusion have been reported to have fewer episodes of fever compared with patients who receive parenteral or epidural pain treatment. Morphine has been shown to depress the oxidative bactericidal function of neutrophils, so the reduction in morphine consumption may lead to a lower risk of immediate postoperative infection [6]. When the recovery of knee function is hampered by pain, patients must be identified, followed up closely, and treated with individualized pain therapy promptly [16].

New Concepts in Pain Management

Although most clinical studies have concentrated on decreasing postoperative pain and acute disability, preemptive analgesia may also provide long-term benefits and either prevent or minimize the severity of chronic pain syndromes [3]. With the preoperative administration of pain therapy (NSAIDs, opioids, neuraxial or regional blocks) and extension of the treatment through surgery and the subsequent postoperative inflammatory response, the sensitization of the dorsal horn neurons may be prevented.

Peripheral neural infiltration techniques or intra-articular blocks can also be valuable adjuncts in pain management. Both single-dose injections of local anesthetics and continuous-infiltration catheter techniques have been described. Injection into the wound requires surgical infiltration of large volumes of concentrated local anesthetic solution into the skin, subcutaneous tissues, or joint capsule. Continuous infiltration techniques use multihole 19-gauge catheters to continuously infuse either 0.125% or 0.25% bupivacaine under the skin and muscle layers of the incision. However, potential infection after implantation remains a concern [3].

No single analgesic technique or drug treatment can be expected to achieve complete abolition of postoperative pain. To avoid high dose requirements and adverse effects, "balanced" or multimodal analgesic regimens have been advocated [3, 9]. At our institution, the regional block is routinely used with systematic administration of acetaminophen (1 g every 6 h) or propacetamol (2 g every 6 h) and perioperative NSAIDs (parecoxib 40 mg daily, ketorolac 15-30 mg every 6 h, or tenoxicam 40 mg daily). We also use a combination of low-dose local anesthetics (levobupivacaine 0.2% at 8 ml/h), lipophilic opioids (sufentanil 0.5 µg/ml), and clonidine (1 µg/ml) in the regional block [1, 6].

After discontinuation of the regional infusion, opioids such as piritramide (0.25 mg/kg every 4 h), a synthetic µ-agonist opioid, or codeine (60 mg every 6 h) are prescribed. Others have used i.v. PCA of morphine (1- to 2-mg bolus with lockout of 6 min) [4, 6, 8] or sustained-release oxycodone PO (20 mg every 12 h) [12]. In the future a form of fentanyl (a synthetic lipophilic opioid), based on a transdermal release patch combined with a small electric current to facilitate dermal migration, but with short onset and duration, will become available. Following the Clinical Practice Guidelines of the USA Veterans Health Administration, intrathecal opioids may be used but intra-articular opioids are not effective. These guidelines also confirm the value of non-pharmacological interventions such as cold therapy, transcutaneous electrical nerve stimulation (TENS), distraction, relaxation, positioning, hypnosis, massage, and exercise. Cold application by means of continuous-flow or cold compression dressings reduces blood loss and pain [17]. TENS may not relieve the most intense aspects of acute pain, but as an analgesic supplement it effectively reduces opioid use [3].

To provide prompt and adequate pain relief, necessary to achieve a rapid functional rehabilitation, and to avoid "analgesic gap" in delivering multimodal pain therapy, inpatient acute pain services can be helpful. The multidisciplinary approach includes caregivers trained to formulate and provide safe and specialized therapy, develop standardized treatment protocols, and optimize methods of drug delivery. It also provides nursing education in assessing patients' pain, in executing standard protocols, and in treating adverse side effects [2].

Appreciation of the severity and character of the pain stimulus and the importance of pain relief in the prevention of a longer rehabilitation or knee stiffness commands that optimal control be provided at each phase of the recovery process. Therapeutic gains are dramatic in patients with underlying cardiovascular and pulmonary disease. Optimally administered regional blockade can suppress the release of catecholamines, maintain hemo-dynamic stability, reduce myocardial oxygen requirements, improve respiratory function, facilitate participation in physical therapy, and reduce length of hospital stay. These advantages outweigh the greater invasiveness, potential side effects, and cost of indwelling catheters, drug preparation, and supervision.

References

1. Singelyn FJ et al (1998) Effects of intravenous patient-controlled analgesia with morphine, continuous epidural analgesia, and continuous three-in-one block on postoperative pain and knee rehabilitation after unilateral total knee arthroplasty. Anesth Analg 87:88-92
2. Strassels SA et al (2002) Postoperative analgesia: economics, resource use, and patient satisfaction in an urban teaching hospital. Anesth Analg 94:130-137
3. Sinatra RS et al (2002) Pain management after major orthopaedic surgery: current strategies and new concepts. J Am Acad Orthop Surg 10:117-129
4. Allen HW et al (1998) Peripheral nerve blocks improve analgesia after total knee replacement surgery. Anesth Analg 87:93-97
5. Rueben SS et al (2002) Evaluation of the safety and efficacy of the perioperative administration of rofecoxib for total knee arthroplasty. J Arthroplasty 17:26-31
6. Chelly JE et al (2001) Continuous femoral blocks improve recovery and outcome of patients undergoing total knee arthroplasty. J Arthroplasty 16:436-445
7. Capdevilla X et al (1999) Effects of perioperative technique on the surgical outcome and duration of rehabilitation after major knee surgery. Anesthesiology 91:8-15
8. Ganapathy S et al (1999) Modified continuous femoral three-in-one block for postoperative pain after total knee arthroplasty. Anesth Analg 89:1197-1202
9. Himmelseher S et al (2001) Small-dose S(+)-ketamine reduces postoperative pain when applied with ropivacaine in epidural anesthesia for total knee arthroplasty. Anesth Analg 92:1290-1295
10. Sinatra RS et al (1992) Acute pain: mechanisms and management. Mosby-Year Book, St. Louis, MO
11. Williams-Russo P et al (1996) Randomized trial of epidural versus general anesthesia: outcomes after primary total knee replacement. Clin Orthop 331:199-208
12. Adams HA et al (2002) Postoperative pain management in orthopaedic patients: no differences in pain score, but improved stress control by epidural anaesthesia. Eur J Anaesthesiol 19:658-665
13. American Society of Regional Anesthesia and Pain Medicine. Consensus statements on neuraxial anesthesia and anticoagulation. Available at http://www.asra.com/
14. Chelly JE et al (2001) Continuous peripheral nerve block techniques. Mosby, London
15. Bogoch ER et al (2002) Lumbar paravertebral nerve block in the management of pain after total hip and knee arthroplasty. J Arthroplasty 17:398-401
16. Ranawat et al (2003) Total knee rehabilitation protocol. J Arthroplasty 18:27-30
17. Webb JM (1998) The use of cold compression dressings after total knee replacement: a randomized controlled trial. Orthopedics 21:59-61

62 Rehabilitation Following Total Knee Arthroplasty

P. Hernigou, A. Poignard, A. Nogier

Summary

Total knee arthroplasty consistently provides favorable outcomes of reduced pain, improved function, and enhanced quality of life for arthritic patients. Although the technical aspects of the operative procedure contribute greatly to the outcome, perioperative rehabilitation remains an important adjunct. Successful rehabilitation involves the collaborative efforts of the surgeon, physical therapist, nursing staff, and patient. Rehabilitation protocols should be specific to reduce ambiguity, yet flexible to accommodate differences in patient characteristics. Critical pathways have been designed to move patients through acute care in a more rapid manner, and in most cases they rely on subacute care facilities to complete patient rehabilitation. This has led to a significant increase in the use of extended care, rehabilitation, and transitional care facilities in order to reduce length of stay and cost while still optimizing the functional outcome after total knee arthroplasty.

Differences in Patient Characteristics Affecting Rehabilitation

Because patient characteristics such as age and preoperative diagnosis have been shown to affect the results of total knee arthroplasty, this information should be used to optimize the rehabilitation protocol and expectations of total knee arthroplasty. Most patients who do not have surgical complications easily accomplish the expected rehabilitation goals of a given postoperative day, resulting in a discharge from the hospital on the scheduled date. However, patients who have surgical complications often do not fare as well.

Patients who experience unexpected perioperative problems or outcomes understandably are disappointed. Patients with low preoperative knee scores or elderly patients should be informed that their hospital stay may be longer than that of most patients, or that they may not be discharged to home. This determination should be made as early as possible. When patients are given an appropriate expectation before surgery, they are better able to cope with unexpected issues that may arise after surgery.

Some preoperative factors can predict patient satisfaction, function, and working capacity. There is a positive association between the duration of preoperative and postoperative sick leave of patients who returned to work. Satisfaction is greater among patients who return to work after surgery. Many investigators have studied correlations between patient age, gender, marital status, body mass index, and co-morbidity and the length of stay in the surgical unit and the need for inpatient rehabilitation [1, 2, 6, 11, 13]. Age was the only factor that correlated with hospital length of stay, while age and diabetes mellitus correlated with the need for inpatient rehabilitation. However, there were no age-related differences in joint pain, function, or quality-of-life measures either before the operation or 6 months after it. Because these patients can be identified preoperatively, one may be able to preempt discharge delays by aggressively treating these patients (physical therapy, occupational therapy, social service, medical consultation). These findings indicate that a single standard allowable length of stay for all patients undergoing total knee arthroplasty is not realistic.

Techniques of Rehabilitation

Although rehabilitation is usually targeted at postoperative recovery, the efficacy of preoperative physical therapy has been investigated in some studies [6, 11, 23]. Some practitioners advocate a preoperative physical therapy program to maximize muscle strength and educate patients about what to expect immediately following surgery. However, no improvement in the outcome of total knee arthroplasty was found when patients had absolved a preoperative physical therapy strengthening protocol for 6 weeks compared with the outcome when patients had had no preoperative exercise [17].

The early postoperative phase of rehabilitation after total knee arthroplasty may be started on the day of surgery, with emphasis on pain control, ankle pumps, gluteal sets, diaphragmatic breathing exercises, and gentle activation exercises for both upper and lower extremities.

Usually, mobility training, dressing, transfers, and ambulation are started within 24-48 h after surgery, depending on surgical procedures and patient co-morbidities.

Continuous Passive Motion Protocol

Continuous passive motion was introduced to the orthopedic community in 1980 by Salter et al. [20] .The biological effect of continuous passive motion on the healing of full thickness defects was studied in the rabbit knee articular cartilage. It was found that continuous passive motion was strikingly beneficial. However, the device described was not suitable for clinical practice. In 1982, Coutts et al. [2] introduced continuous passive motion for the postoperative rehabilitation of patients who underwent total knee arthroplasty. Range of motion (ROM) at day 10 was significantly better and the use of pain medication was decreased [2]. Following this study, the use of continuous passive motion devices following total knee arthroplasty increased dramatically.

At our institution continuous passive motion is started on the morning of postoperative day 1. The nursing staff places the patient's extremity onto the continuous passive motion device 1 h per nursing shift (three times per day), beginning at 0°-30° of flexion. This is increased by 10°-20° per day, based on the patient's level of pain. The patient is also seen by a physical therapist twice a day, beginning on the first postoperative day for gait training with a walker or crutches and active assisted ROM of the knee. The patient is usually discharged late afternoon of postoperative day 6. Outpatient physical therapy is continued two to three times a week for the first 3-4 weeks after discharge. The patients are seen approximately 14 days after surgery for suture removal and to check ROM. If a patient has not progressed to at least 70° flexion at this time, a manipulation is considered.

The effects of continuous passive motion on the range of motion of the knee remain controversial. The reported benefits include decreased need for knee manipulation, fewer instances of deep venous thrombosis, decreased postoperative use of analgesics, and a greater final range of motion. Reported disadvantages include increased wound complications, bleeding, and pain. Patients who undergo continuous passive motion tend to have a greater range of motion at the time of discharge, but this advantage appears to lessen during the subsequent follow-up period.

Alternatives to In-Hospital Continuous Passive Motion

Alternatives to the use of continuous passive motion devices in the hospital have been proposed recently. In a study by Kumar et al., 46 knees for which continuous passive motion was used were compared with 37 knees treated with an early passive flexion protocol ("drop and dangle") [6]. The latter protocol required that the patient be positioned at the side of the bed or in a chair and the foot of the surgically treated leg was placed on the floor by a therapist. With the foot firmly on the floor, the patient moved his or her body forward until 90° knee flexion was achieved. Patients in whom the drop-and-dangle protocol was used had better extension at 6 months. However, manipulation was required in 9% of the group in whom the drop-and-dangle technique was used versus 2.5% in the group of patients who received continuous passive motion. In another prospective randomized study of 80 patients, use of a continuous passive motion device at home was compared with professional home physical therapy visits after total knee arthroplasty [24]. No difference in ROM or extensor lag at 6 months was observed. The cost of continuous passive motion was approximately half that of home physical therapy. In addition, 95% of the patients thought that continuous passive motion use at home was easy and helpful in their rehabilitation.

Manipulation

Manipulation may be necessary after total knee arthroplasty if early postoperative ROM is not adequate. There may be less ultimate ROM at long-term follow-up in knees that do not obtain a satisfactory ROM in the early postoperative period. In the late 1970s and early 1980s manipulation was reported to be necessary after total knee arthroplasty in as many as 54%-60% of patients [4]. Manipulation has been associated with a high incidence of postoperative heterotopic ossification in the quadriceps muscles. Several studies have shown the beneficial effect of continuous passive motion on the rate of manipulation [2, 3, 12, 17, 19, 20]. Coutts et al. [2] reported the results of a multicenter study in 1983: Among patients undergoing total knee arthroplasty, a control group of 129 patients was compared with an experimental group of 137 patients who used constant passive motion. The patients in the continuous passive motion group had no manipulations, whereas 21% of the patients in the control group required manipulation. The indication for manipulation was the inability to achieve 90° of active flexion by 6 weeks after surgery. Manipulation under anesthesia is performed less frequently today than it was 20 years ago. Manipulation rates are now usually below 5% and for some surgeons below 1%. This change in practice reflects the fact that motion may improve spontaneously up to 1 year after the surgery and after manipulation patients may experience complications including hemarthrosis, quadriceps rupture, periprosthetic fracture, implant loosening, and heterotopic bone formation.

62

Prevention of Pain, Wound Healing Complications, Deep Vein Thromboses, and Blood Loss During Rehabilitation

Postoperative Pain Management After Total Knee Replacement

The management of postoperative pain is a challenge that faces surgeons and patients alike after total knee arthroplasty. Many surgeons consider total knee arthroplasty to be much more painful than total hip arthroplasty. Effective pain management can improve the ultimate ROM by allowing earlier achievement of greater flexion.

The value of preemptive analgesia with long-acting oral narcotics delivered on a fixed schedule rather than on an "as-needed" basis has been shown to improve pain control substantially. COX-2 inhibitors have also received attention as an adjunctive form of analgesia that may help to decrease postoperative narcotic requirements. Intra-articular anesthetic injections may provide modest improvements in postoperative pain management for the first few hours following surgery.

Nerve blocks have become increasingly accepted as a form of postoperative pain management. Although the knee is innervated through branches of the femoral, obturator, and sciatic nerves, the individual contributions of each of these nerves to pain patterns after total knee arthroplasty have not been well established. The so-called femoral block in the inguinal region produces a blockade of the femoral, obturator, and lateral femoral cutaneous nerves. Substantial improvements are seen in terms of narcotic use, length of hospital stay, postoperative bleeding, range of motion, and overall complications in patients who receive nerve blocks [6, 7]. Continuous epidural analgesia provides pain relief similar to that with continuous femoral nerve block but is associated with more side effects [6,7]. Usually, the femoral nerve block is given either as a single postoperative injection or as a continuous postoperative infusion.

Wound Healing

Wound complications may occur more frequently in knees that have early continuous passive motion. Maloney et al. compared 95 knees that were immobilized for 4-6 days with 51 knees for which continuous passive motion was begun in the recovery room [10]. There were major wound complications in 2% of knees that were immobilized compared with 12% of knees in which continuous passive motion was begun in the recovery room. The explanation for the increased rate of wound complications after continuous passive motion were partially explained by the study of Johnson, in which the transcutaneous oxygen tension of the midpoint of a total knee arthroplasty incision was measured [5]. In this study of 102 patients who had a pri-

mary total knee arthroplasty, flexion of the knee beyond 40° progressively diminished the viability of the wound edges, particularly the lateral side, for the first 3 days after surgery. Maloney et al. concluded that early vigorous continuous passive motion may increase the chance of skin necrosis or other wound problems [10]. In a randomized study of 54 patients by Nielsen et al., one group received continuous passive motion 4 h/day and the other group received no continuous passive motion [14]. There was no difference in ROM at 14 days after surgery, but there were more wound complications in the group without continuous passive motion.

Deep Vein Thrombosis

The effect of continuous passive motion on the prevalence of deep vein thrombosis after total knee arthroplasty is not clear. In a prospective randomized study of 62 patients who had primary total knee arthroplasty and routine venography, Vince et al. reported a positive venogram in 45% of patients treated with continuous passive motion versus 75% of the control group [22]. No patient had thrombophlebitis of the femoral or pelvic veins and the results of all lung scans were negative. In a review of the prevalence of deep vein thrombosis and pulmonary embolism after total knee arthroplasty using a wide variety of prophylactic measures, Lynch et al. reported a 71% prevalence of venographic deep vein thrombosis and a 22% prevalence of pulmonary embolism in a group of 484 patients [9]. In a separate group of 255 patients in whom continuous passive motion was used, the prevalence of deep vein thrombosis was reduced to 20% and the prevalence of pulmonary embolism was reduced to 6% [15]. These authors concluded that continuous passive motion and pneumatic compression together provided improved prophylaxis against thromboembolism after total knee arthroplasty. However, these data were challenged in another prospective randomized study of 150 patients undergoing total knee arthroplasty, with one group receiving continuous passive motion and a control group doing active assisted exercises of the knee [16]. All patients received aspirin prophylaxis, 650 mg twice a day, beginning on the day of admission. Forty-five percent of the patients who received continuous passive motion had venographically proven calf vein thromboses, compared with 37% of those patients who did not receive continuous passive motion. However, this difference was not statistically significant. No patient had a pulmonary embolism.

Blood Loss After Total Knee Arthroplasty

Continuous passive motion has been reported to increase blood loss after total knee arthroplasty. Lotke et al.

reported on a prospective randomized study of 121 patients with total knee arthroplasties [7]. The greatest blood loss occurred in patients who had intraoperative release of the tourniquet and continuous passive motion begun in the recovery room. Pope et al. performed a prospective randomized study of 57 knees that were divided into three groups [15]. The average blood loss of patients who did not receive continuous passive motion was 956 ml, while patients who received continuous passive motion from 0° to 40° of flexion had a mean blood loss of 1017 ml, and patients who received continuous passive motion from 0° to 70° of flexion had significantly more blood loss (mean: 1558 ml). Findings from these studies indicate that continuous passive motion probably should not be started in the recovery room in order to minimize blood loss.

Influence of Prosthesis Design and Operative Technique on Rehabilitation

Designs of Knee Prostheses

Designs that increase the quadriceps moment arm may reduce quadriceps tension, facilitate activities of daily living, and enhance rehabilitation. Mahoney et al. compared patients who had received a posterior cruciate-substituting prosthesis with patients who had received a design that increased the patellofemoral moment arm by 30% [10]. After the operation, more patients who had received the latter design reported no anterior knee pain and were able to rise from a chair without using their arms. Mobile-bearing knee arthroplasty offers the advantages of increased conformity and greater mobility, which theoretically translates into improved function and range of motion.

Standard Surgical Approach

The medial parapatellar approach and the midvastus approach are used commonly in total knee arthroplasty. Patients managed with both operative approaches during bilateral primary total knee arthroplasty required fewer lateral retinacular releases, had less pain at 1 and 6 weeks, and were more likely to be able to perform straight-leg raises earlier on the side managed with the midvastus approach [6].

We have used a surgical technique which was initiated in 1993 that includes incising and closing the knee in flexion. This may allow earlier return of quadriceps strength and range of motion. A concern with this technique was extension lag. However, our experience has demonstrated that muscle strength is not hindered by closing the knee in flexion.

Minimally Invasive Approach

Minimally invasive approaches have been developed recently. This term implies that there is less disruption of the anatomical structures about the knee. The minimally invasive approach does not violate the skin, extensor mechanism, or suprapatellar pouch as much as conventional approaches do. It may produce less discomfort and a faster recovery.

Patient Expectations at the End of Rehabilitation

Patient-assessed recovery with regard to pain and function after total knee arthroplasty has not been as favorable as that after total hip arthroplasty, even though the quality-of-life improvements recorded after knee arthroplasty matched those recorded after hip arthroplasty [23]. A typical "surgically successful" knee arthroplasty may be considered a failure by the patient because the outcome does not match the patient's expectations. Expectations vary by diagnosis, patient characteristics, and functional status. Regardless of age, patients who have undergone total knee arthroplasty usually do not have comparable overall physical health when matched with the general population for age and gender. In studies comparing functional ability perceived by individuals after total knee arthroplasty with age-matched individuals without knee disability, significantly greater perceived difficulty with walking and stair performance was found in patients with total knee arthroplasty than in controls [6].

The acute care goals are inherently aimed toward hospital discharge, which is achieved when the patient is ambulatory, usually with a walker or cane. This occurs in 5-10 days, and discharge may be to the home, a rehabilitation unit, or a skilled nursing facility. The transition to the intermediate postoperative phase of rehabilitation occurs after 2-3 weeks and continues for 4-12 weeks. The goals are functional independence in all activities of daily living and return to employment, community activities, and recreational pursuits. Ideally, knee ROM of 0°-5° of extension and 110°-120° of flexion will be obtained. Therapeutic exercise should be focused on attaining optimal muscle strength and endurance, ambulation over a variety of surfaces and distances, and safe static and dynamic balance.

One of the most difficult problems at the end of the rehabilitation is the stiff knee. Most patients are content if they have 100° of flexion and can rise from a chair and walk up and down stairs. However, patients who cannot flex beyond 90° will be very aware of the limitation. Manipulation can be offered between 45 days and 8 weeks. However, manipulation beyond 8 weeks may not increase motion and can risk tendon or ligament avulsion, or fracture. Between 3 months and 1 year postoperatively arthroscopic release can be considered.

The end stage of total knee arthroplasty postoperative rehabilitation, from 3 to 12 months, is frequently underemphasized because the patient has had good to excellent pain relief and is walking within 12 weeks. Nevertheless, full physiological and functional recovery usually requires longer than 3 months and may never be attained. Walsh and colleagues compared patients who were 1 year post-total knee arthroplasty with age- and gender-matched controls without knee pathology [23]. Isokinetic peak torque measurements were reduced by more than 25% in the female total knee arthroplasty patients and by 35% in the male patients when compared with controls. The speed of walking and stair climbing was also significantly lower in the total knee arthroplasty patients.

References

1. Colwell CW, Morris BA (1992) The influence of continuous passive motion on the results of total knee arthroplasty. Clin Orthop 276:225-228
2. Coutts RD, Borden LS, Bryan RS, et al (1983) The effect of continuous passive motion on total knee rehabilitation. Orthop Trans 7:535-536
3. Coutts RD, Kaita J, Barr R, et al (1982) The role of continuous passive motion in the postoperative rehabilitation of the total knee patient. Orthop Trans 6:277-278
4. Daluga D, Lombardi AV, Mallory TH, Vaughn BK (1991) Knee manipulation following total knee arthroplasty. J Arthroplasty 6:119-128
5. Johnson DP (1990) The effect of continuous passive motion on wound-healing and joint mobility after knee arthroplasty. J Bone Joint Surg [Am] 72:421-426
6. Kumar PJ, McPherson EJ, Dorr LD, et al (1996) Rehabilitation after total knee arthroplasty. Clin Orthop 331:93-101
7. Lotke PA, Faralli VJ, Orenstein EM, Ecker ML (1991) Blood loss after total knee replacement. Effects of tourniquet release and continuous passive motion. J Bone Joint Surg [Am] 73:1037-1040
8. Lynch AF, Bourne RB, Rorabeck CH, et al (1988) Deep-vein thrombosis and continuous passive motion after total knee arthroplasty. J Bone Joint Surg [Am] 70:11-14
9. Lynch JA, Baker PL, Polly RE, et al (1990) Mechanical measures in the prophylaxis of postoperative thromboembolism in total knee arthroplasty. Clin Orthop 220:24-29
10. Maloney WJ, Schurman DJ, Hangen D, et al (1990) The influence of continuous passive motion on outcome in total knee arthroplasty. Clin Orthop 256:162-168
11. Mauerhan DR, Mokris JG, Ly A, Kiebzak GM (1998) Relationship between length of stay and manipulation rate after total knee arthroplasty. J Arthroplasty 13:896-900
12. McInnes J, Larson MG, Daltroy LH, et al (1992) A controlled evaluation of continuous passive motion in patients undergoing total knee arthroplasty. JAMA 268:1423-1428
13. Montgomery F, Eliasson M (1996) Continuous passive motion compared to active physical therapy after knee arthroplasty. Acta Orthop Scand 67:7-9
14. Nielsen PT, Rechnagel K, Nielsen SE (1988) No effect of continuous passive motion after arthroplasty of the knee. Acta Orthop Scand 59:580-581
15. Pope RO, Corcoran S, McCaul K, Howie DW (1997) Continuous passive motion after primary total knee arthroplasty. Does it offer any benefits? J Bone Joint Surg [Br] 79:914-917
16. Ritter MA, Gandolf VS, Holston KS (1989) Continuous passive motion versus physical therapy in total knee arthroplasty. Clin Orthop 244:239-243
17. Rodgers JA, Garvin KL, Walker CW, et al (1998) Preoperative physical therapy in primary total knee arthroplasty. J Arthroplasty 13:414-421
18. Romness DW, Rand JA (1988) The role of continuous passive motion following total knee arthroplasty. Clin Orthop 226: 34-37
19. Rorabeck CH (1999) Continuous passive motion is a useful postoperative tool. Orthopedics 22:392
20. Salter RB, Simmonds DF, Malcolm BW, et al (1980) The biological effect of continuous passive motion on the healing of full-thickness defects in articular cartilage. J Bone Joint Surg [Am] 62:1232-1251
21. Ververeli PA, Sutton DC, Hearn SL, et al (1995) Continuous passive motion after total knee arthroplasty. Analysis of cost and benefits. Clin Orthop 321:208-215
22. Vince KG, Kelly MA, Beck J, Insall JN (1987) Continuous passive motion after total knee arthroplasty. J Arthroplasty 2:281-284
23. Walsh M, Woodhouse L, Thomas S, Finch E (1998) Physical impairments and functional limitations: a comparison of individuals 1 year after total knee arthroplasty with control subjects. Phys Ther 78:248-258
24. Worland RL, Arredondo J, Angles F, et al (1998) Home continuous passive motion machine versus professional physical therapy following total knee replacement. J Arthroplasty 13:784-787
25. Yashar AA, Venn-Watson E, Welsh T, et al (1997) Continuous passive motion with accelerated flexion after total knee arthroplasty. Clin Orthop 345:38-43

63 Sports and Activity Levels after Total Knee Arthroplasty

P. Aglietti, P. Cuomo, A. Baldini

Summary

Total knee arthroplasty is an effective procedure for relieving symptoms and restoring patients' activities of daily living. Strenuous and vigorous activities after surgery are usually limited and depend on patient preoperative levels and expectations and on implant factors. Modern implant designs are conceived to ensure higher flexion and more physiological kinematics through range of motion. Mobile-bearing knees should meet these expectations. Sports activities after joint replacement are possible and are best indicated for patients who were previously active. High-impact sports should be discouraged, as concern exists about premature polyethylene failure.

Introduction

Total knee arthroplasty (TKA) is a very common and effective procedure for knee osteoarthritis (OA) and other inflammatory diseases. TKA has been documented to relieve pain, improve function, increase social mobility and interaction, and contribute to psychological well being. Furthermore, knee replacement is a cost-effective medical intervention which is associated with significant improvements in quality of life. Ninety percent or more of patients who have knee replacement can expect 10-20 years of satisfactory function [1-4].

Demand for TKA has increased during each of the past 20 years and is expected to increase more in the future. In 1999, over 270,000 TKAs were performed in the United States [5]. In the past decade, indications for TKA have expanded. During the 1970s and 1980s, TKA was performed mostly for pain, disability, or deformity. The expected benefit from the operation was reduction in pain, limb realignment, and functional improvement. However, pain was the primary reason for considering knee replacement surgery. Nowadays, function is a primary reason for knee replacement surgery. Patients are not satisfied with the reduced function that can accompany a stiff, painful, arthritic knee, and they are demanding a TKA to improve their function. Furthermore, total knee replacement patients are younger and more active than patients in previous decades. Increasingly, the desire for improvement in function includes athletic activity. There is considerable debate about the long-term effects of such activities on prosthetic wear, loosening, and revision rates. Many authors advise against a return to sports because of the increased risk of re-operation or component wear. It is tempting to postulate that a return to sports activity increases the likelihood of polyethylene wear, loosening, and revision surgery.

Activity Levels after TKA

Following TKA, patients usually feel better and have increased physical activity. Ries et al. [6] evaluated cardiovascular fitness after knee replacement. Joint reconstruction and rehabilitation were associated with significant improvements in duration of exercise, maximum workload, peak oxygen consumption, and percentage of predicted maximum oxygen uptake. They reported that resumption of physical activity after joint replacement was associated with an improvement in cardiovascular fitness, and patients with arthritic joints treated with joint replacement were more fit than patients with arthritic joints who were treated nonoperatively.

A few studies in the literature aimed to describe in detail the activity level achieved after TKA and whether it meets patients expectations. Weiss and colleagues [7] investigated 176 patients at 1 year after surgery with regard to three categories of activity: (a) activities of daily living, including walking, stair-climbing, sitting, foot care, bathing, and car travel; (b) advanced activities of daily living, including kneeling, squatting, and twisting procedures; and (c) sports activities. All the patients did category 1 activities at least occasionally. Forty-percent of the patients regularly did all the advanced activities while 9% of them did none of these activities on a regular basis. More than two thirds of the patients in the study performed at least a light sport activity such as strengthening or stretching on a regular basis, while only 10% of them were involved in vigorous activities. When activity limitations were investigated, two thirds of the patients reported difficulties in squatting and kneeling and one half of them were particularly limited in turning and cutting maneuvers. Hassaballa [8] and co-workers found in a prospective study as well that most TKA patients were particularly limited in kneeling activities, with only 15% of the patients in the study group able to kneel with little or no difficulty. Furthermore, patients' subjective impressions regarding their ability to perform a particular maneuver may underestimate their real capability to do so. Indeed, the same authors [9] more recently demonstrated that only two thirds of the patients who stated that they were able to kneel could really kneel properly.

Broadbury and colleagues [10] published a retrospective study of 160 patients who received 208 TKAs that analyzed only the return to sports activities. Eighty-one patients had not regularly participated in any sports before surgery, and none of these patients took up sports after surgery. Seventy-nine patients had participated in sports before surgery and 65% of them returned to regular sports after surgery. Patients were more likely to return to low-impact activities such as bowls (91%, returned) than to high-impact activities such as tennis (20% returned).

None of the above-mentioned studies was able to show any relationship between the impact of activity and implant durability.

Sports Activities and TKA

The prerequisites of a TKA allowing participation in sports should be (a) that it restores normal function and (b) that it has long durability.

Normal Function

Normal knee function has been widely described with various techniques and under various activities [11,12]. As previously discussed in this chapter, TKA patients are particularly limited in twisting as well in high flexion activities [7], and for this reason both the surgical procedure and the implant should be aimed at preserving or restoring these functions.

Rotational requirements of the normal knee are consistent and activity dependent. With increasing flexion the tibia internally rotates 4.4° during gait, 7.8° when descending stairs, 16.8° in deep knee bending, and 19.4° when rising from a chair [11], but high interindividual variability has been found. During sports activity rotational requirements of the knee are higher: 50° of internal rotation and 50° of external rotation are required by the lead knee to properly perform a golf swing [13].

Following TKA, femorotibial rotation is usually decreased and the magnitude is highly design dependent.

Posterior stabilized (PS) knees have been shown to have the widest and most reproducible rotational patterns during various activities [14]. Among PS knees, mobile-bearing versions allow higher rotations. With videofluoroscopy, Ranawat and co-workers [15] compared the same PS implant in the fixed and mobile version during deep knee bending and found a significantly higher rotation in the mobile knee. Furthermore, fixed PS knees have an inherent rotational constraint in the cam and post mechanism which is strictly design dependent [16]. Mobile versions also show fewer stresses under torque loads [17].

Maximum knee flexion after TKA has been demonstrated to be multifactorial, and patient, surgical, implant, and rehabilitation features affect the final result. Poor preoperative flexion and a severe deformity are the main patient-related factors which negatively affect final flexion [18,19].

Several factors have been emphasized to improve flexion at surgery [20]. These include: (a) restoration of the posterior recesses of the knee, removal of the posterior osteophytes, preservation of the posterior femoral offset, and removal of posterior capsule adhesions; (b) avoidance of anterior overstuffing, with attention paid to the anteroposterior placement of the components and to the preservation of patellar thickness; (c) proper rotational positioning of the components; (d) preservation of the tibial slope.

Implant design strongly affects maximum flexion. Banks and colleagues [21] found with videofluoroscopy that PS knees reached higher flexion during a lunge activity than both fixed and mobile cruciate-retaining knees. They found a linear correlation with the anteroposterior position of the femur on the tibia at maximum flexion, with an anterior position responsible for an earlier impingement of the femur on the posterior lip of the polyethylene insert with subsequent less flexion. Posterior stability alone seems to be the most important feature, and the addition of the cam and post mechanism to a rotating platform knee in patients who received bilateral implants (mobile version in one knee, fixed in the contralateral) showed no differences in terms of maximum weight-bearing flexion [15].

Knee implants dedicated to restoring high flexion have been designed and manufactured and most of them benefit from thickened posterior femoral condyles and decreased posterior insert height to delay tibiofemoral posterior impingement. A deeper trochlear groove and a polyethylene anterior cut-out enhance patellar tracking and minimize the effects of anterior overstuffing [22].

Long Durability

Long-term effects of high activity levels on TKA durability still need to be exactly defined, and concern exists about the possibility of earlier failures. Several studies have been done to clarify how the success rate is related to the patient's age at initial surgery and have shown different results. Diduch et al.,[23] observed 88 patients younger than 55 years who were treated with TKA and they reported a survival rate of 87% at 18 years. Duffy et al. [24] studied 74 TKAs in 54 patients younger than 55 years and reported an estimated survival rate of 99% at 10 years. Lonner et al. [25] examined 32 patients with osteoarthritis younger than 40 years who were treated with TKAs and reported an aseptic failure rate of 12.5% at 8 years. Ranawat et al. [26] observed 62 patients younger than 55 years who were treated with TKAs and reported a survival rate of 96% at 10 years. These authors all stated that their results were comparable to the survival rate of older patients.

On the other hand, Harrysson et al. [27] analyzed the Swedish Knee Arthroplasty Registry and compared the cumulative revision rates in 21,761 patients older than 60 years and in 1434 patients younger than 60 years treated with a TKA. A higher cumulative revision rate was observed for the group of younger patients (13% at 8.5 years) than for the group of older patients (6% at 8.5 years). Mallon and Callaghan [28] focused on active golfers with a TKA and, at an average follow-up of 4.7 years, found that 79% of the players had radiolucent lines and 50% of them had some pain while or after playing. Lavernia and colleagues [29] performed a study of autopsy-retrieved specimens of 28 polyethylene inserts from primary TKA. All the donors were assigned to a UCLA activity scale category ranging from 0 (wholly inactive) to 10 (impact sports on a regular basis). The specimens were inspected with regard to volumetric and linear wear and the presence of creep. More active patients had statistically significantly higher creep or deformation of implants measured as severity and extent of involvement. UCLA score was the most important predictor of extent of involvement of deformation.

The loads on the knee during vigorous activities may exceed the pressure safety limit that the polyethylene insert can withstand and which has been calculated to be 10 MPa and is generated by a force of about 5 times body weight [30]. Walking and cycling do not seem to be detrimental to the knee joint as the involved forces are less than 4 times body weight. In power walking uphill the involved forces are around 4-5 times body weight and in downhill walking they reach 8 times body weight. Slow jogging is responsible for forces of 8-9 times body weight passing across the knee, and during fast jogging the forces are more than 10 times body weight [31].

After TKA, the pressures on the knee joint occurring during various activities are strongly influenced by the prosthetic design. High tibiofemoral conformity has been shown to decrease stresses. Kuster et al. [32] compared three different total knee designs for loads occurring dur-

ing cycling, power walking, hiking, and jogging using Fuji pressure-sensitive film. The studied designs included a flat tibial inlay, a curved inlay, and a high conforming inlay with mobile bearings. The contact area increased with increasing loads for all three designs. The overall contact area was greater during power walking, downhill walking, or jogging for the mobile-bearing design when compared with the flat or curved designs. The highest contact area was found for the mobile-bearing design during power walking because this design showed full conformity. The overloaded area (area with stress levels above 25 MPa) was computed for each design during cycling, power walking, downhill walking, and jogging. During cycling and power walking the mobile implant showed no overloaded area; in the other designs the overloaded area remained well below 50 mm2. During downhill walking and jogging the overloaded area reached levels as high as 180 mm2 in all designs.

It seems clear that stresses and wear should benefit from high conforming designs, and mobile bearing can offer such an opportunity to active patients even if the advantages remain mainly theoretical and comparative studies have not yet shown differences between mobile and fixed designs. Furthermore, it should be emphasized that not all mobile knees maintain the same high conformity through all range of motion: Many of them are highly conforming only during gait and lose conformity in deep flexion with increasing stresses, thus behaving like fixed-bearing knees whose stresses all exceed the polyethylene safety limit of 10 MPa [33].

Recommended Activities after TKA

Patients should be encouraged to remain physically active for general health and also for the quality of their bone. There is evidence that increased bone quality will improve prosthesis fixation and decrease the incidence of early loosening. Prior to starting any activity it is mandatory to rehabilitate quadriceps and hamstring muscles. Muscular rehabilitation is important for safety and protection of the joint.

The most important question is whether a specific activity is performed for exercise to obtain and maintain physical fitness or whether an activity is recreational only. To maintain physical fitness an endurance activity should be encouraged, to be performed several times a week at high intensity. Since load will influence the amount of wear exponentially, only activities with low joint loads such as swimming, cycling, or possibly power walking should be recommended.

If an activity is carried out at low intensity and therefore at the recreational base, activities with higher joint loads such as skiing or hiking can also be performed. It is unwise to start technically demanding activities after

63

total joint replacement, as the joint loads and the risk of injuries are generally higher for these activities in unskilled individuals. To recommend suitable physical activities after total knee replacement, it is important to consider both the load and the knee flexion angle of the peak load. During activities such as hiking or jogging, high joint loads occur between 40° and 60° of knee flexion, where many knee designs are not conforming and high polyethylene inlay stress will occur. Regular jogging or hiking produces high inlay stress with the danger of delamination and polyethylene destruction for most current total knee prostheses [32].

In 1999, a Knee Society survey was performed with regard to sports activity recommendations following TKA [34]; 58 surgeons took part. Ten activities were recommended: stationary bicycling, croquet, ballroom dancing, golf, horseshoes, shooting, shuffleboard, swimming, doubles tennis, and walking. Seven activities were allowed only if the patient had previous experience: low-impact aerobics, road bicycling, bowling, canoeing, hiking, horseback riding, and cross-country skiing. The following high-impact activities were all discouraged: high-impact aerobics, baseball/softball, basketball, football, gymnastics, handball, hockey, jogging, lacrosse, racquetball, squash, rock climbing, soccer, singles tennis, and volleyball.

Conclusions

Physical activity must be encouraged after TKA to maintain the patient's well being. To recommend a certain activity after total knee arthroplasty, factors such as wear, joint load, intensity, and the type of prosthesis must be taken into account for each patient and sport type. The reduction of wear is one of the main factors in improving long-term results after total joint replacement. Wear is dependent on the load, the number of steps, the design, and the material properties of the implant. Furthermore, the implant should allow normal function resoration, being flexion and rotation friendly. Mobile implants benefit high conformity, which reduces stresses and is rotation friendly.

References

1. Rand JA, Trousdale RT, Ilstrup DM, Harmsen WS (2003) Factors affecting the durability of primary total knee prostheses. J Bone Joint Surg [Am] 85:259-265
2. Aglietti P, Buzzi R, De Felice R, Giron F (1999) The Insall-Burstein total knee replacement in osteoarthritis: a 10-year minimum follow-up. J Arthroplasty 14:560-565
3. Keating EM, Meding JB, Faris PM, Ritter MA (2002) Long-term followup of nonmodular total knee replacements. Clin Orthop 404:34-39
4. Brassard MF, Insall JN, Scuderi GR, Colizza W (2001) Does modularity affect clinical success? A comparison with a minimum 10-year follow-up. Clin Orthop 388:26-32
5. Mendenhall S (2000) Editorial. Orthopedic Network News 11:7
6. Ries MD, Philbin EF, Groff GD, Sheesley KA, Richman JA, Lynch F Jr (1996) Improvement in cardiovascular fitness after total knee arthroplasty. J Bone Joint Surg [Am] 78:1696-1701
7. Weiss JM, Noble PC, Conditt MA, Kohl HW, Roberts S, Cook KF, Gordon MJ, Mathis KB (2002) What functional activities are important to patients with knee replacements? Clin Orthop 404:172-188
8. Hassaballa MA, Porteous AJ, Newman JH, Rogers CA (2003) Can knees kneel? Kneeling ability after total, unicompartmental and patellofemoral knee arthroplasty. Knee 10:155-160
9. Hassaballa MA, Porteous AJ, Newman JH (2004) Observed kneeling ability after total, unicompartmental and patellofemoral knee arthroplasty: perception versus reality. Knee Surg Sports Traumatol Arthrosc 12:136-139
10. Bradbury N, Borton D, Spoo G, et al (1998) Participation in sports after total knee replacement. Am J Sports Med 26:530-535
11. Komistek RD, Dennis DA, Mahfouz M (2003) In vivo fluoroscopic analysis of the normal human knee. Clin Orthop 410:69-81
12. Freeman MA, Pinskerova V (2003) The movement of the knee studied by magnetic resonance imaging. Clin Orthop 410:35-43
13. Gatt CJ Jr, Pavol MJ, Parker RD, Grabiner MD (1998) Three-dimensional knee joint kinetics during a golf swing. Influences of skill level and footwear. Am J Sports Med 26:285-294
14. Dennis DA, Komistek RD, Mahfouz MR, Haas BD, Stiehl JB (2003) Multicenter determination of in vivo kinematics after total knee arthroplasty. Clin Orthop 416:37-57
15. Ranawat CS, Komistek RD, Rodriguez JA, Dennis DA, Anderle M (2004) In vivo kinematics for fixed and mobile-bearing posterior stabilized knee prostheses. Clin Orthop 418:184-190
16. Klein R, Serpe L, Kester MA, Edidin A, Fishkin Z, Mahoney OM, Schmalzried TP (2003) Rotational constraint in posterior-stabilized total knee prostheses. Clin Orthop 410:82-89
17. D'Lima DD, Chen PC, Colwell CW Jr (2001) Polyethylene contact stresses, articular congruity, and knee alignment. Clin Orthop 392:232-238
18. Kawamura H, Bourne RB (2001) Factors affecting range of flexion after total knee arthroplasty. J Orthop Sci 6:248-252
19. Maloney WJ, Schurman DJ (1992) The effects of implant design on range of motion after total knee arthroplasty. Total condylar versus posterior stabilized total condylar designs. Clin Orthop 278:147-152
20. Bellemans J, Banks S, Victor J, Vandenneucker H, Moemans A (2002) Fluoroscopic analysis of the kinematics of deep flexion in total knee arthroplasty. Influence of posterior condylar offset. J Bone Joint Surg [Br] 84:50-53
21. Banks S, Bellemans J, Nozaki H, Whiteside LA, Harman M, Hodge WA (2003) Knee motions during maximum flexion in fixed and mobile-bearing arthroplasties. Clin Orthop 410:131-138
22. Sultan PG, Most E, Schule S, Li G, Rubash HE (2003) Optimizing flexion after total knee arthroplasty advances in prosthetic design. Clin Orthop 416:167-173
23. Diduch D, Insall J, Scott W, Scuderi GR, Font-Rodrigues D (1997) Total knee replacement in young, active patients: long-term follow-up and functional outcome. J Bone Joint Surg [Am] 79:575-582
24. Duffy G, Trousdale R, Stuart M (1998) Total knee arthroplasty in patients 55 years old or younger: 10- to 17-year results. Clin Orthop 356:22-27
25. Lonner JH, Hershman S, Mont M, Lotke PA (2000) Total knee arthroplasty in patients 40 years of age and younger with osteoarthritis. Clin Orthop 380:85-90
26. Ranawat C, Padgett D, Ohashi Y (1989) Total knee arthroplasty for patients younger than 55 years. Clin Orthop 248:27-33
27. Harrysson OLA, Robertsson O, Nayfeh JF (2004) Higher cumulative revision rate of knee arthroplasties in younger patients with osteoarthritis. Clin Orthop 421:162-168
28. Mallon WJ, Callaghan JJ (1993) Total knee arthroplasty in active golfers. J Arthroplasty 8:299-306
29. Lavernia CJ, Sierra RJ, Hungerford DS, Krackow K (2001) Activity level and wear in total knee arthroplasty. J Arthroplasty 4:446-453
30. Collier JP, Mayor MB, Surprenant VA, Surprenant HP, Dauphinais LA, Jensen RE (1990) The biomechanical problems of polyethylene as a bearing surface. Clin Orthop 261:107-113

31. Kuster MS, Wood GA, Stachowiak GW, Gatchter A (1997) Joint load considerations in total knee replacement. J. Bone Joint Surg [Br] 79:109-113
32. Kuster MS, Spalinger E, Blanksby BA, Gatchter A (2000) Endurance sports after total knee replacement: a biomechanical investigation. Med Sci Sports Exerc 721-724
33. Bartel DL, Rawlison JJ, Burstein AH, Ranawat CS, Flynn WF (1995) Stresses in polyethylene components of contemporary total knee replacements. Clin Orthop 317:376-382
34. Healy WL, Iorio R, Lemos MJ (2000) Athletic activity after total knee arthroplasty. Clin Orthop 380:65-71

IX   Future Perspectives

64 Conclusions

M. D. Ries

Summary

Total knee arthroplasty (TKA) is an effective treatment for severe arthrosis of the knee with predictable pain relief and longevity of the arthroplasty. However, late mechanical failure may occur, necessitating revision surgery, and normal range of motion and kinematics are not reliably achieved. Current developments in surgical technique, instrumentation, and implant design including computer-assisted navigation, minimally invasive surgery, use of more durable bearing surface materials, and kinematic implant designs, offer the potential to further improve the function and longevity of TKA.

Current Status of Total Knee Arthoplasty

Reliable improvement in pain and function can be expected following TKA, and survivorship rates of 90%-95% after 10 years have frequently been reported [1-5]. Early failures may result from infection, instability, malalignment, stiffness, reflex sympathetic dystrophy, and patellar problems. Many of these problems can be avoided by proper surgical technique, implant selection, appropriate postoperative pain management, and rehabilitation. Late failures more typically occur from polyethylene wear, and less commonly from implant loosening or periprosthetic fracture. However, elimination of gamma-irradiated in air UHMWPE has reduced the frequency of wear-related failures after TKA.

Although pain and function are dramatically improved after TKA, range of motion may still be slightly limited, causing impairment in activities which require greater knee flexion such as descending stairs or sitting in a low chair. Getting up from a seated position often requires use of the upper extremities to assist active knee extension. While these limitations may not be apparent to patients with relatively sedentary lifestyles, more active patients can experience some functional limitations after TKA.

New Bearing Surface Materials

Failures of fixed-bearing total knee tibial components have usually resulted from fatigue-wear mechanisms which were associated with gamma-irradiated in air UHMWPE. However, gamma-irradiation in air sterilization has not been used by most manufacturers since the mid 1990s, and the typical failure mechanisms previously observed do not appear to be continuing. Use of highly cross-linked polyethylene in total hip arthroplasty is associated with a significant reduction in wear in simulator and early clinical studies [7-12]. However, cross-linking also reduces the mechanical properties of UHMWPE, which limits its utility in high contact stress applications such as fixed-bearing TKA [13, 14]. Impingement-related failures associated with a small contact area between the femoral neck and the acetabular rim have been reported in total hip arthroplasty [15,16]. The bearing surface contact area in the knee is smaller than in the hip and contact stresses are an order of magnitude greater in the knee than in the hip [17]. Currently available highly cross-linked polyethylenes which have reduced mechanical properties compared with non-cross-linked polyethylene may therefore not be suitable for use as an alternative bearing surface in TKA.

During in vivo use, roughening of the cobalt-chrome counterface may also develop. In vitro wear studies of conventional as well as highly cross-linked polyethylene demonstrate an increase in wear when tested against a roughened counterface [18-20]. While wear may be reduced by the use of highly cross-linked polyethylene, its mechanical properties are also reduced. A more appropriate solution to minimize wear caused by in vivo counterface roughening without reducing UHMWPE mechanical properties may be achieved with use of a scratch-resistant ceramic counterface rather than highly cross-linked polyethylene [21, 22].

Minimally Invasive Surgery

TKA performed through a conventional medial parapatellar approach is associated with reliable pain relief, im-

64

provement in function, and 90%-95% 10-year survivorship [1-5]. However, many patients experience significant pain and inflammation which typically occurs to some extent for 6 months after arthroplasty and may limit participation in rehabilitation exercises. Minimally invasive surgery permits TKA to be performed with less soft-tissue trauma. Early reports indicate that minimally invasive surgery is associated with reduced blood loss, less pain, and earlier return of quadriceps function and range of motion [23-25]. However, a minimally invasive approach may compromise surgical exposure and result in an increase in complications. Minimally invasive total hip arthroplasty has been reported to have a higher complication rate than a standard approach [26]. By using small cutting blocks and avoiding dissection of the suprapatellar pouch, reliable results can be achieved with a complication rate which is not greater than conventional TKA [23-25]. Particularly when combined with a pre-operative patient education program and multimodal postoperative pain management, TKA performed through a minimally invasive approach appears to offer significant advantages compared with conventional TKA. However, more muscular patients, those with prior surgery, stiffness, poor skin vascularity, or significant deformity requiring soft-tissue releases may not be appropriate candidates for a minimally invasive approach.

Computer-assisted Surgery

Optimal axial (varus-valgus) alignment, component rotation, anteroposterior positioning, and implant sizing are important technical goals of TKA. Malalignment can compromise the function of the arthroplasty. Conventional intramedullary femoral and intra- or extramedullary tibial instrumentation generally provides satisfactory axial alignment. Direct visualization of the posterior condylar line, epicondylar axis, and anteroposterior axis of the distal femur permits proper rotational orientation of the femoral component. Intraoperative sizing of the distal femur and proximal tibia as well as flexion and extension gaps provides information for implant sizing and positioning. However, many series of TKA performed with conventional instrumentation include occasional cases of implant malalignment which may be sufficient to cause early failure of the arthroplasty or compromise knee function.

Reliable improvement in implant alignment can be achieved with computer-assisted surgery (CAS) to orient the cutting blocks or combined with robotics to perform the bone cuts [27-30]. While most surgeons achieve similar implant alignment with conventional instrumentation, CAS offers a benefit in reducing the number of outliers with occasional malalignment. Although methods of CAS are evolving, currently available systems permit

navigation with either additional fluoroscopic or CT imaging, or imageless techniques [28-30]. CT provides accurate three-dimensional anatomical imaging of the knee, but this method requires preoperative CT scanning and templating of the CT-obtained images. Fluoroscopic-based navigation relies on intraoperative two-dimensional imaging and specific magnification calibration to maintain accuracy of the technique. With the imageless technique, anatomical data points are obtained intraoperatively and a corresponding three-dimensional knee model is chosen by the computer, which matches the data points as closely as possible from a computer library. Each method requires placement of fixation pins in the tibia and femur, and bone and instrument registration with the CAS system. With additional fluoroscopic or CT imaging, further improvement in accuracy may be achieved compared with imageless techniques, although the relative accuracy of these three methods has not been well defined. With any CAS system, additional surgical time is required, as are more nursing and surgeon training and greater costs to implement the system. Availability of CAS in TKA is limited by these issues at many institutions. However, the potential benefits of improvement in implant alignment may outweigh the additional surgical time and cost required for CAS, particularly as more user-friendly and less expensive systems are developed.

New Implant Designs

Incomplete restoration of high-demand functions following TKA is not surprising, since there are many anatomical differences between the normal and the replaced knee. One or both cruciate ligaments and both menisci are removed, the joint-line position is altered, and the articular geometry of the bearing surfaces is changed. Fluoroscopic kinematic studies of TKA patients consistently demonstrate "paradoxical" motion patterns in which the femur is positioned posteriorly on the tibia during knee extension and moves anteriorly during knee flexion. This pattern of motion is the reverse of the normal knee kinematic pattern in which the femur moves posteriorly during flexion. Abnormal kinematics after TKA may limit flexion and decrease quadriceps efficiency. However, kinematics after unicompartmental knee arthroplasty, in which most of the normal anatomical constraints (anterior cruciate ligament, contralateral tibiofemoral compartment, and patellofemoral joint) are preserved, are much closer to that of the normal knee. Knee motion and function after unicompartmental knee arthroplasty also compare favorably to TKA. However, efforts in the past to retain both cruciate ligaments during TKA have resulted in high failure rates due to stiffness and implant loosening. Alternatively, guided-motion implant designs are intended to provide more normal kinematics without retention of the anterior cruciate ligament. The posterior cruciate-substituting cam-and-post mechanism is an example of guided motion, since the engagement of the cam and post during flexion limits anterior translation of the femur and results in a less abnormal knee kinematic pattern than posterior cruciate-retaining TKA [31]. Variation in the tibial bearing surface geometry can also affect tibiofemoral kinematics [32]. Therefore, further improvements in implant design may permit more normal knee kinematics and better knee function, particularly for higher demand activities.

The Future of Total Knee Arthroplasty

TKA is an effective, well-established treatment for severe arthrosis of the knee. However, further improvement in the longevity of the arthroplasty can be achieved with more durable bearing surface materials. Due to the non-conforming shape of the bearing surface, hard-on-hard bearings are unlikely to have a role in TKA and UHMW-PE will remain an important bearing surface material. However, improvements in manufacturing and elimination of gamma-irradiation in air sterilization have already resulted in fewer wear-related problems. Although currently available highly cross-linked polyethylenes decrease the mechanical properties of UHMWPE, which limits their use in TKA, further modifications which improve polymer wear but retain mechanical properties may have an important role in the future.

The introduction of minimally invasive surgery has been well accepted by the general population of arthritic patients, despite the fact that the risks and benefits of the procedure have not been well defined. However, the benefits of earlier return of motion and better pain control may result in improvement in long-term function after TKA. Continued refinement of instrumentation, surgical technique, and indications should result in more predictable outcomes, so it is likely that minimally or less invasive surgery will become a standard technique with well-defined indications and that "conventional" surgical approaches will also have specific indications.

Although computer-assisted surgery offers improvement in implant alignment, the current barriers of increased surgical time, cost, and training limit its application. However, further developments should overcome these barriers to make the techniques of computer navigation more readily available. The extent of implementation of navigation in routine surgical practice is likely to depend on the success of developing user-friendly systems such as non-optical tracking systems which provide reproducible alignment.

Biological treatments to restore arthritic joint surfaces including autologous cartilage transplantation, use of stem cells, and synthetic cartilage may eventually become viable alternatives to TKA. However, continued research will be required for some time before the efficacy of these treatments is defined.

TKA is one of the most cost-effective treatments in medicine, and the number of joint replacement procedures performed in the United States and Europe has been growing steadily in recent years. With the baby-boom population now reaching an age at which arthritic symptoms typically develop, it appears likely that considerably more patients will benefit from TKA in the future.

References

1. Worland RL, Johnson GV, Alemparte J, et al (2002) Ten- to fourteen-year survival and functional analysis of the AGC total knee replacement system. Knee 9:133
2. Laskin RS (2001) The Genesis total knee prosthesis: a 10-year follow-up study. Clin Orthop 388:95
3. Berger RA, Rosenberg AG, Barden RM, et al (2001) Long-term follow-up of the Miller-Galante total knee replacement. Clin Orthop 388:58
4. Buehler KO, Venn-Watson E, D'Lima DD, et al (2000) The press-fit condylar total knee system: 8- to 10-year results with a posterior cruciate-retaining design. J Arthroplasty 15:698
5. Lyback CO, Belt EA, Hamalainen MM, et al (2000) Survivorship of AGC knee replacement in juvenile chronic arthritis: 13-year follow-up of 77 knees. J Arthroplasty 15:166
6. Aglietti P, Buzzi R, De Felice R, et al (1999) The Insall-Burstein total knee replacement in osteoarthritis: a 10-year minimum follow-up. J Arthroplasty 14:560
7. McKellop H, Shen FW, Lu B, et al (1999) Development of an extremely wear-resistant ultra high molecular weight polyethylene for total hip replacements. J Orthop Res 17:157
8. Muratoglu OK, Bragdon CR, O'Connor DO, et al (2001) A novel method of cross-linking ultra-high-molecular-weight polyethylene to improve wear, reduce oxidation, and retain mechanical properties. Recipient of the 1999 HAP Paul Award. J Arthroplasty 16:149
9. Martell JM, Verner JJ, Incavo SJ (2003) Clinical performance of a highly crosslinked polyethylene at two years in total hip arthroplasty: a randomized prospective trial. J Arthroplasty 18 [Suppl 1]:55
10. Digas G, Karrholm J, Thanner J, et al 2003 Highly cross-linked polyethylene in cemented THA: randomized study of 61 hips. Clin Orthop 417:126
11. Digas G, Herberts P, Karrholm J, et al (2004) Crosslinked vs. conventional polyethylene in bilateral hybrid THA. Randomized RSA study. Trans Orthop Res Sec 29:319
12. Heisel C, Silva M, dela Rosa M, et al (2004) Short-term in vivo wear of cross-linked polyethylene. J Bone Joint Surg [Am] 86:248
13. Baker D, Bellare A, L Pruitt (2003) The effects of degree of crosslinking on the fatigue crack initiation and propagation resistance of orthopedic grade polyethylene. J Biomed Mater Res 66:146
14. Baker DA, Hasting RS, Pruitt L (1999) Study of fatigue resistance of chemical and radiation crosslinked medical grade ultrahigh molecular weight polyethylene. J Biomed Mater Res 46:573
15. Halley D, Glassman A, Crowninshield RD (2004) Recurrent dislocation after revision total hip replacement with a large prosthetic femoral head. A case report. J Bone Joint Surg [Am] 86:827
16. Bradford L, Kurland M, Sankaran H, et al (2004) Early failure due to osteolysis in highly crosslinked ultra-high molecular weight polyethylene: a case report. J Bone Joint Surg [Am] 86:1051
17. Bartel DL, Bicknell VL, Wright TM (1986) The effect of conformity, thickness, and material on stresses in ultra-high molecular weight components for total joint replacement. J Bone Joint Surg[Am] 68:1041
18. Ries MD, Salehi A, Widding K, et al (2002) Polyethylene wear performance of oxidized zirconium and cobalt-chromium knee components under abrasive conditions. J Bone Joint Surg [Am] 84:S129

64

19. Widding K, Scott M, Jani S, et al (2003) Crosslinked UHMWPE in knees: Clean versus abrasive conditions. Trans Orthop Res Soc 28:1427

20. Muatoglu O, Burroughs B,Christensen S, et al (2004) In vitro wear of highly crosslinked tibias articulating with explanted rough femoral components. Trans Orthop Res Sec 29:297

21. Laskin RS (2003) An oxidized Zr ceramic surfaced femoral component for total knee arthroplasty. Clin Orthop 416:191

22. Spector M, Ries MD, Bourne RB, et al (2001) Wear performance of ultra-high molecular weight polyethylene on oxidized zirconium total knee femoral components. J Bone Joint Surg [Am] 83:580

23. Laskin RS, Beksac B, Phongkunakorn A, et al (2004) Minimally invasive total knee replacement through a mini-midvastus incision: an outcome study. Clin Orthop 428:74-81

24. Haas SB (2004) Minimally invasive total knee arthroplasty: a comparative study. Clin Orthop 428:68-73

25. Tria AJ, Coon TM (2003) Minimal incision total knee arthroplasty. Clin Orthop 416:185-190

26. Woolson ST, Mow CS, Syquia JF, Lannin JV, Schurman DJ (2004) Comparison of primary total hip replacements performed with a standard incision or a mini-incision. J Bone Joint Surg [Am] 86:1353-1358

27. Van Ham G et al (1998) Machining and accuracy studies for a tibial knee implant using a force-controlled robot. Comput Aided Surg 3:123-133

28. Chauhan SK, Scott RG, Breidahl W, Beaver RJ (2004) Computer-assisted knee arthroplasty versus a conventional jig-based technique. A randomised, prospective trial. J Bone Joint Surg [Br] 86:372-377

29. Stockl B, Nogler M, Rosiek R, Fischer M, Krismer M, Kessler O (2004) Navigation improves accuracy of rotational alignment in total knee arthroplasty. Clin Orthop 426:180-186

30. Victor J; Hoste D (2004) Image-based computer-assisted total knee arthroplasty leads to lower variability in coronal alignment. Clin Orthop 428:131-139

31. Dennis DA, Komistek RD, Mahfouz MR, Haas BD, Steihl JB (2003) Multi-center determination of in vivo kinematics after total knee arthroplasty. Clin Orthop 416:37-57

32. Walker PS, Sathasivam S (2000) Design forms of total knee replacement. Proc Inst Mech Eng 214:101-119

Subject Index